MASTERING
Geriatric Care

MASTERING
Geriatric Care

Springhouse Corporation
Springhouse, Pennsylvania

Staff

Executive Director
Matthew Cahill

Editorial Director
Patricia Dwyer Schull, RN, MSN

Art Director
John Hubbard

Clinical Manager
Judith Schilling McCann, RN, MSN

Senior Editor
H. Nancy Holmes

Editors
Marcia B. Andrews, Shirley Claypool, Peter H. Johnson, Elizabeth Mauro, Doris Weinstock, Patricia A. Wittig

Clinical Editors
Maryann Foley, RN, BSN (project manager); Karen E. Michael, RN, MSN; Beverly Tscheschlog, RN

Copy Editors
Cynthia C. Breuninger (manager), Christine Cunniffe, Mary T. Durkin, Brenna H. Mayer, Patrice Polgar, Pamela Wingrod

Designers
Arlene Putterman (associate art director), Lesley Weissman-Cook (book designer), Amy Litz (project manager), Jacalyn Facciolo, Donald G. Knauss, Kaaren Mitchel

Manufacturing
Deborah Meiris (director), Pat Dorshaw, T.A. Landis, Anna Brindisi

Production Coordinator
Margaret A. Rastiello

Editorial Assistants
Carol Caputo, Beverly Lane, Mary Madden, Jeanne Napier

Printed in the United States of America.
MGC-030598

 A member of the Reed Elsevier plc group

Library of Congress Cataloging-in-Publication Data
Mastering geriatric care.
     p. cm.
   Includes index.
   1. Geriatric nursing. I. Sprinhouse Corporation.
   [DNLM: 1. Geriatric Nursing. WY 152 M423 1996]
RC954.M365 1996
610.73'65 — dc20
DNLM/DLC
ISBN 0-87434-871-4 (alk. paper)   96-28895
                                     CIP

Contents

Contributors & Consultants

Bertha A. Almendarez, RN, MSN
Chairperson, Department of Vocational Nurse
Education
Del Mar College
Corpus Christi, Tex.

Heidi Brush RN,C, BSN
Nursing Supervisor, Home Care Department
Doylestown (Pa.) Hospital

Patricia Cullen, RN, EdD
Associate Professor of Nursing
Gwynedd Mercy College
Gwynedd, Pa.

T.C. England, RN, MSN
Health Occupations Instructor
North Montco Technical Career Center
Lansdale, Pa.

Beverly Sigl Felten, RN, MS, APNP, CS
Gerontological Clinical Nurse Specialist
Gero-Psych Nursing, S.C.
Lannon, Wis.

Cheryl L. George, RN, MS
Director of Education
Sherbrook Community Centre
Saskatoon, Saskatchewan, Canada

Janet E. Gordon, RN, EdD
Associate Professor of Nursing
Gwynedd Mercy College
Gwynedd, Pa.

MaryAnn M. Greenway, RN, MSN, CS, GNP
Gerontologic Clinical Specialist
Philadelphia Geriatric Center

Ginny Wacker Guido, RN, MSN, JD
Professor and Chair, Department of Nursing
Eastern New Mexico University
Portales, N.M.

Mary E. Hujer, RN, MSN, CS
Geriatric Clinical Nurse Specialist
Cleveland Clinic Foundation, Section of Geriatrics

Barbara Jones, RN, DNSc
Associate Professor, Division of Nursing
Gwynedd Mercy College
Gwynedd, Pa.

Mary A. Kaufmann, RN, MSN, LNHA
Director of Skilled Nursing/Hospice/Cancer
Services
Lorain (Ohio) Community–St. Joseph Regional
Health Center

Dr. Margie Maddox, RN, ANP-C, ARNP
Associate Professor, Coordinator of the ANP Track
University of Louisville (Ky.) School of Nursing

Karen E. Michael, RN, MSN
Manager, Concurrent Review/Case Management
QualMed Plans for Health, Inc.
Philadelphia

Penny Stewart Milanovich, RN, MSN, AACHE, CNA
Vice President, Visiting Nurses Association,
Western Pennsylvania
Butler, Pa.

Ruth Mooney, RN, MN, PhD
Director of Clinical Practice and Research for
Nursing
Philadelphia Geriatric Center

Mary Tracy Parsons, RN, MSN
Assistant Professor
Creighton University School of Nursing
Omaha, Neb.

Ann Katherine Patek, RN, MSN
Clinical Instructor
University of Wisconsin–Eau Claire School of
Nursing

Lori Martin Plank, RN, MSN, CS, FNP, GNP
Coordinator, Adult Nurse Practitioner Program
Gwynedd Mercy College
Gwynedd, Pa.

Gail Remus
Associate Professor
University of Saskatchewan College of Nursing
Saskatoon, Saskatchewan, Canada

Joyce L. Ross, RN,C, MSN, CCS, CRNP
Certified Clinical Specialist, Director of Staff
Development
Dunwoody Village
Newtown Square, Pa.

Christine E. Shebest, RN
Clinical Supervisor, Home Care Department
Doylestown (Pa.) Hospital

Sylvia F. Shelly, RN,C
Staff Nurse
Grand View Hospital
Sellersville, Pa.

Grace E. Wert, RN, MSN, CS
Gerontological Clinical Nurse Specialist
Abington (Pa.) Memorial Hospital

Joan Zieja, RN, MPH
Assistant Professor of Nursing
Holy Family College
Philadelphia

Foreword

While the overall U.S. population increased by 45% from 1960 to 1996, the group of adults age 65 and older grew by 100% and the group age 85 and older — the "oldest old"— increased by almost 300%. Indeed, adults age 85 and older make up the fastest-growing segment of the population. Over the next 50 years, their numbers are expected to grow from the current 3 million to 19 million.

These demographics make it clear that health care professionals will need to focus more and more on the health care needs of older adults. Those far-ranging needs include acute care, long-term nursing care, subacute care, home care, adult day care, and inpatient and outpatient rehabilitative and psychiatric care. And as older adults live longer and are more productive, those of us who care for them will also need to emphasize health promotion and maintenance — for instance, ensuring adequate nutrition and physical activity, eliminating physical and psychological stresses, and teaching proper use of prescription medications.

Unfortunately, many nurses are ill-equipped to deal with older adults' complex problems and highly specialized needs. That's where *Mastering Geriatric Care* helps beyond measure. This practical, hands-on reference provides solid gerontologic information for nurses practicing in all care settings as well as for nursing students — and, indeed, for anyone who cares for elderly patients.

In Chapter 1, you'll find an overview of the geriatric population, including demographics, societal attitudes toward the elderly, normal physiologic changes associated with aging, and age-related adjustments and transitions. Chapter 2 focuses on assessing the older adult. It describes useful tools for functional assessment and provides systematic guidelines for adapting the physical examination and psychosocial assessment to distinguish your patient's illness from typical aging processes.

Keeping older adults healthy is the focus of

Chapter 3, which discusses the importance of exercise, nutrition, sleep, elimination, and sexual function in maintaining health and well-being. It also touches on the need for preventive health measures, such as regular checkups and immunizations, as Americans look increasingly to managed care systems to meet their health care needs.

Chapter 4 addresses the mental and emotional needs of your older patients. It provides assessment tools and nursing interventions for common mental disorders affecting this age-group, such as anxiety, depression, and dementia. It also examines the effects of various drugs on mental status and provides useful information on available outpatient treatment options.

In Chapter 5, you'll learn what you can do to prevent falls — a major health risk for older people. You'll discover the most common risk factors for falls as well as the steps you can take — and teach to caregivers — to eliminate or minimize risks. Chapter 6 looks at two other common age-related problems — declining hearing and vision — and their impact on both the older adult and the caregiver.

Chapters 7 through 13 discuss specific disorders that commonly affect older people, categorized by body system. Chapters 7 and 8 deal with cardiovascular and respiratory diseases, such as coronary artery disease, myocardial infarction, peripheral vascular disease, pneumonia, and adult respiratory distress syndrome. Chapters 9 and 10 look at the common neurologic and musculoskeletal diseases, including Alzheimer's disease, stroke, Parkinson's disease, osteoarthritis, and hip fractures.

Chapter 11 addresses three common problems — incontinence, benign prostatic hyperplasia, and urinary tract infection. Incontinence, the most misunderstood of the three, affects about 30% of elderly people but is often overlooked by health care providers and by older adults themselves, who regard it as an inevitable part of growing old. You'll learn how to assess this aggravating problem and how to help your patients overcome it.

In Chapters 12 and 13, you'll find a comprehensive discussion of cancer and diabetes, two diseases that are prevalent in older adults and that require sophisticated health care interventions. Drug and alcohol abuse, problems not recognized often enough in older adults, are addressed in Chapter 14. You'll learn why some elders abuse alcohol and misuse prescribed medications, and you'll discover useful strategies to help patients deal with this growing problem.

Chapter 15 addresses another problem that's becoming more prevalent: elder abuse and neglect. It identifies strategies for assessing physical and mental abuse as well as interventions you can perform when you suspect abuse. You'll learn how to report abuse, the legal requirements for doing so, the recommended institutional policies, and the route to take when you suspect a co-worker of abusing patients.

Chapter 16 deals with the important subject of proper drug use. Older adults take more prescribed medications than any other age-group, yet they often take them incorrectly, changing either the dosage or the frequency of administration. You'll discover how best to assess your patient for this problem and how to improve his compliance. You'll also learn how age-related changes affect drug metabolism and how complex coexisting medical conditions can affect drug use.

Chapter 17 deals with specific procedures for reestablishing bowel and bladder control after illness or surgery or despite normal physiologic decline. In Chapter 18, you'll learn how age-related changes in skin, such as decreased elasticity, affect skin integrity and wound care. Control of chronic pain is frustrating for most caregivers. Chapter 19 explains theories of pain and provides practical interventions for helping your patients deal with chronic pain.

Chapter 20 covers the sensitive legal and ethical concerns associated with older adults, such as living wills, informed consent, guardianship, and the use of physical and chemical restraints. An invaluable appendix discusses the many community services available to older adults, provides an extensive list of specific resources, and lists selected titles for further reading.

In summary, *Mastering Geriatric Care* is a comprehensive, practical resource for nurses in all settings who are caring for an ever-growing population of older adults. Understanding the physiologic changes and special needs of older patients will focus your skills, increase your confidence, and result in improved care for your older patients.

Mary Knapp, MSN, CRNP, NHA, FAAN
President
The Whitman Group, National Aging Specialists
Huntingdon Valley, Pa.

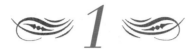

Understanding the geriatric population

Chances are that many, if not most, patients in your practice are or will soon be older adults. Studies show that people age 65 or older require health care services more frequently than any other age-group. In fact, they account for 30% of all hospital discharges and 36% of the country's personal health care expenditures.

When caring for older patients, use the same techniques you would use for any other adult, but with certain important modifications: You need to take into account the physiologic and biological changes that normally occur during aging and to understand older adults' special health requirements. Among other things, they may need help learning to access community services, avoid falls, and deal with age-related problems such as incontinence. You also need to understand the effects of drugs on older patients and the options available in long-term care. Equally important, you need to examine personal feelings about elderly people to make sure that common misconceptions about aging aren't affecting the quality of care you provide.

SOCIETAL ATTITUDES AND BELIEFS

Older adults make up the most stereotyped age-group. Normal aging and the changes associated with it are rarely viewed as positive — or even natural. We describe most changes as losses, such as a loss of tissue elasticity or a decrease in blood flow. We regard aging as a series of inevitable, negative events that a person must tolerate. In addition, we often mention aging changes and disease conditions in the same breath.

Some of the myths, misconceptions, and negative stereotypes about older people stem from our culture's values and beliefs. Our youth-oriented society values intelligence, strength, self-reliance, and productivity — characteristics rarely attributed to older adults. Many people perceive older adults as senile, sick, and making few worthwhile contributions to society. Portrayals of elderly people in movies, television, advertisements, and other media compound this image.

While seemingly harmless, such images perpetuate negative ideas about aging that can affect health care workers and the quality of health care that older adults receive. Stereotyping can affect all aspects of care planning and implementation — for example, a nurse regularly delaying response to an older patient's call bell. It can influence salaries — nurses working in nursing homes typically make less money than those working in other facilities. It can also affect policy and program development. (See *Dispelling common myths about aging,* page 2.)

Fear of aging

Most people don't know enough about the realities of aging; they fear death and, therefore, fear growing

Dispelling common myths about aging

Here are some common misconceptions about aging and the facts to help dispel them.

Most older people are senile or demented.

Senility is an inaccurate term used to refer to dementing conditions that are always caused by pathologic changes. Most people age 65 and older aren't mentally disturbed. Significant, progressive, cognitive impairments are a consequence of disease that affects less than 5% of people ages 65 to 74 and about 25% of people older than age 85.

Most old people feel miserable and depressed most of the time.

Studies of happiness, morale, and life satisfaction reveal that most older people are just as happy as when they were younger. Only about one-third of older people show signs of depression.

Older people can't work as effectively as younger people.

On the contrary, studies show that older workers produce more consistent output and have less job turnover, fewer accidents, and less absenteeism than younger workers.

Older people can't learn complex new skills and experience decline in intellectual ability.

Older adults are capable of learning new things, but the speed at which they process information is slower. Healthy older adults show no decline and sometimes show improvement in some cognitive skills such as wisdom, judgment, creativity, and common sense. Most show a slight and gradual decline in other cognitive skills, such as abstraction, calculation, and verbal comprehension.

Most older people are sick and need help with daily activities.

In fact, 80% of older people are healthy enough to carry on their normal lifestyle. About 15% have chronic health conditions that interfere with their daily lives, and another 5% are institutionalized.

Older people are set in their ways and can't change.

People tend to become more stable in their attitudes as they age, but they adapt to many social changes and changes in lifestyle. In fact, older people may be required to change more frequently than when they were younger because of major events in their lives.

older. *Gerontophobia* refers to this fear and the refusal to accept older people into the mainstream of society.

Anyone — regardless of age — can experience gerontophobia, which sometimes causes strange behavior, such as teenagers buying antiwrinkle cream, 30-year-olds considering facelifts, 40-year-olds having hair transplants, and long-term marriages dissolving so that one spouse can pursue someone younger.

The extreme forms of gerontophobia are ageism and age discrimination. Like other forms of prejudice, they result from ignorance about a group of people who are different from ourselves.

Ageism, the dislike of aging and older persons, rests on a belief that aging makes people unattractive, unintelligent, and unproductive; it's an emotional prejudice.

Age discrimination goes beyond emotion; it's the practice of treating people differently simply because of their age. Refusing to hire older people, barring them from bank loans, and limiting the types or amounts of health care provided, despite laws prohibiting such actions, are examples of age discrimination.

Definitions of aging

The words "aging" and "old age" are highly subjective. "Aging" is defined as the time from birth to the present for a living individual, as measured in specific units. "Old" is defined as having lived for a long time and is often synonymous with negative terms, such as "ancient," "antiquated," and "timeworn."

The meanings of old and aging depend to a great extent on how old the speaker is and that person's experiences. Children don't describe themselves as aging, but they happily proclaim how old they are. For adults, aging is negatively associated with being old, and old age is commonly described as any age several years beyond the speaker's.

The process of aging is a complex one that can be described chronologically, physiologically, and functionally.

Chronologic age refers to the number of years a person has lived. Easy to identify and measure, it's the most commonly used objective method. In addition, chronologic age serves as criteria in society for certain activities, such as driving, employment, and the collection of retirement benefits. With the passage of the Social Security Act and the establishment of Medicare, age 65 became the minimum age of eligibility for retirement benefits. In the United States, therefore, 65 is the accepted age for becoming a senior citizen. Many people, however, are challenging this determination.

Physiologic age refers to the determination of age by body function. Although age-related changes affect everyone, it's impossible to pinpoint exactly when these changes occur. That's why physiologic age isn't useful in determining a person's age.

Functional age refers to a person's ability to contribute to society and benefit others and himself. It's based on the fact that not all individuals of the same chronologic age function at the same level. Many people may be chronologically older but remain physically fit, mentally active, and productive members of society. Others may be chronologically young, but physically or functionally old.

Chronologic categories
In an attempt to further define the aging population, old age has been divided into chronologic categories. One such classification uses three categories:
• young-old (ages 65 to 74)
• middle-old (ages 75 to 84)
• old-old (age 85 and older).
The fastest growing segment of the older population is over age 75. Those who require help are called the frail elderly. Of those noninstitutionalized adults ages 75 to 84, about 25% need help with daily activities. Of those age 85 and older, nearly one-half need help with daily activities.

Characteristics common to the frail elderly include:
• poor mental and physical health
• low socioeconomic status
• predominantly female
• possibly isolated living conditions
• more and longer hospital stays with more money spent on health care and drugs

• more frequent visits to the doctor
• more use of nursing home beds than hospital beds.

Demographics of aging
The older adult population is growing rapidly. In 1990, 31 million older adults accounted for approximately 12.5% of the U.S. population. By the year 2030, older adults are projected to make up about 22% of the U.S. population.

Since 1900, the percentage of older adults in the population has tripled. The greatest increase occurred in the 65-to-74 age-group, which is eight times larger now than in 1900. The current 75-to-84 age-group is 13 times larger, and the age-85-and-older group is 24 times larger. Between the ages of 65 and 69, women outnumber men by a ratio of 120 to 100; over age 85, the ratio is 258 to 100. According to projections, the growth of the elderly population will peak in 2030. The most rapid increase will occur from 2005 to 2030, as the baby boom generation reaches age 65.

THE NORMAL AGING PROCESS

Aging is a normal part of human development. The patterns of aging — what happens, how, and when — vary greatly among older people. Although specific changes are identified as part of the normal aging process, each person ages in his own way. As the years accumulate, people become more diverse rather than more alike, each influenced by physical, social, and environmental factors. How a person ages depends on life experiences, available support systems, and previous coping skills. In addition, not all body systems age from the same functional level or at the same rate.

Theories of aging
Various theories have been proposed to explain the process of normal aging and help dispel some of the myths. A set of biological, psychosocial, and developmental theories of aging provides guidelines to

determine how well a patient is adjusting to aging. These theories also identify areas that need to be assessed and provide a basis for interventions and rationales in nursing care. No single theory of aging is universally accepted. *Biological theories* attempt to explain physical aging as an involuntary process, which eventually leads to cumulative changes in cells, tissues, and fluids. Intrinsic biological theory maintains that aging changes arise from internal, predetermined causes. Extrinsic biological theory maintains that environmental factors lead to structural alterations, which, in turn, cause degenerative changes.

Psychological theories of aging attempt to explain age-related changes in cognitive function, such as intelligence, memory, learning, and problem solving, while *sociologic theories* attempt to explain changes that affect socialization and life satisfaction. Sociologic theories maintain that as social expectations change, people assume new roles, which leads to changes in identity. Finally, *developmental theories* describe specific life stages and tasks associated with each stage. (See *Reviewing selected theories of aging.*)

NORMAL PHYSIOLOGIC CHANGES OF AGING

The loss of some body cells and reduced metabolism in other cells characterize aging. These processes cause a decline in bodily function and changes in body composition.

Although an older person's body tends to work less efficiently than a younger person's, illness doesn't inevitably accompany old age. Certainly a person's heart, lungs, kidneys, and other organs will be less efficient at age 60 than they were at age 20. However, you shouldn't equate aging with the unavoidable breakdown of body systems. It's important for you to recognize the gradual changes in body function that normally accompany aging, so you can adjust your assessment techniques accordingly. It's equally important for you to recognize that even laboratory test values will change to reflect the aging process. Values considered abnormal in younger adults may be perfectly normal in older adults (see *How lab values change in elderly patients,* pages 7 to 9). Understanding the normal aging process can help you understand why a person's risk of developing certain diseases and sustaining injuries increases over time. (See *Illness and injury: Why the risks increase with age,* page 10.)

Nutrition

A person's protein, vitamin, and mineral requirements usually remain the same as he ages, whereas caloric needs are lessened. Diminished activity may lower energy requirements by about 200 calories per day for men and women ages 51 to 75, 400 calories per day for women over age 75, and 500 calories per day for men over age 75.

Other physiologic changes that can affect nutrition in an older patient include:
- decreased renal function, causing greater susceptibility to dehydration and formation of renal calculi
- loss of calcium and nitrogen (in patients who aren't ambulatory)
- diminished enzyme activity and gastric secretions
- reduced pepsin and hydrochloric acid secretion, which tends to diminish the absorption of calcium and vitamins B_1 and B_2
- decreased salivary flow and diminished sense of taste, which may reduce the person's appetite and increase his consumption of sweet and spicy foods
- diminished intestinal motility and peristalsis of the large intestine
- thinning of tooth enamel, causing teeth to become more brittle
- decreased biting force
- diminished gag reflex.

Some common conditions found in older people can affect nutritional status by limiting the patient's mobility and, therefore, his ability to obtain or prepare food or feed himself.

Diminished intestinal motility typically accompanies aging and may cause GI disorders such as constipation. Fecal incontinence may also occur. Nutritionally inadequate diets of soft, refined foods low in dietary fiber, physical inactivity, emotional stress, or certain medications can also cause consti-

Reviewing selected theories of aging

This chart discusses some of the common biological and psychosocial theories of aging.

THEORY	SOURCES	RETARDANTS
BIOLOGICAL THEORIES		
Cross-link theory Strong chemical bonding between organic molecules in the body causes increased stiffness, chemical instability, and insolubility of connective tissue and deoxyribonucleic acid.	Lipid, protein, carbohydrate, and nucleic acids	Restricting calories and lathyrogens (antilink agents)
Free-radical theory Increased unstable free radicals produce effects harmful to biological systems, such as chromosomal changes, pigment accumulation, and collagen alteration.	Environmental pollutants; oxidation of dietary fat, protein, carbohydrate, and elements	Improving environmental monitoring; decreasing intake of free-radical-stimulating foods; increasing intake of vitamins A and C (mercaptans) and vitamin E
Immunologic theory An aging immune system is less able to distinguish body cells from foreign cells; as a result, it begins to attack and destroy body cells as if they were foreign. This may explain the adult onset of conditions such as diabetes mellitus, rheumatic heart disease, and arthritis. Theorists have speculated on several erratic cellular mechanisms capable of precipitating attacks on various tissues through autoaggression or immunodeficiencies.	Alteration of B and T cells of the humoral and cellular systems	Immunoengineering — selective alteration and replenishment or rejuvenation of the immune system
Wear and tear theory Body cells, structures, and functions wear out or are overused through exposure to internal and external stressors. Effects from the residual damage accumulate, the body can no longer resist stress, and death occurs.	Repeated injury or overuse; internal and external stressors (physical, psychological, social, and environmental), including trauma, chemicals, and buildup of naturally occurring wastes	Reevaluating and possibly adjusting lifestyle
PSYCHOSOCIAL THEORIES		
Activity theory Successful aging and life satisfaction depend on maintaining high level of activity.	Quality and meaningfulness of activities more important than quantity; life satisfaction related to involvement in life	Increasing activities in other areas when activities in one area decrease
Continuity theory Individual remains essentially the same, despite life changes; focuses more on personality and individual behavior over time.	Assumed stability of individual patterns or orientation over time	Taking into account the impact of major societal changes, which can alter individual expectations and behaviors

(continued)

Reviewing selected theories of aging (continued)

THEORY	SOURCES	RETARDANTS
PSYCHOSOCIAL THEORIES *(continued)*		
Disengagement theory		
Progressive social disengagement occurs with age.	Decreased participation in society resulting from age-related changes in health, energy, income, and social roles	Taking into account diversity of individual outlook and lifestyle and social structure variables, such as economy and social organizations
Social exchange theory		
Social behavior involves doing what is valued and rewarded by society.	Diminished resources and increased dependency, leading to unequal contribution to society and reduced power and value; decreased number of roles available in society	Assuming new roles and friendships with other older adults to help socialize person and help person adjust to age-related norms

---

pation. Laxative abuse results in the rapid transport of food through the GI tract, decreasing digestion and absorption.

Socioeconomic and psychological factors that affect nutritional status include loneliness, decline of the older person's importance in the family, susceptibility to nutritional quackery, and lack of money or transportation to buy nutritious foods.

Skin, hair, and nails

Skin changes, such as facial lines around the eyes (crow's feet), mouth, and nose, noticeably show aging. These lines result from subcutaneous fat loss, dermal thinning, decreasing collagen and elastin, and a 50% decline in cell replacement. With the decreased rate of skin cell replacement, an older person's wound may heal more slowly and he may be more susceptible to infection. Women's skin shows signs of aging about 10 years earlier than men's because it's thinner and drier. Very old people's skin loses its elasticity until it may seem almost transparent. The supraclavicular and axillary regions, the knuckles, and the hand tendons and vessels are more prominent, as are fat pads over bony prominences.

Mucous membranes become dry, and sweat gland output lessens as the number of active sweat glands declines. Body temperature becomes more difficult to regulate because of the decrease in size, number, and function of sweat glands and the loss of subcutaneous fat. Although melanocyte production decreases as a person ages, localized melanocyte proliferations are common and cause brown spots (senile lentigo) to appear, especially in areas regularly exposed to the sun.

Hair pigment decreases with age, and hair may turn gray or white. Hair also thins as the number of melanocytes declines; by age 70, it's baby fine again. Hormonal changes cause pubic hair loss. Facial hair often increases in postmenopausal women and decreases in aging men.

Aging also may alter nails. They may grow at different rates, and longitudinal ridges, flaking, brittleness, and malformations may increase. Toenails may discolor.

Other common hyperplastic skin conditions in older people include senile keratosis (dry, harsh skin) and senile angioma (a benign tumor of dilated blood vessels caused by weakened capillary walls).

How lab values change in elderly patients

Standard normal laboratory values reflect the physiology of 20 to 40 year olds. However, normal values for older patients often differ because of age-related physiologic changes.

Certain tests, though, remain unaffected by age. These include partial thromboplastin time (PTT), prothrombin time (PT), serum acid phosphatase, serum carbon dioxide, serum chloride, serum glutamic-oxaloacetic transaminase (SGOT), and total serum protein. You can use this chart to interpret other, changeable test values in your elderly patients.

TEST VALUES AT 20 TO 40 YEARS	AGE-RELATED CHANGES	CONSIDERATIONS
BLOOD TESTS		
Albumin 3.5 to 5.0 g/dl	Under age 65: Higher in men Over age 65: Levels equalize, then decrease at same rate	Increased dietary protein intake needed in older patients if liver function is normal; edema a sign of low albumin level
Alkaline phosphatase 13 to 39 IU/L	Increases 8 to 10 IU/L	May reflect liver function decline or vitamin D malabsorption and bone demineralization
β-globulin 2.3 to 3.5 g/dl	Increases slightly	Increases in response to decrease in albumin if liver function is normal; increased dietary protein intake needed
Blood urea nitrogen (BUN) Men: 10 to 25 mg/dl Women: 8 to 20 mg/dl	Increases, possibly to 69 mg/dl	Slight increase acceptable in absence of stressors, such as infection or surgery
Cholesterol 120 to 220 mg/dl	Men: Increases to age 50, then decreases Women: Lower than men until age 50, increases to age 70, then decreases	Rise in cholesterol level (and increased cardiovascular risk) in women as a result of postmenopausal estrogen decline; dietary changes, weight loss, and exercise needed
Creatine kinase (CK) 17 to 148 U/L	Increases slightly	May reflect decreasing muscle mass and liver function
Creatinine 0.6 to 1.5 mg/dl	Increases, possibly to 1.9 mg/dl in men	Important factor to prevent toxicity when giving drugs that are excreted in urine
Creatinine clearance 104 to 125 ml/min	Men: Decreases; formula:(140 - age x kg body weight)/72 x serum creatinine Women: 85% of men's rate	Reflects reduced glomerular filtration rate; important factor to prevent toxicity when giving drugs that are excreted in urine

(continued)

How lab values change in elderly patients *(continued)*

TEST VALUES AT 20 TO 40 YEARS	AGE-RELATED CHANGES	CONSIDERATIONS
BLOOD TESTS		
Glucose tolerance (fasting plasma glucose) 1 hr: 160 to 170 mg/dl 2 hr: 115 to 125 mg/dl 3 hr: 70 to 110 mg/dl	Rises faster in first 2 hrs, then drops to baseline more slowly	Reflects declining pancreatic insulin supply and release and deminishing body mass for glucose uptake. Rapid *rise* can quickly trigger hyperosmolar hyperglycemic nonketotic syndrome. Rapid *decline* can result from certain drugs, such as alcohol, beta blockers, and MAO inhibitors.
Hematocrit (HCT) Men: 45% to 52% Women: 37% to 48%	May decrease slightly (unproven)	Reflects decreased bone marrow and hematopoiesis, increased risk of infection (fewer and weaker lymphocytes, and immune system changes that diminish antigen-antibody response)
Hemoglobin (HGB) Men: 13 to 18 g/100 ml Women: 12 to 16 g/100 ml	Men: Drops 1 to 2 g/100 ml Women: Unknown	Reflects decreased bone marrow, hematopoiesis, and (for men) androgen levels
High-density lipoproteins (HDL) 80 to 310 mg/100 ml	Levels higher in women than in men; levels equalize with age	Compliance with dietary restrictions required for accurate interpretation of test results
Lactate dehydrogenase (LDH) 45 to 90 U/L	Increases slightly	May reflect declining muscle mass and liver function
Leukocytes 4,300 to 10,800/mm^3	Drop to 3,100 to 9,000/mm^3	Decrease proportionate to lymphocytes
Lymphocytes T: 500 to 2,400/mm^3 B: 50 to 200/mm^3	Decrease	Decrease proportionate to leukocytes
Platelets 150,000 to 350,000/mm^3	Change in characteristics: decreased granular constituents, increased platelet-release factors	May reflect diminished bone marrow, increased fibrinogen levels
Potassium 3.5 to 5.5 mEq/L	Increases slightly	Requires avoidance of salt substitutes composed of potassium, food-label vigilance, and knowledge of hyperkalemia's signs and symptoms

How lab values change in elderly patients (continued)

TEST VALUES AT 20 TO 40 YEARS	AGE-RELATED CHANGES	CONSIDERATIONS
BLOOD TESTS *(continued)*		
Thyroid-stimulating hormone (TSH) 0.3 to 5.0 microIU/l	Increases slightly	Suggests primary hypothyroidism or endemic goiter at much higher levels
Thyroxine (T$_4$) 4.5 to 13.5 mcg/100 ml	Decreases 25%	Reflects declining thyroid function
Triglycerides 40 to 150 mg/100 ml	Range widens: 20 to 200 mg/100 ml	Suggests abnormalities at any other levels, requiring additional tests such as serum cholesterol
Tri-iodothyronine (T$_3$) 90 to 220 ng/100 ml	Decreases 25%	Reflects declining thyroid function
URINE TESTS		
Glucose 0 to 15 mg/100 ml	Decreases slightly	May reflect renal disease or UTI; unreliable check for older diabetic patients, as glycosuria may not occur until plasma glucose level exceeds 300 mg/100 ml
Protein 0 to 5 mg/100 ml	Increases slightly	May reflect renal disease or UTI
Specific gravity 1.032	Decreases to 1.024 by age 80	Reflects 30% to 50% decrease in number of nephrons available to concentrate urine

Eyes and vision

Eye structure and visual acuity change with age. The eyes sit deeper in their sockets and the eyelids lose their elasticity, becoming baggy and wrinkled. The conjunctiva becomes thinner and yellow, and pingueculae — fat pads that form under the conjunctiva — may develop. As the lacrimal apparatus gradually loses fatty tissue, the quantity of tears decreases and evaporation occurs more quickly.

With age, the cornea loses its luster and flattens, while the iris fades or develops irregular pigmentation. Increased connective tissue may cause sclerosis of the sphincter muscles. The pupil becomes smaller, which decreases the amount of light that reaches the retina; older adults need about three times as much light as a younger person to see objects clearly. Aging diminishes night vision and depth perception.

The sclera becomes thick and rigid, and fat deposits cause yellowing. The vitreous can degenerate over time, revealing opacities and floating vitreous debris, and can also detach from the retina.

Illness and injury: Why the risks increase with age

The normal aging process places older adults at risk for certain diseases and injuries. Here are some examples.
- Decreased cerebral blood flow increases risk of stroke.
- An older person's spinal cord is tightly encased in vertebrae that may be studded with bony spurs or shrunken around the cord. Even a minor fall can cause severe cord damage.
- In older women, osteoporosis can cause compression fractures even without a history of trauma.
- Brittle bones make an older person especially prone to fractures. Falling on an outstretched arm or hand or experiencing a direct blow to the arm or shoulder is very likely to fracture the shoulder or humerus.
- Diminished cardiac rate and stroke volume place an older person at risk for developing congestive heart failure, hypertensive crisis, arterial occlusion, and myocardial infarction.
- Weakened chest musculature reduces an older person's ability to clear lung secretions and increases his risk of developing pneumonia, tuberculosis, and other respiratory diseases.
- In older men, prostatic hypertrophy is a common cause of urinary tract obstruction and acute urine retention.
- A weakened immune system increases an older, debilitated person's risk of acquiring almost any infection he's exposed to.

Through the ophthalmoscope, the vitreous, detached from the area of the optic disk, looks like a dark ring in front of the disk. With age, the lens enlarges and loses transparency. Accommodation decreases because of impaired lens elasticity (presbyopia).

Older adults often experience impaired color vision, especially in the blue and green ranges, because cones in the retina deteriorate. They also experience decreased reabsorption of intraocular fluid, which predisposes them to glaucoma.

Ears and hearing

Many older people lose some degree of hearing. Sometimes, the gradual buildup of cerumen in the ear is the cause. Usually, however, hearing loss results from the slowly progressing deafness of aging, called presbycusis or senile deafness. This irreversible, bilateral, sensorineural hearing loss usually starts during middle age, slowly worsens, and affects men more than women.

Presbycusis appears in four forms. The most common form, sensory presbycusis, is caused by atrophy of the organ of Corti and the auditory nerve. The accompanying hearing loss occurs mostly in the high-pitch ranges. By age 60, most adults have difficulty hearing above 4,000 Hz. (The normal range for speech recognition is 500 to 2,000 Hz.) Older adults can't easily distinguish the high-pitched consonants: s, z, t, f, and g.

Aging causes degenerative structural changes in the entire auditory system. The incidence of hearing loss in older people is probably higher than statistics indicate. Often, an older person isn't immediately aware of a hearing defect's onset or progression. He may recognize the problem but, accepting it as a natural aspect of aging, may not seek medical help.

Respiratory system

Age-related anatomic changes in the upper airways include nose enlargement from continued cartilage growth, general atrophy of the tonsils, and tracheal deviations from changes in the aging spine. Possible thoracic changes include increased anteroposterior chest diameter, as a result of altered calcium metabolism, and calcification of costal cartilages, which reduces mobility of the chest wall. Kyphosis advances with age because of such factors as osteoporosis and vertebral collapse.

Also, pulmonary function decreases in older people because of respiratory muscle degeneration or atrophy. Ventilatory capacity diminishes for several reasons. First, the lungs' diffusing capacity declines. Decreased inspiratory and expiratory muscle strength diminishes vital capacity. Second, lung tissue degeneration causes a decrease in the lungs' elastic recoil capability, which results in an elevated residual volume. Thus, aging alone can cause emphysema.

Last, the closing of some airways produces poor ventilation of the basal areas, resulting in both a decreased surface area for gas exchange and reduced partial pressures of oxygen (PO_2). The normal partial pressures of oxygen in arterial blood (PaO_2) decreases to 70 to 85 mm Hg. Oxygen saturation decreases by 5%. The lungs become more rigid, and the number and size of alveoli decline with age. In addition, a 30% reduction in respiratory fluids heightens the risk of pulmonary infection and mucus plugs. Thus, maximum breathing capacity, forced vital capacity, vital capacity, and inspiratory reserve volume diminish with age, leaving the older patient with lowered tolerance for oxygen debt.

Cardiovascular system

As a person ages, his heart usually becomes slightly smaller and loses its contractile strength and efficiency (although exceptions occur in people with hypertension or heart disease). By age 70, cardiac output at rest has diminished by about 30% to 35% in many people. Fibrotic and sclerotic changes thicken heart valves and reduce their flexibility, leading to rigidity and incomplete closure of the heart valves, which may result in systolic murmurs. In addition, the thickness of the left ventricular wall increases by 25% between the ages of 30 and 80. Older people may also develop obstructive coronary disease and fibrosis of the cardiac skeleton.

As the myocardium of the aging heart becomes more irritable, extra systoles may occur, along with sinus arrhythmias and sinus bradycardias. In addition, increased fibrous tissue infiltrates the sinoatrial node and internodal atrial tracts, which may cause atrial fibrillation and flutter. The veins also dilate and stretch with age, and coronary artery blood flow decreases 35% between the ages of 20 and 60. The aorta becomes more rigid, causing systolic blood pressure to rise disproportionately higher than the diastolic, resulting in a widened pulse pressure. Electrocardiogram (ECG) changes include increased PR, QRS, and QT intervals, decreased amplitude of the QRS complex, and a shift of the QRS axis to the left.

The heart's ability to respond to physical and emotional stress also may decrease markedly with age. Heart rate takes longer to return to normal after exercise. Usually, aging also contributes to arterial and venous insufficiency as the strength and elasticity of blood vessels decrease. All these factors contribute to older people's increased incidence of cardiovascular disease, particularly coronary disease.

GI system

The physiologic changes that accompany aging usually prove less debilitating in the GI system than in most other body systems. Normal changes include diminished mucosal elasticity and reduced GI secretions, which, in turn, modify some processes — for example, digestion and absorption. GI tract motility, bowel wall and anal sphincter tone, and abdominal muscle strength also may decrease with age. Any of these changes may cause complaints in an older patient, ranging from loss of appetite to constipation.

Normal physiologic changes in the liver include decreased liver weight, reduced regenerative capacity, and decreased blood flow to the liver. Because hepatic enzymes involved in oxidation and reduction markedly decline with age, the liver metabolizes drugs and detoxifies substances less efficiently.

Renal system

After age 40, a person's renal function may diminish; if he lives to age 90, it may have decreased by as much as 50%. This change is reflected in a decline in the glomerular filtration rate caused by age-related changes in renal vasculature that disturb glomerular hemodynamics. Renal blood flow decreases 53% from reduced cardiac output and age-related atherosclerotic changes. In addition, tubular reabsorption and renal concentrating ability decline because the size and number of functioning nephrons decrease. As a person ages, his bladder muscles weaken, which may result in incomplete bladder emptying and chronic urine retention — predisposing the bladder to infection.

Other age-related changes that affect renal function include diminished kidney size, impaired renal clearance of drugs, reduced bladder size and capacity, and decreased renal ability to respond to

---

Characterizing the male climacteric

This list reviews the physiologic changes that characterize the male climacteric.
- Testosterone production declines.
- Pleasure sensations become less genitally localized and more generalized.
- Erections require more time and stimulation to achieve.
- Erections aren't as full or as hard.
- The prostate gland enlarges and its secretions diminish.
- Seminal fluid decreases.
- Ejaculatory force diminishes.
- Contractions in the prostate gland and penile urethra during orgasm vary in length and quality.
- The refractory period following ejaculation may lengthen from minutes to days.

---

variations in sodium intake. By age 70, blood urea nitrogen levels rise by 21%. Residual urine, frequency, and nocturia also increase with age.

Male reproductive system

Physiologic changes in older men include reduced testosterone production, which, in turn, may cause a decrease in libido. A reduced testosterone level also causes the testes to atrophy and soften and decreases sperm production by 69% to 48% between the ages of 60 and 80. Normally, the prostate gland enlarges with age and its secretions diminish. Seminal fluid also decreases in volume and becomes less viscous. During intercourse, older men experience slower and weaker physiologic reactions. However, these changes don't necessarily weaken a man's sex drive or lessen his sexual satisfaction. (See *Characterizing the male climacteric.*)

Female reproductive system

Declining estrogen and progesterone levels cause numerous physical changes in an aging woman. Significant emotional changes also take place during the transition from childbearing years to infertility. A postreproductive woman will benefit from

counseling and instruction on the changes she'll experience during the latter third of her life. She'll also need to know the best way to cope with these changes if she's to continue leading a full and satisfying life.

Because a woman's breasts and her internal and external reproductive structures are estrogen-dependent, aging takes a more conspicuous toll on the female than the male. As estrogen levels decrease and menopause approaches, usually at about age 50, the following changes occur.

Ovaries

Ovulation usually stops 1 to 2 years before menopause. As the ovaries reach the end of their productive cycle, they become unresponsive to gonadotropic stimulation. With aging, the ovaries atrophy and become thicker and smaller.

Vulva

This structure atrophies with age. Changes include pubic hair loss and flattening of the labia majora. Vulval tissue shrinks, exposing the sensitive area around the urethra and vagina to abrasions and irritation — for example, from undergarments. The introitus also constricts, tissues lose their elasticity, and the epidermis thins from 20 layers to about 5.

Vagina

Atrophy causes the vagina to shorten and the mucous lining to become thin, dry, less elastic, and pale as a result of decreased vascularity. In this state, the vaginal mucosa is highly susceptible to abrasion. In addition, the pH of vaginal secretions increases, making the vaginal environment more alkaline. The type of flora also changes, increasing the older woman's chance of vaginal infections.

Uterus

After menopause, the uterus shrinks rapidly to half its premenstrual weight, then continues to shrink until the organ reaches approximately one-fourth its premenstrual size. The cervix atrophies and no longer produces mucus for lubrication, and the endometrium and myometrium become thinner.

Breasts

Glandular, supporting, and fatty tissues atrophy. As Cooper's ligaments lose their elasticity, the breasts become pendulous. The nipples decrease in size and become flat. Fibrocystic disease that may have been present at menopause usually diminishes and disappears with increasing age. The inframammary ridges become more pronounced.

Pelvic support structures

Relaxation of these structures occurs commonly among postreproductive women. Initial relaxation usually occurs during labor and delivery, but clinical effects often go unnoticed until the process accelerates with menopausal estrogen depletion and loss of connective tissue elasticity and tone. Signs and symptoms include pressure and pulling in the area above the inguinal ligaments, low backache, a feeling of pelvic heaviness, and difficulty in rising from a chair. Urinary stress incontinence may also become a problem if urethrovesical ligaments weaken.

Neurologic system

Aging affects the nervous system in many ways. Neurons of the central and peripheral nervous systems undergo degenerative changes. Nerve transmission slows down, causing the older person to react sluggishly to external stimuli. After about age 50, the number of brain cells decreases at a rate of about 1% per year. Yet clinical effects usually aren't noticeable until aging is more advanced.

As a person ages, the hypothalamus becomes less effective at regulating body temperature. The cerebral cortex undergoes a 20% neuron loss. The corneal reflex becomes slower, and the pain threshold increases. An older person experiences a decrease in stages III and IV sleep, causing frequent awakenings; rapid-eye-movement sleep also decreases.

Musculoskeletal system

Adipose tissue stores usually increase with age; lean body mass and bone mineral contents usually diminish. The most apparent change is decreasing height. This results from exaggerated spinal curvatures and narrowing intervertebral spaces, which

shorten the trunk and make the arms appear relatively long. Other changes include decreased bone mass, muscle mass (which may result in muscle weakness), and collagen formation, which causes loss of resilience and elasticity in joints and supporting structures. Synovial fluid becomes more viscous, and the synovial membranes become more fibrotic.

In addition, aging may cause difficulty in tandem walking. Usually the person walks with shorter steps and a wider leg stance to achieve better balance and stable weight distribution.

Immune system

Immune function starts declining at sexual maturity and continues declining with age. During this decline, the immune system begins losing its ability to differentiate between self and nonself, and the incidence of autoimmune disease increases. The immune system also begins losing its ability to recognize and destroy mutant cells, which presumably accounts for the increase in cancer among older people.

Decreased antibody response in older people makes them more susceptible to infection. Tonsillar atrophy and lymphadenopathy commonly occur. Total and differential leukocyte counts don't change significantly with age. However, some people over age 65 may exhibit a slight decrease in the leukocyte count. When this happens, the number of B cells and total lymphocytes decreases, and T cells decrease in number and become less effective. Also, the size of the lymph nodes and spleen reduces slightly.

Fatty bone marrow replaces some active blood-forming marrow — first in the long bones and later in the flat bones. The altered bone marrow can't increase erythrocyte production as readily as before in response to such stimuli as hormones, anoxia, hemorrhage, and hemolysis. With age, vitamin B_{12} absorption may also diminish, resulting in reduced erythrocyte mass and decreased hemoglobin and hematocrit.

Endocrine system

A common and important endocrine change in older people is a decreased ability to tolerate stress.

The most obvious and serious indication of this diminished stress response occurs in glucose metabolism. Normally, fasting blood glucose levels aren't significantly different in young and old adults. But when stress stimulates an older person's pancreas, the blood glucose concentration increases more and remains elevated longer than in a younger adult. This diminished glucose tolerance occurs as a normal part of aging, a good point to keep in mind when evaluating an older person for diabetes.

In women, ovarian senescence at menopause causes permanent cessation of menstrual activity. Changes in endocrine function during menopause vary from woman to woman, but normally estrogen levels diminish and follicle-stimulating hormone production increases. This estrogen deficiency may result in either or both of two key metabolic effects: coronary thrombosis and osteoporosis. Remember, too, that some symptoms characteristic of menopause (such as depression, insomnia, headaches, fatigue, palpitations, and irritability) may also be associated with endocrine disorders.

In men, the climacteric stage lowers testosterone levels and seminal fluid production.

Other normal variations in endocrine function include reduced progesterone production, a 50% decline in serum aldosterone levels, and a 25% decrease in cortisol secretion rate.

AGE-RELATED ADJUSTMENTS AND TRANSITIONS

Aging is associated with many role changes and transitions. Some roles — such as spouse, friend, or employee — may be lost, while new roles — such as widow or volunteer — may arise. Such changes require role adjustment. Factors that influence role adjustment include age, sex, culture, beliefs, attitudes, income, health, and past experiences. Although change may be a single event, the effect is interactive with all areas of life.

Role changes

With aging, changes in the marital role may occur. After retirement, the division of labor and household management may change. One spouse may become the primary caregiver if the other becomes ill. If a spouse dies, social relations for the survivor may change. As a result, spouses may need to renegotiate household roles as well as leisure and social activities.

If an older adult becomes more dependent, a reversal of parent-child roles often takes place. Associated with increased dependence is a loss of power, status, and decision-making, forcing adjustments in the older person himself and in his relationships. By age 70, most people take on a grandparenting role; this role usually is a supportive, companionship role.

Gradual erosion of the independent-adult role is linked to the aging person's growing need for assistance. It's also linked to stereotypes about older people. For example, health care professionals may view older adults as unreliable historians and thus discount their self-reports.

In addition, the older person may cross over to a "sick" role because of the multiple interactive health problems that can arise and his limited power to negotiate care.

Retirement

Retirement brings a major role change because it alters the way a person manages time and daily activities. The retiree must adapt to a nonworker role; others also must adjust. For example, the spouse may view retirement as a threat to territoriality and authority.

Retirement alters identity, power, status, and friendships. The retiree may need to find new relationships and activities. Retirement also is viewed as the beginning of old age.

Research has demonstrated that a person's income, health, and desire to retire predict his satisfactory adjustment to retirement. People with more income and education seem better prepared for retirement. Some organizations now offer preretirement counseling. For example, employees may be able to cut back on work hours gradually to retire in stages. Adjusting to retirement may be easier if the person begins postretirement activities before retiring.

Multiple losses

Aging is associated with major physical, psychological, and sociologic losses as well as a reduced ability to adapt to and compensate for stressors. Older adults may lose a sense of control because of such factors as physical decline, status and role changes, negative cultural attitudes and mass media portrayals, and crime victimization. Loss of loved ones, income, and perhaps decent transportation and housing, added to multiple or chronic diseases and their resulting limitations, can increase the older adult's sense of vulnerability and deplete coping resources.

Loneliness

Any loss that creates a deficit in intimacy and interpersonal relationships can lead to loneliness. Even sensory deprivation increases the risk. And loneliness can provoke or aggravate physical symptoms, sleep disturbances, and shortened survival.

Of course, not all loneliness can be avoided. For example, the death of a spouse is a major cause of loneliness. Retirement, poor health, and inactivity also may contribute to loneliness. The older adult needs caring, personal contact, and confidants in other age groups. It takes a satisfying relationship with frequent contact to prevent loneliness. However, some older people do choose to be alone.

Depression and suicide

More likely in the older adult, depression increases in frequency and intensity with age. Changes in neurotransmitters, multiple losses, and decreased internal and external resources contribute to its incidence. Depression may be associated with complaints of physical symptoms and sleep disturbance. It also may occur in early stages of dementia, making depression the most common psychiatric problem among older adults.

Risk factors for depression include a recent major loss, feelings of rejection by or isolation from family or friends, feelings of hopelessness, absence of an identifiable role in life, and loss of a partner or sexual function. Depression is the most common psychological consequence of disability, and with depression comes the increased risk of suicide.

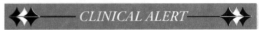 CLINICAL ALERT

The suicide rate for older adult men is seven times that for older adult women. Risk factors for suicide include alcoholism, bereavement (especially within 1 year after a loss), loss of health, living alone, and children who have married and moved away. Suicide among older adults rarely is an impulsive act; most suicide attempts are not gestures or threats.

Fear of death

While most other people avoid the topic, older adults commonly think and talk about death. Perhaps because they've already lost a lot, they usually have less fear of death than younger people. Their greater fears are dependency, pain, and loss of function and control.

However, fear of the process of dying, the ultimate loss of self, and the unknown may lead to denial. Fear of death also may involve such concerns as separation from loved ones and questions about judgment and afterlife. But denying death can prevent a person from valuing life. And preparation for death can be a positive experience and a major developmental task of adulthood.

CHANGING ATTITUDES

Some societies devalue older adults, viewing them as obsolete and expendable, making older adults feel worthless. Others, as in Japan, revere their aged, presuming and esteeming their advanced knowledge, wisdom, and skills.

Our own society is slowly adjusting its attitudes about aging as the number of older adults increases

ANA standards of professional gerontological nursing performance

The American Nurses Association (ANA) has developed eight standards to help focus your care of older adults.

Standard I: Quality of care
The gerontological nurse systematically evaluates the quality of care and effectiveness of nursing practice.

Standard II: Performance appraisal
The gerontological nurse evaluates his or her own nursing practice in relation to professional practice standards and relevant statutes and regulations.

Standard III: Education
The gerontological nurse acquires and maintains current knowledge in nursing practice.

Standard IV: Collegiality
The gerontological nurse contributes to the professional development of peers, colleagues, and others.

Standard V: Ethics
The gerontological nurse's decisions and actions on behalf of clients are determined in an ethical manner.

Standard VI: Collaboration
The gerontological nurse collaborates with the aging person, significant others, and health care providers in providing client care.

Standard VII: Research
The gerontological nurse uses research findings in practice.

Standard VIII: Resource utilization
The gerontological nurse considers factors related to safety, effectiveness, and cost in planning and delivering client care.

Reprinted with permission from *Scope and Standards of Gerontological Clinical Nursing Practice*, American Nurses Association, 1995.

and new roles for them emerge. We see the individual as continually evolving, and increasingly we devote attention to self-development and obligations to others. More positive attitudes about old age now exist among older people themselves and among many younger people, better educated people, and people who've had contact with healthy older adults.

Among health care professionals, attitudes about aging are changing as well. A good example is the American Nurses Association's (ANA's) emphasis on holistic care and treatment of older patients. The new attitude recognizes the need for nurses to address not only age-related diseases, but associated aspects and problems — physiologic, pathologic,

psychological, economic, and sociologic — to maximize their nursing capabilities. The ANA's standards of gerontological nursing provide general guidelines for the nursing care of older adults. The standards address the nursing process and emphasize the patient's involvement in decision making and goal setting (see *ANA standards of professional gerontological nursing performance*).

People are beginning to view aging as a normal part of the developmental process, a lifelong continuum that begins at conception and culminates with death. As a health care professional, you're in a prime position to help make this final phase rewarding and meaningful for the older adults in your care.

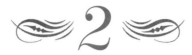

Tailoring your assessment

*F*or a patient of any age, your thorough assessment and the diagnosis you reach are the crucial foundation of care. With older patients, your assessment is particularly important because of the complexity of their needs and the wide variation in their function. To identify your patient's problems and needs, you must integrate a sound theoretical knowledge of the gerontologic population with your assessment skills.

ADAPTING YOUR ASSESSMENT

In assessing elderly patients, you'll find that they differ not only from other age-groups, but also from other people of the same age. Although all older adults experience a diminishing ability to respond to stress, an increasing number of losses, and the physiologic changes associated with aging, these changes affect individuals at different times, rates, and degrees. To assess an older person effectively, you should adapt your assessment to take into account common age-related changes, role transitions, and psychological adjustments that may be affecting your patient.

Although not synonymous with disease or disability, aging is commonly associated with an increased incidence of chronic disease. But disease findings may be difficult to distinguish from those that represent normal age-related changes. What's

more, the older patient often has vague symptoms that are not clearly characteristic of a disorder. Therefore, assessing both physical and psychosocial function can provide key information about your patient's status.

Currently, no definitive norms exist for a healthy older adult. For example, though certain laboratory values represent normal ranges for younger adults, your older patient with the same values may have a serious problem. Specifically, hemoglobin may decline with age, but a low hemoglobin level in an older adult isn't normal.

Similarly, no definitive norms exist for many pathologic conditions. For example, controversy exists over what represents normal blood pressure for older people. Is an elevated systolic pressure merely an age-related change, or does it warrant treatment? Often, developmental norms are lumped together under the broad category of "old age" or "over 65," even though a 65-year-old may be greatly different from a 75-year-old. So it's crucial for you to rely on your older patient's previous patterns as a basis for determining his current status.

Variables affecting assessment
Your assessments may take place in a variety of settings: acute care facility, home, senior center, adult day care center, and long-term care facility. While the setting and the patient's age don't affect the methods you use to collect data, other factors can interfere. The time you allow for the assessment, your patient's energy level, the environment, the

patient's consent, language or communication deficits, the patient's attitude and, very importantly, your own attitude about aging — all affect the overall atmosphere of trust, caring, and confidentiality.

Your attitude

Communicating with an older adult may challenge you to confront your personal attitude about aging and older people. Examine your feelings and decide in advance how you'll handle them. Any prejudices you reveal will probably interfere with your efforts to communicate, because older people are especially sensitive to others' reactions and can easily detect negative attitudes and impatience.

Your patient's attitude

As you assess your patient, try to determine his attitude toward his body and health. An older person may have a distorted perception of his health problems, dwelling on them needlessly or dismissing them as normal signs of aging. He may ignore a serious problem because he doesn't want his fears confirmed. If your older patient is seriously ill, the subjects of dying and death may come up during the health history interview. Listen carefully to any remarks he makes about dying. Be sure to ask about his religious affiliation and spiritual needs; many older people find comfort in their religious beliefs and practices. Also ask whether he has or wants help with a living will. The health history can serve as a life review for the older person by allowing him to recount his history in a purposeful, systematic manner.

Language

The language you use when you assess an older patient should be tailored to that individual. Consider his educational level, culture, and other languages he may speak.

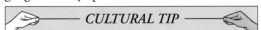

— CULTURAL TIP —

Be aware that in times of stress, a person may revert to using his native language because it provides comfort and security and he may be able to express himself better.

Deficits

Sensory deficits, such as hearing and vision losses, are common in older people. Other impairments, such as musculoskeletal or neurologic deficits, appear frequently. All of these can significantly interfere with accurate data collection. With sensory or neurologic deficits, the older person may misinterpret a question or not hear it at all. With musculoskeletal deficits, discomfort or pain may keep him from focusing on your questions or instructions. As a result, he may respond incorrectly or inappropriately. If these deficits aren't taken into consideration, they can cause inaccuracies in the assessment and the conclusions you draw.

Consent

Informed consent, always essential, is crucial for the older patient. He has the right to know why you're doing the assessment, what procedures it involves, and what types of information you need. He has the right to refuse to answer any questions or to participate in any aspect of the assessment. (*Note:* If he's able to clothe, feed, and take basic care of himself, he's likely to be considered competent.)

Time and energy level

Be sure to allow enough time for your assessment. The older adult possesses a wealth of information but generally processes information more slowly than a younger adult. Your patient may need extra time, or even several shorter sessions if problems such as fatigue or discomfort limit the amount of time he can participate meaningfully.

Environment

You may need to modify the environment to suit an older patient, taking into account any sensory or musculoskeletal changes.

Tools for a functional assessment

You can use functional assessment to evaluate the older adult's overall well being and self-care abilities. It will help you identify individual needs and care deficits, provide a basis for developing a plan of care that enhances the abilities of the older adult with coexisting disease and chronic illness, and provide feedback about treatment and rehabilitation. You can use the information to identify and match the older adult's needs with such services as housekeeping, home health care, and day care to help the patient maintain independence. Numerous tools are available to help you perform a methodical functional assessment.

Katz index

A widely used tool for evaluating ability to perform daily personal care activities is the Katz Index of Activities of Daily Living. This tool ranks the person's ability to perform six functions: bathing, dressing, toileting, transfer, continence, and feeding. It describes his functional level at a specific point in time and objectively scores his performance on a three-point scale. (See *Katz index of activities of daily living,* page 20.)

Lawton scale

Another widely used tool is the Lawton Scale for Instrumental Activities of Daily Living (IADL). This tool evaluates the ability to perform more complex personal care activities. It addresses the activities needed to support independent living, such as the ability to use the telephone, cook, shop, do laundry, manage finances, take medications, and prepare meals. The activities are rated on a three-point scale, ranging from independence, to needing some help, to complete disability. (See *Lawton scale for instrumental activities of daily living,* page 21.)

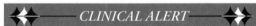
✦✦ CLINICAL ALERT ✦✦

When using the IADL scale, make sure to evaluate your patient in terms of safety. For example, a person may be able to cook a small meal for himself but leaves the stove burner on after cooking.

FANCAPES

Known by its acronym, FANCAPES focuses more on assessing physiologic function. The letters stand for:

- fluids (state of hydration and factors contributing to maintenance of adequate hydration)
- aeration (adequacy of oxygen exchange)
- nutrition (mechanical and psychological factors, amounts and types of food consumed)
- communication (sight and sound; voice quality; adequate functioning of tongue, teeth, pharynx and larynx; ability to read words and understand spoken language)
- activity (activities of daily living [ADLs], coordination, balance, strength)
- pain (pressure, discomfort, losses)
- elimination (bladder and bowel elimination, assistive devices)
- socialization (giving and receiving love, function in society, feelings of self worth).

FANCAPES provides helpful information about a person's ability to meet his own needs and the amount of assistance he may need.

Barthel index and scale

The Barthel Index also is used to assess ability for self care. It evaluates 10 items: feeding, moving from wheelchair to bed and returning, performing personal toilet, getting on and off the toilet, bathing, walking on a level surface or propelling a wheelchair, going up and down stairs, dressing and undressing, maintaining bowel continence, and controlling the bladder. Each item is scored according to the degree of assistance needed; over time, results reveal improvement or decline. (See *Barthel index,* pages 22 and 23.)

A similar scale, called the Barthel Self-Care Rating Scale, is a more detailed scale to evaluate function. Both tools provide information to help you determine the type of assistance needed. They're used more often in rehabilitation and long-term care settings as tools to document improvement in a patient's abilities.

OARS

The Older Americans Research and Service Center (OARS) is an assessment tool developed at Duke University in 1978. A multidimensional tool, it evaluates level of function in 5 areas: social resources, economic resources, physical health, mental health, and ADLs. Each area is scored on a scale of 1 to 6. At the end of the assessment, a cumulative

CHARTING GUIDE

Katz index of activities of daily living

Evaluation Form   Name *James Collins*   Date *November 4, 1996*

For each area of functioning listed below, check the description that applies. (The word "assistance" means supervision, direction, or personal assistance.)

Bathing: Sponge bath, tub bath, or shower.

| ☑ Receives no assistance (gets into and out of tub by self if tub is the usual means of bathing). | ❏ Receives assistance in bathing only one part of the body (such as the back or a leg). | ○ Receives assistance in bathing more than one part of the body (or not bathed). |

Dressing: Gets clothes from closets and drawers, including underclothes and outer garments, and uses fasteners, including suspenders if worn.

| ☑ Gets clothes and gets completely dressed without assistance. | ❏ Gets clothes and gets dressed without assistance except for tying shoes. | ○ Receives assistance in getting clothes or in getting dressed, or stays partly or completely undressed. |

Toileting: Goes to the room termed "toilet" for bowel movement/urination, cleans self afterward, and arranges clothes.

| ☑ Goes to toilet room, cleans self and arranges clothes without assistance. (May use object for support such as cane, walker, or wheelchair and may manage night bedpan or commode, emptying it in morning.) | ○ Receives assistance in going to toilet room or in cleaning self or arranging clothes after elimination or in use of night bedpan or commode. | ○ Doesn't go to toilet room for the elimination process. |

Transfer

| ☑ Moves into and out of bed as well as into and out of chair without assistance. (May use object such as cane or walker for support.) | ○ Moves into or out of bed or chair with assistance. | ○ Doesn't get out of bed. |

Continence

| ❏ Controls urination and bowel movement completely by self. | ☑ Has occasional accidents. | ○ Supervision helps keep control of urination or bowel movement, or catheter is used, or is incontinent. |

Feeding

| ☑ Feeds self without assistance. | ❏ Feeds self except for assistance in cutting meat or buttering bread. | ○ Receives assistance in feeding or is fed partly or completely through tubes or by IV fluids. |

Evaluator: *P. Rasteni, RN*

Index   ❏ **Indicates independence**   ○ **Indicates dependence**

A: Independent in all six functions.
B: Independent in all but one of these functions.
C: Independent in all but bathing, and one additional function.
D: Independent in all but bathing, dressing, and one additional function.

E: Independent in all but bathing, dressing, toileting, and one additional function.
F: Independent in all but bathing, dressing, toileting, transferring, and one additional function.
G: Dependent in all six functions.

Other: Dependent in at least two functions but not classifiable as C, D, E, or F.

Adapted with permission from Katz, S., et al. "Studies of Illness in the Aged: The Index of ADL — A Standardized Measure of Biological and Psychosocial Function," *JAMA* 185:914-19, 1963. © 1963, American Medical Association.

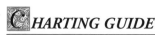HARTING GUIDE

Lawton scale for instrumental activities of daily living

Name *Julia Lippey*   Rated by *Katherine Mitchell, RN*   Date *November 18, 1996*

1. Can you use the telephone?
without help .... ③
with some help 2
completely unable 1

2. Can you get to places beyond walking distance?
without help .... ③
with some help 2
not without special arrangements 1

3. Can you go shopping for groceries?
without help .... ③
with some help 2
completely unable 1

4. Can you prepare your own meals?
without help .... ③
with some help 2
completely unable 1

5. Can you do your own housework?
without help 3
with some help .... ②
completely unable 1

6. Can you do your own handyman work?
without help 3
with some help .... ②
completely unable 1

7. Can you do your own laundry?
without help .... ③
with some help 2
completely unable 1

8a. Do you take medicines or use any medications? ......
Yes (If yes, answer Question 8b.) .... ①
No (If no, answer Question 8c.) 2

8b. Do you take your own medicine?
without help (in the right doses at the
right times) .... ③
with some help (if someone prepares it for
you and/or reminds you to take it) 2
completely unable 1

8c. If you had to take medicine, could you do it?
without help (in the right doses at the
right time) 3
with some help (if someone prepared it for
you and reminded you to take it) 2
completely unable 1

9. Can you manage your own money?
without help .... ③
with some help 2
completely unable 1

The IADL scale evaluates more sophisticated functions than the ADL index. Patients or caregivers can complete the form in a few minutes. The first answer in each case — except for 8a — indicates independence; the second indicates capability with assistance; and the third, dependence. In this version the maximum score is 29, although scores have meaning only for a particular patient, as when declining scores over time reveal deterioration. Questions 4 to 7 tend to be gender specific; modify them as necessary.

Adapted with permission from Lawton, M.P., and Brody, E.M. "Assessment of Older People: Self-Maintaining and Instrumental Activities of Daily Living," *The Gerontologist* 9(3):179-186, Autumn 1969.

impairment score is determined. The lower the score, the less the impairment.

Minimum Data Set

In an attempt to improve the quality of care in extended care facilities, the federal government instituted major reforms through the Omnibus Budget Reconciliation Acts (OBRA). A standardized assessment tool called the Minimum Data Set was developed to make the assessment more consistent and reliable throughout the country. The use of this method is required in all extended care facilities that receive federal funding. (See *Minimum data set*, pages 25 to 28.)

To stress the importance of timely assessment, time limits have been established by most institu-

HARTING GUIDE

Barthel index

Date <u>*October 7, 1996*</u>

Patient's name <u>*Joseph Porter*</u>

Evaluator <u>*Janice Wu*</u>

Action	With help	Independent
1. Feeding (if food needs to be cut up = help)	5	⑩
2. Moving from wheelchair to bed and return (includes sitting up in bed)	5 to 10	⑮
3. Personal toilet (wash face, comb hair, shave, clean teeth)	0	⑤
4. Getting on and off toilet (handling clothes, wipe, flush)	5	⑩
5. Bathing self	0	⑤
6. Walking on level surface (or, if unable to walk, propel wheelchair)	0*	5 or 15
7. Ascending and descending stairs	⑤	10
8. Dressing (includes tying shoes, fastening fasteners)	⑤	10
9. Controlling bowels	⑤	10
10. Controlling bladder	⑤	10

Definition and Discussion of Scoring

A person scoring 100 is continent, feeds himself, dresses himself, gets up out of bed and chairs, bathes himself, walks at least a block, and can ascend and descend stairs. This doesn't mean that he's able to live alone; he may not be able to cook, keep house, or meet the public, but he's able to get along without attendant care.

1. Feeding

   10 = Independent. The person can feed himself a meal from a tray or table when someone puts the food within his reach. He must be able to put on an assistive device if needed, cut up the food, use salt and pepper, spread butter, and so forth. Also, he must accomplish these tasks in a reasonable time.

   5 = The person needs some help with cutting up food and other tasks, as listed above.

2. Moving from wheelchair to bed and return

   15 = The person operates independently in all phases of this activity. He can safely approach the bed in his wheelchair, lock brakes, lift footrests, move safely from bed, lie down, come to a sitting position on the side of the bed, change the position of the wheelchair, if necessary, to transfer back into it safely, and return to the wheelchair.

   10 = Either the person needs some minimal help in some step of this activity, or needs to be reminded or supervised for safety in one or more parts of this activity.

   5 = The person can come to a sitting position without the help of a second person but needs to be lifted out of bed, or needs a great deal of help with transfers.

3. Handling personal toilet

   5 = The person can wash hands and face, comb hair, clean teeth, and shave. He may use any kind of razor but he must be able to get it from the drawer or cabinet and plug it in or put in a blade without help. A female must put on her own makeup, if any, but need not braid or style her hair.

4. Getting on and off toilet

   10 = The person is able to get on and off the toilet, unfasten and refasten clothes, prevent soiling of clothes, and use toilet paper without help. He may use a wall bar or other stable object for support, if needed. If he needs to use a bed pan instead of toilet, he must be able to place it on a chair, use it competently, and empty and clean it.

   5 = The person needs help to overcome imbalance, handle clothes, or use toilet paper.

5. Bathing self

   5 = The person may use a bath tub or shower or give himself a complete sponge bath. Regardless of method, he must

CHARTING GUIDE

Barthel index (continued)

be able to complete all the steps involved without another person's presence.

6. Walking on a level surface

15 = The person can walk at least 50 yards without help or supervision. He may wear braces or prostheses and use crutches, canes, or a walkerette, but not a rolling walker. He must be able to lock and unlock braces, if used, get the necessary mechanical aids into position for use, stand up and sit down, and dispose of the aids when he sits. (Putting on, fastening, and taking off braces is scored under Dressing).

5 = If the person can't ambulate but can propel a wheelchair independently, he must be able to go around corners, turn around, maneuver the chair to table, bed, toilet, and other locations. He must be able to push a chair at least 150' (45.7 m). Don't score this item if the person receives a score for walking.

7. Ascending and descending stairs

10 = The person can go up and down a flight of stairs safely without help or supervision. He may and should use handrails, canes, or crutches when needed, and he must be able to carry canes or crutches as he ascends or descends.

5 = The person needs help with or supervision of any one of the above items.

8. Dressing and undressing

10 = The person can put on, fasten, and remove all clothing (including any prescribed corset or braces) and tie shoe laces (unless he requires adaptations for this). Such special clothing as suspenders, loafers, and dresses that open down the front may be used when necessary.

5 = The person needs help in putting on, fastening, or removing any clothing. He must do at least half the work himself and must accomplish the task in a reasonable time.

Women need not be scored on use of a brassiere or girdle unless these are prescribed garments.

9. Controlling bowels

10 = The person can control his bowels without accidents. He can use a suppository or take an enema when necessary (as in spinal cord injury patients who have had bowel training).

5 = The person needs help in using a suppository or taking an enema or has occasional accidents.

10. Controlling bladder

10 = The person can control his bladder day and night. Spinal cord injury patients who wear an external device and leg bag must put them on independently, clean and empty the bag, and stay dry, day and night.

5 = The person has occasional accidents, can't wait for the bed pan or get to the toilet in time, or needs help with an external device.

The total score is less significant or meaningful than the individual items, because these indicate where the deficiencies lie.

Any applicant to a chronic hospital who scores 100 should be evaluated carefully before admission to see whether such hospitalization is indicated. Discharged patients with scores of 100 should not require further physical therapy but may benefit from a home visit to see whether any environmental adjustments are needed.

*Score only if unable to walk.

Adapted with permission from Mahoney, F.I., and Barthel, D.W. "Functional Evaluation: The Barthel Index," *Maryland State Medical Journal* 14:62, 1965.

tions. According to OBRA, the physical portion of the assessment must be complete by a licensed nurse within 24 hours of a patient's admission. The entire assessment must be completed within 4 days.

OBRA also mandates that the total assessment be revised and updated whenever a significant change occurs in a resident's mental or physical condition.

PERFORMING THE HEALTH ASSESSMENT

A comprehensive health assessment of the older person focuses on current health status, including a review of systems, medical history, and ability to function in the environment. This information establishes the person's baseline health status, allowing you to evaluate any improvement or decline in his condition over time and to determine the need for support services.

Obtaining the health history

The health history and interview, the first phase of the health assessment, provide a subjective account of the older adult's present and past health status. They also initiate your relationship and establish the patient's well-being as your primary concern. The information you obtain from the health history alerts you to key areas of focus for the physical examination. Talking with the older person about health concerns increases his health awareness and helps you identify any knowledge deficits and launch your patient teaching. Because the patient may overlook some important health information, you must interview methodically and also gather information from family members or friends.

Preparing for the interview

Approaching an older patient for a health history needn't be difficult if you anticipate his special needs. Keep the following points in mind.

Timing. If possible, plan to talk with an older person early in the day, when he's likely to be most alert. Many older people experience the "sundown syndrome," which means their capacity for clear thinking diminishes by late afternoon or early evening. Some may even become disoriented or confused late in the day.

During the assessment, watch for signs of possible fatigue, such as sighing, grimacing, head and shoulder drooping, irritability, slouching, or leaning against something for support. If one long session is too taxing for your patient, schedule additional times and take advantage of other interaction, such as bathing, grooming, and meals, to elicit additional data and validate existing data. Clarify inconsistencies and possible inaccuracies by assessing your patient more than once and at different times of the day.

Environment. Choose an area that's private, comfortable, warm enough (75° F [23.9° C] is usually comfortable for the older person), and draft-free. Make sure the area provides ample space, especially if the person uses assistive devices. Avoid bright fluorescent lighting or direct sunlight. Instead, use diffused lighting.

Have water or other fluids available, and make sure your patient is close to a bathroom. Have a comfortable chair available for the patient (if he isn't on bed rest), especially if the interview may be lengthy. Because arthritis and other orthopedic disabilities may make sitting in one position for a long time uncomfortable, encourage an older person to change his position in the chair (or bed) and to move around as much as he wants during the interview.

Deficits. If your patient wears glasses, make sure he has them before the interview begins. Pull shades and block any bright light from the patient's view. Reduced visual acuity or environmentally induced blindness from bright lights, shiny floors, or direct sunlight can cause squinting or poor eye contact in an older person. During the interview, face the patient closely at eye level.

To help compensate for a hearing impairment, close the door to the room to minimize background noise, such as passing foot traffic, paging systems, televisions, radios, ringing telephones, or outside conversation. An older person with a hearing impairment may have difficulty understanding fast-paced speech; you may notice that he seems distracted, fails to follow the conversation, or looks puzzled by your questions. Make sure the room is well lit, so the patient can read your lips, if necessary. Ascertain which ear is his better ear and speak toward it. If the patient wears a hearing aid, make

(Text continues on page 29.)

HARTING GUIDE

Minimum data set

This federal regulatory form, known as the Minimum Data Set, is a standardized assessment tool that must be filled out for every person admitted to a long-term care facility. Different sections of the form must be completed and signed by various staff members, such as doctors, nurses, and social workers.

MINIMUM DATA SET FOR NURSING HOME RESIDENT ASSESSMENT AND CARE SCREENING (MDS)
(Status in last 7 days, unless other time frame indicated)

SECTION A. IDENTIFICATION AND BACKGROUND INFORMATION

1. ASSESSMENT DATE
1 2 — 0 7 — 1 9 9 6
Month   Day   Year

2. RESIDENT NAME
Amy   J.   Gaston
(First)   (Middle Initial)   (Last)

3. SOCIAL SECURITY NO.
0 4 1 — 2 4 — 0 0 0 0

4. MEDICAID NO. (If applicable)

5. MEDICAL RECORD NO.
M M 0 0 0 9 9 2 2 6 8

6. REASON FOR ASSESSMENT
1. Initial admission assess.   5. Significant change in status
2. Hosp/Medicare reassess.   6. Other (e.g., UR)
3. Readmission assessment
4. Annual assessment   → 2

7. CURRENT PAYMENT SOURCE(S) FOR N.H. STAY
(Billing Office to indicate; check all that apply)
Medicaid — a.   VA — d.
Medicare — b. X   Self pay/Private insurance — e. X
CHAMPUS — c.   Other — f.

8. RESPONSIBILITY/ LEGAL GUARDIAN
(Check all that apply)
Legal guardian — a.   Family member responsible — d. X
Other legal oversight — b.   Resident responsible — e.
Durable power attrny./ health care proxy — c. X   NONE OF ABOVE — f.

9. ADVANCED DIRECTIVES
(For those items with supporting documentation in the medical record, check all that apply)
Living will — a.   Feeding restrictions — f.
Do not resuscitate — b.   Medication restrictions — g.
Do not hospitalize — c.   Other treatment restrictions — h.
Organ donation — d.   NONE OF ABOVE — i. X
Autopsy request — e.

10. DISCHARGE PLANNED WITHIN 3 MOS.
(Does not include discharge due to death)
0. No   1. Yes   2. Unknown/uncertain   → 0

11. PARTICIPATE IN ASSESSMENT
a. Resident   b. Family
0. No   0. No
1. Yes   1. Yes
2. No family   → a. 1 b. 1

12. SIGNATURES
Signature of RN Assessment Coordinator
Christine Saslo RN MSN
Signatures of Others Who Completed Part of the Assessment
James Shaw RN BSN
Susan Rowe MSW

SECTION B. COGNITIVE PATTERNS

1. COMATOSE
(Persistent vegetative state/no discernible consciousness)
0. No   1. Yes (Skip to SECTION E)   → 0

2. MEMORY
(Recall of what was learned or known)
a. Short-term memory OK—seems/appears to recall after 5 minutes
0. Memory OK   1. Memory problem   → a. 1
b. Long-term memory OK—seems/appears to recall long past
0. Memory OK   1. Memory problem   → b. 1

3. MEMORY/ RECALL ABILITY
(Check all that resident normally able to recall during last 7 days)
Current season — a.   That he/she is in a nursing home — d.
Location of own room — b.   NONE OF ABOVE are recalled — e. X
Staff names/faces — c.

□ = Code the appropriate response   □ = Check all the responses that apply

SECTION C. COMMUNICATION/HEARING PATTERNS (right column continuation of Section A area)

4. COGNITIVE SKILLS FOR DAILY DECISION-MAKING
(Made decisions regarding tasks of daily life)
0. Independent—decisions consistent/reasonable
1. Modified Independence—some difficulty in new situations only
2. Moderately Impaired—decisions poor; cues/supervision required
3. Severely Impaired—never/rarely made decisions   → 2

5. INDICATORS OF DELIRIUM—PERIODIC DISORDERED THINKING/ AWARENESS
(Check if condition over last 7 days appears different from usual functioning)
Less alert, easily distracted — a.
Changing awareness of environment — b.
Episodes of incoherent speech — c.
Periods of motor restlessness or lethargy — d.
Cognitive ability varies over course of day — e.
NONE OF ABOVE — f. X

6. CHANGE IN COGNITIVE STATUS
Change in resident's cognitive status, skills, or abilities in last 90 days
0. No change   1. Improved   2. Deteriorated   → 2

SECTION C. COMMUNICATION/HEARING PATTERNS

1. HEARING
(With hearing appliance, if used)
0. Hears adequately—normal talk, TV, phone
1. Minimal difficulty when not in quiet setting
2. Hears in special situations only—speaker has to adjust tonal quality and speak distinctly
3. Highly impaired/absence of useful hearing   → 1

2. COMMUNICATION DEVICES/ TECHNIQUES
(Check all that apply during last 7 days)
Hearing aid, present and used — a.
Hearing aid, present and not used — b.
Other receptive comm. techniques used (e.g., lip read) — c.
NONE OF ABOVE — d. X

3. MODES OF EXPRESSION
(Check all used by resident to make needs known)
Speech — a. X   Signs/gestures/sounds — c.
Writing messages to express or clarify needs — b.   Communication board — d.
Other — e.
NONE OF ABOVE — f.

4. MAKING SELF UNDERSTOOD
(Express information content—however able)
0. Understood
1. Usually Understood—difficulty finding words or finishing thoughts
2. Sometimes Understood—ability is limited to making concrete requests
3. Rarely/Never Understood   → 1

5. ABILITY TO UNDERSTAND OTHERS
(Understanding verbal information content—however able)
0. Understands
1. Usually Understands—may miss some part/intent of message
2. Sometimes Understands—responds adequately to simple, direct communication
3. Rarely/Never Understands   → 2

6. CHANGE IN COMMUNICATION/ HEARING
Resident's ability to express, understand or hear information has changed over last 90 days
0. No change   1. Improved   2. Deteriorated   → 0

SECTION D. VISION PATTERNS

1. VISION
(Ability to see in adequate light and with glasses if used)
0. Adequate—sees fine detail, including regular print in newspapers/books
1. Impaired—sees large print, but not regular print in newspapers/books
2. Highly Impaired—limited vision; not able to see newspaper headlines; appears to follow objects with eyes
3. Severely Impaired—no vision or appears to see only light, colors, or shapes   → 0

2. VISUAL LIMITATIONS/ DIFFICULTIES
Side vision problems—decreased peripheral vision (e.g., leaves food on one side of tray, difficulty traveling, bumps into people and objects, misjudges placement of chair when seating self) — a.
Experiences any of following; sees halos or rings around lights; sees flashes of light; sees "curtains" over eyes — b.
NONE OF ABOVE — c. X

3. VISUAL APPLIANCES
Glasses; contact lenses; lens implant; magnifying glass
0. No   1. Yes   → 1

(continued)

CHARTING GUIDE

Minimum data set (continued)

SECTION E. PHYSICAL FUNCTIONING AND STRUCTURAL PROBLEMS

1. **ADL SELF-PERFORMANCE**—*(Code for resident's PERFORMANCE OVER ALL SHIFTS during last 7 days—Not including setup)*

   0. *INDEPENDENT* — No help or oversight — OR — Help/oversight provided only 1 or 2 times during last 7 days

   1. *SUPERVISION* — Oversight, encouragement or cueing provided 3+ times during last 7 days — OR — Supervision plus physical assistance provided only 1 or 2 times during last 7 days

   2. *LIMITED ASSISTANCE* — Resident highly involved in activity; received physical help in guided maneuvering of limbs or other nonweight bearing assistance 3+ times — OR — More help provided only 1 or 2 times during last 7 days

   3. *EXTENSIVE ASSISTANCE* — While resident performed part of activity, over last 7-day period, help of following type(s) provided 3 or more times:
      — Weight-bearing support
      — Full staff performance during part (but not all) of last 7 days

   4. *TOTAL DEPENDENCE* — Full staff performance of activity during entire 7 days

2. **ADL SUPPORT PROVIDED** — *(Code for MOST SUPPORT PROVIDED OVER ALL SHIFTS during last 7 days; code regardless of resident's self-performance classification)*

   0. No setup or physical help from staff
   1. Setup help only
   2. One-person physical assist
   3. Two+ persons physical assist

			(1) SELF-PERF.	(2) SUPPORT
a.	BED MOBILITY	How resident moves to and from lying position, turns side to side, and positions body while in bed	3	3
b.	TRANSFER	How resident moves between surfaces—to/from: bed, chair, wheelchair, standing position (EXCLUDE to/from bath/toilet)	4	3
c.	LOCO-MOTION	How resident moves between locations in his/her room and adjacent corridor on same floor. If in wheelchair, self-sufficiency once in chair	4	2
d.	DRESSING	How resident puts on, fastens, and takes off all items of street clothing, including donning/removing prosthesis	4	3
e.	EATING	How resident eats and drinks (regardless of skill)	2	2
f.	TOILET USE	How resident uses the toilet room (or commode, bedpan, urinal); transfer on/off toilet, cleanses, changes pad, manages ostomy or catheter, adjusts clothes	4	3
g.	PERSONAL HYGIENE	How resident maintains personal hygiene, including combing hair, brushing teeth, shaving, applying makeup, washing/drying face, hands, and perineum (EXCLUDE baths and showers)	4	2

3. **BATHING** — How resident takes full-body bath/shower, sponge bath, and transfers in/out of tub/shower (EXCLUDE washing of back and hair. *Code for most dependent in self-performance and support. Bathing Self-Performance codes appear below.*

   0. Independent—No help provided
   1. Supervision—Oversight help only
   2. Physical help limited to transfer only
   3. Physical help in part of bathing activity
   4. Total dependence

a.	b.
4	3

4. **BODY CONTROL PROBLEMS** — *(Check all that apply during last 7 days)*

Balance—partial or total loss of ability to balance self while standing	a. X		Hand—lack of dexterity (e.g., problem using toothbrush or adjusting hearing aid)	g. X
Bedfast all or most of the time	b.		Leg—partial or total loss of voluntary movement	h.
Contracture to arms, legs, shoulders, or hands	c. X		Leg—unsteady gait	i. X
Hemiplegia/hemiparesis	d.		Trunk—partial or total loss of ability to position, balance, or turn body	j.
Quadriplegia	e.		Amputation	k.
Arm—partial or total loss of voluntary movement	f.		NONE OF ABOVE	l.

5. **MOBILITY APPLIANCES/ DEVICES** — *(Check all that apply during last 7 days)*

Cane/walker	a.		Other person wheeled	d. X
Brace/prothesis	b.		Lifted (manually/ mechanically)	e. X
Wheeled self	c.		NONE OF ABOVE	f.

6. **TASK SEG-MENTATION** — Resident requires that some or all of ADL activities be broken into a series of subtasks so that resident can perform them
   0. No   1. Yes | 0 |

7. **ADL FUNC-TIONAL REHABILI-TATION POTENTIAL**

Resident believes he/she capable of increased independence in at least some ADLs	a.
Direct care staff believe resident capable of increased independence in at least some ADLs	b.
Resident able to perform tasks/activity but is very slow	c.
Major difference in ADL Self-Performance or ADL Support in mornings and evenings (at least a one category change in Self-Performance or Support in any ADL)	d.
NONE OF ABOVE	e. X

8. **CHANGE IN ADL FUNCTION** — Change in ADL self-performance in last 90 days
   0. No change   1. Improved 2. Deteriorated | 0 |

SECTION F. CONTINENCE IN LAST 14 DAYS

1. **CONTINENCE SELF-CONTROL CATEGORIES** *(Code for resident performance over all shifts)*

   0. CONTINENT — Complete control
   1. USUALLY CONTINENT — BLADDER, incontinent episodes once a week or less; BOWEL, less than weekly
   2. OCCASIONALLY INCONTINENT — BLADDER, 2+ times a week but not daily; BOWEL, once a week
   3. FREQUENTLY INCONTINENT — BLADDER, tended to be incontinent daily, but some control present (e.g., on day shift); BOWEL, 2-3 times a week
   4. INCONTINENT — Had inadequate control. BLADDER, multiple daily episodes; BOWEL, all (or almost all) of the time

| a. | BOWEL CONTI-NENCE | Control of bowel movement, with appliance or bowel continence programs, if employed | 4 |
| b. | BLADDER CONTI-NENCE | Control of urinary bladder function (if dribbles, volume insufficient to soak through underpants), with appliances (e.g., foley) or continence programs, if employed | 4 |

2. **INCONTIN-ENCE RELATED TESTING** — *(Skip if resident's bladder continence code equals 0 or 1 AND no catheter is used)*

Resident has been tested for a urinary tract infection	a. X
Resident has been checked for presence of a fecal impaction, or there is adequate bowel elimination	b. X
NONE OF ABOVE	c.

3. **APPLIANCES AND PROGRAMS**

Any scheduled toileting plan	a.		Pads/briefs used	f. X
External (condom) catheter	b.		Enemas/irrigation	g.
Indwelling catheter	c.		Ostomy	h.
Intermittent catheter	d.		NONE OF ABOVE	i.
Did not use toilet room/ commode/urinal	e.			

4. **CHANGE IN URINARY CONTINENCE** — Change in urinary continence/appliances and programs in last 90 days
   0. No change   1. Improved 2. Deteriorated | 0 |

SECTION G. PSYCHOSOCIAL WELL-BEING

1. **SENSE OF INITIATIVE/ INVOLVE-MENT**

At ease interacting with others	a. X
At ease doing planned or structural activities	b.
At ease doing self-initiated activities	c.
Establishes own goals	d.
Pursues involvement in life of facility (e.g., makes/keeps friends; involved in group activities; responds positively to new activities; assists at religious services)	e.
Accepts invitations into most group activities	f. X
NONE OF ABOVE	g.

2. **UNSETTLED RELATION-SHIPS**

Covert/open conflict with and/or repeated criticism of staff	a.
Unhappy with roommate	b.
Unhappy with residents other than roommate	c.
Openly expresses conflict/anger with family or friends	d. X
Absence of personal contact with family/friends	e.
Recent loss of close family member/friend	f.
NONE OF ABOVE	g.

3. **PAST ROLES**

Strong identification with past roles and life status	a.
Expresses sadness/anger/empty feeling over lost roles/status	b. X
NONE OF ABOVE	c.

CHARTING GUIDE

Minimum data set (continued)

SECTION H. MOOD AND BEHAVIOR PATTERNS

1.	SAD OR ANXIOUS MOOD	(Check all that apply during last 30 days)	
		VERBAL EXPRESSIONS of DISTRESS by resident (sadness, sense that nothing matters, hopelessness, worthlessness, unrealistic fears, vocal expressions of anxiety or grief)	a.
		DEMONSTRATED (OBSERVABLE) SIGNS of mental DISTRESS	
		— Tearfulness, emotional groaning, sighing, breathlessness	b.
		— Motor agitation such as pacing, handwringing or picking	c.
		— Failure to eat or take medications, withdrawal from self-care or leisure activities	d.
		— Pervasive concern with health	e.
		— Recurrent thoughts of death—e.g., believes he/she about to die, have a heart attack	f.
		— Suicidal thoughts/actions	g.
		NONE OF ABOVE	h. X
2.	MOOD PERSISTENCE	Sad or anxious mood intrudes on daily life over **last 7 days** — not easily altered, doesn't "cheer up" 0. No 1. Yes	0
3.	PROBLEM BEHAVIOR	(Code for behavior in last 7 days) 0. Behavior not exhibited in last 7 days 1. Behavior of this type occurred less than daily 2. Behavior of this type occurred daily or more frequently	
		WANDERING (moved with no rational purpose, seemingly oblivious to needs or safety)	a. 0
		VERBALLY ABUSIVE (others were threatened, screamed at, cursed at)	b. 0
		PHYSICALLY ABUSIVE (others were hit, shoved, scratched, sexually abused)	c. 0
		SOCIALLY INAPPROPRIATE/DISRUPTIVE BEHAVIOR (made disrupting sounds, noisy, screams, self-abusive acts, sexual behavior or disrobing in public, smeared/threw food/feces, hoarding, rummaged through others' belongings)	d. 0
4.	RESIDENT RESISTS CARE	(Check all types of resistance that occurred in the last 7 days)	
		Resisted taking medications/injection	a.
		Resisted ADL assistance	b.
		NONE OF ABOVE	c. X
5.	BEHAVIOR MANAGEMENT PROGRAM	Behavior problem has been addressed by clinically developed behavior management program. (Note: Do not include programs that involve only physical restraints or psychotropic medications in this category) 0. No behavior problem 1. Yes, addressed 2. No, not addressed	0
6.	CHANGE IN MOOD	Change in mood in **last 90 days** 0. No change 1. Improved 2. Deteriorated	0
7.	CHANGE IN PROBLEM BEHAVIOR	Change in problem behavioral signs in **last 90 days** 0. No change 1. Improved 2. Deteriorated	0

SECTION I. ACTIVITY PURSUIT PATTERNS

1.	TIME AWAKE	(Check appropriate time periods over last 7 days) Resident awake all or most of time (i.e., naps no more than one hour per time period) in the:	
		Morning a. X Evening	c.
		Afternoon b. X NONE OF ABOVE	d.
2.	AVERAGE TIME INVOLVED IN ACTIVITIES	0. Most—more than ²/₃ of time 2. Little—less than ¹/₃ of time 1. Some—¹/₃ to ²/₃ of time 3. None	2
3.	PREFERRED ACTIVITY SETTINGS	(Check all settings in which activities are preferred)	
		Own room a. X Outside facility	d.
		Day/activity room b. X NONE OF ABOVE	e.
		Inside NH/off unit c.	

4.	GENERAL ACTIVITY PREFERENCES (adapted to resident's current abilities)	(Check all PREFERENCES whether or not activity is currently available to resident)				
		Cards/other games	a.	Spiritual/religious activities	f. X
		Crafts/arts	b.	Trips/shopping	g.
		Exercise/sports	c. X	Walking/wheeling outdoors	h.
		Music	d. X	Watch TV	i. X
		Read/write	e.	NONE OF ABOVE	j.
5.	PREFERS MORE OR DIFFERENT ACTIVITIES	Resident expresses/indicates preference for other activities/choices 0. No 1. Yes				1

SECTION J. DISEASE DIAGNOSES

Check only those diseases present that have a relationship to current ADL status, cognitive status, behavior status, medical treatments, or risk of death. (Do not list old/inactive diagnoses.)

1.	DISEASES	(If none apply, CHECK the NONE OF ABOVE box)			
	HEART/CIRCULATION		**PSYCHIATRIC/MOOD**	
	Arteriosclerotic heart disease (ASHD)	a.	Anxiety disorder	p.
	Cardiac dysrhythmias	b.	Depression	q. X
	Congestive heart failure	c.	Manic depressive (bipolar disease)	r.
	Hypertension	d.	**SENSORY**	
	Hypotension	e.	Cataracts	s.
	Peripheral vascular disease	f. X	Glaucoma	t.
	Other cardiovascular disease	g.	**OTHER**	
	NEUROLOGICAL		Allergies	u.
	Alzheimer's	h.	Anemia	v. X
	Dementia other than Alzheimer's	i.	Arthritis	w.
	Aphasia	j.	Cancer	x.
	Cerebrovascular accident (stroke)	k.	Diabetes mellitus	y.
	Multiple sclerosis	l.	Explicit terminal prognosis	z.
	Parkinson's disease	m.	Hypothyroidism	aa. X
	PULMONARY		Osteoporosis	bb.
	Emphysema/Asthma/COPD	n.	Seizure disorder	cc.
	Pneumonia	o.	Septicemia	dd.
			Urinary tract infection—in last 30 days	ee. X
			NONE OF ABOVE	ff.

2.	OTHER CURRENT DIAGNOSES AND ICD-9 CODES	a. *Hypertension* 4 0 2 . 1 1
		b.
		c.
		d.
		e.
		f.

SECTION K. HEALTH CONDITIONS

1.	PROBLEM CONDITIONS	(Check all problems that are present in last 7 days unless other time frame indicated)			
		Constipation	a.	Pain—resident complains or shows evidence of pain daily or almost daily	j.
		Diarrhea	b. X		
		Dizziness/vertigo	c.		
		Edema	d. X	Recurrent lung aspirations in last 90 days	k.
		Fecal impaction	e.	Shortness of breath	l.
		Fever	f.	Syncope (fainting)	m.
		Hallucinations/delusions	g.	Vomiting	n.
		Internal bleeding	h.	NONE OF ABOVE	o.
		Joint pain	i.		
2.	ACCIDENTS	Fell in **past 30 days**	a.	Hip fracture in **last 180 days**	c.
		Fell in **past 31-180 days**	b. X		
				NONE OF ABOVE	d.

(continued)

𝒞HARTING GUIDE

Minimum data set (continued)

3.	STABILITY OF CONDITIONS	Conditions/diseases make resident's cognitive, ADL, or behavior status unstable—fluctuating, precarious, or deteriorating	a. X
		Resident experiencing an acute episode or a flare-up of a recurrent/chronic problem	b.
		NONE OF ABOVE	c.

SECTION L. ORAL/NUTRITIONAL STATUS

1.	ORAL PROBLEMS	Chewing problem	a.
		Swallowing problem	b.
		Mouth pain	c.
		NONE OF ABOVE	d. X

2.	HEIGHT AND WEIGHT	Record height (a.) in inches and weight (b.) in pounds. Weight based on most recent status in **last 30 days**; measure weight consistently in accord with standard facility practice—e.g., in a.m. after voiding, before meal, with shoes off, and in nightclothes. HT (in.) a. 710 WT (lb.) b. 180
		c. Weight loss (i.e., 5%+ in **last 30 days**; or 10% in **last 180 days**) 0. No 1. Yes . 0

3.	NUTRITIONAL PROBLEMS	Complains about the taste of many foods a.	Regular complaint of hunger d.
		Insufficient fluid; dehydrated b.	Leaves 25%+ food uneaten at most meals e.
		Did **NOT** consume all/almost all liquids provided **during last 3 days** c.	*NONE OF ABOVE* f. X

4.	NUTRITIONAL APPROACHES	Parenteral/IV a.	Dietary supplement between meals f.
		Feeding tube b.	Plate guard, stabilized built-up utensil, etc. g.
		Mechanically altered diet c.	*NONE OF ABOVE* h.
		Syringe (oral feeding) d.	
		Therapeutic diet e. X	

SECTION M. ORAL/DENTAL STATUS

1.	ORAL STATUS AND DISEASE PREVENTION	Debris (soft, easily movable substances) present in mouth prior to going to bed at night	a.
		Has dentures and/or removable bridge	b. X
		Some/all natural teeth lost—does not have or does not use dentures (or partial plates)	c.
		Broken, loose, or carious teeth	d.
		Inflamed gums (gingiva); swollen or bleeding gums; oral abscesses, ulcers or rashes	e.
		Daily cleaning of teeth/dentures	f. X
		NONE OF ABOVE	g.

SECTION N. SKIN CONDITION

1.	STASIS ULCER	(open lesion caused by poor venous circulation to lower extremities) 0. No 1. Yes	0
2.	PRESSURE ULCERS	(Code for highest stage of pressure ulcer) 0. No pressure ulcers	1
		1. Stage 1 A persistent area of skin redness (without a break in the skin) that does not disappear when pressure is relieved	
		2. Stage 2 A partial thickness loss of skin layers that presents clinically as an abrasion, blister, or shallow crater	
		3. Stage 3 A full thickness of skin is lost, exposing the subcutaneous tissues—presents as a deep crater with or without undermining adjacent tissue	
		4. Stage 4 A full thickness of skin and subcutaneous tissue is lost, exposing muscle and/or bone	
3.	HISTORY OF RESOLVED/CURED PRESSURE ULCERS	Resident has had a pressure ulcer that was resolved/cured in **last 90 days** 0. No 1. Yes	0

4.	SKIN PROBLEMS/CARE	Open lesions other than statis or pressure ulcers (e.g., cuts)	a.
		Skin desensitized to pain, pressure, discomfort	b.
		Protective/preventive skin care	c. X
		Turning/repositioning program	d. X
		Pressure relieving beds, bed/chair pads (e.g., egg crate pads)	e. X
		Wound care/treatment (e.g., pressure ulcer care, surgical wound)	f. X
		Other skin care/treatment	g. X
		NONE OF ABOVE	h.

SECTION O. MEDICATION USE

1.	NUMBER OF MEDICATIONS	*(Record the number of different medications used in the last 7 days; enter "0" if none used)*	0 7
2.	NEW MEDICATIONS	Resident has received new medications during the **last 90 days** 0. No 1. Yes	0
3.	INJECTIONS	*(Record the number of days injections of any type received during the last 7 days)*	7
4.	DAYS RECEIVED THE FOLLOWING MEDICATION	*(Record the number of days during last 7 days; enter "0" if not used; enter "1" if long-acting meds. used less than weekly)*	
		Antipsychotics	a. 0
		Antianxiety/hypnotics	b. 0
		Antidepressants	c. 7
5.	PREVIOUS MEDICATION RESULTS	*(SKIP this question if resident currently receiving antipsychotics, antidepressants, or antianxiety/hypnotics—otherwise code correct response for last 90 days)* Resident has previously received psychoactive medications for a mood or behavior problem, and these medications were effective (without undue adverse consequences) 0. No, drugs not used 1. Drugs were effective 2. Drugs were not effective 3. Drug effectiveness unknown	

SECTION P. SPECIAL TREATMENT AND PROCEDURES

1.	SPECIAL TREATMENTS AND PROCEDURES	SPECIAL CARE—Check treatments received during the last 14 days	
		Chemotherapy a.	IV meds f. X
		Radiation b.	Transfusions g.
		Dialysis c.	O_2 h.
		Suctioning d.	Other ___ i.
		Trach. care e.	*NONE OF ABOVE* j.
		THERAPIES—**Record the number of days** each of the following therapies was administered (for at least 10 minutes during a day) in the last 7 days:	
		Speech—language pathology and audiology services	a. 0
		Occupational therapy	b. 0
		Physical therapy	c. 0
		Psychological therapy (any licensed professional)	d. 0
		Respiratory therapy	e. 0
2.	ABNORMAL LAB VALUES	Has the resident had any abnormal lab values during the **last 90 days**? 0. No 1. Yes 2. No tests performed	1
3.	DEVICES AND RESTRAINTS	Use the following codes for last 7 days: 0. Not used 1. Used less than daily 2. Used daily	
		Bed rails	a. 2
		Trunk restraint	b. 0
		Limb restraint	c. 0
		Chair prevents rising	d. 2

sure it's in place and working properly.

Speak clearly and distinctly in a normal tone of voice. Don't shout because shouting raises the pitch of your voice and may make understanding you harder, not easier. Because hearing loss from aging (presbycusis) affects perception of high-pitched tones first, speaking in a low voice will help reduce its effects. Repeat facts periodically during the interview.

Communication. Always address an older patient as Miss, Mrs. or Mr. and the surname, unless he or she requests otherwise. Experts also recommend the use of touch. For example, shake the patient's hand when you say hello, then hold it briefly to convey concern. Use body language, touch, and eye contact to encourage participation. Act patient, relaxed, and unhurried.

Talk *to* the person, not *at* him. Tell him how long the process will take. If language poses a problem, enlist the aid of an interpreter, family member, or friend as appropriate.

Early in the interview, try to evaluate your patient's ability to communicate and his reliability as a historian. If you have any doubts about these matters before the interview begins, ask him if a family member or a friend can be present. Don't be surprised if your older patient *requests* that someone assist him; he, too, may have concerns about getting through the interview on his own. Having another person present gives you a chance to observe your patient's interaction with this person and provides more data for the history. However, this may prevent the patient from speaking freely, so plan to talk with him privately sometime during your assessment.

Provide carefully structured questions to elicit significant information. Keep your questions concise, rephrase those he doesn't understand, and use nonverbal techniques, such as facial expressions, pointing, or touching to enhance your meaning.

Use terms appropriate to the patient's level of understanding; avoid using jargon and complex medical terms. Offer explanations in lay terms, and then use the related medical terms, if appropriate, so the patient can become familiar with them.

To foster your older patient's cooperation, take a little extra time to help him see the relevance of your questions. You may need to repeat an explanation several times during the interview, but don't repeat unnecessarily. Give the patient plenty of time to respond to your questions and directions. Remain silent to allow him to collect his thoughts and ideas before responding.

Patience is the key to communicating with an older adult who responds slowly to your questions. But don't confuse patience with patronizing behavior. Your patient will easily perceive such behavior and may interpret it as lack of genuine concern.

Consent. Initial contact with the older patient should focus on ensuring that he knows the purpose of the assessment and how he can help during the history taking — an important step in establishing a trusting relationship.

Review all parts of the assessment including the kinds of information you need. Explain how the information will be used and with whom you'll share it. Ask only for information that's relevant to the patient's condition. For example, you wouldn't obtain a detailed obstetric history from a 75-year-old woman who doesn't have a gynecologic problem. If the patient refuses to answer questions or to participate, document the refusal appropriately.

Once you've obtained an older adult's cooperation, you may have some trouble getting him to keep his story brief. He has a lot of history to relate and may reminisce during the interview. Try to find time to let him talk; you may obtain valuable clues about his current physical, mental, and spiritual health. If you must keep the history brief, remind him how much time you have available for the interview, and offer to come back another time to chat with him informally.

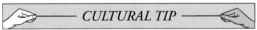

CULTURAL TIP

Be alert to your patient's cultural background during the interview. Don't confuse cultural differences with abnormal behavior. For example, a Southeast Asian patient may not look you in the eye when speaking and may answer "yes," inappropriately, to a direct question, both out of deference and fear of giving offense. Using first names, touching, and other methods useful with most patients, may be considered inappropriate by a Southeast Asian patient, who may react negatively or not respond at all. Before drawing conclusions, try to evaluate the effect of any cultural differences and react accordingly.

Current health status

The first part of the interview explores the person's chief complaint and his current health status.

● Begin by asking the patient his full name, address, age, date of birth, birthplace, and contact persons in case of an emergency. Record your information on an appropriate patient history form.

● Although mental status is usually assessed toward the end of the physical examination, you can assess certain aspects of it in a nonthreatening way during the general conversation. Asking the patient to state his name and date of birth and then to calculate his age tests his ability to calculate and his remote, recent, and immediate memory.

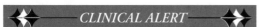
CLINICAL ALERT

To avoid false assessments of his ability to calculate, ascertain the patient's educational level to ensure that he has learned to perform the calculation.

● Record the reason for admission, or the chief complaint, in the person's own words. Evaluate each complaint in terms of onset, location, duration, timing, intensity, any aggravating or alleviating factors, any treatment measures, and the impact on lifestyle.

● Ask the patient about any current medications, both prescription and nonprescription, including the name, dosage, frequency, and reason for the medication. Older people often use multiple medications, placing them at risk for adverse reactions to drugs. If the person has brought any of his medications with him, ask to see them.

● Next, ask about any treatments he's receiving, such as pulmonary treatments, wound care, or pain control.

● Finally, list any devices that the person uses, such as a cane, walker, corrective lenses, or hearing aid. Ask if he uses any home safety devices, such as grab rails in the shower or tub, smoke alarms, nonskid floor surfaces, and strong lighting.

Medical history

The medical history includes an overview of the person's general health status, a history of his adult illnesses, a record of past hospitalizations and their purpose, the frequency of doctor's visits, and previous use of medications and treatments and their purpose.

● Before asking specific questions about medical history, ask an open-ended question such as "How would you describe your overall health?" This can provide specific information about the health history and reveal how the patient perceives his health status.

● Try to determine the patient's reaction to any previous hospitalizations. Someone who has had a bad experience may fear readmission and thus withhold important information.

● Ask about a history of any cardiac, respiratory, or neurologic disorders; cancer; surgery; trauma; falls; or fractures. The patient's detailed recall of all major illnesses, surgical procedures, and injuries is necessary for you to complete the history. For example, fractures he experienced early in life may figure significantly now in osteoporosis. As you record his past history, try to get an idea of the amount of stress he has had recently and the way he has handled previous health problems. Don't be concerned if he can't relate this medical history chronologically; just be sure to record his age at the time each medical condition occurred. Try to obtain a chronological report, including the event, date, treatment received, and the doctor involved. Because the older patient usually has been treated by many doctors, eliciting their names, reasons for treatment, and dates can yield important clues.

● Pay special attention to your patient's medication history because he probably takes medication routinely. Find out what medications (over-the-counter and prescription) he has taken in the past and the dosage for each.

Review of systems

The review of systems for the older person involves asking questions that keep in mind the physiologic changes considered normal in the aging process. Remember that the older person often has an atypical disease presentation. For example, subtle changes in appetite and mental status may be his only symptoms.

Begin reviewing specific body areas and systems, using either a head-to-toe approach or the major body system method. Either provides a systematic and organized framework, so choose the method that works best for you. The example below, using the body system approach, demonstrates the information you need to elicit.

Skin, hair, and nails

● Ask about any unhealed sore or mole or an irregularly shaped lesion.
● Ask the patient whether his skin is dry, oily, or normal.
● Does he experience itching, easy bruising, rashes, calluses, or bunions? Rashes may be side effects of certain medications. Contact allergies, calluses, and bunions can interfere with ambulation and other ADLs.
● Your patient may report typical age-related changes: that his skin seems thinner and looser (less elastic) than before, that he perspires less, and that his scalp feels dry. His fingernails may have thickened and changed color slightly. Find out if he can take care of his own nails.

Eyes

● Has the patient noticed any increased tearing, or diminished near vision (presbyopia)?
● Ask about changes, especially night vision or any double or blurred vision. Does he need more light than usual when reading? Does he have any difficulty driving?
● Also ask about corrective lenses, glaucoma, and the date of his most recent eye examination.

Ears and hearing

● Question the patient about ear pain. He should be free of any pain.

● Ask about tinnitus, which has been present in older people without hearing impairment. In the absence of other clinical symptoms, tinnitus is considered benign.
● Ask about cerumen, ear discharge, and hearing problems. Older people often have difficulty hearing high-pitched sounds such as those produced by smoke alarms. Conductive hearing loss can be attributed to cerumen plugs; unilateral hearing loss should be investigated further to rule out acoustic neuroma. In general older people are expected to have diminished hearing. Noting which ear is affected helps you improve communication by targeting your speech toward the good ear. It also enables you to plan for a hearing aid, if appropriate.

Respiratory system

● Ask about lung or breathing problems. Remember that hypoventilation and hypoperfusion from respiratory disease can produce confusion or slowed mental function in the older person.
● Ask if he experiences any shortness of breath on exertion or when lying down. Older people commonly experience dyspnea on exertion; it can also result from lung infections, such as bronchitis or pneumonia.
● Does the patient get an annual influenza immunization? When was his last one?
● If he reports trouble breathing, explore the precipitating circumstances. To assess his tolerance level, note the distances he says he can travel and the type of exertion that normally produces dyspnea.
● Does he cough excessively? Does the cough produce a lot of sputum. If so, what color is it?
● Does he report bleeding from mucous membranes? Has his sense of smell decreased?
● If your patient is retired, record any possible exposure to harmful substances by asking about his former occupation.

Cardiovascular system

● Ask your patient whether he's gained weight recently, if his belts or rings feel tight, or if he's noticed his ankles swelling. In addition, find out if he tires more easily now than previously, if he has trouble breathing, and if he becomes dizzy when he rises from a chair or bed. These are chief indicators of congestive heart failure; more than half of all older people suffer from some degree of this disorder.

- Check level of consciousness, noting any confusion or slowed mental status; occasionally, these are early signs of inadequate cardiac output.
- Question him about chest pain. Any pain could be angina pectoris. However, remember that his chief complaint may be dyspnea or palpitations rather than the more definitive chest pain, because aging contributes to coronary artery plaque development but also promotes collateral circulation to areas deprived of perfusion. Also keep in mind that these signs and symptoms in older people may indicate pathology in many systems other than cardiovascular, including the urinary, endocrine, musculoskeletal, and respiratory systems.

Because an older person is less sensitive to deep pain, keep in mind that he may describe his chest pain as heavy or dull, whereas a younger person would describe the same pain as sharp. Even if he's having a myocardial infarction, he may only experience confusion, vomiting, faintness, and dizziness.

- Ask about ADLs, any signs or symptoms associated with these activities, and his response to physical and emotional exertion. Reduced cardiac reserve limits the older person's ability to respond to conditions such as infection, blood loss, hypoxia-induced arrhythmias, and electrolyte imbalances.
- Try to correlate your assessment of the patient's ADLs and his mental status with any eating and sleeping difficulties.
- Determine if he has a history of smoking, frequent coughing, wheezing, or dyspnea, which may indicate chronic lung disease. Pulmonary hypertension resulting from pulmonary disease is a chief cause of left ventricular heart failure.
- Ask about any adverse reactions your patient may be experiencing from prescribed medication. Weakness, bradycardia, hypotension, and confusion may indicate elevated potassium levels. Weakness, fatigue, muscle cramps, and palpitations may indicate inadequate levels of potassium. Anorexia, nausea, vomiting, diarrhea, headache, rash, vision disturbances, and mental confusion may indicate an overdose of digitalis glycosides or antiarrhythmic medications.

GI system
- Ask about any change in his sense of taste. An older person may complain about a foul taste in his mouth, which may be a result of decreased saliva production.
- If he wears dentures, find out how comfortable they are and how well they work. An improper fit may explain a report of declining appetite.
- If he reports difficulty in swallowing, ask if he has the same degree of difficulty swallowing both solid foods and liquids. Does food lodge in his throat? Does he experience pain after eating or while lying flat?
- Question him about weight loss, rectal bleeding, and elimination habits. About 50% of older adults develop diverticulosis. Ask if he has experienced any crampy abdominal pain in the left lower quadrant. Remember that abdominal disorders often present atypically in the older adult. For example, diffuse abdominal pain may indicate fecal impaction. Fecal incontinence is abnormal at any age. In an older person it's commonly seen with laxative abuse, advanced dementia, and cerebrovascular disease.
- Note the presence of any devices, such as a feeding tube, parenteral nutrition, or an ostomy.

GU system
- Investigate any report of incontinence. When incontinence occurs, does your patient feel the loss of control, or does he sense the urge to urinate? Ask if he uses pads or experiences enuresis. If he urinates in the middle of the night, find out if the urge awakens him.

Most older adults think that urinary incontinence is a result of aging, but common causes of urinary incontinence include fecal impaction, prostatic obstruction, atrophic vaginitis, infection, and certain medications.

- Ask an older male about any frequent urinary infections, urinary incontinence, dribbling after urination, and decrease in the size and force of the urine stream; all are common manifestations of prostatic obstruction.

• Ask an older female if she experiences vaginal itching, discharge, or pain. Ask if she performs monthly breast self-examination and, if so, whether she has detected any abnormalities. Postmenopausal bleeding and breast masses are abnormal and require prompt evaluation.

Neurologic system
• Inquire about changes in coordination, strength, or sensory perception.
• Has your patient had any difficulty controlling his bowels or his bladder?
• Does he have headaches or seizures?
• Has he experienced any temporary losses of consciousness? Syncope (loss of consciousness) may represent a cardiac, neurologic, or metabolic disorder. Common complaints are a feeling of "blacking out" or complete amnesia of events during a specific time period. Ask about events that preceded the syncopal episode as well as the initial events remembered once he regained consciousness.
• Has he felt dizzy (a sensation of unsteadiness and movement within the head or of light-headedness) or felt vertigo (a sensation that the room is rotating around the person or that the person himself is rotating)? Vertigo in the aged may be attributed to inner ear disorders, such as labyrinthitis, Ménière's disease, and benign positional vertigo, or to posterior circulatory diseases, such as vertebrabasilar insufficiency or cerebrovascular accident.
• Question your patient about any memory loss or forgetfulness.

Musculoskeletal system
• If the chief complaint is pain associated with a fall, determine if the pain preceded the fall. Pain present before a fall may indicate a pathologic fracture.
• Ask if your patient has noticed any vision or coordination changes that may make him more susceptible to falling.
• Is he afraid of falling? If so, why? Unsteady gait may explain an older adult's fear of falling.
• Does he have a deformity or wear a prosthesis?
• Ask if he has any joint pain, low back pain or weakness or stiffness in an extremity. Osteoarthritis commonly accounts for older adults' complaints of pain, stiffness, or limitation in weight-bearing joints. Focal pain may occur in individuals who have another rheumatoid disease, such as rheumatoid or gouty arthritis or carpal tunnel syndrome.
• When recording your patient's history of illness, determine if he has asthma or arthritis, because treatment with steroids can lead to osteoporosis. Arthritis also produces joint instability and pernicious anemia. In pernicious anemia, inadequate absorption of vitamin B_{12} leads to loss of vibratory sensation and proprioception, resulting in falls. Cancer of the breast, prostate, thyroid, kidney, or bladder may metastasize to bone. Hyperparathyroidism leads to bone decalcification and osteoporosis. Hormone imbalance can result in postmenopausal osteoporosis.

Hematologic and immune systems
• Ask if your patient experiences joint pain, weakness, or fatigue. Does he take walks? If so, for how long? Does he have any difficulty using his hands? Do his knees bother him?
• Determine your patient's typical daily diet. Does he live alone and cook for himself? Because of limited income, limited resources, and decreased mobility, older people may have diets deficient in protein, calcium, and iron — nutrients essential to hematopoiesis. Even with an adequate diet, nutrients may not be metabolized because of reduced enzymes. (About 40% of people over age 60 have iron deficiency anemia.)
• Ask about current medications, and note which ones produce adverse effects similar to signs and symptoms of hematologic and immune disorders. For instance, digitalis may cause anorexia, nausea, and vomiting; aspirin can produce mucosal irritation and GI bleeding; excessive laxative use can prevent absorption of dietary nutrients.

Psychosocial assessment
• Begin the psychosocial history by asking about use of alcohol and tobacco. Note the quantity and type of alcoholic beverages consumed. For example, one ounce of brandy with dinner or one fifth of scotch per week. Document tobacco use in "pack years," the number of packs smoked per day multiplied by

the numbers of years your patient has smoked.

● Ask if he has any difficulty sleeping, unresolved problems, sadness, depression, or loss of interest in usual activities. A person with a major depressive disorder commonly has difficulty sleeping and changes in appetite.

● Ask an older person, regardless of his mood, about his sleeping habits. When does he go to bed and when does he wake up? Does he use any sleeping aids, such as medications or alcohol, to help him get to sleep? Does he take naps during the day?

● What is his employment status? If he's employed, ask about his job and whether his health problems will interfere with his returning to work. Talk with him about his plans for retirement, if he has any, and his attitude toward this phase of his life.

● If he expresses financial concerns, explore them further in a financial history. Ask if his income meets his monthly expenses for food, rent, household items, clothing, and other bills. A person whose income falls below his monthly expenses should be referred to social services for assistance. Remember to ask your patient if he receives any pensions or Social Security payments.

● How does the patient spend his time? What are his hobbies? How often does he see people socially? Has his activity level decreased lately?

● Does he live alone or with a spouse, family member, or friend? Does he own a home, rent, or live in a retirement, boarding, or nursing home?

● Make a point of talking with your older patient about his family and friends. Find out what significant relationships he has because these play a central role in his overall health and well-being. This part of the assessment can yield vital information about his support network.

Despite popular belief, families provide a substantial amount of help to their older members. So assessing family involvement is crucial. If your patient is hospitalized and seriously ill, or must transfer to another type of facility (such as a nursing home), he'll need the emotional support of family and friends. If he's returning home after an illness, he may need their help.

● Does your patient rely on assistance from family or friends to perform his usual daily activities?

● What person is primarily responsible for his care? Is this person overwhelmed or stressed?

● If your patient doesn't have a family or any friends on whom he can depend for support, record this for referring him to a social service agency later. Record the names of his next of kin.

● Note any use of community resources, such as meal service, reduced-fare or free transportation for seniors, adult day care, and home health services. Without your intervention, loneliness may discourage an older patient from getting well.

● Inquire about your patient's sexual activity. Don't ignore the subject because of the patient's age. Approach this aspect of the psychosocial history with the same sensitivity and respect for privacy that you would show with a younger person. Be especially sensitive to the patient's cultural background and moral values. This is especially true for a person who may be a generation or more older than you. If your patient is reluctant to discuss his sexual activity, don't press him for information. By inquiring, you've indicated your openness to discuss sexual issues. While patients may not disclose information immediately, they often bring it up at a later time.

ADL assessment

● Ask for a description of a typical day at home, including activities, eating habits, and sleep patterns. An older person's daily activities may affect his health, and his health problems may, in turn, threaten his ability to function independently.

● Ask your patient if he has decreased his activities recently; inactivity increases the risk of osteoporosis. Also ask him to describe his usual diet. Older people often have an inadequate calcium or vitamin intake, which can cause osteoporosis and muscle weakness.

● Because his eating habits may suggest other significant lines of questioning, find out how much of an appetite he usually has, how he prepares his food (does he use a lot of salt?), and how much fluid he normally consumes. You can put this information into a chart, showing which foods he eats at which times during the day.

● Ask about matters related to mobility. Is he able to move around at home easily and safely? Can he handle his basic food, clothing, and shelter needs?

Does he drive to the supermarket, use public transportation, or rely on a friend or relative to drive him?

● Ask if he expects to be able to continue with his routine after he is discharged from the hospital.

● To gain further information about your patient's functional status, use any of the assessment tools discussed earlier.

● Evaluate the safety of your patient's environment for performing ADLs to determine if he needs to change his residence to accommodate his physical changes. For example, ask about stairs and location of bathrooms. Does his home have adequate lighting, heating, and air conditioning; secured carpeting; smoke alarms; enough telephones; and safe electrical wiring?

Performing the physical examination

The physical examination is the second component of the health assessment. Together with the health history, it helps you identify and evaluate your patient's strengths, weaknesses, capabilities, and limitations. Use inspection, palpation, percussion, and auscultation to gather objective patient data, which provides new information and helps you validate the subjective data you obtained during the health history.

Preparing for the physical examination

Organization and planning are the keys to a successful physical examination. Because an older person may become easily fatigued during the physical examination, it is important to have all the necessary equipment within easy reach and in proper working order. In addition, you should anticipate your patient's needs by being prepared for modifications and additional comfort measures as necessary. Keep the following points in mind.

● Respect your patient's need for modesty; make sure that the examination area is private and explain how to put on the gown and drape.

● Ensure his comfort throughout the examination; have pillows and blankets available for added warmth and assistance in positioning.

● Anticipate any problems with mobility or strength that might require assistance from another person, use of alternative positions, or changes in the usual sequence of the examination.

The general survey

Begin the physical examination with a general, head-to-toe observation to gain an overall impression of your patient's status. This survey should include observations about:

● overall appearance, including skin, hygiene, grooming, and body build

● general mobility status

● level of consciousness, affect, and mood

● any overt signs of distress.

Vital signs

Before taking vital signs, make sure that the patient has rested for about 10 minutes. If the measurements, especially the pulse and respiratory rates are taken immediately after physical exertion, false readings may occur.

Temperature. Obtain a temperature orally or tympanically, depending on your facility's policy. If your patient is a mouth breather or dyspneic, use the tympanic, rectal, or axillary route instead of the oral route.

Normal temperature in an older adult can range from 96° F to 98.6° F (35.6° C to 37° C). However, the aging process alters temperature regulation, making temperature an unreliable sign of infection. The older adult is at high risk for infection because of age-related changes in immunity and increased incidence of hospitalization, which can lead to nosocomial infections. Yet even with a clinical infection, an older person may register no fever. Hypothermia, however, is a medical emergency and must be evaluated immediately.

Pulse. To obtain the most accurate pulse rate, count the apical pulse for 1 minute. Measure all pulses in terms of rate, rhythm, strength, and equality.

The resting pulse rate remains fairly constant through old age, ranging from 60 to 100 beats per minute. However, after exercise, an older person's pulse rate may take longer to return to the baseline.

The incidence of arrhythmias increases with age. Irregular rhythms should be reported immediately.

Respirations. Obtain a respiratory rate. Also assess the depth, rhythm, and quality of respirations. In the older adult respiratory rate, rhythm, and quality remain constant during rest but a period of apnea followed by deep breaths may occur during sleep. With exercise, the respiratory rate will increase and take longer to return to the baseline.

The respiratory rate may be a reliable sign of infection and congestive heart failure in older people, especially if the resting respiratory rate is tachypneic.

Blood pressure. Obtain blood pressure readings in both arms (see *Measuring an older person's blood pressure*). Changes in blood pressure may reflect several physiologic, age-related changes: a gradual increase in systolic and diastolic values, widening of pulse pressure influenced by an increase in arterial rigidity and a decrease in vessel resiliency, and a tendency to develop orthostatic hypotension. Changes may also be pathologic, such as with hypertension.

Height and weight

The best way to determine an older adult's height is to use a tape measure, measuring from the crown to the rump and then from the rump to the heels. This technique will account for changes in the curvature of the spine, such as senile kyphosis or widow's hump. Height usually decreases about 2" to 3" (5 to 2.6 cm) with age.

Obtain your patient's weight, noting whether it is with shoes or without. Any subsequent weight checks should be done using the same scale, at the same time of day, and with the patient clothed in the same way.

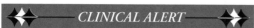

CLINICAL ALERT

If the patient has difficulty standing, use a chair scale; if he is bedridden, use a bed scale.

Sudden or profound weight changes are not a normal result of aging. However, a gradual weight

gain over the years may occur if the person continues to consume the same amount of calories as when he was younger and more active. Certain diseases, such as congestive heart failure and depression, may produce weight gain. Weight loss of more than 10% of the person's typical weight in a short period, such as 6 months, necessitates further follow up; it may indicate depression, a physiologic disorder, or a mechanical problem with eating.

Skin

Inspect the skin of the scalp, head, neck, trunk, and limbs. Note the color, temperature, texture, tone, turgor, thickness, and moisture.

Skin color normally varies from whitish pink to ruddy olive or yellow tones to shades of brown from light to blue-black. Areas such as the knees or elbows may appear relatively darker because of sun exposure. Calloused areas may appear yellow.

Disease may change skin color. Typical discolorations include redness, pallor, jaundice, ashen gray color, cyanosis, and bronze or brawny color. Brawny discoloration of the legs typically signifies chronic venous insufficiency. Ecchymosis and petechiae can occur from vitamin C deficiency.

Skin temperature can be described as cool, cold, warm, or hot. Use the ball of the hand to get an accurate assessment and to feel for symmetrical changes in temperature. Unilateral changes along with other clinical findings suggest a problem.

Skin typically becomes thicker with age. If corns occur, they usually appear on the dorsal portion of the small toes. Aging skin also becomes translucent, friable, and more susceptible to breakdown from trauma. The gradual decrease in total body water and sebum production leads to dry skin, particularly of the legs.

Skin texture may be smooth or rough. Increased dryness, with flaking and scaling, particularly on the extremities is not uncommon.

Skin turgor may be an unreliable sign of hydration in older people because of the reduction in the amount of subcutaneous tissue. Check turgor by pinching the subcutaneous tissue at the forehead or over the xiphoid process and watching for a quick return to baseline.

Measuring an older person's blood pressure

To achieve the most accurate results when taking an older patient's blood pressure, follow these guidelines:

- Allow this person to sit quietly for a few minutes before taking the reading. More time is required for the older adult to adjust to a baseline function, even after a minor stress such as walking into the examination room. A physically deconditioned patient will require even more time.
- Use the appropriate size cuff for accurate results. A regular adult cuff may be too small or too large. For small arms, use a pediatric cuff. Use a large adult cuff or leg cuff for an obese older adult.
- Don't be fooled by the auscultatory gap often found in older adults. Palpate the bracial artery as you inflate the cuff in increments of 10 mm Hg. Inflate the

cuff 20 to 30 mm Hg past the point at which the pulse disappears. As you deflate the cuff, listen for sounds. The first sound may be followed by a "gap" of 20 to 30 mm Hg before the sounds are heard again.
- Take readings on both arms, especially if this is the first encounter with the patient. A difference of more than 10 mm Hg in the right arm may indicate arteriosclerotic plaque in the right subclavian artery. The correct reading will be obtained from the left arm.
- Take readings with the patient in lying, sitting, and standing positions to monitor for orthostatic hypotension, especially if he's taking antihypertensive medications.

Adapted with permission from Anderson, M. *Caring for the Elderly Client.* Philadelphia: F.A. Davis Co., 1995.

Inspect the skin for the presence of tears, lacerations, scars, lesions, and ulcerations. As the distance between the outer layer of the skin surface the underlying bones becomes reduced from the loss of subcutaneous tissue, the protective effects of the fat pads and subcutaneous tissue diminish, increasing the likelihood of pressure ulcers. Look for early signs, such as local redness over pressure sites. Stasis ulcers of the legs, also common in older people, usually reflect chronic venous insufficiency.

Be alert to the common benign skin lesions found in older people. These must be differentiated from precancerous or malignant lesions. Note the size, pattern of distribution, shape, color, consistency, borders, and when they appeared. Any suspicious lesion warrants further evaluation.

Hair and nails. Inspect and palpate your patient's hair, noting color, quantity, distribution, and texture — fine, silky, or coarse. Hair thinning and sparseness are readily observed around the axilla and symphysis pubis. A disease such as hypothyroidism and hyperthyroidism produce changes in both hair texture and distribution.

Inspect fingernails and toenails, noting color,

shape, thickness, presence of lesions, and capillary refill.

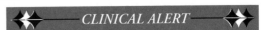
CLINICAL ALERT

Nail beds normally appear pink, but dark-skinned individuals may have pigment deposits and yellowed nails, a normal finding.

Some distortion of the normal flat or slightly curved nail surface is normal, but other changes in color, shape, or angle may indicate pathology. For example, people with anemia often have pale nail beds and slow capillary refill. Hypertrophy of the nails is a common clinical condition causing thickness and a hooked, clawlike deformity. Fungal infection of the nails commonly produces thickened, friable nails and a yellow discoloration. Ingrown nails often cause infection and mobility problems for the older adult. Infection at the bed of the nail appears as redness and possibly with heat, drainage and, if severe, bulging at the nail base. Respiratory distress or heart disease may produce cyanotic nail beds and clubbing of the fingers.

Head and face. Inspect the head, noting size, contour, and symmetry. The size and shape of the skull should not change with age. Soft tissue swelling or bulging of the cranium may indicate recent head trauma.

Palpate the skull, noting tenderness, masses, or lesions. Point tenderness or localized enlargement of the cranium requires further evaluation.

Inspect the face and neck area for color and proportion. Color should be evenly distributed. Facial features should be in proportion to head size. Observe facial expression and movements. Your patient should look alert and interested, with smooth expressive movements. The presence of a masklike or blank face often accompanies Parkinson's disease and certain psychiatric disorders.

Nose and mouth. Examine the external portion of the nose, noting any asymmetry or abnormality such as a structural deformity. Inspect the internal mucosa, noting color and any discharge, swelling, bleeding, or lesions. The area should be pink and moist with clear mucus and without any crusting or lesions.

Palpate the frontal and maxillary sinuses for tenderness, which should not be present.

Inspect the mouth, beginning with the lips. Note color, symmetry, any lesions or ulceration, and hydration status. Dry, parched lips indicate dehydration.

Note the presence of any dental appliances. Inspect the mouth with the appliance in place, noting the fit and observing for any sores or abscesses that may occur from friction. Poorly fitting dentures may produce fissures or cracks at the corners of the mouth (cheilosis); vitamin B complex deficiencies produce cheilosis with reddened lips.

Inspect the mucosa, noting color texture, hydration status, and any exudate. Poor oral hygiene can cause a white exudate coating the mucosa or tongue.

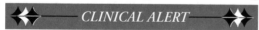

The mucosa and gums should be pink, smooth, and moist, but the mucosa of a dark-skinned person may be slightly bluish, a normal finding.

Palpate for lesions or nodules, noting any tenderness, pain, or bleeding. Inspect the gums for color,

inflammation, lesions, and bleeding. They should be pink and moist. If your patient has his natural teeth, note the number and condition.

Observe the tongue, noting its color, size, texture, and coating. The tongue normally is pink to red, smooth, and free of involuntary movement. However, extrapyramidal side effects of psychotropic drugs can cause involuntary movements, such as lip smacking, tongue protrusion, and slow rhythmic movements of the tongue, lips, or jaws. An enlarged tongue may be seen in a person with hypothyroid disease.

Assess the tongue's position. Deviation to the right or left suggests a neurologic disorder. Sublingual varicosities may be a result of iron deficiency anemia.

Observe the pharynx for signs of inflammation, discoloration, exudate, and lesions. The area should be pink to pale pink without discharge or lesions.

Eyes

When you examine an older person's eyes, keep in mind that ocular signs of aging can affect the appearance of the entire eye. You may see that the eyes sit deeper in the bony orbits, a normal finding that results from age-induced fatty tissue loss. Check eyebrow symmetry and distribution of hair.

Compare eyelid color to facial skin color; the lid should be free of any color changes such as redness. Check for lesions or edema, and note the direction of the eyelashes. Determine whether the upper eyelid partially or completely covers the pupil, which indicates ptosis, an abnormal finding. Common conditions affecting the eyelids in the aged include entropion and ectropion.

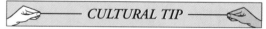

Asian people may have eyelids with epicanthal folds.

Inspect the lacrimal apparatus, noting any discharge, redness, edema, excessive tearing, or tenderness. Aging can affect the lacrimal apparatus in several ways. For example, the delicate canaliculi and nasolacrimal ducts may become plugged or kinked, resulting in constantly watering eyes. Such a blockage can also decrease tear production, causing dryness of an older person's eyes. Assess for keratitis sicca — burning, dry, or irritated eyes from decreased tearing.

Examine the sclera and conjunctiva. The sclera usually appears creamy white in color.

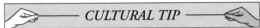

CULTURAL TIP

Dark-skinned individuals may have small spots on the sclera, a normal finding.

Because of the presence of fat, however, the sclera and conjunctiva may appear yellow. One common observation in older people is a yellow-tinged thickening of the bulbar conjunctiva, triangular in shape and occurring on the inner and outer margins of the cornea.

When you inspect the conjunctiva, be aware that its luster may appear dimmed, and it may be drier and thinner than in a younger person. This dryness may trigger frequent episodes of conjunctivitis.

When you inspect the corneas, you may note lipid deposits on the periphery, known as arcus senilis. In people who are at least age 50, these deposits usually have no pathologic effect. The cornea also flattens with age, sometimes causing astigmatism.

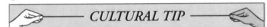

CULTURAL TIP

A grey-blue cornea is a normal finding in dark-skinned individuals.

Inspect the pupils. Note pupil size, shape, and reaction to light. An older adult's pupils may be abnormally small, if he's taking medication to treat glaucoma. If an intraocular lens was implanted in the pupillary space after cataract removal, the pupil may be irregularly shaped. Cataracts readily appear as opacification in the pupil and may obscure the transmission of light to the macula. When you examine the macula with an ophthalmoscope, you may note that the foveal light reflex is not as bright as in younger patients, a normal finding.

Inspect the iris, noting any margin aberrations. You may see bilateral irregular iris pigmentation, with the normal pigment replaced by a pale brown color. If your patient has had an iridectomy to treat glaucoma, the iris may have an irregular shape.

Test visual acuity with and without any corrective lenses, noting any differences. Perform an ophthalmoscopic examination to inspect the internal eye structures. The structure may be difficult to see in a person with senile miosis; to improve visualization, use a bright light in a dimly lit room. During the examination, observe for the larger, dark red veins; small, bright red arteries; yellowish, oval optic disk; and avascular macula. Background eye changes, characteristic of diseases common in older people, can be seen.

Ears

Inspect the auricle, noting color and any temperature changes, discharge, or lesions. Palpate the auricle for tenderness. Inspect the internal ear structures with an otoscope. Examine the external canal and tympanic membrane and observe for the light reflex. Note any lesion, bulging of the tympanic membrane, cerumen accumulation, or (in an older male) hair growth.

Inspection and palpation of the auricles and surrounding areas should yield the same findings as in the younger adult, with the exception of the normally hairy tragus in an older man. Examination with the otoscope yields similar results. Remember that the eardrum in some older adults may normally appear dull and retracted instead of pearl gray, but this can also be a clinically significant sign. (Cerumen buildup may make otoscopic examination impossible until the ears are cleaned.)

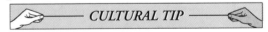

CULTURAL TIP

Cerumen is yellow in light-skinned patients and dark orange or brown in dark-skinned patients.

To detect hearing loss early in an older person, always perform the Weber and Rinne tuning fork tests.

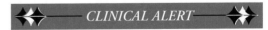

CLINICAL ALERT

Be particularly careful when you perform the Weber test, because an older person may become confused if he hears the tone better in his affected ear. As a result, he may falsely report that he hears the tone better in his other ear.

Also evaluate the patient's ability to hear and understand speech, in case you need to recommend rehabilitative therapy.

If your patient wears a hearing aid, inspect it carefully for proper functioning. Check how well the aid fits. Examine the earpiece, sound tube, and any connecting tubing for cracks and for the presence of dust, cerumen, or other sound-obstructing matter. Check that the batteries are installed correctly. Suspect that the aid isn't functioning properly if your patient reports that what he hears through it sounds fluttery or garbled.

Suspect presbycusis if an older adult complains of gradual hearing loss over many years but has no history of ear disorders or severe generalized disease.

In most people, the physical examination shows no abnormalities of the ear canal or eardrum. The Rinne test is positive — that is, the patient hears the air-conducted tone longer than the bone-conducted tone, with air conduction about equal in both ears. If your patient has a positive history of vertigo, ear pain, or nausea, suspect some pathology other than presbycusis. Any hearing or vestibular function abnormality requires immediate referral for audiometric testing.

Neck

Inspect the neck, noting scars, masses, and asymmetry. If masses are evident, gently palpate them, noting the consistency, size, shape, mobility, and tenderness. Repeat this for the lymph nodes.

Check the trachea for alignment. The trachea is normally located midline at the suprasternal notch. Note displacement and the presences of any masses. Inspect the thyroid gland while your patient takes a sip of water. Note any masses or bulging. Normally, the thyroid is invisible.

Try to palpate the thyroid; normally, it's not palpable. Note any masses nodules or enlargement.

Chest and respiratory system

Inspect the chest's shape and symmetry both anteriorly and posteriorly. Note the anteroposterior-to-lateral diameter. The older patient's thorax should be symmetrical despite the normal, age-related change in anteroposterior-to-lateral diameter.

Observe for rib retraction along the intracostal spaces as the patient inhales deeply; observe for bulging of the intracostal spaces as he exhales. An older patient with asthma or emphysema, secondary to chronic obstructive pulmonary disease, will typically show intracostal retraction or bulging. During respirations, listen for inspiratory or expiratory wheezes which may be audible from the oral airways.

◆◆ ── *CLINICAL ALERT* ── ◆◆

As you inspect an older person's thorax, be especially alert for degenerative skeletal changes, such as kyphosis.

Palpate the anterior and posterior chest for tenderness, masses, or lumps. Localized tenderness over the costochondral junctions suggests costochondritis, a frequent cause of chest pain in older patients. Assess diaphragmatic excursion. Palpating for diaphragmatic excursion may be more difficult because of loose skin covering the older adult's chest. Therefore, when you position your hands, slide them toward his spine, raising loose skin folds between your thumbs and the spine. In the older patient, excursion should be symmetrical, but lung expansion may be reduced because of decreased elasticity of the rib cage.

Palpate the anterior and posterior chest symmetrically for tactile fremitus. Fremitus is usually most evident near the tracheal bifurcation.

Percuss the patient's lung fields anteriorly and posteriorly from bases to apices. Make certain to percuss in a symmetrical fashion for comparison. Normal lung fields will sound resonant on percussion. Bony prominences, organs, or consolidated tissue will sound dull. When you percuss the chest, remember that loss of elastic recoil capability in an older person stretches the alveoli and bronchioles, producing hyperresonance.

Auscultate from the bases to the apices, anteriorly and posteriorly. Ask the patient to take some deep breaths, in and out, with his mouth open. During auscultation, carefully observe how well your patient tolerates the examination. He may tire easily because of low tolerance to oxygen debt. Also, taking deep breaths during auscultation may produce light-headedness or syncope faster than in a younger person. You may hear diminished sounds at the lung bases because some of his airways are closed. Inspiration will be significantly more audible than expiration on auscultation of the lungs.

In the absence of disease, crackles at the bases can be attributed to reduced mobility. If you hear crackles, ask the patient to cough. Crackles secondary to congestive heart failure will not clear with coughing; crackles caused by physical immobility may clear. Older adults with pulmonary fibrosis or interstitial lung disease often exhibit "Velcro type" crackles. Rhonchi or wheezes signify bronchospasm and necessitate further evaluation.

If the patient shows evidence of adventitious breath sounds with dullness on percussion, check for consolidation, and then check for egophony to help confirm consolidation.

During your assessment, keep in mind that older adults have a greater risk of developing respiratory disorders than do younger adults. Also, they may not experience the same signs and symptoms as a younger person (see *Recognizing respiratory disorders in older adults,* page 42).

Cardiovascular system

Inspect and palpate the point of maximal impulse (PMI). In a young person, the PMI is located around the fifth or sixth, left intercostal space at the midclavicular line. In an older person, the PMI may be displaced downward to the left.

Using the ball of your hand, palpate over the aortic, pulmonic, and mitral areas for thrills, heaves, or vibrations. You may detect a palpable thrill in a person with valvular heart disease.

Auscultate the heart over the aortic, pulmonic, tricuspid, and mitral areas, and Erb's point. Listen for S_1 and S_2 over each area, noting the intensity and splitting of S_1. Also listen for extra diastolic heart sounds, S_3 and S_4, which you may be able to detect in an older adult. An S_3 heart sound is heard between S_1 and S_2, usually at the lower sternal border, and indicates ventricular decompensation. In an older adult, S_3 is not a reliable indicator of congestive heart failure; it may be physiologic or it may occur in response to an increased diastolic flow. An S_4 heart sound is heard after S_2 and before S_1. S_4 sounds are most audible over the heart's apex.

◆ CLINICAL ALERT ◆

Kyphosis and scoliosis, common in older people, distort the chest wall and may displace the heart slightly. Thus, your patient's apical impulse and heart sounds may be slightly displaced.

Auscultate for cardiac murmurs. A murmur does not necessarily indicate an abnormality. Listen to the heart rate over the apex, counting for one full minute. Note the rate and rhythm. A common rhythm abnormality is atrial fibrillation, exhibited as an irregular rhythm. Bradycardia and tachycardia are abnormal findings. Widespread variations in rhythm are common among older people.

Assess the vessels of the head, neck, trunk, and extremities. Palpate the carotid arteries one at a time, pressing lightly to avoid obliterating the carotid pulse. Because of increased sensitivity of the baroreceptors as well as atherosclerotic changes in the vessels, palpation of the carotid arteries can result in narrowing of the arterial lumen (pulse may be more difficult to palpate). Note the rate, rhythm, strength, and equality of both pulses. Remember that palpating both at once can cause bradycardia.

Auscultate each carotid artery for bruits, usually high-pitched sounds representing a narrowing of either the arterial or venous lumen.

Assess for jugular vein distention. Identify the level of venous pulsation and measure its height in relation to the sternal angle. A height exceeding 3 cm is considered abnormal and indicates right-sided heart failure.

Palpate the peripheral arteries, noting the rate, rhythm, strength, and equality of pulses. Also note the presence of any bruits. In the older adult, expect arteries to be tortuous and appear kinked; they also may feel stiffer. However, the pulses should be symmetrical in strength.

Inspect the legs, noting color, temperature,

edema, trophic changes of the toes, and any varicosities. Color variations may include pallor, erythema, or pink, red, mottled, cyanotic, or brawny discoloration. Pallor, cyanotic, or mottled discoloration is seen in people with arterial insufficiency. Brawny discolorations are seen in people with long-standing chronic venous insufficiency. An older person should have no significant color deterioration attributed to age alone.

Using the ball of the hand, assess the temperature of the extremities; it should be equal bilaterally. Thrombosis is usually associated with a feeling of heat, but this response may be reduced in the older adult.

Check for edema, which is best assessed over bony prominences or the sacrum and typically pronounced in the most dependent areas of the body. Edema may result from numerous causes, so further evaluation is needed. Ascertain if the edema is pitting or non-pitting and grade the degree of edema.

GI system

Assessing an older adult's GI system is similar to examining a younger adult's, with these differences:

Abdominal palpation is usually easier and the results more accurate, because the older adult's abdominal wall is thinner (from muscle wasting and loss of fibroconnective tissue) and his muscle tone is usually more relaxed. A rigid abdomen occurs less commonly in an older person. Abdominal distention is more common.

Inspect the belly, noting shape and symmetry and any scars, masses, pulsations, distention, or striae. The abdomen may be described as obese, scaphoid, or distended.

Auscultate all four quadrants for bowel sounds. Listen over the abdominal aorta for bruits.

Percuss to determine the presence of air or fluid, the size of the liver, and any bladder distention. Air in the large bowel will sound tympanic, whereas fluid will sound dull. Bowel obstruction can occur secondary to long standing fecal impaction. On percussion, this presents as a distended and tympanic abdomen. If impaction is present, percussion will reveal dullness.

Percuss the liver. The normal liver size at the midclavicular line is 2 ¼" to 4 ¾" (6 to 12 cm) in diameter. Also, percuss over the symphysis pubis toward the umbilicus, noting any change in percussion. Dullness in this area may indicate bladder distention.

Palpate the belly, noting any masses or tenderness on light or deep palpation. Watch for any peritoneal signs such as rigidity or rebound tenderness. Masses in the lower quadrants may be impacted stool. Try to palpate the liver; normally it's not palpable.

GU system

When you assess an older adult's GU system, you'll use the same basic technique you would with a younger patient. Because of degenerative changes affecting body functions, older people are more susceptible than younger adults to certain renal disorders. Susceptibility to infection, for example, increases with age, and kidney infection from obstruction is a common cause of hospitalization among older adults. An older person who is immobilized is especially vulnerable to infection from urinary stasis or poor personal hygiene. A urinary tract infection in an older adult is frequently asymptomatic, or the symptoms are vague and ill defined; if untreated, it may progress to renal failure.

Altered cardiac output (such as in congestive heart failure) lowers renal perfusion and may result in azotemia. The kidneys compensate by retaining sodium and increasing edema. Medications to improve myocardial contractility and therapy with diuretics may increase renal function temporarily, but prerenal azotemia from depletion of intravascular volume often results.

Poor musculature from childbearing and from aging may predispose older women to cystocele. This condition can result in frequent urination, urgency, incontinence, urine retention, and infection. Obstruction in an older woman may result from uterine prolapse or pelvic cancer.

Keep in mind that cancer risk is higher in older people. Bladder cancer, common after age 50, is more prevalent in men than in women. Symptoms of bladder cancer include frequency, dysuria, and hematuria.

Almost all men over age 50 have some degree of prostatic enlargement. In men with benign prostatic hypertrophy or advanced prostate cancer, however, the gland becomes large enough to compress the urethra and sometimes the bladder, obstructing urine flow. If not treated, benign prostatic hypertrophy can impair renal function, causing initial signs and symptoms such as urinary hesitancy and intermittency, straining, and a reduction in the diameter and force of the urine stream. As the gland continues to enlarge, urinary frequency increases and nocturia occurs, possibly with hematuria. All these signs and symptoms may also be caused by a urinary system disorder.

When assessing the male genitalia, inspect the pubic hair, glans of the uncircumcised penis, penile shaft, scrotum and inguinal canals for bulging masses, lesions, inflammation, edema, or discoloration. The pubic hair becomes sparse and gray with age. Palpate any lesions noting size, shape, consistency, and tenderness.

Palpate the testes for size, shape, consistency and tenderness. Normally, in an older adult, the testes may be slightly smaller than adult size but they should be equal, smooth, freely movable, and soft

without nodules. Inspect and palpate the inguinal canal; you shouldn't observe any bulging.

When assessing the female genitalia, inspect the perineum for rash, lesion, or nodule. Examine the area for color, size, and shape. Inspect the vaginal orifice and observe for any bulging of tissues or organs.

Perform an internal pelvic examination, if qualified. Take care to maximize your patient's comfort, because the atrophic changes of the vaginal mucosa in the older female increase her discomfort during the pelvic examination. When you begin, remember to use a small speculum because of the decreased vaginal size in older women. To facilitate insertion, dampen the speculum with warm water; don't use a lubricant, because it may alter Pap smear results. Proceed slowly. Abrupt insertion of the speculum can damage sensitive degenerating tissue. When you perform the bimanual examination, remember that the ovaries normally regress with age, and you may not be able to palpate them. Obtain a Pap smear to screen for cervical cancer.

To examine the rectum, place the female patient in a side-lying position and the male patient bent over. Inspect the anus and overall skin surface characteristics. The area should be smooth and uninterrupted with coarse skin and slightly increased pigmented areas around the anus. Note any masses, nodules, lesions, or hemorrhoids.

Palpate the rectum using a gloved, lubricated finger, noting muscle tone. After withdrawing the finger, test any stool for blood. For males, assess the prostate gland. Note the size, consistency, shape, surface, and symmetry, and record any tenderness. The gland should be round, soft, nontender, free of masses, and about ¾" to 1 ½" (2 to 4 cm) in diameter.

Musculoskeletal system

Assessing the musculoskeletal system is vital in determining an older adult's overall ability to function. Limitations in range of motion, difficult ambulation, and diffused or localized joint pain can be detected easily during the physical examination.

Remember that older people may need more time or assistance with tests, such as range of motion or

Quick checks of balance and gait

Testing balance and gait are important parts of the physical examination. If time is limited, consider the methods below to gain this important information quickly.

Method #1

Tell the patient to walk in a straight line and turn 180 degrees.
• Can the patient move steadily and turn without difficulty?
Ask the patient to stand for a few seconds without support.
• Do you notice any swaying?
While the patient is standing, push lightly on the patient's sternum.
• Can the patient resist without losing control?

Method #2

Use this method if time is severely limited. Ask the patient to sit in an armless chair without upholstery, get up without using the hands, walk to the end of the hallway, turn around, and walk back to the starting point.
  Simply note the difficulties the older patient experiences during the exercise, including any inappropriate stance and limited ability to lift the feet or swaying the arms

Adapted with permission from Beck, J., et al., "Geriatric Assessment: Focus on Function," *Patient Care* 28:10-32, February 28, 1994.

gait assessment, because of weakness and decreased coordination. During your assessment, be alert for signs of motor and sensory dysfunction: weakness, spasticity, tremors, rigidity, and various types of sensory disturbances. Keep in mind that an uncertain gait and balance problems may cause damaging falls. Be sure to differentiate gait changes caused by joint disability, pain, or stiffness from those caused by neurologic impairment or another disorder.

Observe your patient's walk, noting gait and posture. Gait reflects the integration of reflexes as well as motor function. Older adults tend to take smaller steps, reduce the height of their steps, reduce their arm swing, and flex their elbows and knees. Gait disorders may occur if the patient limps or drags a foot from paresis. Posture may reveal kyphotic changes of the spine. To avoid injury, the patient with this condition must compensate by tilting his head back.

Assess static balance and station by gently pushing on the patient's shoulders while he's standing. The normal response includes bending at the waist, knees, ankles, and shoulders to create a forward flexion of the body. An abnormal response, in which the patient falls forward without bending, may indicate musculoskeletal or neurologic dysfunction.

Observe your patient's tandem walking to watch for any exaggerated ataxia and to observe the position of the head and neck in relation to shoulders and legs (see *Quick checks of balance and gait*). Note whether the patient turns quickly and whether the head, neck, and shoulders move as one unit or separately.

To assess calf and ankle muscles for weakness, have the patient walk on his toes, and then on his heels. Observe his spine from the side. Assess the height of the hips; both hips should be equally aligned. People who have had hip fractures or hip surgery may have a shortened leg.

Elicit Romberg's sign to evaluate posture and balance; it is positive if the patient sways.

Inspect the joints of the hands, wrists, elbows, shoulders, neck, hips, knees, and ankles. Note any joint enlargement, swelling, tenderness, crepitus, temperature changes, or deformities. A person with degenerative joint disease will complain of pain with motion and have enlarged joints due to bone changes, stiffness with range of motion, tenderness, crepitus, joint deformities, and palpable osteophytes.

Assess the foot for common deformities. These include hallux valgus, prolapsed metatarsals, and hammer toes.

Inspect each muscle group for atrophy, fasciculations, involuntary movements, and tremor. Move the joints through passive range-of-motion exercises, and palpate the muscles for tone and strength. Note any crepitus during the range of motion exercises. Resistance to passive range of motion indicates hypertonicity, whereas flaccidity indicates hypotonicity.

Assess for rigidity and spasticity. Rigidity can be detected best in the wrist or elbow joint. Cogwheel rigidity commonly occurs secondary to diseases involving the basal ganglia and side effects of certain neuroleptic drugs.

Throughout the physical examination, ask the patient to show you how he buttons or zippers his clothing, allowing you to directly observe his ability to perform selected ADLs. Observe him grasping items, such as the doorknob or water faucets.

Neurologic system

The neurologic examination includes assessment of level of consciousness or awareness, affect and mood, cognition, orientation, speech, general knowledge, memory, reasoning, object recognition and higher cognitive functions, cranial nerves, motor and sensory systems, and reflexes.

When you perform a neurologic examination of an older adult, use the same technique you would for a younger adult. However, you'll usually detect an alteration in one or more senses.

Begin by observing your patient's general appearance, including mood, affect, and grooming. Note whether he is appropriately dressed, responds appropriately to questions, and is oriented to person, time, and place. Changes in the environment, such as admission to an acute care facility, can cause marked confusion in an older person who was previously alert and oriented.

Note your patient's affect. A flat affect signals a disorder of the basal ganglia, such as Parkinson's disease. An older patient who seems depressed may require further evaluation; a number of assessment tools are available including the Geriatric Depression Scale. For more information, see Chapter 4, Meeting Mental and Emotional Needs.

Note the patient's speech. Speech disorders usu-ally occur in response to circulatory disorders and can readily be detected during casual conversation.

Assess vocabulary and general knowledge level by discussing current news items or family events.

Assess the patient's memory — his immediate, recent, and remote recall. Assess immediate recall by naming a certain number of objects or reciting a group of numbers and having the patient repeat them immediately. To elicit recent memory, ask the patient about events that occurred in the past 24 to 48 hours. To assess remote memory, ask the patient to recall significant events that occurred many years ago.

Assess the patient's ability to reason. Ask him questions requiring judgment, insight, and abstraction.

Assess object recognition. Point to two objects and ask the patient to identify each. The response is graded as normal or agnosia (the inability to name objects).

A number of screening tools are available to assess an older adults's cognitive status. One example is the Mini-Mental State Examination, which tests attention, recall, and language (see *Mini-mental state examination,* pages 46 and 47).

Cranial nerves. Assess each cranial nerve sequentially, beginning with cranial nerve I and progressing to cranial nerve XII. Few changes occur among older adults as a normal byproduct of aging, except for the following:
- olfactory nerve (I) — progressive loss of smell
- optic nerve (II) — decreased visual acuity, presbyopia, limited peripheral vision
- facial nerve (VII) — decreased perception of taste, particularly sweet and salty; drooping or relaxation of the muscles in the forehead and around the eyes and mouth
- auditory nerve (VIII) — presbycusis or loss of high-tone hearing, later generalized to all frequencies
- glossopharyngeal nerve (IX) — sluggish or absent gag reflex
- hypoglossal nerve (XII) — unilateral tongue weakness (may also be caused by malnutrition or structural malformation of the face).

(Text continues on page 48.)

HARTING GUIDE

Mini-mental state examination

Of the many assessment tools available for testing a patient's psychological condition, the Mini-Mental State Examination offers a quick and simple way to quantify cognitive function and screen for cognitive loss. The examination tests the patient's orientation, registration, attention, calculation, recall, and language and motor skills. Each section of the test involves a related series of questions or commands. The patient receives one point for each correct answer, and you add up the points and use the total score to get a general idea of the patient's mental state.

To administer the examination, seat the patient in a quiet, well-lighted room. Ask him to listen carefully and to answer each question as accurately as he can.

Don't time the test, but do score it right away. To score, add the number of correct responses. In the section on attention and calculation, include either items 14 to 18 or item 19, not both. The patient can receive a maximum total score of 30 points. Usually, a score below 24 indicates cognitive impairment, although this may not be an accurate cutoff for highly or poorly educated patients. A score below 20 usually appears in patients with delirium, dementia, schizophrenia, or affective disorder, and not in normal elderly people or in patients with neurosis or personality disorder.

THE MINI-MENTAL STATE EXAMINATION

Patient's Name _Elizabeth Snead_

Date _October 12, 1996_

Orientation

Ask the patient for the date. Then ask for any missing information (year, month, day of the week). Ask if he knows what season it is. Ask him to name the hospital and the floor he's currently on. Finally, ask for the town or city, the county, and the state. Give a point for each right answer (maximum score: 10).

1. Date ___/___
2. Year ___/___
3. Month ___/___
4. Day ___/___
5. Season ___/___
6. Hospital ___/___
7. Floor ___0___
8. Town or city ___/___
9. County ___/___
10. State ___/___

Registration

Tell the patient that you'd like to test his memory. Then say "ball," "flag," and "tree" clearly and slowly, taking about 1 second to say each word. After you've said all three words, ask him to repeat them. The first repetition determines the score (0 to 3), but keep saying the words (up to six trials) until he can repeat all three. If he doesn't eventually say all three, recall can't be meaningfully tested.

11. Ball ___/___
12. Flag ___0___
13. Tree ___/___
Number of trials __2__

Attention and calculation

You may perform this section of the test in one of two ways. Begin by asking the patient to count backward from 100 by sevens. Stop after he's said 5 numbers (93, 86, 79, 72, 65). Score one point for each correct number.

14. 93 ___/___
15. 86 ___/___
16. 79 ___/___
17. 72 ___0___
18. 65 ___0___

CHARTING GUIDE

Mini-mental state examination (continued)

OR
If the patient can't or won't perform this task, ask him to spell "world" backward (D, L, R, O, W). Assign one point for each correctly placed letter. For example, DLROW=5, DLORW=3. Record how the patient spelled "world" backward: _____

_____

19. Number of correctly placed letters _____

Recall
Ask the patient to recall the three words you previously asked him to remember (in the registration section). Give a point for each correct answer.

20. Ball _/_____
21. Flag _0_____
22. Tree _0_____

Language and motor skills
This section of the assessment has six parts.

Naming
Show the patient a wristwatch and ask, "What is this?" Repeat the question when holding a pencil. Give one point for each object named correctly.

23. Watch _/_____
24. Pencil _/_____

Repetition
Ask the patient to repeat "No ifs, ands, or buts." Allow only one try, and give one point for correct repetition.

25. Repetition _/_____

Three-stage command
Hand the patient a piece of blank paper and say, "Take the paper in your right hand, fold it in half, and put it on the floor." Score one point for each action performed correctly.

26. Takes in right hand _/_____
27. Folds in half _/_____
28. Places on floor _0_____

Reading
On a blank piece of paper, print "close your eyes" in letters large enough for the patient to see clearly. Ask him to read it and do what it says. Score one point only if he actually closes his eyes.

29. Closes eyes _/_____

Writing
Give the patient a blank piece of paper, and ask him to make up a sentence and write it. Evaluate whether the sentence contains a subject and a verb, and makes sense. Correct grammar and punctuation aren't necessary.

30. Writes sentence _/_____

Copying
On a clean piece of paper, draw intersecting pentagons, with each side about 1" long. Ask the patient to copy your drawing exactly as it appears. All 10 angles must be present and two must intersect to receive a point. Ignore tremor and rotation.
Example:

31. Draws pentagons _0_____

Total score _22_____

Adapted with permission from Folstein, M.F., et al. "Mini-Mental State: A Practical Method for Grading the Cognitive State of Patients for the Clinician," *Journal of Psychiatric Research* 12(3):189-98, November 1975. © 1975, Elsevier Science Ltd., Oxford, England.

Motor and sensory systems. Evaluate muscle and joint function. Also assess for rapid, rhythmic, alternating movements, which determine coordination. Observe your patient for the ability to repeat maneuvers and for smoothness in executing them. Expect the speed of response in an older person to be reduced.

Also check your patient's ability to perceive pain, using the sharp and dull end of a safety pin; temperature, using hot and cold substances; touch, using a light touch of the hand; and vibration, using a vibrating tuning fork. Also evaluate two-point discrimination and position sense. Perception should be accurate and symmetrical.

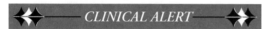

CLINICAL ALERT

Be aware that people over age 70 may show a decrease in vibratory sensation over the ankle.

Reflexes. You should assess an older adult's reflexes in the same manner as in other age-groups. The plantar and Babinski's reflexes are important in assessing for upper motor neuron disease. Any hyperactive, diminished, or asymmetrical responses are abnormal.

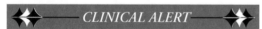

CLINICAL ALERT

Keep in mind that the Achilles tendon reflex may be difficult to elicit in the older patient.

Hematologic and immune systems

Assessing hematologic and immune function is the same for an older adult as for a younger adult. However, when obtaining certain diagnostic tests, be alert to the possibility of changes related to age. And when evaluating vital signs, remember that the older patient will have a diminished febrile response to infection.

Endocrine system

Many endocrine disorders cause signs and symptoms in older people that resemble changes that normally occur with aging. For this reason, these disorders are easily overlooked during assessment. For example, an adult with hypothyroidism experiences mental status changes and physical deterioration, including weight loss, dry skin, and hair loss. Yet these same signs and symptoms characterize normal aging.

Other endocrine abnormalities may complicate your assessment because their signs and symptoms are different in older people. For example, hyperthyroidism usually causes anxiety, but some older adults may instead experience depression or apathy (a condition known as apathetic hyperthyroidism of the elderly). What's more, an older person with hyperthyroidism may initially have signs and symptoms of congestive heart failure or atrial fibrillation rather than the classic manifestations associated with this disorder.

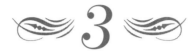

Maintaining physical health

From a geriatric care perspective, older people fall into two broad groups: those who are living in the community and can satisfy most of their basic needs, and those who are frail and living in long-term care settings. Although nursing care requirements differ for each group in important respects, older people all require special attention in the following areas: exercise, nutrition, rest and sleep, elimination, sexual function, and preventive medical care. You'll find information about each in this chapter.

MEETING MOBILITY AND EXERCISE NEEDS

Mobility, the ability to perform unrestricted movement, is essential to one's independence and freedom. Older people experience loss of mobility, and the functional loss and lowered activity level that go with it, from normal age-related changes in major body systems (see *Age-related changes affecting mobility,* page 50). Impaired mobility may also result from organic disease such as multiple sclerosis or severe depression; pain; or prolonged treatments such as traction or the use of a cast. In an institutional setting, older people may experience impaired mobility because of medications, activity restrictions, or the use of restraints. Additionally, many older people feel that they have worked all their lives

and should now be taken care of. Finally, our youth-oriented culture does not encourage or value functional independence in older people — an attitude that is counterproductive to healthy physical aging.

The health benefits of exercise are obvious and well-known, yet less than 50% of all adults exercise for the minimum recommended period of 20 minutes three times per week. Musculoskeletal inactivity or immobility adversely affects all body systems. A recent report of the United States Preventive Services Task Force linked physical inactivity with the development of several premorbid health conditions, including hypertension, coronary artery disease, non-insulin-dependent diabetes mellitus, and osteoporosis. Other experts add obesity and falls to this list.

Benefits of aerobic exercise
The need for lifelong exercise in maintaining good health has become evident to health care professionals. The benefits of exercise include increased energy and independence, a sense of well-being and relaxation, reduced stress and fatigue and, in some cases, weight loss and improved patterns of rest and sleep. And experts have singled out *aerobic exercise* — physical exertion that's sustained long enough (more than 2 or 3 minutes) to cause a marked temporary increase in respiratory and heart rates — as the key factor in achieving healthy aging.

Studies have shown that to provide benefits, exercise must be performed at regular intervals over

Age-related changes affecting mobility

The following major physical changes in five body systems affect the mobility of older people.

Musculoskeletal
- Alterations in joint surfaces, ligaments, tendons, and connective tissues
- Decreased bone density (increases vulnerability for fractures)
- Decreased number and size of muscle fibers
- Atrophy of muscle tissue; replaced with fibrous tissue

Pulmonary
- Loss of elastic lung recoil
- Increased airway resistance
- Reduced vital capacity
- Decreased chest wall compliance
- Decreased gas exchange

Cardiovascular
- Increased blood pressure
- Decreased stroke volume
- Decreased cardiac reserve (ability to respond to stress)

Integumentary
- Decreased subcutaneous adipose tissue
- Decreased elasticity of connective tissue
- Loss of sweat and sebaceous glands

Central nervous
- Reduced nerve conduction speed
- Decreased rate and magnitude of reflex response
- Decreased sensory activity
- Decreased myoneural transmission
- Decreased muscle contraction speed
- Increased postural sway (contributes to balance problems)

Adapted with permission from Chenitz, W.C., et al. *Clinical Gerontological Nursing*. Philadelphia: W.B. Saunders Co., 1991.

obtain an aerobic benefit. However, more recent research that's especially germane to older adults has found that three 10-minute exercise sessions per day confer the same fitness benefits as one 30-minute session. What's more, people who haven't exercised at all appear to gain most significantly in reduced risk of cardiovascular problems from small increases in activity.

Many community-dwelling older people can reach an aerobic fitness level. Frail older persons can also do well by maintaining or increasing minimal levels of mobility.

Planning an exercise program

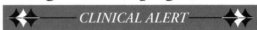
CLINICAL ALERT

You'll need to obtain medical clearance before planning an exercise program for an older person.

The scope of this evaluation will be determined by the primary care provider and may include a history and physical examination (focusing on the cardiovascular, pulmonary, musculoskeletal, and neurologic systems), diagnostic tests of renal and liver function, an electrocardiogram (ECG), and possibly an exercise stress test. This last test provides valuable information on maximum aerobic capacity, which can then be used to tailor an exercise program to the individual. The evaluation is less thorough for frail older people, whose exercise goals are more modest.

The individualized exercise program aims to maintain or increase flexibility, strength, endurance, range of motion, balance, and coordination. It should include a 10-minute warmup of stretching exercises, followed by the actual conditioning activity, and end with a 10-minute cool-down session of slow walking and stretching. To ensure success and compliance, involve the individual in planning realistic and enjoyable exercises and explain their specific health benefits. (See *How to exercise safely*.)

Other factors that encourage compliance include convenient or on-site location, group participation, scheduling that fits into one's current lifestyle, low

time. Most experts believe fitness results are negligible if a person exercises fewer than three times a week. Conversely, a person seems to gain no additional benefit if he exercises more than five times per week. For a time, a regimen of 20 to 30 minutes of continuous activity per day was deemed necessary to

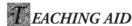 *EACHING AID*

How to exercise safely

Dear Patient:

The following tips will help you to exercise safely. Remember that your goal is to pace yourself, not to overdo it.

What you should do
● If you've been inactive for a long time, return to exercise gradually.
● Take part in fitness activities, such as walking and swimming, rather than competitive sports, such as tennis.
● Wait 2 to 3 hours after a heavy meal before exercising. Also avoid hot or cold showers immediately before or after exertion.
● Wear comfortable, lightweight clothing and shoes with adequate support. Dress in layers and remove articles of clothing as you warm up.
● Perform warm-up exercises to stretch muscles and loosen joints; this will lessen the risk of muscle strain or ligament damage. A good warm-up offers psychological benefits as well. Use this time to focus on the activities ahead and to get rid of tension. First, take your pulse and then do 5 to 10 minutes of stretching exercises and light calisthenics.
● Gradually work toward your optimal aerobic training level. Take your pulse two or three times, and adjust your pace according to your pulse rate and how you feel. If you exceed your target heart rate, or if you have chest discomfort, breathlessness, or palpitations, slow down *gradually.* Don't stop immediately unless your symptoms continue or worsen.
● Gradually decrease the pace of your exer-cise for 5 to 10 minutes to "cool down." Then do 5 minutes of light calisthenics and simple stretching exercises. At this point, your pulse should be not more than 15 beats above your resting pulse rate. If you feel dizzy or faint after exercise, you may need a longer cool-down period.
● Keep an exercise diary listing the date and time, activity and its duration, your pulse rate, and any symptoms that you experienced. Tracking your progress will help to keep you motivated, and the record you develop will help you and your doctor.

What you shouldn't do
● Don't exercise in extreme heat or cold, windy weather, high humidity, or heavy pollu-tion or at high altitudes.
● Don't exercise if you have a fever or don't feel well.
● Don't stop exercising abruptly. If you do, the amount of blood circulating back to the heart, which is still beating rapidly, won't be ad-equate to meet your body's needs.

When to slow down
● If you have any symptoms of muscle cramps, a side "stitch," or excessive shortness of breath or fatigue, slow down and stop.
● If you experience any chest pain, a cold sweat, dizziness, nausea or vomiting, heart palpitations, fluttering, or an abnormal heart rhythm, stop immediately and call your doctor.

cost, and absence of special equipment requirements. In addition, some managed care insurance plans provide financial incentives for participating in ongoing exercise programs.

Determining target heart rate

Before your patient begins an exercise program, you'll need to document baseline functional status, resting blood pressure, and resting pulse rate.

For a patient who has been sedentary most of his life to derive aerobic benefit from exercise, he must attain a minimum level of exercise intensity. The American College of Sports Medicine has recently identified three levels of exercise intensity: low intensity, categorized as <50% of maximum aerobic capacity; moderate intensity, 50% to 70%; and high intensity, >70%. The minimum exercise level required for cardiovascular benefit is 40% to 50% of maximum aerobic capacity.

You can calculate maximum aerobic capacity by using the results of the exercise stress test or by using this formula:

220 − (age) = maximum predicted heart rate.

Then calculate the *target heart rate* by multiplying the maximum predicted heart rate by the percentage of the maximum rate desired for the particular patient (see *Heart rates according to age*). For example, for a 70-year-old sedentary patient who will be exercising at 55% of maximum aerobic capacity (moderate intensity), calculate the target heart rate as follows:

220 − 70 = 150 (maximum predicted heart rate)
150 x 0.55 = 82 (target heart rate).

Teach the individual to monitor his pulse rate during exercise to avoid exceeding the target heart rate and overstressing the heart. Advise him to monitor the pulse during the cool-down phase for return to resting heart rate.

This method is contraindicated for those who are taking medications that alter the resting heart rate. A practical, safe alternative (if concurrent cardiovascular monitoring is unavailable) is to institute a low-intensity exercise program that includes normal everyday activities, such as walking, gentle stretching, and gardening.

Nursing interventions

Regardless of the setting in which you work, you can take steps to see that your patient becomes — and stays — physically active.

Community-based settings

If you work in a senior center, adult day-care center, or community health center, you can create exercise programs for individuals or groups. (See the Selected References at the end of this book for resources that can help you set up a program.) Check community resources, too: Many YMCAs and fitness centers offer programs tailored to older people. Some programs include patients with special needs, such as those with arthritis or who are physically challenged. Many shopping malls open early for senior walkers, thereby providing a safe, protected environment for walking at all times of the year. Hospitals are also beginning to reach out to community-dwelling older people who have fragile support systems.

If your patient says he can't exercise because of lack of time, fear of injury, or fatigue, provide helpful encouragement to motivate him (see *Overcoming barriers to exercise,* page 54).

Institutional settings

If you're working with frail older people in a long-term care setting, you can intervene on several levels to maintain and enhance residents' physical activity. At the administrative or staff development level, you can emphasize functional mobility as a priority for staff members and educate them in specific measures to facilitate this. Staff nurses need to establish a baseline functional assessment for each patient and implement a program to maintain or improve this level, including periodic reassessment.

For independently mobile patients, offer a group exercise program three to five times a week, and provide opportunities for independent or supervised walking, which may be combined with physical, occupational, or recreational therapy (for example, group outings to a park, nature center, or mall). Another option is a therapeutic aquatic program, either on-site or at the local YMCA (with transportation provided). Physically active, wheelchair-

Heart rates according to age

The table below is useful for calculating maximum aerobic capacity when determining a target heart rate for your older patient's exercise program. For example, if you start at the lowest level of fitness (column 2, 55% of maximum), the figures in that column provide the target heart rate.

Age (years)	55% maximum [a]	60% of maximum [b]	90% of maximum [c]	Maximum [d]
50	93	102	153	170
55	91	99	149	165
60	88	96	143	160
65	85	93	140	155
70	82	90	135	150
75	80	87	132	145
80	77	84	129	140

[a] Minimum exercise heart rate for health benefit designated by American College of Sports Medicine (ACSM)
[b] Minimum exercise heart rate for fitness designated by ACSM
[c] Maximum exercise heart rate designated by ACSM
[d] Maximum average heart rate adjusted for age (according to formula: maximum = 220 - [age]). This formula is only an approximation of any individual's response and will not apply if certain rate-altering medications are taken, such as beta blockers and some calcium antagonists.

Adapted with permission from American College of Sports Medicine, Preventive and Rehabilitative Exercise Committee. *Guidelines for Exercise Testing and Prescription,* 4th ed. Baltimore: Williams & Wilkins, 1991.

bound individuals can also be included in group exercises for upper extremity strengthening — such as working out on the pulleys in the physical therapy department.

Frail older people who need help to ambulate can participate in a daily walking program to improve mobility, maintain or improve endurance, and prevent falls. For example, the patient can walk to and from the dining room or the bathroom with the help of nursing assistants. The staff also benefits because their physical care burden is decreased and the potential for back injury is reduced. Other studies show patient benefits (improved mobility, decreased falls) from such activities as tai chi (an ancient Chinese system of exercises), yoga, flexibility exercises, and endurance and resistance exercises.

Ambulatory patients with dementia tend to wander. Provide a safe area for such patients to move about, and make sure they don't physically exhaust themselves. Also, monitor their nutritional and hydration status.

If you're working with older patients in an acute care facility, perform an admission assessment to determine preadmission functional levels, current level of performance, and postdischarge goals to promote physical activity and independence. Because dramatic and rapid changes can occur in this population, evaluate activities of daily living (ADL) capabilities and mobility daily. If the treatment plan calls for bed rest, reassess the need for this continuously.

Beginning discharge planning and rehabilitation therapies early can help the patient regain functional ground. Teaching patients bed exercises, such as quadriceps strengthening and preventive measures for footdrop, can help to prepare for this. Carrying out or supervising patient transfers and ambulation orders is also critical. A restorative nursing program

Overcoming barriers to exercise

Patients have lots of excuses for not exercising. Here are some ways to counteract your patient's negative attitudes toward exercise.

REASONS FOR NOT EXERCISING	SUGGESTED RESPONSES
"Exercise is hard work."	"Pick an activity that you enjoy and that's easy for you."
"I don't have the time."	"It will only take about three 20-minute sessions a week."
"I'm usually too tired to exercise."	"Tell yourself, 'This activity will give me more energy.'"
"I hate to fail, so I won't start."	"Exercise isn't a test; start off slowly and choose something that you like."
"I don't have anyone to work out with."	"Ask someone like a neighbor or coworker who might be a willing partner. Or choose an activity that you can do by yourself."
"There's no convenient place to exercise."	"Pick an activity that you can do in a convenient place; for example, walk around the neighborhood, or do exercises at home using a videotape."
"I'm afraid I'll get hurt."	"Try walking; it's very safe and an excellent exercise."
"The weather is bad."	"There are many activities that you can do in your own home even when the weather is bad."
"Exercise is boring."	"Listen to music or a book on tape to keep your mind occupied. Walking, running, or biking can take you past many interesting places."
"I'm too overweight."	"You can benefit regardless of your weight. Pick an activity that you're comfortable with, like walking."
"I'm too old."	"It's never too late to start; people of any age can benefit from exercise."

Adapted with permission from Project PACE. *Physician-Based Assessment and Counseling for Exercise.* San Diego: San Diego State University, 1991.

tailored to the patient's needs may also be indicated.

Teach nonprofessional staff as well as patients the importance of maintaining or restoring functional abilities. For example, if you're working with a stroke patient who's paralyzed on the dominant side, teach staff how to position a wheelchair for transfer so that the patient's unaffected side can lead and he or she can help with the transfer. Staff can also teach the patient to use his or her the unaffected arm in bathing, feeding, and dressing.

Recommend follow-up measures that promote a return to optimal functioning and create a supportive environment, such as home health services with physical or occupational therapy, specific instruc-tions for exercises for the patient to perform at home, or an outpatient rehabilitation program (such as cardiac rehabilitation).

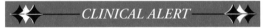
CLINICAL ALERT

Because older adults have reduced thirst perception, they're at increased risk for dehydration. So monitoring hydration status and replacing fluids are critical before, during, and after exercise.

You'll need to teach healthy older people to drink fluids frequently and offer fluids frequently to frail older people.

MEETING NUTRITIONAL NEEDS

Eating is a complex biological, social, cultural, and behavioral phenomenon. One's dietary preferences and eating habits profoundly affect nutritional status and health. Of course, good nutrition is essential no matter what your patient's age. But because of a variety of interrelated factors — inactivity, low income, lack of transportation, need for special diets, and the disappearance of the corner grocery store — older people are especially vulnerable to malnutrition.

Assessing nutritional status

In many ambulatory care settings, nutritional assessment consists primarily of obtaining a 24-hour dietary recall and comparing it to the Food Pyramid, but this obtains at best a cursory assessment of food intake in a limited time period. Nutrition assessments in the acute care setting are usually a part of the nurse's admission assessment and are rather superficial — they're sometimes limited to food preferences and allergies. Daily food intake is documented on flow sheets and the dietitian is consulted as needed.

Few assessment instruments are specific to older persons. A nutritional component is included as part of the assessment and care screening minimum data set (MDS) for nursing home residents. The Nutrition Screening Initiative (NSI), a joint venture of the American Academy of Family Physicians, the American Dietetic Association, and the National Council on Aging, includes screening methods and interventions to prevent and remedy nutritional deficiencies specifically in older adults. The NSI is widely used in outpatient settings. This program begins with a self-administered questionnaire that highlights areas of known risk for nutritional deficiencies. After the questionnaire is scored, at-risk patients are referred for more extensive screening. This includes another questionnaire (Screen 1) administered by a health professional. It further explores the known risk areas using the mnemonic device DETERMINE:

- Disease
- Eating poorly
- Tooth loss or mouth pain
- Economic hardship
- Reduced social contact and interaction
- Multiple medications
- Involuntary weight loss or gain
- Need for assistance with self-care
- Elder at an advanced age.

A second screening test (Screen 2) elicits in-depth information about nutritional status as well as specific biochemical, clinical, and diagnostic test data using the mnemonic device ABCDEF:

- Anthropometric: height and weight. Some studies have found an association between weight loss over time and mortality (the greater the weight loss, the higher is the mortality risk), particularly in cognitively impaired older patients with self-care deficits. The question of what is the most appropriate scale for height/weight/age-related measurements in older persons is still unsettled.
- Biochemical: A serum albumin level less than 3.5mg/dl is a good nonspecific indicator of poor nutritional status, as are low hemoglobin, hematocrit, and serum cholesterol. Serum vitamin B_{12} level can rule out B_{12} deficiency.
- Clinical, physical, and medical history.
- Dietary history: A food diary (list of all food and drink consumed in a 24-hour period), including use of supplements, sources for obtaining food, food storage, and cooking facilities.
- Empathy: Active listening, probing about diet, allowing the patient ample time to divulge problems.
- Functional assessment: Patients who are dependent on others for help with ADLs or instrumental ADLs (IADLs), including shopping and meal preparation, or who are cognitively impaired and at risk for nutritional problems.

Once you've assessed your patient's nutritional status, you can begin to formulate interventions.

Learning about dietary recommendations

Most national educational programs on the subject of nutrition, including Healthy People 2000,

Dietary Guidelines for Americans, and the Food Guide Pyramid, are aimed at the general population, not specifically at older adults.

The Food Guide Pyramid, introduced by the U.S. Department of Agriculture (USDA) in 1992, offers visual as well as written information on recommended daily allowances of six food groups; it supersedes the older Basic Four Food Groups recommendations, which did not address the issues of fat, cholesterol, sodium, or essential minerals in the diet. Although the pyramid includes information on portion sizes as well as the suggested number of servings for older adults, this data is often omitted or presented on a separate page. As a result, many consumers disregard portion size under the impression that they're following a healthy diet as long as they follow the basic guidelines shown in the picture. (See *Guide to daily food choices,* page 57.)

A more pertinent USDA source, *Food Facts For Older Adults,* applies established dietary guidelines to community-dwelling older adults and includes healthy recipes, shopping and food preparation tips, and further nutrition resources.

Even the system of Recommended Dietary Allowances (RDAs) formulated by the National Research Council, which offers specific caloric guidelines for older people, groups this information under a single "age 51-plus" category. Thus, health care providers who work with older adults should consult a nutritionist if they suspect a problem in this area. Beyond this, there is little information available on RDAs specifically for older people. (See *Recommended dietary allowances,* page 58.)

Nursing interventions
Interventions are determined based on the nutritional assessment findings and the setting in which the older person lives. In general, you'll need to focus on the following areas: preventing dehydration, ensuring adequate calcium and fiber intake, preventing drug interactions with foods, dealing with feeding problems (such as food preparation, use of utensils, oral and dental hygiene, and swallowing difficulties), and educating the patient and caregivers about nutritional requirements.

Preventing dehydration
The institutionalized elderly are at particularly high risk for dehydration because of their diminished thirst perception and any combination of physical, cognitive, speech, mobility, and visual impairment. You can take a number of steps to avoid dehydration in such patients (see *Preventing dehydration in your patients,* page 59).

First and foremost, advise your patient to drink plenty of fluids — at least 30 ounces (1,000 ml) per day, unless contraindicated. If your patient is taking prescription diuretics, warn him not to decrease fluid intake, even if he feels that frequent elimination restricts his mobility or ability to socialize. Also advise him that drinking alcoholic or caffeinated beverages increases diuresis, thereby increasing the need for fluids.

If your patient has urinary incontinence, make sure he doesn't purposely limit fluid intake in an attempt to reduce incontinence episodes. Finally, advise the mobile patient to drink extra fluids during activity in hot weather to replace losses due to perspiration and evaporation.

Ensuring adequate calcium and fiber intake
Calcium, found in dairy products, tofu, leafy green vegetables, oysters, salmon, and sardines, is essential for maintaining bone density and preventing osteoporosis. You can easily boost your patient's dietary calcium by adding 1 or 2 teaspoons of nonfat dry milk to regular milk, cereals, and yogurt. Adequate fiber is important in promoting regular bowel movements and may help prevent colon cancer. Some dietary fiber sources (such as oat bran) also lower cholesterol. Significant sources of dietary fiber are whole grain cereals and breads, raw fruits, leafy vegetables, and legumes. Over-the-counter products that add fiber to the diet, such as FiberCon crackers and Metamucil, are also available. When using these products, adequate fluid intake is essential to prevent intestinal obstruction.

Preventing drug interactions with foods
Because your patient may be taking many different drugs to treat a variety of conditions, the risk of drug-nutrient interactions is high. Drugs can affect

EACHING AID

Guide to daily food choices

Dear Patient:

Use the guide below to help you eat more healthfully. Try to have at least the lowest number of suggested servings from each of these food groups every day. (The lower numbers of servings are suggested for older women; the higher numbers are suggested for older men.)

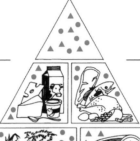

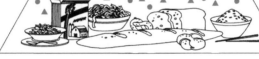

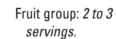

Fats, oils, and sweets group: *Use sparingly.*

Milk, yogurt, and cheese group: *2 servings.*

Meat, poultry, fish, dry beans, eggs, and nuts group: *2 servings.*

Vegetable group: *3 to 4 servings.*

Fruit group: *2 to 3 servings.*

Bread, cereal, rice, and pasta group: *6 to 9 servings.*

What counts as 1 serving?

Breads, cereals, rice, and pasta:
1 slice of bread
½ cup of cooked rice or pasta
½ cup of cooked cereal
1 oz of ready-to-eat cereal

Fruits:
1 piece of fruit or melon wedge
¾ cup of juice
½ cup of canned fruit
¼ cup of dried fruit

Vegetables:
½ cup of chopped raw or cooked vegetables
1 cup of leafy raw vegetables

Milk, yogurt, and cheese:
1 cup of milk or yogurt
1 ½ to 2 oz of hard cheese
2 cups of cottage cheese

Meat, poultry, fish, dry beans, eggs, and nuts:
2 ½ to 3 oz of cooked lean meat, poultry, or fish
Count ½ cup of cooked beans or 1 egg or 2 tbs of peant butter as 1 oz of lean meat (about ⅓ serving)

Fats, oils, and sweets:
Limit calories from these, especially if you need to lose weight.

Key: ● Fat naturally occurring and added   ▲ Sugars added
These symbols show that fat and added sugars come mostly from fats, oils, and sweets, but can be part of or added to foods from the other food groups as well.

Adapted from *Food Facts for Older Adults,* U.S. Department of Agriculture, Human Nutrition Information Service, Home and Garden Bulletin #251.

Recommended dietary allowances

The table below lists recommended daily allowances of major vitamins and nutrients for people age 51 and older. The figures are intended for most normal people living in the United States under usual environmental stresses. Individual diets should consist of a variety of common foods in order to provide other nutrients whose daily requirements are less well defined.

Nutrient	Males	Females
Protein (grams)	63	50
Vitamin A (µg)	1,000	800
Vitamin D (µg)	5	5
Vitamin E (mg)	10	8
Vitamin K (µg)	80	65
Vitamin C (mg)	60	60
Thiamine (mg)	1.2	1.0
Riboflavin (mg)	1.4	1.2
Niacin (mg)	15	13
Vitamin B_6 (mg)	2.0	1.6
Folate (µg)	200	180
Vitamin B_{12} (µg)	2.0	2.0
Calcium (mg)	800	800
Phosphorus (mg)	800	800
Magnesium (mg)	350	280
Iron (mg)	10	10
Zinc (mg)	15	12
Iodine (µg)	150	150
Selenium (µg)	70	55
Copper (mg)	1.5 to 3.0	1.5 to 3.0
Manganese (mg)	2.0 to 5.0	2.0 to 5.0
Fluoride (mg)	1.5 to 4.0	1.5 to 4.0
Chromium (µg)	50 to 200	50 to 200
Molybdenum (µg)	75 to 250	75 to 250
Sodium (mg) minimum	500	500
Chloride (mg) minimum	750	750
Potassium (mg) minimum	2000	2000

Adapted with permission from *Recommended Dietary Allowances*, 10th ed. © 1989 by the National Academy of Sciences. Courtesy of the National Academy Press, Washington, D.C.

the patient's nutritional status by altering nutrient absorption, metabolism, utilization, or excretion. Likewise, various foods, beverages, and mineral or vitamin supplements can affect the absorption and effectiveness of drugs. These interactions must be considered when evaluating your patient's medication regimen. (See *Effects of selected drugs on nutrients,* pages 60 and 61.)

Dealing with feeding problems

In dealing with nutritional problems, your interventions will vary, depending on the type of facility.

Acute care settings. For patients in acute care settings, you'll need to monitor nutritional status, hydration status, and the effects of medical treatments daily. Some older patients initially have food or fluid restrictions and require parenteral supplementation.

If a patient is anorectic, consider asking family members and other visitors to bring special foods from home that may improve the patient's appetite. In addition, encouraging the family to collaborate in feeding a dependent patient can help promote the patient's recovery, enhance his feeling of well-being, and stimulate him to eat more.

Before discharge, teach the patient and family about desirable nutritional practices and any prescribed therapeutic diets. Note the patient's dietary needs and preferences as well as special feeding techniques or assistive devices on the transfer form or postdischarge referral form to ensure continuity of care.

Long-term care settings. Frail older people in group residential and long-term care settings pose a different set of nutritional challenges. Research shows that these older adults are interested in food preparation, service, and quality. They usually look forward to mealtimes and are easily disappointed if food does not meet their expectations.

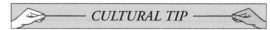

CULTURAL TIP

People of different ethnic and cultural backgrounds have specific dietary preferences. In many cases, appropriate dietary adjustments

Preventing dehydration in your patients

To maintain adequate hydration, your elderly patient needs between 1,000 and 3,000 ml of fluid a day. Less than 1,000 ml daily may lead to constipation, which can contribute to urinary incontinence. It may also result in more concentrated urine, which predisposes the patient to urinary tract infections. Follow these guidelines to make sure your patient is adequately hydrated.

Monitoring and assessment
- Monitor intake and output. Ensure an intake of at least 1,500 ml of oral fluids and urine output of 1,000 to 1,500 ml per 24 hours.
- Assess skin turgor and mucous membranes.
- Monitor vital signs, especially pulse rate, respiratory rate, and blood pressure. An increase in pulse and respiratory rates with decreased blood pressure may indicate dehydration.
- Monitor laboratory test results, such as serum electrolyte, blood urea nitrogen, and creatinine levels; hematocrit; and urine and serum osmolarity. Also check for signs of acidosis.
- Weigh the patient at the same time daily, using the same scale, and with the patient wearing the same type of clothes.
- Auscultate bowel sounds for any increase in activity. Also monitor stools for character: Hard stools may indicate dehydration; loose, watery stools indicate loss of water.

- Be aware of diagnostic tests that affect intake and output (for example, laxative or enema use, which cause fluid loss), and replace any lost fluids.

Providing fluids
- Provide fluids frequently throughout the day, for example, every hour and with a bedtime snack.
- Provide modified cups that the patient can handle; help those who have difficulty.
- Offer fluids other than water; find out the types of beverages the patient likes and the preferred temperatures (for example, ice cold or room-temperature drinks).
- Monitor coffee intake; coffee acts as a diuretic and may cause excessive fluid loss.
- If the patient is unable to take oral fluids, request an order for I.V. hydration.

can determine whether the patient will eat at all. If you can't arrange for a special diet, encourage family members or friends to bring in suitable foods that can be heated and served at mealtimes.

Oral health concerns, such as poor oral hygiene, loose or missing teeth, or absent or ill-fitting dentures, can also contribute to feeding problems. Make every effort to secure needed dental care for your patient and to replace lost or ill-fitting dentures. If this isn't possible because of profound disability or economic constraints, the patient will need a pureed diet.

Dysphagia (difficulty swallowing) can seriously compromise an older person's nutritional status.

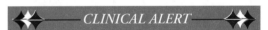
CLINICAL ALERT

Be alert for signs of dysphagia, such as coughing while eating or while drinking a thin liquid such as water, eating slowly, difficulty swallowing, weight loss, recurrent pneumonia, or a gurgling voice during or after eating. The patient with dysphagia may try to compensate by turning away or refusing further food, which can easily be misinterpreted as lack of appetite.

To help the patient with dysphagia, instruct him or her in "chin-tuck and swallow" technique; add thickeners to liquids, or provde thicker liquids such as tomato juice, or give pureed foods. If indicated, have the patient evaluated for swallowing problems by a speech therapist.

Effects of selected drugs on nutrients

Certain drugs can affect specific nutrient absorption or excretion by the body, producing nutrient toxicity or deficiency. Below is a list of selected drugs and their effects on nutrients.

DRUG	NUTRIENT	DRUG EFFECT
Adrenocorticosteroids	Vitamin D	Decrease metabolism
	Zinc, vitamin C, potassium, magnesium	Increase urine excretion
	Calcium	Decrease absorption; increase urine excretion
	Phosphorus, vitamin A, vitamin B_6	Decrease absorption
	Glucose, triglycerides, cholesterol	Increase blood levels
Antacids	Vitamin D, iron, thiamine	Interfere with absorption and use
	Phosphorus	Interfere with absorption and use; increase excretion
Anticonvulsants	Folic acid	Interfere with absorption and use
	Vitamins D, K	Interfere with metabolism
Aspirin	Folic acid	Interferes with absorption and use; promotes faster folate excretion
	Vitamin C	Increases urine excretion
	Vitamin K	Depletes body stores; increases urine excretion
Chlorothiazides	Calcium	Increase absorption
	Carbohydrate	Decrease tolerance
	Riboflavin, potassium, zinc, magnesium	Increase excretion
Chlorthalidone	Zinc	Increases excretion
Cholestyramine	Vitamins A, D, E, K, and B_{12}; folic acid; iron	Interferes with absorption and use
	Calcium	Increases excretion
Colchicine	Vitamins A and B_{12}, fat, lactose	Interferes with absorption and use
	Sodium, potassium	Increases excretion
Digitalis	Glucose	Interferes with absorption and use
	Magnesium	Increases excretion
Ethacrynic acid	Potassium, sodium, magnesium, calcium	Increases excretion
Hydrochlorothiazide	Magnesium, potassium, zinc, riboflavin	Increases urine excretion
Isoniazid	Vitamin B_6	Decreases metabolism
	Iron	Increases absorption
Laxatives	Vitamins D and K, glucose, calcium	Interfere with absorption and use
	Potassium, sodium, calcium, magnesium, water-soluble vitamins	Increase excretion

Effects of selected drugs on nutrients *(continued)*

DRUG	NUTRIENT	DRUG EFFECT
Levodopa	Vitamin B_{12}	Interferes with absorption and use
	Sodium, potassium	Increases excretion
Methotrexate	Vitamin B_{12}	Interferes with absorption
	Fat, carotene, lactose, cholesterol	Causes malabsorption
Mineral oil	Vitamins A, D, E, and K; phosphorus; calcium	Interferes with absorption and use
Monoamine oxidase (MAO) inhibitors	Tyramine, tyrosine	Block metabolism
Neomycin	Vitamins A, B_{12}, and K; protein; fat; lactose; calcium; iron	Interferes with absorption and use
	Sodium, potassium	Increases excretion
Penicillin G potassium	Vitamin K	Decreases synthesis
	Potassium	Increases excretion
	Folic acid, vitamin B_{12}, calcium, magnesium, glucose, carotene, cholesterol	Decreases absorption
Phenobarbital	Vitamin D, thiamine, folic acid, calcium	Interferes with absorption and use
	Vitamin C	Increases excretion
Phenytoin	Calcium	Interferes with absorption and use
	Vitamins C and D	Increases excretion
	Folic acid	Decreases mucosal uptake
Potassium chloride	Vitamin B_{12}	Interferes with absorption
Primidone	Calcium, folic acid, vitamins B_6 and B_{12}	Decreases absorption
Sulfonamides	Folic acid, iron, vitamin B_{12}, calcium	Decrease absorption
	Vitamin K	Reduce synthesis
Tetracyclines	Folic acid, calcium, vitamin B_{12}, magnesium, copper, iron, cobalt, manganese, zinc	Decrease absorption
	Vitamin K	Decrease synthesis
	Vitamin B_6	Inactivate the vitamin
Thyroxine	Riboflavin	Interferes with absorption and use
Triamterene	Folic acid	Interferes with absorption and use
	Calcium	Increases excretion
Warfarin	Vitamin K	Decreases synthesis

Finally, many patients in long-term care settings need help in feeding themselves. Typically, this is carried out by nursing assistants and supervised by the nurse. Setting up a feeding table, providing modified utensils and cups, helping the patient open containers, and cutting up food may be sufficient.

Try not to do more than the patient needs; this can encourage dependence and promote functional loss, especially in cognitively impaired patients.

One study of functional feeding of patients with dementia found the following measures were sufficient to promote self-feeding without prolonging mealtimes:

- reducing interruptions and distractions
- placing residents at a dining table
- using placemats and namecards
- using finger foods
- placing food directly in front of the patient
- maintaining consistency in mealtime activities
- prompting and cueing.

Patient teaching

As a health care provider, you'll need to educate your patients about the crucial role of nutrition in maintaining their physical health. In selecting written materials, consider the ethnic background, educational level, visual capabilities, and primary language of the intended reader.

If the patient has recently been discharged from an acute-care or rehabilitation facility, contact the dietitian there to find out if the patient has special dietary needs.

If you work in a community setting, find out about available nutrition support resources, such as congregate meals (provided at a church or senior center, for example, under auspices of the Older Americans Act); home-delivered meals (such as Meals on Wheels); and in-home services for meal preparation.

For the older person who lives alone but is mobile, encourage meal sharing or swapping with similar people in the vicinity to improve nutrition for all involved and increase socialization.

As appropriate, use other community programs, such as case management by the area Agency on Aging; social services to help poor people obtain food stamps; surplus food distribution programs; food pantries; church-related groups; and nutrition services provided by local or state health departments.

MEETING REST AND SLEEP NEEDS

The importance of rest and sleep in maintaining physical health in older people is often discounted or ignored, particularly in institutional settings, where routines are so important. Rest and sleep serve a restorative function both physiologically and psychologically. Physiologically, body organs are rested, energy is conserved, biorhythms are preserved, and mental alertness and neurologic efficiency are restored. Psychologically, tension is reduced, and a feeling of well-being emerges. This restorative function is especially important to older people, who require more time to adjust to changes. Older people deprived of sleep may become forgetful, disoriented, or confused; cognitively impaired persons will exhibit increased restlessness, wandering behavior, and "sundowner syndrome" (ocurrence or exacerbation of confusion, agitation, and disruptive behavior during late afternoon and early evening hours). The quality of sleep may be affected by age-related changes as well as organic or mental disorders.

Sleep patterns in the elderly

Normal sleep consists of REM (rapid eye movement) and non-REM components. Non-REM sleep is subdivided into four stages: Stage I encompasses dropping off to sleep; during this stage, the person is easily aroused and doesn't realize that he has been asleep. Muscle twitching or jerking signals relaxation during this stage. Stages II and III include progressively deeper sleep. In Stage IV, the deepest level, arousal is difficult. From here, the person progresses to REM sleep.

REM sleep occurs several times during the nightly sleep cycle but is most prominent in the early morning. In REM sleep, activity and vital signs accelerate, resulting in mounting excitement and tension release, manifested as tossing and turning, muscle twitching, and increases in respiratory rate, heart rate, and blood pressure. Increased respiratory and heart rates may adversely affect patients who have chronic cardiorespiratory problems. Otherwise, REM sleep helps release tension and aids central nervous system metabolism. Deprivation of REM sleep has been shown to cause irritability and anxiety.

Stage IV, the deepest level of non-REM sleep, is essential in maintaining physiologic health. Sleep experts know that this stage is notably decreased in older people, but they haven't determined the effects of this decrease. Sleep patterns of older people are marked by frequent awakenings, diminished stage III and IV non-REM time, more time spent awake during the night as a whole, and more frequent daytime naps. Most healthy older adults report no symptoms related to these changes other than not getting enough sleep or sleeping poorly. Studies suggest that daytime napping may reduce nocturnal sleep time and quality in some older people. If indicated, advise your patients to monitor the effects of napping on their nighttime sleep and on their feelings of well-being during the day.

Assessing sleep patterns

Perform a detailed assessment of your patient with a sleep disturbance, including direct observation, questioning the patient and family members about his sleep patterns, and possibly having the patient keep a sleep diary for 3 to 4 weeks.

When assessing your patient's sleep patterns, determine the following through observation and direct questioning:
- how well the older person sleeps at home
- bedtime and waking time
- bedtime rituals
- preferred nighttime environment (amount of light and ventilation, room temperature, door open or closed, music, type of bedclothes)
- frequency and duration of awake time
- activities usually performed in the early evening hours
- leisure activities, hobbies
- medications taken, including sleep aids
- tendency to sleep alone or with a partner
- perceived health status and satisfaction with life
- food or fluids consumed shortly before bedtime
- number of nightly trips to the bathroom.

In addition, have the patient record the following data in a sleep diary, if possible:
- time that he wakes up
- time and amount of sleep medication given, including times of repeated doses
- episodes of disorientation or confusion
- frequency of need for pain medications or for help with toileting
- time spent out of bed.

Nursing interventions

After determining the patient's sleep patterns, you'll develop an individualized plan of care that balances the patient's needs with those of the health care facility. Staff-initiated noise (such as talking outside the patient's room) can be kept to a minimum and lighting adjusted appropriately. Late risers can complicate the morning schedule, but offering two sittings at breakfast may remedy the problem.

Care measures such as comfortable positioning of patients who need assistance with mobility or ADLs, a backrub or massage, and soft music can help induce sleep.

If indicated, administer analgesics to a patient in pain. Teach deep breathing, progressive relaxation exercises, and guided imagery to promote relaxation and sleep.

Schedule treatments and procedures during waking hours, and eliminate nighttime vital sign assessments as soon as the patient's condition permits. Finally, consider administering sleep aids temporarily when other methods have failed. Commonly prescribed drugs used to induce sleep include the antihistamine diphenhydramine (Benadryl) and the benzodiazepines triazolam (Halcion) and temazepam (Restoril). Monitor the patient for possible adverse reactions to these drugs (such as rebound insomnia, nightmares, and confusion).

Patient teaching

Regardless of setting, you can teach your patient certain helpful measures to promote healthy sleep (see *Dealing with sleep disturbances,* page 64.)

Dealing with sleep disturbances

Difficulty falling or staying asleep is a common problem of older adults, whether they live at home or in a nursing home. If your patient has a sleep problem, advise him to:
- maintain the same daily schedule for waking, resting, and sleeping
- get up at his usual time even if his sleep has been disturbed or his bedtime changes temporarily
- establish a bedtime ritual and stick to it
- exercise everyday but avoid vigorous exercise at night
- limit naps to 1 to 2 hours per day, at the same time each day
- take a warm bath in late afternoon or early evening
- avoid caffeine-containing beverages and products
- practice relaxation methods, such as deep breathing, music, rocking, massage, or reading calm material
- avoid alcoholic beverages or limit his intake to small amounts each day
- eat a light snack of carbohydrates and fat before bed
- use the bed for sleep only
- if he's awake at night for longer than 30 minutes, get out of bed and engage in a nonstimulating activity such as reading.

ENCOURAGING PROPER ELIMINATION

Many older adults have problems with elimination of body wastes. These difficulties usually stem not from age-related physiologic changes per se, but from environmental, social, cognitive, and mobility factors that affect physical processes. Many older people, family members, caregivers, and even health care workers view incontinence as a normal part of the aging process. But urinary and fecal incontinence are not inevitable consequences of aging. As a health care provider, you can spread this message to older people in all settings and teach patients and caregivers specific measures that promote normal elimination. (For more information on bowel and bladder training, see Chapter 17.)

Elimination in older patients

Age-related changes in urinary and bowel elimination include diminished bladder capacity and reduced renal concentration of urine, which lead to urinary frequency and nocturia; weakened pelvic floor muscles (in women); enlarged prostate (in men); and loss of bladder and rectal sphincter control. Constipation, a frequent complaint among older people, may result from many causes, including weakened anal sphincter control, diminished defecation reflex, inactivity and immobility, diminished peristalsis, inadequate dietary fiber, adverse effects of drugs, and laxative dependence.

Nursing interventions

Promoting proper elimination is an essential part of caring for older persons, who must cope with normal age-related changes that interfere with urinary and bowel elimination.

Promoting urinary elimination

Changes in bladder function mean more frequent trips to the bathroom for urination, a smaller amount of urine per episode, and less time between the urge to void and the actual act. Making changes in elimination routines based on this knowledge can help promote normal bladder function in healthy older adults.

Evaluate the patient's environment for barriers to continence, and suggest needed modifications. For example, identify the location of the bathroom nearest to where the patient spends most of his time. And consider the effect of barriers, such as stairs, lack of privacy, impaired mobility, and dependence in ADLs.

The patient's medical history can also yield valuable clues for promoting optimal bladder function. For example, advise a patient who's taking diuretics to drink adequate fluids and to take his medication in the morning to avoid nocturia.

Avoiding constipation

If your older patient complains of constipation, first make sure he's aware that a daily bowel movement is not necessarily the norm for every person. Inform him that every individual has his own pattern of regularity, which may vary from three times per day to once every 3 to 5 days, depending on his bowel muscle tone, activity level, and food intake.

Then teach him steps he can take to help prevent this problem, such as:
- including high-fiber foods (fresh, uncooked fruits and vegetables, bran, and other whole grain products) in his daily diet (temporary bloating or flatulence may occur after increasing fiber consumption)
- drinking at least 10 glasses of liquids, such as water and fruit juice, each day
- avoiding laxatives and enemas, if possible, but using a bulk-forming laxative to help maintain bowel regularity if necessary (this type is least likely to cause problems, especially if he drinks enough liquids)
- never ignoring the urge to defecate (trying to respond as soon as he gets the urge)
- trying to exercise regularly. Exercise increases bowel activity.

Promoting bowel elimination

If you work with older people, you probably hear numerous complaints about bowel elimination problems, especially about constipation. Many people think they're constipated if they miss only one bowel movement. If your patient complains of constipation, try to confirm it by asking the following:
- Has the patient experienced a decrease in the normal frequency of bowel movements?
- Does the patient have difficulty defecating because of hard stools?
- Are both of these factors present? (Interventions may differ according to which problem is evident.)

Once you've determined that your patient has constipation, you can assess the situation further. Ask the patient about his usual dietary habits, including fiber content and fluid intake; changes in eating pattern (quantity, variety, frequency, setting); activity and exercise level; medications, including over-the-counter preparations; use of laxatives or cathartics; presence of hemorrhoids; changes in bowel function (such as excessively hard or loose stools, frequent constipation or diarrhea); pain or bleeding on defecation; and frequency of bowel movements. An abdominal assessment and a digital rectal examination can help to confirm or rule out a physiologic problem.

To manage constipation resulting from decreased mobility and dependence in institutionalized older patients, many facilities routinely administer a mixture of bran, fruit, and fruit juice to promote regular bowel elimination. An example of such a mixture is PAB, a combination of 1 cup of prune juice, 1 cup of applesauce, and 1 cup of All-Bran cereal. Patients who take such a supplement must drink adequate fluids and be monitored for abdominal pain, diarrhea, and signs of distress.

In addition, you can teach healthy older adults steps that will help them alleviate or prevent constipation themselves (see *Avoiding constipation*).

DEALING WITH SEXUALITY

Many people feel that advanced age makes a person physically and psychologically incapable of having sex or of maintaining a loving sexual relationship with another person. Older people are viewed as being sexually undesirable, disinterested in sex, and unable to perform functionally. But research gives a very different picture — most men and women continue to maintain sexual interest and activity well into their 70s and 80s. Men and women of all ages say they need the intimacy, pleasure, and tenderness that sexual expression provide to maintain a healthy state of mind and body.

Sexual responses and aging

Research has shown that older people experience sex-specific changes, such as decreased speed and duration of erection in men, and diminished vaginal lubrication in women. However, in their landmark 1979 study of men and women ages 51 to 78, Kolodny, Masters, and Johnson found that male and female sexual responses did not decrease significantly with age, nor did the capacity to experience orgasm. They further found that prolonged abstinence from sexual activity increases the risk of genital atrophy from disuse.

Besides physiologic changes, other factors that may inhibit sexual activity include cultural taboos, rigid moral principles, negative self-image, loss of privacy and independence, drug side effects, and illnesses, such as arthritis, neuropathy, and peripheral vascular disease. There's also the fact that women live longer than men and are therefore more likely to find themselves without a partner.

Nursing interventions

Many couples develop sexual problems later in life because they are uninformed about age-related physiologic changes. A man may perceive a diminishing ability to achieve an erection as evidence that he's becoming impotent. A woman may interpret this sign as evidence that the man no longer finds her attractive or that he's just too old for sex.

As a nurse, you can help educate older people about normal changes in sexual response and about modifications that may be necessary. Your first step, though, should be a thorough assessment.

Obtaining the sexual history

When developing a sexual history, be sensitive to the patient's cultural background and moral values, especially because he or she may be a generation or more older than you. If the patient is uncomfortable discussing sexual matters, respect the person's right not to do so, and don't press the topic. He or she may broach the subject at a later time.

To elicit the availability of a partner, ask the patient about marital status and living arrangements. Ask about the status of the relationship and the health of the partner. Determine if the couple is monogamous.

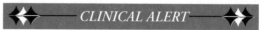

CLINICAL ALERT

Many older people are not aware that they may be at risk for sexually transmitted diseases, including AIDS, if they have more than one partner.

Determine the patient's need for screening; for example, Pap smears and mammograms for women and prostate examinations for men. Note any past genitourinary or gynecologic surgeries, infections, or chronic illnesses, all of which can have a significant physical or psychosocial impact on sexual function.

Carefully review the patient's medications. Many drugs adversely affect sexual function.

Patient teaching

When developing a teaching plan, you'll need to consider the presence or absence of health issues that may affect sexuality. Also consider the patient's self-image and perception of overall health; knowledge of the aging process and its effects on sexual responses; and level of sexual interest, activity, and satisfaction.

You can suggest ways for the patient to increase self-esteem and provide information about sexuality and aging to increase knowledge and dispel sexual myths. Because many older patients don't understand age-related sexual changes, explain the following points, as appropriate:

● Many postmenopausal women are multiorgasmic.
● To achieve orgasm, women require some form of clitoral contact and stimulation.
● The woman's pleasure can be enhanced by improved ejaculatory control, which allows for prolonged intercourse.
● The older man requires increased or direct genital contact to achieve arousal and orgasm.
● Coital positions can be varied for maximum enjoyment. All positions are socially acceptable.
● Afterplay (hugging, caressing) enhances emotional satisfaction.

● Consuming more than moderate amounts of alcohol before sex may impair sexual performance. If appropriate, suggest a variety of sexual activities other than intercourse that can help fulfill the need for sexual contact — for example, oral or manual genital stimulation, kissing, hugging, and hand-holding.

Sexuality, aging, and AIDS
Because society considers the elderly population asexual and presumably not at risk for HIV infection, AIDS researchers and educators have largely ignored them. However, the Centers for Disease Control and Prevention reports that people age 50 and older make up 10% of total AIDS cases nationwide and that the incidence of HIV infection and AIDS among older adults is increasing.

The need for patient education is obvious. Although many older people have satisfying monogamous sex lives, they may seek sexual expression with others after divorce or the death of a partner. Because older adults believe it unnecessary to pro-tect against pregnancy, they may also fail to protect themselves against disease. But new partners could be infected with HIV from unprotected sex, blood transfusions, or I.V. drug use. Therefore, all older people should be educated about HIV transmission, testing, and treatment and about the symptoms of opportunistic infections. Health care professionals also should be careful to avoid making assumptions when elderly people experience certain symptoms. For example, assuming that an older adult with dementia has Alzheimer's disease (rather than possibly HIV-related dementia) or that an opportunistic infection is due to chronic diseases (rather than possibly AIDS) can prevent timely and appropriate treatment.

Sexual activity in the nursing home
Although nursing home residents may be chronically ill or cognitively impaired, they have the same need for sexual expression and intimacy as other older adults. Yet sexual behavior by nursing home residents is frowned upon by society at large and often by staff and family members as well. With over 50% of nursing home residents affected by Alzheimer's and related diseases, health care professionals need to consider the sexual needs of cognitively impaired patients in formulating the plan of care (see *Managing sexual activity in the nursing home,* page 68).

PROVIDING PREVENTIVE MEDICAL CARE

For older people, preventive medical care — such as periodic general checkups, vision and hearing tests, monitoring of blood pressure and serum cholesterol levels, and immunizations — helps prevent small problems from escalating into life-threatening ones and facilitates early treatment of serious conditions. Dental care and good oral hygiene help the patient retain his teeth and avoid the reduced self-esteem and discomfort associated with losing them.

Health screenings
Older people should be screened routinely for the following major health parameters:
● *Blood pressure.* This should be measured ideally at each doctor's visit but at least every 2 years. The American College of Physicians recommends yearly measurements in patients who have diastolic pressure between 85 and 89 mm Hg, are of African-American descent, are moderately or extremely obese, have a history of hypertension, or have a first-degree relative with hypertension.
● *Height and weight.* These should be measured periodically as part of a comprehensive physical examination. The impact of these recommendations on patients in long-term care settings is minimal, because policies provide for much more frequent monitoring in this population. (The minimum data set for nursing home resident assessment and care screening, which must be regularly updated, includes height and weight measurements.)
● *Cholesterol.* Cholesterol levels (both total and high-density-lipoproteins) should be measured every 5 years; a lipoprotein analysis should be done on all patients with known coronary artery disease.

Managing sexual activity in the nursing home

In dealing with sexual activity in nursing homes, staff members must balance two competing responsibilities: they must protect cognitively impaired or otherwise vulnerable patients from sexual coercion, but must try to promote patient independence and autonomy. Staff and family members of residents also tend to be troubled by overt sexual behavior, such as masturbation, genital exposure, and sexual remarks by older patients. One study found that staff identified public masturbation as among the behaviors they find "seriously disturbing."

Policy considerations

It's not known how many facilities have adapted formal policies on residents' sexual behavior. Usually, institutional ethics committees address problems individually. Any decisions regarding a patient's sexual behavior and competence to participate in a sexual relationship should be considered by an interdisciplinary treatment team that includes the nursing assistants and therapists who work with the patient daily.

General guidelines

Although there are no set rules for handling problematic sexual behavior, some problems may be avoided with careful forethought:
- Consider the patient's sexual needs before admission to the nursing home. Some homes have a more flexible approach than others. Some older women complain about the lack of available men in nursing homes because of the survival differential; this concern should be considered in the decision to institutionalize the patient. If the patient has been engaging in overt sexual behavior, discuss this with nursing home officials before admission.
- Assess the competence and sexual function of patients interested in pursuing sexual relationships.
- Develop a plan for dealing with patients who masturbate or expose their genitals in public areas. The staff might remind such a patient of the need for privacy and then move the patient to his or her room.
- Make private time available for patients. Consider having a room available for residents who want to be intimate. If an extra room is not available, consider scheduling private times for patients to use their rooms when their roommates are engaged elsewhere. In intermediate care facilities, allow patients to leave the facility for a few hours, if medically feasible.
- Discuss the patient's sexual behavior with the treatment team, particularly those involved in his or her daily care. Reinforce the idea that sexual behavior is normal and that acknowledging a patient's sexuality helps to affirm that patient's humanity. Don't automatically construe sexual overtures or remarks by an elderly resident as sexual harassment. Such remarks may be patient's only remaining form of sexual expression.
- Address truly disruptive problems, such as physical combativeness, with behavioral methods. Use physical or pharmaceutical restraints as a last resort.
- Educate families about sexuality, reinforcing the concept that sexual expression is normal, even for their aging relatives.

Adapted with permission from Galindo, D., et al. "Sexual Health after 60," *Patient Care* 29(7):25-38, April 15, 1995.

- *Dental health.* A checkup should be performed at least once a year.
- *Vision.* A vision screening that includes a glaucoma test should be done every 2 years. In the interim, you can evaluate a patient's functional reading ability (if he has no cognitive deficits) by having him read the newspaper. Make sure the patient is wearing glasses or contacts if they're normally worn.

- *Hearing.* The older patient's hearing should be evaluated periodically. Because of the expense and time involved in a formal hearing evaluation, no specific timeline has been established.

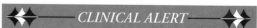

CLINICAL ALERT

When dealing with a patient who seems to have difficulty hearing, first inspect the ear canals for cerumen impaction, remove the

Guidelines for periodic cancer screening

This list summarizes the recommendations for cancer screening of older adults developed by major cancer organizations and study groups.

BREAST

American Cancer Society (ACS), National Cancer Institute (NCI)
Annual breast examination and mammogram for women over age 50
American Geriatric Society (AGS)
Annual breast exam; mammogram every 1 to 2 years
U.S. Preventive Services Task Force (USPSTF)
Annual breast examination; mammogram every 1 to 2 years until age 75

CERVIX

ACS, NCI
Annual Pap smear; may be done less often after three normal smears
AGS, USPSTF
Pap smears every 1 to 3 years, stopping at age 65 if several tests are normal; continue in those without previous screening
Canadian Task Force on the Periodic Health Examination (CTFPHE)
Pap smears every 5 years for ages 36 to 74

PROSTATE

ACS (1993)
Annual digital rectal exam (DRE) and prostate-specific antigen (PSA) test for men over age 50
USPSTF
PSA and transrectal ultrasonography (TRUS) not recommended; insufficient evidence for DRE

COLON AND RECTUM

ACS
Annual fecal occult blood test (FOBT) and flexible sigmoidoscopy every 3 to 5 years after two examinations 1 year apart over age 50
NCI
Annual FOBT and flexible sigmoidoscopy every 3 to 5 years; air-contrast barium enema or colonoscopy for high-risk people
USPSTF
Insufficient evidence for FOBT or sigmoidoscopy; screen high-risk patients

MOUTH

ACS, NCI
Annual examination over age 40
CTFPHE
Annual examination over age 65
USPSTF
Screening needed only for people who find suspicious lesion on self-examination or those at high risk

SKIN

SACS, NCI
Annual complete skin examination over age 40
CTFPHE, USPSTF
Skin examination only for those at high risk

Adapted with permission from Noe, C.A., and Barry, P. "Healthy Guidelines for Cancer Screening and Immunizations," *Geriatrics* 51(1):75-83, January 1996. ©1996, Advanstar Communications, Inc.

cerumen if present, and then evaluate hearing before recommending a workup.

● *Cancer screening.* Recommended tests include examination of the colon and rectum, mouth and skin, breasts and cervix (in women), and prostate (in men). The recommended frequency of such tests varies (see *Guidelines for periodic cancer screening*). Before recommending these tests, you may want to determine what Medicare will reimburse, especially if finances are a concern.

You'll also need to encourage female patients to conduct their own breast self-examinations every month. This may be a delicate teaching assignment for some older women, who may be uncomfortable touching themselves.

Immunizations

When the topic of immunizations is raised, older adults are frequently excluded, except for influenza. In fact, older people need continuing protection against tetanus and pneumococcal infections as well.

Influenza

Approximately 80% to 90% of flu-related deaths occur in people over age 65. Influenza vaccines can prevent 30% to 40% of flu cases and 80% of flu-related deaths in older people. All older adults should receive a yearly influenza immunization unless contraindicated, ideally from mid-October to mid-November in anticipation of the flu season. The vaccine is widely available and covered by Medicare.

Explain that fever, malaise, and myalgia may occur from 6 to 48 hours after the vaccination. Also emphasize that any respiratory illness that occurs after the vaccination is usually coincidental, not vaccine-related.

Be aware that patients who have had an *anaphylactic reaction* to eggs should not receive the influenza vaccine. Those who have a documented *IgE-mediated hypersensitivity* to eggs may also be at risk for reactions. People who have fever should not be vaccinated until their symptoms resolve.

Tetanus

Tetanus almost always occurs in nonimmunized or partially immunized people, and adults over age 60 account for 60% of cases. Everyone should receive the primary tetanus (Td) series in childhood and a booster every 10 years. However, if a person sustains a "dirty" wound any time after completing the primary series, he should get a booster if more than 5 years has elapsed since the primary dose.

Older patients who never started the primary series should receive three Td vaccinations. The second vaccination should be given 4 to 8 weeks after the first, and the third, 6 to 12 months after the second. If the patient started the primary series but never completed it, he can receive the remaining vaccinations without restarting.

Pneumococcal infections

Older adults are also at risk of dying from pneumococcal infections, such as pneumococcal pneumonia and bacterial meningitis. All adults over age 65 should receive one dose of this vaccine. Those who are considered at high risk (immunocompromised, asplenic or on dialysis) should be revaccinated 6 years after the initial dose.

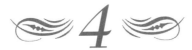

Meeting mental and emotional needs

The health of an older person is a composite of the person's lifestyle, physical health, social support network, coping skills, and cognitive abilities. As people age, issues they've grappled with their entire lives (or possibly tried to ignore), such as alcoholism, family dysfunction, abuse, and other stressors, tend to impact their health. If a dementia process begins, long-buried issues may suddenly take on major significance. Mental health problems in older adults often contribute to decreased self-esteem, diminished quality of life, and impaired social functioning.

Good mental health implies a capacity to manage life stresses to achieve a state of emotional homeostasis. Consider the life crises the older person may face: retirement, with accompanying loss of status and independence; loss of spouse and other loved ones; sensory losses; and possibly, disease, pain, surgery, dependence, and institutionalization. Depending on the person's coping mechanisms, any one of these could precipitate psychological problems. The cumulative effect could overwhelm even an emotionally strong, healthy person.

Many older adults who seek mental health services have an underlying physical illness. Keep in mind that the far-reaching physical changes of aging often have profound psychological effects. And emotional difficulties also may cause physical symptoms.

STRESSFUL LIFE EVENTS

The following review will help you understand the losses and other stressful life events that older people face, how they respond to these losses, and how you can help them deal with these situations.

Loss
As adults reach advanced age, their social support network begins to break apart as friends die or move away. The strength and comfort that these friends provided, which helped the individual to buffer or cope with loss, is no longer there. Loss can be a catalyst to developing physical and mental illness in late life. Response to loss is very individual. Examples of nontraditionally defined loss that may result in a grieving process or progress to depression include death of a pet, sale of a home, and admission to a long-term care facility. Ill-fitting dentures and being forced to give up driving have prompted serious suicide attempts in older adults.

Retirement
People often define themselves by how they make their living; this image affects their lifestyle, friends, social network, and financial dealings. Retirement often precipitates changes in spousal relationships and use of leisure time. Couples who enjoyed satisfying relationships while being separated for most of the working day may now need to adjust to

being together for longer periods. Troubled relationships may now become much more difficult. Lack of productive work and the absence of a social network outside the workplace often add to a negative outlook after retirement.

The earlier a person has prepared for retirement, the better his outlook and quality of life should be. If you have an older patient who's preparing for retirement, be sure to keep in mind the following teaching needs:

- structuring leisure time
- planning to live within a limited budget
- getting to know one's spouse again now that retirement approaches
- meeting new friends outside of work, such as through clubs, volunteer work, religious affiliations, and hobbies.

Widowhood

One of the most profound losses a person can experience is the death of a spouse. In addition, widowhood can seriously affect a person's financial status, social network, and physical and mental health. When the loss of spouse occurs late in life, the person has a much greater risk of developing depression, anxiety, and substance abuse than a younger person because of decreased resiliency, a higher incidence of chronic illness, and the breakdown of social support networks. Older men have an even higher risk of physical and mental illness than older women.

In addition to the loss of marital companionship, unsettled issues may remain for years after the death of a spouse. A long marriage doesn't necessarily mean a happy one. Unresolved guilt feelings related to infidelity, physical or substance abuse, and financial problems after widowhood are a few examples of issues that can fester and lead to serious mental illness, sometimes decades after the death of a spouse. Family and spousal caregivers especially may have unresolved issues that can fester.

Make your older patient aware of counseling services, support groups, and other resources that are available to help him cope with the loss of a spouse. If the affected person is a caregiver, inform her about respite care services that are available.

Death of an adult child

Adult children are an important part of the older adult's social support network. Ethnic and cultural groups such as Jewish, Native American, and Asian families place a high value on intergenerational relationships. The death of an adult child can be even more devastating to the older adult than the death of a spouse because parents expect their children to outlive them and be a support in advancing age. Refer an older patient who must cope with the loss of an adult child to an appropriate community resource, such as Interfaith, a clergyman, or a grief therapist.

Family estrangement

Older people may become estranged from family members for many reasons, such as drug or alcohol abuse and disagreements over religion, sexual orientation, choice of marriage partner, inheritance issues, or business dealings. Estrangement from grandchildren and great-grandchildren can be especially painful. As the years go by, an older adult may yearn to reestablish family ties that were broken years before. Referring such a patient to family therapy can be very effective.

Changes in body image

Older adults may go through the grieving process and may become depressed after experiencing alterations in body image due to trauma, serious illness such as stroke or coronary artery disease, surgery, or a decrease in functional ability. What's more, physical changes that impact lifestyle can be devastating to the older adult's self-esteem and sexuality. You can assess your patient's response to a changed body image by encouraging discussion. If indicated, refer him to a psychotherapist for follow-up.

Financial loss

Many older people face serious financial hardships after retirement, especially if they must depend on Social Security as their primary, or sole, source of income. And older people today are especially vulnerable to financial scams. After experiencing serious economic hardship during the Depression in the 1930s, some older people have developed a lasting mistrust of financial institutions and may have large sums of money hidden in their homes. Con artists, aware of these possibilities, are adept at preying on older people. Some family members may also try to steal from their elderly relatives.

To forestall abuses of this kind, most states have a mechanism for a trusted individual, or guardian, to manage the financial affairs of an older person who's mentally or physically incapacitated. Usually the mechanism is a power of attorney. The authority of the power of attorney and the guardian vary by state. Report suspected abuses to the local Office on Aging or county department of human services. (For additional information on power of attorney, see Chapter 20.)

COMMON PSYCHIATRIC PROBLEMS

Older adults don't usually develop new mental illness late in life; most mental illnesses in older people are chronic, having started earlier in life. Some forms of mental illness run in families, such as depression and schizophrenia. You may find an older adult suffering from depression along with an adult child and perhaps a grandchild. With support from family and friends, a person with a mental health problem can develop coping skills that allow him to function for years, sometimes without treatment.

Discussed below are various mental health disorders that commonly strike older adults.

Anxiety
Many psychosocial stressors, such as an impending serious diagnostic test, a sudden financial reversal, or the severe illness of a family member, can trigger a normal anxiety reaction. In many cases, the symptoms of anxiety resemble those of depression; a person who's depressed is likely to be anxious as well. Many physical disorders are marked by symptoms of anxiety (see *Disorders associated with*

anxiety, page 74). Finally, because many older adults take several different medications, you need to be aware of drugs that may cause anxiety symptoms.

Assessment
Skillful assessment is essential because older patients with anxiety tend to have many physical complaints that can lead to actual physical disorders if left untreated.

The Hamilton Anxiety Rating Scale is a useful tool for assessing anxiety (see *Hamilton anxiety rating scale,* pages 75 and 76). Sharing the information from this scale with the doctor and other health care team members can determine the progress of treatment interventions.

Remember to ask your patient about the drugs he's taking. Anxiety symptoms can result from the use of various drugs, including caffeine, thyroid hormone, aminophylline, oral antidiabetic drugs, nonsteroidal anti-inflammatory drugs (NSAIDs), steroids, digitalis glycosides, and selective serotonin re-uptake inhibitors (SSRIs). Asking the doctor to substitute another drug with fewer anxiety-producing adverse effects is preferable to adding additional drugs just to treat anxiety symptoms.

CLINICAL ALERT
Alcohol is a common method of self-treatment for anxiety, but not a benign one. Be sure to ask your patient about his alcohol use — what type he drinks (beer, wine, whisky), approximately how much per day, and for how long. One martini a day for 30 years may easily have serious consequences.

Nursing interventions
The best way to assist the anxious older adult is to refer him to an available mental health professional, chaplain, or social worker.

Depression
Depression is the most common psychiatric illness affecting older adults, but regarding it as a normal response to aging is a mistake. In addition, it's often underdiagnosed and untreated in this age-group.

The term "depression" is used to describe a

Disorders associated with anxiety

The table below highlights some of the more common disorders associated with anxiety.

Pulmonary	Metabolic	Nutritional	Cardiovascular	Gastrointestinal	Sensory
Pulmonary embolism	Electrolyte imbalances	Vitamin B_{12} deficiency	Myocardial infarction	Irritable bowel syndrome	Pain
Chronic obstructive pulmonary disease	Hyperthyroidism or hypo-thyroidism	Trace element deficiency	Congestive heart failure	Constipation	Impaired vision
			Stroke	Diarrhea	Impaired hearing
Pneumonia			Arrhythmias	Ulcers	Headache
			Mitral valve prolapse		

mood, a symptom, or a disease. Physical, hormonal, psychological, and social factors profoundly contribute to its development in older people. However, the first episode of a primary major depressive disorder in people over age 50 usually has a specific medical cause requiring a thorough diagnostic evaluation. For example, Parkinson's disease is strongly associated with depression because of the imbalance in brain chemicals it causes. Urinary tract infections also are strongly associated with depression. Several non-psychotropic drugs may produce depression as an adverse effect, including beta blockers (such as propranolol and atenolol), methyldopa, and corticosteroids. Stress, too, is strongly associated with the development of depression in older people.

Assessment

If you suspect your patient may be depressed, evaluate his symptoms carefully. Several assessment tools are available, including the Hamilton Depression Rating Scale and the Geriatric Depression Scale (see *Geriatric depression scale (short form)*, page 77).

Major depression is marked by a persistent depressed mood and diminished interest or pleasure in daily activities. Other symptoms include sleep disturbances, inappropriate guilt, loss of energy, poor concentration, changes in appetite, psychomotor retardation or agitation, a passive wish for death, and suicidal thoughts or attempts.

Be aware that suicide among older adults is a serious problem. Basic signs of suicidal thinking that warrant further investigation include sudden hoarding of medications, giving away possessions, a sudden interest in guns, and despondent comments. An older person at risk needs an immediate thorough assessment by an experienced mental health professional.

CLINICAL ALERT

Older adults at highest risk of suicide are at least 85 years old, depressed, with high self-esteem, and a need to control life. Even a frail nursing home resident with these characteristics may have the strength required to accomplish the act.

Thorough assessment of a depressed patient helps to rule out possible underlying causes, such as adverse reactions to medications, hypothyroidism, and other disorders. Depression also should be differentiated from dementia, although they may coexist.

HARTING GUIDE

Hamilton anxiety rating scale

Patient's name _Edward Moses_   Date of first report _12/1/96_

Therapy _To be determined_   Date of this report _12/1/96_

Instructions:
Use this checklist to record your patient's degree of anxiety and progress toward recovery. Fill in the appropriate rating for each item, using this scale:

0 None   **1** Mild   **2** Moderate   **3** Severe   **4** Extreme

ITEM	RATINGS
Anxious mood Worry, anticipation of the worst, irritability	1
Tension Tension, restlessness, inability to relax, fatigability, trembling, easy startle response, easy movement to tears	1
Fear Fear of dark, strangers, being left alone, animals, traffic, crowds	0
Insomnia Difficulty falling asleep, broken sleep, unsatisfying sleep and fatigue on waking, dreams, nightmares, night terrors	2
Cognition Difficulty concentrating, poor memory	0
Depressed mood Loss of interest, lack of pleasure in hobbies, depression, early waking, daily mood swings	1
Behavior at interview Fidgeting, restlessness or pacing, tremor of hands, furrowed brow, strained face, sighing or rapid respiration, pallor, swallowing, belching, brisk tendon jerks, dilated pupils, exophthalmos	1
Sensory symptoms Tinnitus, blurred vision, hot and cold flushes, feeling of weakness, picking sensation	0
Cardiovascular symptoms Tachycardia, palpitations, chest pain, throbbing of vessels, faintness feelings	1
Respiratory symptoms Chest pressure or constriction, choking feeling, sighing, dyspnea	1
Gastrointestinal symptoms Difficulty swallowing, flatus, abdominal fullness or pain, burning sensations, stomach growling, nausea, vomiting, loose bowels, constipation, weight loss	2
Genitourinary symptoms Urinary frequency or urgency, amenorrhea, menorrhagia, loss of libido, premature ejaculation, impotence, frigidity	2

(continued)

C HARTING GUIDE

Hamilton anxiety rating scale (continued)

ITEM	RATINGS
Autonomic symptoms Dry mouth, flushing, pallor, tendency to sweat, giddiness, tension headaches, hair standing on end	*1*
Somatic (muscular) symptoms Aches and pains, twitching, stiffness, myoclonic jerking movements, grinding of teeth, unsteady voice, increased muscle tone	*2*
Total score	*15*

Interpretation
15: Indicates anxiety; doesn't necessarily warrant therapy
18 or more: Moderate to severe anxiety; consider therapy

Adapted from Hamilton, M. "Diagnosis and rating of anxiety." In Lader, M. D., ed. "Studies of Anxiety," British Journal of Psychiatry 3:76-79, 1969.

Nursing interventions

The biopsychosocial nature of depression presents multiple challenges for caregivers of older adults. However, you can carry out many nursing interventions without a doctor's order that can help your depressed older patient. Exercise, such as walking and swimming, is a natural means of treating depression; it helps replace certain depleted brain chemicals, such as serotonin and norephinephrine. Gardening therapy is also effective for treating people with mental illness. Even manipulating the intensity and sources of environmental sound and music can make a difference.

Bipolar disorder

Also known as manic depressive illness and cyclical depression, bipolar disorder is characterized by cyclical mood changes from very high (elation, euphoria) to deep depression.

Assessment

The older adult with bipolar disorder may exhibit markedly changing mental status, confusion, agitation, and depression. As the patient swings from hyperexcited euphoria to a moderate state, then to depression and psychomotor retardation, changes in medications must be made.

Nursing interventions

Managing an older adult with bipolar disorder requires close monitoring because of his slower metabolism and extended clearance of medications. The drug of choice is lithium, but this drug can cause renal damage and thyroid impairment in older adults, especially those with other medical problems.

Obsessive compulsive disorder

Obsessive compulsive disorder (OCD) can begin at any stage in adulthood. It's marked by repetitive performance of acts or rituals, such as hand washing, house cleaning, checking doorknobs, and making lists. A person with OCD may have a very rigid personality and will insist on performing everyday tasks in an unvarying order. This rigid behavior, which usually develops over a lifetime, can be exacerbated if the person experiences a serious stressful event.

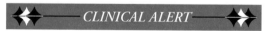 *CLINICAL ALERT*

If the patient is prevented or distracted from his pattern of ritual activity, he may become anxious or agitated. Any environmental alteration (such as transfer to a nursing home or a visit from a stranger in the patient's home care setting) may trigger a need for treatment.

ℭHARTING GUIDE

Geriatric depression scale (short form)

Patient name _Michael Jeffries_   Date: _11/15/96_

Answer the following questions by circling the answer that best describes how you felt over the past week.

	Yes	No
1. Are you basically satisfied with your life?	(Yes)	No
2. Have you dropped many of your activities and interests?	Yes	(No)
3. Do you feel that your life is empty?	Yes	(No)
4. Do you often get bored?	Yes	(No)
5. Are you in good spirits most of the time?	(Yes)	No
6. Are you afraid that something bad is going to happen to you?	Yes	(No)
7. Do you feel happy most of the time?	Yes	(No)
8. Do you often feel helpless?	Yes	(No)
9. Do you prefer staying at home to going out and doing new things?	(Yes)	No
10. Do you feel that you have more problems with memory than most people?	Yes	(No)
11. Do you think it's wonderful to be alive now?	Yes	(No)
12. Do you feel pretty worthless the way you are now?	Yes	(No)
13. Do you feel full of energy?	Yes	(No)
14. Do you feel that your situation is hopeless?	Yes	(No)
15. Do you think that most people are better off than you?	Yes	(No)

Scoring
Score one point for each of the following answers:

1. No	4. Yes	7. No	10. Yes	13. No
2. Yes	5. No	8. Yes	11. No	14. Yes
3. Yes	6. Yes	9. Yes	12. Yes	15. Yes

Interpretation

0 to 5 - Normal   Score _____

6 or more - Depression possible   Examiner _____   Date _____

Adapted with permission from Sheikh, J.I., and Yesavage, J.A. "Geriatric Depression Scale (GDS): Recent Evidence and Development of a Shorter Version," *Clinical Gerontologist* 5(1/2):165-73, June 1986. ©1986, The Haworth Press, Inc., Binghamton, N.Y.

Assessment

Nursing assessment of the OCD patient should focus on identifying the patient's repetitive acts or rituals. In older adults, these rituals are commonly manifested as morbid fears and obsessions with bodily functions. The patient performs the rituals out of a need for control and order and as a means of coping with anxiety.

Nursing interventions

Clomipramine (Anafranil) is a tricyclic antidepressant used to treat OCD. If the doctor prescribes this drug for your patient, be especially alert for cardiac problems and possible hallucinations. Fluvoxamine maleate (Luvox), an SSRI, is also approved for treating OCD, although most of the SSRI drugs should be effective.

Delirium

Also called acute confusional state, acute encephalopathy, and altered mental status, delirium isn't a disease but a symptom of an underlying problem. It can develop from infection, blood sugar imbalance, pain, or head injury; after a surgical procedure, anesthesia, or a sudden change in physical surroundings; or from a drug interaction or withdrawal.

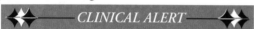
CLINICAL ALERT

If your patient suddenly develops a change in mental status, assess him for cardiovascular problems, such as fluid shift or arrhythmias; infections, including urinary tract and pulmonary infections; unrelieved pain; electrolyte imbalance; and drug toxicity.

Assessment

The symptoms of delirium can be the same as those of depression or psychosis. To determine the underlying problem, perform a thorough physical assessment, including vital signs and assessment for pain and sensory deprivation.

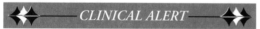
CLINICAL ALERT

To rule out drug toxicity as the cause of the patient's behavior, obtain diagnostic blood levels if the patient takes drugs with overdose potential, such as alcohol, salicylates, theophylline, digoxin, thyroid hormone, or a benzodiazepine.

Nursing interventions

● Have someone stay with the patient while you notify the doctor of the change in mental status.
● Obtain most recent lab results and specimens for any newly ordered lab tests. Review the patient's current medications with the pharmacist for possible delirium-inducing interactions.
● Reassure the patient by speaking in a calm voice, moving slowly and deliberately, and explaining your actions.
● Reorient the patient. Decrease noise, light, and other environmental stimuli.
● Provide for the patient's safety by having someone sit by his bed, perhaps a family member. Use restraints, if necessary.
● If your facility has a psychiatric liaison team, alert team members for assistance with immediate patient management, care planning, and staff support.

Dementia

There are many forms of dementia, or cognitive loss. Alzheimer's disease is one form, although it's not considered a psychiatric disorder, according to the National Alzheimer's Association. Many types of dementia are reversible, such as the dementia that occurs with pernicious anemia and responds to vitamin B_{12} therapy. Other types of dementia aren't reversible.

Between 60% and 75% of nursing home residents have some form of dementia, and a sizable portion of them are receiving psychotropic drugs inappropriately or excessively. As a result of the Omnibus Budget Reconciliation Act of 1987 (OBRA), efforts have been made to reduce the use of such chemical restraints. OBRA regulates this use of neuroleptics and benzodiazepines in long-term care facilities. Several research studies have indicated that about one third of these patients could do without neuroleptics and benefit instead from nursing, environmental, and other multidisciplinary interventions.

Assessment

Decreased intellectual function, personality changes, impaired judgment, and change in affect are common manifestations of dementia. A thorough nursing assessment is essential in making a definitive diagnosis.

Nursing interventions

● Decrease environmental stimuli, such as noise,

excessive artificial light, and television use.
- Speak to your patient in a soft, calm, low-pitched voice.
- Redirect him to appropriate activities when behavior problems occur.
- Avoid placing the patient in large rooms with large numbers of people, such as dining rooms or group activity rooms; small, private gathering places are less overwhelming.
- Referral to health care professionals skilled in caring for these patients is often appropriate.
- If appropriate, suggest that family members consult a mental health professional for help in coping with caregiver stress, financial pressures, and other related issues. Also refer them to other community resources as appropriate.

TREATING MENTAL ILLNESS

Until comparatively recently, people with mental or emotional illnesses bore a stigma of shame, fear, and weakness; family members kept them out of sight. This environment began to change in the 1950s with the advent of major psychotropic drugs, such as chlorpromazine and imipramine, which gave a new level of relief from the debilitation of mental illness. Electroconvulsive therapy was developed into a safe, effective treatment for depression. Thanks to new drugs and other treatments, most mentally ill patients today are not institutionalized and can be treated in many different settings.

Public attitudes toward mental illness have changed, too, as a result of media exposure and community education programs held at local senior centers, hospitals, and churches. Depression and Anxiety Screening Day programs encourage older adults and families to learn more about mental health and help bring people together with skilled practitioners for treatment.

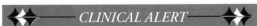

CLINICAL ALERT

Many community and psychiatric specialty hospitals offer free educational programs on psychiatric issues, such as family dynamics, depression, and anxiety, for the public and for health care professionals. Some programs even carry free continuing education credits. Contact your area hospital public relations department for details. To find out about your local psychiatric community resources, referral sources, local retirement campuses, and other support groups, visit your local public library, or call the local Department on Aging or the nearest chapter of the Alliance for the Mentally Ill.

Mental health care team approach

Older people are no longer passive recipients of psychiatric services with no choice in making mental health decisions. They're now the focus of a new entity, the geriatric mental health treatment team. In this team approach to treatment, patients and families join with multidisciplinary caregivers to set goals and make decisions regarding the type of treatment and its implementation.

The nurse works with the physical therapist, social worker, dietitian, doctor, chemical dependency counselor, psychologist, pharmacist, and professionals in other disciplines, as needed, to best meet the needs of the older adult. Because no single professional discipline can meet the needs of every older adult with emotional needs, referrals should be made early in the treatment process.

Older adults, like all patients with mental health needs, have a right to confidentiality in all matters related to their health care. You must obtain a signed informed consent from the patient or family before sharing information with other professionals or facilities, and the patient's actual name and identity should never be disclosed to the public.

Geropsychiatric nursing

Nurses who work with mentally ill older adults must have a firm background in the behavioral and social sciences, the normal aging process, pathophysiology, psychiatric disorders, as well as pharmacology and psychopharmacology. Geropsychiatric nursing, one of the newest and most rapidly growing nursing specialties, fills this need. It blends expertise from four nursing specialties: gerontologic, psychiatric, medical-surgical, and community health nursing.

The geropsychiatric nurse is a registered nurse working as part of the mental health team. Typically, this nurse gives the most direct hands-on care and works as a case manager or a shift supervisor.

The geropsychiatric nurse must also be familiar with community resources that can help the older adult maintain the highest level of wellness. Older adult dementia evaluation centers, geropsychiatric outpatient therapy clinics, group homes, nutritional services, transportation, and home maintenance services are just a few examples of the specialized community services available for older adults with mental health needs.

Advanced practice nursing

Advanced practice nurses (APNs) provide a variety of specialty services to older adults with physical and mental health needs. APN credentials usually include a master's degree in nursing and advanced certification in a specialty area, such as clinical nurse specialist or nurse practitioner. In most states, APNs have some form of prescriptive authority, working in a doctors' group practice, a hospital, or independent practice.

The geriatric APN is a resource in the care of the older adult with mental health needs. She can see the older adult on site and intervene with research-based, advanced nursing clinical skills. A geropsychiatric APN combines a strong background in medical-surgical nursing and patient education, may be certified to provide psychotherapy, and may be able to prescribe medications.

Because of their accessibility, APNs are sometimes better able than other health care professionals to meet older adults' special mental health needs. Specially trained, board-certified geropsychiatrists aren't available in all settings, such as nursing homes, or in all geographic areas. In addition, older adults may have preconceived, negative ideas about working with psychiatrists.

Management options

Various strategies can be used to help the older adult meet his mental and emotional needs. Among these strategies are stress management, outpatient therapy, and support groups.

Stress management

Patterns of coping with stress are learned behavior. Children observe a parent's method of reacting to stress and copy the same behavior, effective or not. Eventually, ineffective coping strategies can result in depression, family dysfunction, violence, and substance abuse. Because mental health issues interfere with many aspects of life, older adults and their families can improve their quality of life by dealing with these issues. Many older adults aren't referred for psychotherapy because of a mistaken belief that they wouldn't benefit. However, breaking the cycle of dysfunctional coping behavior can be accomplished with people of all ages through various types of talk therapy.

Outpatient therapy

Psychotherapy can be very effective in helping older adults learn to cope with stressful life events. Outpatient therapy is usually provided by experienced mental health professionals, such as psychologists, psychotherapists, social workers, psychiatric APNs, geropsychiatric APNs, and psychiatrists. A multidisciplinary team approach that provides comprehensive care is most effective. Therapy can be provided to individuals, couples, families, or groups. Insurance covers most short-term outpatient psychotherapy costs.

Support groups

Support groups give older people a chance to discuss how an illness affects their life and lets them help each other by sharing workable solutions. This form of mental health treatment differs from psychotherapy in that the support group consists of peers or family members who have experienced a common problem, and the group may or may not have a mental health professional as a facilitator to monitor and focus the discussion. Support groups often meet in churches, senior centers, hospitals, schools, and other public meeting places. Alcoholics Anonymous and Narcotics Anonymous are examples of well-known, nationally organized support groups. Such groups may be free or may require a nominal fee.

Settings for providing mental health care

Mental health problems are no longer treated only in the hospital. Nurses must be prepared to meet the psychiatric needs of their older patients in outpatient surgery, home care, short-term rehabilitation, adult day-care, nursing homes, clinics, and every other setting where health care is provided.

Home care

Home care is one of the newest delivery settings for geropsychiatric nursing. Services provided in the home are expanding rapidly and currently include detoxification, dementia care, psychotherapy, and medication management.

As inpatient hospital stays get shorter in all areas of geriatric care, the geropsychiatric nurse must be prepared to draw on her medical-surgical, community health, and psychiatric nursing expertise to meet the patient's needs. An older home care patient may be returning home after a hospital stay or from a partial hospitalization program, a rehabilitation center, or a group home; or he may just need psychiatric nursing care to remain in the home.

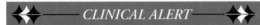

CLINICAL ALERT

To successfully meet the needs of the older psychiatric home care patient, you need to be flexible, respect the patient's right to choose his own lifestyle, and keep in close touch with other treatment team members.

The geropsychiatric home care nurse must have knowledge of physical assessment; movement disorders; crisis deescalation; cardiac, hypertensive, and psychiatric medications and their interactions (especially important because of the older patient's tendency to polypharmacy); and community protective services for the elderly. Because this patient may be receiving services from a community mental health clinic, a case management firm, and a community support program simultaneously, the home care nurse's coordinating skills are also very important.

Finally, the older home care patient is vulnerable to criminal and abusive acts. If you learn of threats to the patient or any other unusual situations, report them to the police. The patient's descriptions of bizarre threatening situations may in fact have a base in reality.

Nursing homes

Admission to a nursing home may cause situational depression in the older adult. The nurse, social worker, and mental health consultant should be alert for this development and be prepared to help the patient adjust to the change of environment. Even temporary nursing home admission can cause depression. Patients brought to nursing homes for short-term rehabilitation programs are much younger than the typical resident. Many of these patients will not become residents, but may stay for only a few weeks. It's important to remind these "younger older" patients that their stay is only temporary and that their goal is to return home.

Psychiatric services provided to older adults in long-term care facilities are regulated by OBRA. These regulations, and subsequent updates, mandate the monitoring of physical and chemical restraints (psychotropic drugs) in skilled nursing facilities. OBRA guidelines require older nursing home residents who are diagnosed with a primary psychiatric disorder to be treated for that disorder by a mental health professional. In addition, new residents in skilled nursing facilities must be screened for mental illness prior to admission.

Skilled nursing facilities are required to have professional mental health consultants available to monitor behavior, work with staff, and manage psychotropic medications. Many nursing homes have one nursing staff member designated as the first-line, in-house mental health nursing specialist. This nurse is readily accessible on short notice to help with a specific nursing home resident or answer a complicated question, but doesn't have the depth of knowledge, background, or experience of an APN. If the clinical problem continues, worsens, or requires in-depth assessment, the patient is referred to the APN consultant for telephone consultation or monthly rounds.

Geropsychiatric clinical nurse specialists are increasingly working as nursing home consultants, sharing their expertise with attending doctors, other nursing staff, and families. In many cases, this clinical nurse specialist can successfully manage behavior problems in the nursing home without help from a psychiatrist. Some families may prefer to have their loved one seen by a geropsychiatric APN in the nursing home rather than by a psychiatrist in an unfamiliar office.

Emergency departments

Research shows that older adults living in the community are less apt to use the emergency department (ED) for primary care than other age-groups. However, they may be escorted to the ED by the police or other health care personnel after an episode of violent or threatening behavior, or a suicide attempt. Unfortunately, once in the ED, they may no longer exhibit the threatening behavior. Any geriatric patient with a history of acting-out behavior requires a thorough physical assessment with baseline diagnostics, including electrocardiography, complete blood count with differential, chemistry panel, and urinalysis. The objective is to keep the patient from harming himself or others, provide rapid tranquilization or sedation, and avoid over-medication and toxicity.

Older adults are at severe risk for oversedation, particularly with violent behavior, because their diminished kidney and liver function increases the time needed to metabolize and excrete medications. Hence, they may not respond to a sedative immediately, resulting in more medication being administered. The effect of drug accumulation can range from a hangover feeling to near-coma as they slowly metabolize and excrete the sedative.

The crisis-oriented environment of an ED is very frightening to the older adult, especially one who has impaired vision or poor hearing or who doesn't understand why he's at the hospital. Some delirious older patients may speak out in their native language; if you can find a coworker who speaks the language, you may find the patient is making perfect sense in that language.

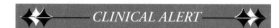

Have a portable hearing aid available to make sure the older patient can hear your assessment questions and cooperate with treatment.

Some hospitals have addressed the problems associated with providing quality care for the mentally ill in the ED by developing a community liaison nurse. Working collaboratively with other staff, this nurse is the link between crisis intervention, outreach, and continuity of care. This nurse can provide valuable information to the intervention team and facilitate rapid referrals.

Inpatient geropsychiatric units

This inpatient setting is used to evaluate dementia and to stabilize aggressive or suicidal patients. Efforts focus on rapid evaluation to rule out physical illness, rapid stabilization of mood, and discharge planning. Inpatient geropsychiatric hospital stays are brief, reflecting trends toward community-based health care. (Long inpatient psychiatric stays are no longer reality, even in public institutions.)

Discharge planning for the geropsychiatric patient is a complex process because of possible financial implications, such as health insurance limitations and the choices available for care. The patient, family, and interdisciplinary team must be in constant communication during the inpatient stay. Note that geropsychiatric patients don't follow a predetermined discharge routine from inpatient hospitalization to partial hospitalization to home care. Decisions about discharge are based on insurance coverage, patient and family preferences, availability of transportation, and the patient's function level and ability to interact in therapeutic social groups.

Partial hospitalization

Psychiatric partial hospitalization provides intense, structured, multidisciplinary therapy for patients who have more acute needs than outpatients. Partial programs have been set up as an adjunct when patients have used up their allotted insurance coverage for inpatient days but still require intense treatment. Many partial hospitalization programs are associated with specialty psychiatric and chemical abuse programs. Patients are usually picked up in vans and taken to the partial hospitalization site, then driven home at night.

Psychologists, occupational therapists, chemical dependency counselors, dietitians, nurses, psychiatrists, and pharmacists make up the multidisciplinary team. The team establishes individual treatment goals and plans interventions to meet specific needs.

Nursing care prepares the older patient and his family to adapt to living with mental illness and to stabilize lifestyle changes to stay well. Patients are taught to apply new coping skills learned in the hospital to the real world. Some of these skills include medication management, stress management, and activities of daily living.

General hospital units

Older patients on nonpsychiatric units in general hospitals need to have health care providers who are knowledgeable in all aspects of geriatric health needs, not just the problem presenting at the time of admission. Because acute care stays are so short, there is little time to get to know the geriatric patient and help him safely adjust to the environment.

Many hospitals have established multidisciplinary liaison-psychiatric intervention teams to assist in rapid expert assessment and interventions. These teams can help deescalate crisis situations, educate hospital staff on specific interventions, counsel families, and make referrals for postdischarge specialty care. Multidisciplinary team members typically include a geropsychiatric clinical nurse specialist, pharmacist, physical therapist, psychiatrist, psychologist, chemical dependency counselor, chaplain, and social worker.

Acute care admission assessments are a vital step in rapidly evaluating the older adult. Be sure to consult old patient records, if available, for accuracy. On admission, verify medication lists with the family and caregivers. Again, you'll need a thorough knowledge of drug interactions, because new drugs may have been added before hospitalization, increasing the risk of side effects.

Behavioral problems in hospitalized geriatric patients can lead to serious complications because the staff is usually not trained to recognize psychiatric problems early. Anxious and agitated patients have a much greater risk of falls. The use of physical restraints, even if applied properly, can result in broken bones and skin tears.

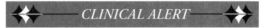
CLINICAL ALERT

The use of physical restraints (including inappropriate use of side rails) on older patients has been associated with pressure ulcers, infections, incontinence, functional impairment, cardiac stress, altered nutrition, and agitation. Strangulation, accidental death, and serious injuries have also been reported as well as precipitation of posttraumatic stress disorder reactions.

Guidelines on long-term care of the federal government and the Joint Commission on Accreditation of Healthcare Organizations mandate careful consideration before restraining an individual. Restraints should be placed at the joint, not in the middle of a limb. Side rails should be used appropriately.

The use of psychotropic medications, such as antidepressants, major tranquilizers, sedatives, and lithium, in older patients with concomitant medical and mobility problems profoundly increases the likelihood of falls. Discontinuing medications before surgery, then reordering them a few days later, may cause withdrawal symptoms for a patient receiving benzodiazepines or other psychotropic medications. The older patient with congestive heart failure who is managing bipolar disorder with lithium needs skilled care to prevent lithium toxicity with diuretics. Postanesthesia delirium is a frightening but common condition in postsurgical geriatric patients. Be sure to educate the older adult and family about these possibilities.

Managed care systems

The change to managed care is yet another step in the evolution of health care from fee-for-service reimbursement, with little incentive for prevention, to a capitated delivery system with built-in cost and quality measures. Psychiatric care of older adults in a managed care system aims to provide services in the least restrictive environment and the most cost-effective manner. Examples include partial hospitalization programs and psychiatric-focused home care.

Third-party reimbursement has created a new health care decision maker with an increasingly strong say in the types of services that are reimbursed. Success in working with managed care systems means survival. Those providers that can document short inhospital stays, low rates of readmission, fewer unscheduled repeat clinic visits, and customer satisfaction will stay in the business of health care. Nonprofit and for-profit systems must provide identical quality outcomes. Older adults, families, and health care workers can best adapt to this system by keeping informed about choices, learning to speak the new language of capitation, and developing negotiation skills.

If you're asked to speak to a representative of a managed care firm about your patient, follow these pointers:
• Make sure the representative has a signed consent form for disclosure of information.
• Answer questions honestly but briefly; share only objective information, and don't volunteer information.
• Answer questions related to treatment goals, objectives, and progress toward those goals.
• Don't offer your personal opinion, even when asked.

Psychopharmacologic treatment

Psychotropic drugs act in certain areas of the brain to alter mood and behavior. Drugs such as chlorpromazine and imipramine have revolutionized psychiatric treatment. However, because older people typically take several medications concurrently for other illnesses, they're at great risk for drug interactions and adverse effects; the risk is increased further because older people metabolize drugs more slowly. As a rule, dosages for older adults should start at 25% of the dose for younger adults and be increased gradually. (For more information on drug metabolism, see Chapter 16.)

Different groups of psychotropic drugs tend to cause distinctive arrays of adverse reactions in older adults. This can be used to evaluate treatment response and identify emerging adverse effects.

Neuroleptics

Neuroleptics, also called antipsychotics or major tranquilizers, were one of the first classes of psychiatric drugs. Examples of commonly used neuroleptics include chlorpromazine, clozapine (Clozaril), haloperidol (Haldol), thioridazine hydrochloride (Mellaril), thiothixene (Navane), risperadone (Risperdal), loxapine hydrochloride (Loxitane), fluphenazine enanthate (Prolixin), perphenazine (Trilafon), trifluoperazine (Stelazine), and prochlorperazine (Compazine).

Although very effective, neuroleptic drugs can cause serious adverse effects, such as tardive dyskinesia (TD), an irreversible movement disorder. The DISCUS Scale is an assessment tool that can be used to monitor movement disorders such as TD (see *Dyskinesia identification sytem: Condensed user scale [DISCUS]*).

Benzodiazepines

Benzodiazepines are used to treat anxiety and seizure disorders. They're addictive, tend to interact with many medications, and shouldn't be discontinued abruptly because withdrawal may occur. Examples of benzodiazepines include alprazolam (Xanax), diazepam (Valium), lorazepam (Ativan), oxazepam (Serax), temazepam (Restoril), clorazepate (Tranxene), chlordiazepoxide (Librium), and midazolam (Versed).

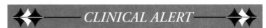

◆◆──── CLINICAL ALERT ────◆◆

Benzodiazepines with long half-lives tend to accumulate in the system and may cause oversedation. Benzodiazepines are sometimes given along with narcotics to add to the analgesic effect or as a preanesthetic. Be aware that an older adult patient may take longer to recover from anesthesia if these combinations are used.

Antidepressants

Antidepressants, as the name suggests, are used to

CHARTING GUIDE

Dyskinesia identification system: Condensed user scale (DISCUS)

The DISCUS scale shown below is a standard assessment tool used to evaluate movement disorders, such as tardive dyskinesia, that sometimes are a side effect of neuroleptic drugs. It also comes with an instruction sheet that includes prerequisites for diagnosis.

Name __Harold Marcus__

__Mill Valley Hospital__
(facility)

**Dyskinesia Identification System:
Condensed User Scale (DISCUS)**

Current psychotropics/anticholinergic
and total mg/day

__Haldol, 0.5 mg po__ ___1__mg

_____ ____mg

_____ ____mg

Exam type (check one)
- ☑ 1. Baseline
- ☐ 2. Annual
- ☐ 3. Semi-annual
- ☐ 4. D/C — 1 month
- ☐ 5. D/C — 2 month
- ☐ 6. D/C — 3 month
- ☐ 7. Admission
- ☐ 8. Other

Cooperation (check one)
- ☐ 1. None
- ☑ 2. Partial
- ☐ 3. Full

Scoring

0 - Not present (movements not observed, or some movements observed but not considered abnormal)

1 - Minimal (abnormal movements difficult to detect, or movements easy to detect but occurring only once or twice in a short, nonrepetitive manner)

2 - Mild (abnormal movements easy to detect and occurring infrequently)

3 - Moderate (abnormal movements easy to detect and occurring frequently)

4 - Severe (abnormal movements easy to detect and occurring almost continuously)

NA - Not assessed (or not able to assess)

Assessment

DISCUS item and score (circle one score for each item)

Face	1. Tics	0	①①	2	3	4	NA
	2. Grimaces	⓪	1	2	3	4	NA
Eyes	3. Blinking	⓪	1	2	3	4	NA
Oral	4. Chewing/lip smacking	⓪	1	2	3	4	NA
	5. Puckering/sucking/ thrusting lower lip	⓪	1	2	3	4	NA
Lingual	6. Tongue thrusting/ tongue in cheek	⓪	1	2	3	4	NA
	7. Tonic tongue	⓪	1	2	3	4	NA
	8. Tongue tremor	⓪	1	2	3	4	NA
	9. Athetoid myokymic/ lateral tongue	⓪	1	2	3	4	NA
Head/ Neck/ Trunk	10. Retrocollis/torticollis	⓪	1	2	3	4	NA
	11. Shoulder/hip torsion	⓪	1	2	3	4	NA
Upper limb	12. Athetoid/myokymic finger-wrist-arm	⓪	1	2	3	4	NA
	13. Pill rolling	⓪	1	2	3	4	NA
Lower limb	14. Ankle flexion/ foot tapping	⓪	1	2	3	4	NA
	15. Toe movement	⓪	1	2	3	4	NA

Comments

_____

_____

_____

15-item score ___1__

Rater's signature
and title __Barbara Rice, RN__

Exam date __7/22/96__
Next exam
date __1/22/97__

Evaluation

1. Greater than 90 days' neuroleptic exposure   Yes No
2. Scoring/intensity level met   Yes No
3. Other diagnostic conditions?   Yes No
 (If yes specify)

_____

4. Last exam date _____
 Last total score _____
 Last conclusion _____

Preparer's signature and title for items 1 to 4
(if different from doctor)

_____

5. Conclusion (circle one)
A. No tardive dyskinesia (TD); if scoring prerequisite met, list other diagnostic condition or explain in comments
B. Probable TD
C. Masked TD
D. Withdrawal TD
E. Persistent TD
F. Remitted TD
G. Other (specify in comments)

6. Comments

_____

_____

_____

Doctor's
signature _____
Date _____

(continued)

CHARTING GUIDE

Dyskinesia identification system: Condensed user scale (DISCUS) *(continued)*

SIMPLIFIED DIAGNOSES FOR TARDIVE DYSKINESIA

Prerequisites

The 3 prerequisites for diagnosing tardive dyskinesia (TD) are as follows, although exceptions may occur.

1. A history of at least 3 months' total cumulative neuroleptic exposure. (Include amoxapine and metoclopramide in all categories below as well.)
2. Scoring/intensity level. Total score of 5 or more. Also be alert for any change from baseline or scores below five which have at least a moderate (3) or severe (4) movement on any item or at least two mild (2) movements on two items located in different body areas.
3. Other conditions are not responsible for the abnormal involuntary movements.

Diagnoses

The diagnosis is based on the current exam and its relation to the last exam. It can shift depending on whether movements are present or not, whether movements are present for 3 months or more (6 months for a semi-annual assessment), and whether neuroleptic dosage changes occur and affect movements.

- No TD (Movements not present on this exam, or movements present but caused by some other condition. The last diagnosis must be *No TD, Probable TD,* or *Withdrawal TD.)*
- Probable TD (Movements present on this exam for the first time, or for the first time in 3 months or more. The last diagnosis must be *No TD* or *Probable TD.)*
- Persistent TD (Movements present on this exam and have been present for 3 months or more with this exam or present at some point in the past. The last diagnosis can be any except *No TD.)*
- Masked TD (Movements not present on this exam, but this is due to a neuroleptic dosage increase or restart after an earlier exam when movements were present. Or movements not present due to the addition of a non-neuroleptic medicaton to treat TD. The last diagnosis must be *Probable TD, Persistent TD, Withdrawal TD,* or *Masked TD.)*
- Remitted TD (Movements are not present on this exam, but persistent TD has been diagnosed and no neuroleptic dosage increase or restart has occurred. The last diagnosis must be *Persistent TD* or *Remitted TD.* If movements re-emerge, the diagnosis shifts back to *Persistent TD.)*
- Withdrawal TD (Movements are not present while patient receives neuroleptics or at the last dosage level, but are seen within 8 weeks after neuroleptic reduction or discontinuation. The last diagnosis must be *No TD* or *Withdrawal TD.* If movements continue for 3 months or more after neuroleptic reduction or discontinuation, the diagnosis shifts to *Persistent TD.* If movements do not continue for 3 months or more after the reduction or discontinuation, the diagnosis shifts to *No TD.)*

INSTRUCTIONS

1. The rater completes the Assessment according to the standardized exam procedure. If the rater also completes the Evaluation items 1 to 4, he/she must also sign the preparer box. The form is given to the physician. Or the doctor may perform the assessment.
2. The physician completes the Evaluation section. The physician is responsible for the entire Evaluation section and its accuracy.
3. A doctor should examine any person who meets the three prerequisites or has movements not explained by other factors. He should obtain any neurologic assessments or differential diagnostic tests that may be needed.
4. File form according to policy or procedure.

Other conditions (partial list)

1. Age
2. Blind
3. Cerebral palsy
4. Contact lenses
5. Dentures, no teeth
6. Down's syndrome
7. Drug intoxication (specify)
8. Encephalitis
9. Extrapyramidal side effects (specify)
10. Fahr's syndrome
11. Heavy metal intoxication (specify)
12. Huntington's chorea
13. Hyperthyroidism
14. Hypoglycemia
15. Hypoparathyroidism
16. Idiopathic torsion dystonia
17. Meige syndrome
18. Parkinson's disease
19. Stereotypies
20. Syndenham's chorea
21. Tourette's syndrome
22. Wilson's disease
23. Other (specify)

treat depression. When used in older adults, they require careful administration and evaluation. For example, older adults have a greater chance of developing heart disease than younger adults, and all antidepressants pose a risk of cardiovascular problems (although the risk is greater with some, such as tricyclic antidepressants and monoamine oxidase [MAO] inhibitors, compared with the newer SSRIs). Specific vascular problems that have been associated with antidepressants include heart failure, hypertension, hypotension, arrhythmias, and conduction problems.

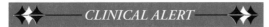

Watch for evidence of cardiac symptoms in an older depressed patient receiving any type of antidepressant, especially combinations such as an SSRI and a tricyclic, because of the risk of drug interactions.

Tricyclic antidepressants. The tricyclic antidepressants (TCAs), developed in the 1950s and 1960s, are highly effective and less costly than newer antidepressants. However, they can increase the heart rate, which can be a problem if your older adult patient has a cardiovascular condition. Other adverse effects include dry mouth, sedation, mydriasis, dizziness, constipation, confusion, tachycardia, delirium, urine retention, and thermoregulatory impairment.

Commonly used TCAs include amitriptyline (Elavil), imipramine (Tofranil), doxepin (Sinequan), nortriptyline (Pamelor), desipramine (Norpramin), clomipramine (Anafranil), and maprotiline (Ludiomil).

Serotonin-specific reuptake inhibitors (SSRIs). This class of antidepressants has fewer anticholinergic side effects and is less cardiotoxic than the older TCAs. However, they should still be used cautiously in older patients. The SSRIs are energizing antidepressants; in an older patient, this energizing effect may increase agitation, especially with long-term use. Because these drugs may also suppress appetite, another antidepressant may be a better choice for the older patient who's already

underweight or has a poor appetite.

Commonly used SSRIs include fluoxetine (Prozac), sertraline (Zoloft), paroxitine (Paxil), and fluvoxamine maleate (Luvox).

Other new antidepressants. Two new antidepressants, nefazodone (Serzone) and venlafaxine (Effexor), target the action of both serotonin and norepinephrine. They don't suppress appetite like the SSRIs, but they may cause bradycardia and decreased blood pressure. When given in reduced dosages to older patients, nefazodone has a lower incidence of cardiovascular effects.

Other psychotropic drugs

Other drugs used to treat mental health and psychiatric problems include bupropion, buspirone, and lithium.

Bupropion. The antidepressant bupropion (Wellbutrin) isn't pharmacologically related to either TCAs or SSRIs. However, its side effects in older patients, including agitation and insomnia, are similar to those of the SSRIs.

Buspirone. The only drug in the azapirone class that has been approved for use in the United States, buspirone (BuSpar) isn't addictive. It has a subtle onset and a relatively benign side effect profile. It may take 2 to 4 weeks to be effective, but doesn't require an OBRA-mandated dosage reduction. Buspirone should not be given on an as-needed basis because its effectiveness is not related to time of administration but to the development of a therapeutic blood level.

Lithium. The drug of choice for treating bipolar disorder, lithium is a salt that's metabolized and excreted as the body manages fluids. In older adults, lithium may increase the risk of dehydration when used with diuretics.

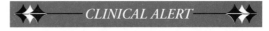

Always be sure to notify the prescriber when an older adult taking lithium and diuretics develops any condition affecting fluid and electrolyte levels, such as nausea, vomiting, or diarrhea. Older people can quickly develop life-threatening lithium toxicity with dehydration.

Treatment of an older adult with bipolar disorder should be managed by a special geriatric mental treatment team because of the complexity and interaction of medical conditions, polypharmacy, and psychiatric issues.

Cytochrome P-450 drug interactions

The cytochrome P-450 system is an enzyme system in the liver that detoxifies and metabolizes certain drugs and other substances. This system determines the speed at which certain drugs are eliminated from the body. Inhibition of excretion through the enzyme system can result in drug accumulation in the body, leading to toxicity. The SSRI drugs, plus venlafaxine and nefazodone, interfere with this enzyme system, thereby inhibiting the excretion of some commonly prescribed drugs used by the elderly, such as nortriptyline (Pamelor), amitriptyline (Elavil), warfarin, aminophylline, beta blockers, calcium channel blockers, and some antibiotics. The result is increased blood levels of the inhibited drug, sometimes to toxic levels, with serious adverse — if not lethal — effects.

◆◆ ——— *CLINICAL ALERT* ——— ◆◆

The best way to make sure any combination of drugs is safe for an older adult is to consult a pharmacist first. You might prevent a lethal drug interaction.

Never assume that a doctor who has prescribed a drug is fully aware of all the potential problems associated with it. When multiple prescribers are treating older adults, the need for collaboration on drug use is even greater.

Be sure to keep medication lists up to date. The geriatric nurse is in the best position to ensure that the care team coordinates its efforts to administer drugs safely and effectively.

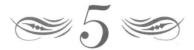

5

Reducing risk of falls

One of the primary goals of those who care for the elderly is to help their patients maintain as much independence as possible for as long as possible in a safe environment. According to Maslow, a safe environment is one that offers stability, protection, order, and freedom from fear, anxiety, and chaos. For older patients, safety and security are as important as basic physiologic needs, such as food and water.

An elderly person's feelings of danger or insecurity may be based on real or perceived threats. And those fears can affect the person's behavior and responses to attempted health care interventions. For example, a person who feels threatened may impose limitations on himself and become rigid and isolated, refusing help from others. Many older people become immobilized by fear of falling or of being the victim of a crime. For such people, providing basic physiologic needs can be a challenge. On the other hand, a perceived threat can motivate a person to adopt behaviors that promote safety and wellness, such as walking only on well-lit streets if he's afraid of falling or of crime.

In addition to facing physical threats, elderly people are often threatened by multiple losses that compromise their ability to maintain their independence and self-determination. By looking at the situation through the eyes of the elderly person, you'll be better able to provide interventions that increase the patient's safety, both real and perceived.

As a person ages, his likelihood of suffering an injury from an accident and becoming disabled

increases. Physiologic changes of aging, underlying disease processes, and psychological, social, and economic stresses all can increase a person's risk of accidents and injury. Among people over age 65, injuries from accidents are the fifth leading cause of death. Accidents occur more frequently in extended-care facilities because residents have disabling conditions, are in an unfamiliar environment, and are more dependent on others for care. Yet, as with accidents in other age-groups, most accidents that the elderly suffer are preventable.

FALLS: INCIDENCE AND IMPACT

Falls are a leading predictor of morbidity and mortality in the elderly population, accounting for about two-thirds of all accidents in this age-group. Nearly one-third of older adults who live outside a nursing home fall at least once a year, and an estimated one-half of those fall more than once. The incidence of falls is about 25% for persons age 70; it increases to 35% for people age 75 and older. About 85% of falls occur in the home, usually in the afternoon or evening.

In acute care hospitals, 85% of all inpatient incident reports are related to falls; of those who fall, 10% fall more than once and 10% experience a fatal fall. Between one-half and two-thirds of institutionalized elderly people experience falls every year.

Risk factors for hip fractures in falls

Although hip fractures account for only 2% of injuries, they lead to increased dependence in 85% of patients and death in 27%. The risk of sustaining a hip fracture depends on the following factors:

- distance fallen (the greater the distance, the greater the risk)
- presence or absence of protective reflexes (the greater the loss, the greater the risk)
- amount of body fat and muscle padding (the less fat and padding, the greater the risk)
- bone strength (the weaker the bones, the greater the risk)
- impact of surface (the harder the surface, the greater the risk).

Adapted with permission from Tideiksaar, R. *Falls in Older Persons: Prevention and Management in Hospitals and Nursing Homes.* Boulder, Colo.: Tactilitics, Inc., 1993.

About 40% of those who fall experience more than one fall and, for those over age 85, 20% of falls prove fatal. In one study at a rehabilitation center, 37% of the falls were found to occur during the busiest times of the day, especially around shift changes, and were related to patients' needs for elimination, food or fluid, or sleep. More falls occurred during the first week and after the third week of institutionalization.

In all settings, the majority of falls take place in the bedroom or bathroom and are related to going to or from the bathroom, transferring to or from bed, or leaning out of chairs. Active people fall more often than inactive people, but those who are frail and have difficulty with activities of daily living (ADLs) have more repeat falls.

Impact

Falls, especially patterns of repeated falls, are one of the leading causes of institutionalization in the older population. Up to 15% of falls result in physical injury, usually fractures or soft-tissue damage. Hip fractures account for only about 2% of injuries but lead to death within 1 year in 27% of cases, partly because of underlying disease and the consequences of immobility. (See *Risk factors for hip fractures in falls.*) About 85% of people with hip fractures suffer functional losses leading to increased dependence. Other common injuries resulting from falls include bruises, lacerations, and subdural hematomas. Acute or chronic pain is another consequence of injuries that should not be overlooked or minimized.

In addition to causing physical injuries, falls may take a psychological toll as well. For example, an elderly person may become more worried about the future — specifically, about his ability to remain independent — because of cognitive or functional losses suffered during hospitalization. The person may experience a loss of self-esteem or a fear of falling again, of being unable to perform ADLs, or of social rejection, which in turn can lead to depression and withdrawal. The result is decreased activity, a further decline in functional abilities, and an increased risk for falls. (See *Consequences of falls.*)

The reactions of family members after a fall can also affect an older person's outlook. For example, family members may become overprotective, trying to limit the older person's activities or making decisions for him. Such actions only increase the person's feelings of incompetence and fear of becoming dependent.

Falls also have a direct impact on health care resources by increasing the use of emergency department services for diagnosis and treatment of injuries and by increasing hospital admissions and length of hospital stay to treat injuries from falls and resulting complications. Falls cost the United States about $100 billion every year in both direct and indirect costs.

FOCUS ON PREVENTION

By focusing your efforts on preventing falls, you can make tremendous gains in preserving life; helping your patients maintain their functional abilities, independence, and quality of life; and conserving health care dollars. One study has shown that proactive interventions to meet the needs of geriatric patients in an acute care setting could reduce falls by more than 80%. To be effective, a prevention program must consist of an accurate analysis of the problem, clearly stated goals, practical and efficient interventions, and a strong commitment by all participants to make it work.

Assessment findings

By learning the causes of falls and assessing an older person for risk factors, you can predict and thus prevent falls in many instances. Whether you practice in the community, a clinic or doctor's office, or an acute, subacute, or long-term care setting, you'll need to compile and analyze data on the incidence of falls and any information related to those falls for the specific patient population involved. Individual data should always be a part of the elderly patient's record and should be updated frequently. This information is critical in detecting trends and patterns and in providing a basis for setting reasonable and measurable goals for both patients and the facility. Your assessment of the individual elderly patient must be comprehensive because it will provide baseline information, help you assess the patient's present status, and identify risk factors.

History of falls

Document the patient's history of falls or near-falls, including the specific activity the patient was engaged in at the time of the fall, any symptoms he experienced at the time of or just before the fall, the time and location of the fall, and any injuries sustained. Many people will minimize or even forget falls if no injuries resulted. They may also be reluctant to share this information if they perceive a threat to their independence or the possibility of having to undergo uncomfortable or costly diagnostic procedures or treatments.

Medication review

Find out which medications the patient is taking, either from the patient himself or, if that's not possible, from his caregiver. Some people consider medications to be only drugs that are prescribed by

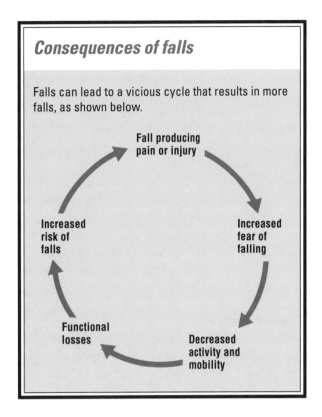

Consequences of falls

Falls can lead to a vicious cycle that results in more falls, as shown below.

Fall producing pain or injury → Increased fear of falling → Decreased activity and mobility → Functional losses → Increased risk of falls →

a doctor, so be sure to ask about over-the-counter drugs, homeopathic remedies, and drugs borrowed from others. A good question to ask is, "What do you do when you . . . (have a headache, are constipated, have a cough, etc.)?"

For example, a 75-year-old man may complain of tinnitus and bruises on his extremities. When asked what medications he takes, he may reply only that he takes one generic aspirin a day for prevention of stroke, as prescribed by his doctor. But further questioning may reveal that he also takes another over-the-counter aspirin four times a day for arthritis pain, a buffered aspirin frequently for headaches, and an occasional effervescent aspirin for upset stomach, suggesting the possibility of aspirin toxicity. Without thorough questioning, you could easily overlook this diagnosis.

Also, determine the reason for taking the medication, how much of it the patient takes, and how often he takes it. And find out if he's taking prescribed medications as often as he should and in the correct dosages. Socioeconomic factors, such as a limited budget or limited access to a pharmacy, can cause elderly people to cut down on their drug dosage or take the drug less often than they should. Cultural factors, such as suspicion of Western medicine, can also affect the patient's compliance with prescribed drug therapy. You'll need to be sensitive and nonjudgmental in eliciting such information.

Medical history

The medical history should include outcomes of past events. For instance, it's important to know that a patient who had abdominal surgery the previous year became acutely confused when given morphine for pain relief or experienced anesthesia-induced delirium. Such knowledge can help you identify risk factors and plan preventive interventions.

Cognitive status

Assessment of cognitive status is particularly important in the elderly, who often have atypical and nonspecific presenting symptoms, such as a change in mental status or repeated falls. When assessing a patient's cognitive abilities, avoid using vague terms, such as "confused," which provide no useful information with which to make comparisons. Instead, be as specific as possible in your descriptions so you'll be able to identify subtle changes that may occur later. For instance, you might note that before admission to a nursing home, a patient was "oriented to person only and had marked short-term memory loss" but that she was "pleasant and seemed content with her surroundings." With this type of objective information, you'll be able to recognize that a change has occurred if the patient later becomes suspicious and agitated.

Whenever possible, use common assessment tools that are objective as well as easy to understand and administer, such as the Mini-Mental State Examination (see Chapter 2), the Delirium Rating Scale, and the Geriatric Depression Scale (see Chapter 4).

Social history

A social history is important in identifying risk factors. An older person who lives alone, has experienced significant losses (especially recently), and has few social supports is at greater risk than

average for depression and cognitive impairment, which can lead to functional losses. Try to obtain information about self-care abilities and instrumental activities of daily living (IADLs) from the patient whenever possible, and have it validated by someone who has observed the patient functioning at home. Quite often, if no family member is available, the primary doctor, a visiting nurse, or a close neighbor can provide this information.

Nutritional status

In evaluating a patient's nutritional status, pay particular attention to hydration status and protein values. Dehydration can cause confusion and hypovolemia; hypovolemia can cause light-headedness or orthostatic hypotension, a primary cause of falls. Depleted protein stores (especially albumin) increase the incidence of drug interactions and adverse reactions, which also increase the incidence of falls.

Also consider the patient's overall appearance, and include measurements of height and weight, routine blood chemistry studies, and urinalysis. Assessment by a dietitian or nutritionist, including a record of the patient's usual eating and drinking patterns, can provide valuable information.

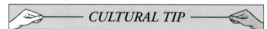
CULTURAL TIP

A patient's strong cultural beliefs and preferences may directly influence his eating habits and, in some cases, his compliance with treatment regimens. For example, a hospitalized patient from a non-Western culture may have difficulty adapting to Western-style hospital food, which can affect his nutritional status. And he may have difficulty adhering to special diets (such as for heart or renal failure) or food-related medication regimens (such as for treatment of diabetes) after he's been discharged from the hospital.

Elimination patterns

Don't forget to assess your patient's elimination patterns. Getting to and from the bathroom and transferring to and from the toilet have been identified as major factors in falls, so be sure to document the patient's usual patterns of bowel and bladder elimination along with any related ongoing problems. You'll need objective information to identify changes from baseline status as well as risks. For example, if a patient who is receiving narcotics for pain has not had a bowel movement in 3 days, you should know whether such a pattern is normal for this patient or an indication that an intervention is needed.

Environmental assessment

Assess your elderly patient's environment — the setting in which he lives — no matter how large or small it might be. Look for environmental "traps," such as loose carpeting, steep stairs, or poor lighting; broken or missing windows, doors, or locks, which may threaten the patient's personal security; inadequate and inaccessible heat, water, and toilet; and inappropriate food and clothing. If the person lives in the community, survey the surrounding neighborhood for potential threats to safety and security, environmental hazards, and adequacy of resources. Pay special attention to common and obvious hazards that have the potential to cause a fall, such as high curbs and uneven walkways.

Present status

To determine an elderly patient's present status, you'll need good listening skills and good physical assessment skills. In many cases, you'll get more information from the patient's stories than from his answers to your questions. Telling a story is not necessarily a diversionary technique (although it may be). Rather, it may be the patient's way of describing symptoms that are vague and difficult to describe succinctly. Also, don't overlook the patient's body language, which can provide clues to his condition, especially if he has cognitive or neurologic deficits.

Your primary focus should be the patient's functional abilities (ADLs, IADLs). Many assessment tools are available to help you obtain objective information: the Barthel Index, the Katz Index of Activities of Daily Living, and the Lawton Scale for Instrumental Activities of Daily Living (see Chapter 2). Compare the data you collect from these tools to data from previous assessments so you can identify, report, and record trends and risks.

Risk identification

Identifying risk factors, followed by timely and appropriate interventions, is the key to a successful program of preventing falls. Whenever you perform an assessment, be alert for risk factors — the "little red flags" that should warn you about potential problems. By anticipating problems before they occur, you can take preventive action and avoid negative outcomes.

Risk assessment tools can help quantify risk for falls and serve as a basis for interventions. But such tools should never be used instead of a full assessment. (See *Risk assessment scale for falls,* page 94.)

Risk factors for falls are usually classified as intrinsic (physiologic, or within the body), extrinsic (external, or outside the body), or iatrogenic (resulting from medical care or treatment). Unclassified or idiopathic falls are those with no identifiable cause. In the older population, falls usually result not from a single risk factor but from a combination. Although the categories overlap, they help to identify which factors can be eliminated or reduced and which can only be managed.

Intrinsic factors

The following physiologic factors increase the risk of falls.

Age and sex. The incidence of falls increases markedly at age 75, with people ages 80 to 89 at the highest risk. Most studies have found that women are at higher risk than men.

Sensory deficits. Vision and hearing problems are a major contributing factor in falls. Aging affects the eyes' ability to adapt quickly to changes in lighting levels. Eye diseases and neurologic conditions can produce restricted vision; for example, a stroke can produce visual field cuts, and glaucoma can impair peripheral vision. Elderly people are more likely to slip or trip when hazardous items are outside their visual fields or when their depth perception has been compromised. Sidewalks, grass, other uneven

HARTING GUIDE

Risk assessment scale for falls

This standardized assessment tool can help you evaluate your patient's risk for falls and plan preventive measures if needed. A score above 4 indicates the need for interventions.

PARAMETERS	PATIENT FALL RISK SCORES				Patient Score		
					TIME		
	4	**3**	**2**	**1**	0800	1600	2400
Age	—	80+	70 to 79	—	2	2	2
Mental status	Intermittent confusion or impulsiveness (or both)	—	Confused (baseline)	—	4	4	4
Elimination	"Can't wait/ won't wait"	Independent and incontinent	Needs assistance	Indwelling catheter	2	2	2
History of falling	History of multiple falls (3 or more)	—	Has fallen 1 or 2 times	—	2	2	2
Gait and balance	Unsteady, poor balance standing or walking	Orthostatic hypotension	—	Needs supervision or assistance with equipment	1	1	1
Medications (By drug class below)	3 or more drug classes	2 drug classes	1 drug class	—	1	1	2
TOTAL RISK SCORES					14	14	15

Drug classes:
1. **Cardiovascular** (antihypertensives, vasodilators, antiarrhythmics, nitrates)
2. **Psychoactive** (sedatives, hypnotics, barbiturates, anxiolytics, antihistamines, anticonvulsants, antidepressants)
3. **Pain** (narcotics, PCA, epidural)
4. **Diuretics/cathartics**
5. **Anesthetics** (first 24 hours post-op)

Total risk scores:
9-20 = extremely high risk
5-8 = high risk
0-4 = low risk
If score is > 4, falls prevention protocol should be implemented.

TIME	NAME
0800	J. Kuka, RN
1600	H. Cane, RN
2400	P. Seria, RN.

Adapted with permission from Abington Memorial Hospital Department of Nursing, Abington, Pa.

surfaces, and brightly patterned floors are also visual hazards and are particularly difficult to maneuver. Loss of color perception can make it difficult to distinguish objects in a pathway, such as a blue footstool on a gray carpet.

Hearing loss can impair an older person's ability to distinguish sounds that ordinarily signal danger, such as verbal warnings from another person, alarms, traffic noise, and so forth. Unaccommodated vision and hearing deficits can also contribute to delirium, especially in an acute care setting. And decreased sensation in the hands and feet is another significant risk factor for falls.

Medical conditions. Many neurologic, cerebro-vascular, cardiovascular, and musculoskeletal conditions cause seizures, drop attacks, and syncopal episodes that result in falls. People with cancer or other progressive, debilitating diseases have a high risk of falling, as do those with multiple or chronic conditions. People with psychiatric conditions or cognitive losses are at risk, especially if they lack attentiveness or insight. Proprioceptive difficulties, orthostatic hypotension, arrhythmias, vertigo, dehydration, electrolyte disorders, urinary and bladder dysfunction, limitations in mobility, and pain are a few of the common medical problems that increase the risk of falls in the elderly.

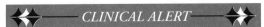

CLINICAL ALERT

A fall can be the sole indicator that an elderly person has an acute illness or is suffering an exacerbation of a chronic illness.

Gait and balance changes. Gait and balance disorders are the second most common cause of falls, after environmental hazards. As a person ages, lean muscle mass decreases, and tendons and ligaments begin to calcify, causing increased rigidity and decreased flexibility, especially in the legs and back. Posture tends to become stooped because of degenerative changes in the spine (markedly so with osteoporosis), causing a change in the center of gravity. Women develop a narrow base of support and a waddling gait, whereas men tend to have a wider base and a short-stepped, shuffling gait.

Degenerative changes in the cerebellum and the vestibular system, slowed neurologic response times, and the altered center of gravity all affect the older person's ability to maintain balance when challenged. Decreased muscle strength and range of motion, bowing of the legs, and less elevated footsteps may compound the problem. Foot problems that cause discomfort, such as corns, bunions, or overgrown toenails, may also affect walking.

Many tools are available to assist in evaluating gait and balance. A simple way to assess balance is to find the functional reach measure. (See *Functional reach measure,* page 96.) In the Tinetti Balance and Gait Evaluation, gait and mobility are measured separately, then the two scores are added together. A total score of 12 to 20 is associated with recurrent falls, as is a gait score of less than 9 or a balance score of less than 10. (See *Tinetti Balance and Gait Evaluation,* pages 97 and 98.)

Whenever possible, a physical or occupational therapist should provide a full mobility and functional assessment of any patient who has gait or balance problems or who is at high risk for them.

Extrinsic factors
The following external factors increase the risk of falls.

Environmental traps. The most common cause of falls is environmental factors — objects or barriers in the person's surroundings. Electric cords, throw rugs, loose carpeting, toys, pets, stools, or other low furniture or objects in a person's pathway can cause him to trip. Wet floors, bathtubs, or showers and objects left on the floor can lead to a slip. Low lighting, light that causes a glare, uneven or highly patterned floors, and stairs that are too steep or that lack a handrail all pose a danger to elderly people.

Environmental barriers — such as bed rails — are another common risk factor. People who fall while attempting to climb out of bed over the side rails sustain some of the most serious injuries. Beds left in an elevated position or with the wheels unlocked, chairs that are too low or unstable, and toilets that are too low all increase the danger of falls during transfers.

Functional reach measure

Keeping a patient's frequently used items within "functional reach"— the distance that he can comfortably reach without straining — can help prevent falls. You can determine a patient's functional reach as follows:

● Have the patient stand upright with one shoulder about 6" (15 cm) away from the wall and his face parallel to the wall.

● Put a piece of tape on the wall to mark the position of the front of the shoulder at the joint.

● With his arms outstretched from the shoulder and parallel to the floor, have the patient reach out as far as he can comfortably, while remaining balanced and not moving either foot.

● Have the patient make a fist while remaining in this position, and mark the wall again at that point.

● Measure the distance between the two marks to find the functional reach measure.

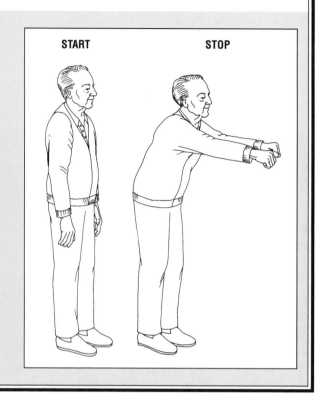

Clothing can also be an environmental trap. Long, loose clothing can catch on furniture, door-knobs, or objects that have fallen onto the floor. Shoes that fit loosely or that have slippery or sticky soles are also hazardous.

Assistive devices. Many falls are associated with the improper use of assistive devices, such as canes and walkers. Many elderly people buy such devices without learning how to use them and fail to maintain them properly (for example, replacing worn rubber tips on canes or walkers).

Alcohol abuse. Alcohol abuse is a significant cause of falls in the elderly, especially those who live alone. Symptoms of alcohol abuse are easy to overlook because of their similarity to other medical problems. Such symptoms include GI disorders, malnutrition, hypoglycemia, poor sleep patterns, peripheral neuropathies, tremors, abnormal gait, and cognitive impairments and depression, which often lead to self-neglect.

Iatrogenic factors

Medications. Although they're necessary for the treatment of disease, medications — whether prescription drugs, over-the-counter drugs, homeopathic remedies, or borrowed drugs — pose a significant danger to the elderly population. Because aging causes major changes in the pharmacokinetics and pharmacodynamics of drugs, older people often require changes in the types of drugs they take and in drug dosages.

Be sure to document all medications that the patient is taking, including form (tablet, liquid), dosage, route, and frequency. Include any that have been newly prescribed (or self-prescribed) within the previous 7 days and any change in the frequency or dosage of a medication already in use. Also record

CHARTING GUIDE

Tinetti Balance and Gait Evaluation

This tool can be used to evaluate how successfully a patient remains at rest or moves about in ordinary activities. It takes 5 to 15 minutes to administer. To prepare, you'll need an armless upholstered chair, a walking space (such as a large room or a hallway), and any of the patient's walking aids (such as a cane or a walker).

Observe the patient during each of the maneuvers listed below, and select the number that best describes his performance. The maximum score is 28; the lowest is zero. The higher the score, the better the patient's gait and balance. You can assess any deterioration in his condition by periodically repeating the evaluation and comparing later scores to the baseline score.

BALANCE

Instructions: Seat the patient in a hard, armless chair and test the following maneuvers:

1. Sitting balance
0 = Leans or slides in chair
1 = Steady, safe

2. Arising
0 = Unable without help
1 = Able but uses arm to help
2 = Able without use of arms

3. Attempts to arise
0 = Unable without help
1 = Able but requires more than one attempt
2 = Able to arise with one attempt

4. Immediate standing balance (first 5 seconds)
0 = Unsteady (staggers, moves feet, marked trunk sway)
1 = Steady but uses walker or cane or grabs other object for support
2 = Steady without walker, cane, or other support

5. Standing balance
0 = Unsteady
1 = Steady but wide stance (medial heels more than 4" apart) or uses walker, cane, or other support
2 = Narrow stance without support

6. Nudge (Patient at maximum position with feet as close together as possible. Examiner pushes lightly on patient's sternum with palm of hand three times.)
0 = Begins to fall
1 = Staggers, grabs, but catches self
2 = Steady

7. Eyes closed (at maximum position, as in number 6)
0 = Unsteady
1 = Steady

8. Turn 360 degrees
0 = Discontinuous steps
1 = Continuous steps
0 = Unsteady (grabs, staggers)
1 = Steady

9. Sit down
0 = Unsafe (misjudged distance, falls into chair)
1 = Uses arms or not a smooth motion
2 = Safe, smooth motion

_____ /16   **BALANCE SCORE**

(continued)

CHARTING GUIDE

Tinetti Balance and Gait Evaluation (continued)

GAIT

Instructions: Patient stands with examiner. He then walks down hallway or across room, first at his usual pace, then back at a rapid but safe pace (using usual walking aid, such as walker or cane).

10. Initiation of gait (immediately after told to go)
0 = Any hesitancy or multiple attempts to start
1 = No hesitancy

11. Step length and height (right foot swing)
0 = Does not pass left stance foot with step
1 = Passes left stance foot
0 = Right foot does not clear floor completely with step
1 = Right foot completely clears floor

12. Step length ad height (left foot swing)
0 = Does not pass right stance foot with step
1 = Passes right stance foot
0 = Left foot does not clear floor completely with step
1 = Left foot completely clears floor

13. Step symmetry
0 = Right and left step length not equal (estimate)
1 = Right and left step length appear equal

14. Step continuity
0 = Stopping or discontinuity between steps
1 = Steps appear continuous

15. Path (Estimated in relation to floor tiles 12" wide. Observe excursion of one foot over about 10' of course.)
0 = Marked deviation
1 = Mild to moderate deviation or uses a walking aid
2 = Straight without walking aid

16. Trunk
0 = Marked sway or uses walking aid
1 = No sway but flexes knees or back or spreads arms out while walking
2 = No sway, no flexion, no use of arms, and no walking aid

17. Walk stance
0 = Heels apart
1 = Heels almost touching while walking

____ /12 **GAIT SCORE**

____ /28 **TOTAL MOBILITY SCORE (BALANCE AND GAIT)**

Adapted with permission from Galindo, D.J., et al. "Gait Training and Falls in the Elderly," *Journal of Gerontological Nursing* 21(6):15-16, June 1995.

any adverse reactions to medications. Certain medications are known to increase the risk of falls for various reasons. (See *Medications associated with falls.*)

Assess the patient's knowledge of each medication (or his caregiver's knowledge, if appropriate). Many patients who fail to comply with their medication regimen do so unintentionally; they simple don't know or understand how to take the medication correctly. You need to be aware of such knowledge deficits if your interventions are to be effective.

Medical devices. Indwelling urinary catheters, I.V. tubes and poles, and feeding tubes all must be considered risk factors for falls. As with medications, these devices are sometimes unavoidable in treating elderly people, but they should be discontinued as soon as possible.

When used in an acute care setting, all these devices increase the risk of falls. When the patient is trying to move around, I.V. tubes and poles can lead to trips, and spills from urine drainage bags can lead to slips. A nasogastric tube can interfere with a patient's vision, particularly if it's secured in a way that won't allow him to wear his eyeglasses. Indwelling catheters can lead to urinary tract infections or to incontinence for a time after removal, both of which may increase the risk of falls when the patient tries to get to the bathroom.

Restraints. The use of physical restraints to prevent falls has been the subject of considerable debate. Although preventing falls is important, recent studies have shown that restraints do not prevent serious injuries and can actually do more harm than good. Restraining an elderly person to a bed or chair puts him at risk for a host of complications, including muscle weakness and atrophy, bone demineralization, loss of balance, pressure ulcers, orthostatic hypotension, hypostatic pneumonia, urine retention, incontinence, constipation, decreased appetite, agitation, delirium, and depression. And the use of restraints often exacerbates or compounds the problem for which the person was originally restrained, such as agitation or restlessness. The risk of falling then increases rather than decreases, creating additional risk factors.

Of course, restraints are necessary at times, but they should be used only when all other alternatives have been tried and have failed. In many cases, the cause of agitated behavior is an unmet basic need, such as toileting or pain relief. Determining the cause of the patient's behavior can lead to a simple alternative measure, such as changing his position, providing a bedpan, or administering an analgesic. Information on alternatives to restraints is widely available. If you can't avoid using restraints, make sure you take appropriate steps to decrease the patient's risk of complications and further falls.

Medications associated with falls

This chart highlights some classes of drugs that are commonly prescribed for elderly patients and the possible adverse effects of each that may increase a patient's risk of falling.

DRUG CLASS	ADVERSE EFFECTS
Diuretics	Hypovolemia
	Orthostatic hypotension
	Electrolyte imbalance
	Urinary incontinence
Antihypertensives	Hypotension
Tricyclic antidepressants	Orthostatic hypotension
Antipsychotics	Orthostatic hypotension
	Muscle rigidity
	Sedation
Benzodiazepines and antihistamines	Excessive sedation
	Confusion
	Paradoxical agitation
	Loss of balance
Narcotics	Hypotension
	Sedation
	Motor incoordination
	Agitation
Hypnotics	Excessive sedation
	Ataxia
	Poor balance
	Confusion
	Paradoxical agitation
Antidiabetic drugs	Acute hypoglycemia
Alcohol	Intoxication
	Motor incoordination
	Agitation
	Sedation
	Confusion

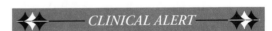

CLINICAL ALERT

The Joint Commission on Accreditation of Healthcare Organizations and the federal government require health care professionals in long-term care facilities to use restraints judiciously — only as a last resort — and to closely monitor a patient when restraints are used.

Delirium. A common problem in hospitalized elderly patients, delirium is associated with an increase in mortality rate, length of hospital stay, nursing home placement, and risk for falls. Like repeated falls, delirium can signal the onset of an acute illness or the exacerbation of a chronic condition (in which case, it would be considered an intrinsic factor).

Medications are the most common cause of iatrogenic delirium. The most common offenders include, but are not limited to, psychotropic drugs and benzodiazepines, antihistamines (including H_2-receptor antagonists), anticholinergics and drugs with anticholinergic adverse effects, narcotics and hypnotics, antibiotics, and nonsteroidal anti-inflammatory drugs. Delirium can also result from rapid withdrawal from benzodiazepines or alcohol. Other non-drug-related causes of delirium include dehydration and, according to one study, the stress of hospitalization itself.

Care planning

Encourage your elderly patient or the person providing or managing his care (nurse, family member, or significant other) to take an active part in developing the care plan. Prioritize problems based on baseline and assessment data, and then negotiate solutions with the patient to obtain the best possible outcomes. Give the patient the teaching handout, *Coping with falls.*

You'll need to update your care plans continually as you review risk factors and outcomes of interventions. Be sure to document interventions or techniques that work well and that motivate and reassure both the patient and the caregiver.

Nursing interventions

After you've identified risk factors, you'll need to rank them according to priority, starting with those requiring the most immediate intervention and those easiest to reduce or eliminate. Address medical issues first to rule out or treat underlying disorders. Next, review baseline information to determine which risks are new and which have been present for some time. Try to ascertain from the data how long-standing risks were addressed previously, what the outcomes were, and whether or not further or different interventions are needed.

Dealing with medical conditions

Make sure that all assessment data are recorded and reported. Investigate and follow up on new complaints, particularly any evidence or reports of falls or a change in mental status.

Minimizing sensory deficits

Ensure that eyeglasses and hearing aids are clean, in working order, and within the patient's reach. Check the patient's ears for impacted cerumen, and take the necessary steps to remove it. Consult with an ophthalmologist or audiologist as necessary.

Make sure lighting is bright enough to compensate for visual deficits, without producing a glare. Venetian blinds or sheer curtains on windows can help. See that floors and furniture are not highly polished. Install nightlights in the bedroom and bathroom, and place light switches where the patient can reach them without having to walk through the dark. Also provide a bright flashlight.

Monitoring nutrition

The importance of adequate nutrition and fluids cannot be overemphasized. Because the sensation of thirst is often diminished or absent in the elderly, you can't rely on it to signal the need to increase fluids when dehydration is a threat. Unless medically contraindicated, offer your elderly patient fluids frequently. The patient may tolerate small, frequent meals better than large meals. Also, encourage the patient to add more high-fiber foods, such as fruits and vegetables, to his diet.

Begin alternative methods of nutrition early for people who can't take oral nutrition for any length of time, especially elderly trauma patients. Alert the social worker if the patient isn't eating properly because of financial constraints or an inability to shop for or prepare food.

Coping with falls

Dear Patient:

If you fall, don't panic. Roll onto your stomach, turning your head in the direction of the roll. If you feel sharp pain, don't move. Call for help.

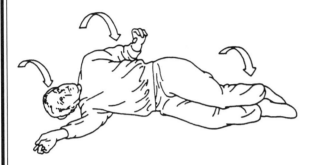

If you're free of pain, crawl to the nearest chair or sofa. Place both hands on the seat, bending slightly forward so that your hands support your weight.

Now, bend one knee, and place your foot flat on the floor. Then push yourself up with your hands while swiveling to sit in the chair. After you've rested a few minutes, call a family member or your doctor for help.

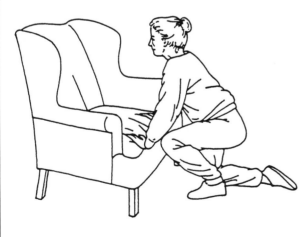

Preventing a fall

Take special care to avoid falls. Some falls result from dizziness, poor coordination, or muscle weakness. But most result from poor safety practices at home. Follow these guidelines to reduce your risk of falls.

Provide good lighting

● Place light switches or lamps near the entrance to each room, at the top and bottom of all stairways, and next to your bed.
● Replace low-wattage light bulbs with 75- or 100-watt bulbs.
● Use nightlights in your bedroom and bathroom.
● Outline the edges of steps with brightly colored paint or tape so they'll be easier to see.

Adapt your home

● Remove clutter, especially in hallways and on stairs. Arrange furniture to provide clear pathways, and secure electrical cords.
● Install handrails on both sides of all stairways as well as near the tub and toilet.
● Place frequently used clothing and other items where you can reach them easily. Avoid climbing up on stepladders or chairs for items out of your reach.

Assisting with elimination

If the elderly person lives at home, make sure that bathroom facilities are in working order and accessible. Help the patient obtain a raised toilet seat and grab bars, if needed, and encourage regular routines to facilitate elimination. In the hospital or nursing home, try to maintain elimination patterns that the person followed at home, such as getting up at 6 a.m., having a cup of coffee, and then going to the bathroom.

Take a proactive approach to toileting. Because most falls occur during the busiest times of the day and are related to elimination, try to take patients who need help with toileting to the bathroom before the busy periods. Patients who are receiving diuretics or I.V. hydration may need to go to the bathroom frequently, especially at night. If you think a patient is going too frequently (for instance, if he just got off the commode and feels he needs to go again), have him evaluated for a urinary tract infection.

Keep a commode close to the bedside and lower the bed rail to eliminate episodes of climbing over bed rails and subsequent incontinence. Teach the patient safe ways to transfer from bed to chair and from bed to commode, and have him practice as often as necessary.

Encourage the patient to use the bathroom whenever possible to provide comfort and privacy. The bathroom should be conveniently located and well lit and have all necessary items within easy reach. A portable commode is preferable to a bedpan when the patient is not allowed to ambulate. If a patient appears to be constipated or is receiving drugs that are constipating, begin a bowel elimination program and continue it until a regular pattern is established.

Assisting with gait and balance

Obtain a physical therapy evaluation for a patient who has gait and balance problems or who has been on bed rest for more than 3 days (except for a patient with long-standing problems that have been addressed who shows no evidence of deterioration). Trauma patients and others who require extended bed rest should get physical therapy at the bedside as soon as they are medically stable. Try to get such patients out of bed early and often.

To help decrease the incidence of orthostatic hypotension and balance disorders, use the stand-and-pivot method of transferring patients between the chair and bed whenever possible. Weight-bearing, even for a very short time, promotes peripheral circulation and can slow down the bone demineralization that takes place in bedridden elderly patients. Evaluate transferring procedures frequently. Encourage the patient to ambulate whenever possible, and monitor his safety when he does. Examine the patient's feet regularly and consult a podiatrist if you detect any problems.

In the nursing home and at home, encourage elderly people to participate in activities that promote mobility and functional independence. Many senior centers and nursing homes have walkers clubs or exercise groups to provide socialization and the incentive to be active.

Eliminating environmental hazards

For elderly people living in the community, local visiting nurse associations, hospitals, or health or fire departments can arrange for home safety checks to be performed. They can also teach family members or other caregivers how to check for and eliminate hazards in the home.

If you're doing a home safety check, look for the following:
- Are frequently used objects placed within functional reach of the elderly person? (Objects used infrequently should be put away and retrieved by someone other than the patient whenever they're needed.)
- Are pots and pans and other kitchen equipment light enough so that an older person can handle them easily even when they contain food?
- Are assistive devices for housekeeping, personal hygiene, and dressing readily available? And has the patient been taught how to use them properly?
- Is lighting adequate?
- Have throw rugs been removed and loose tiles or floor boards repaired?
- Do stairways have good indirect or diffused lighting and a secure handrail? If stairs are uneven,

in poor repair, or very steep, see that they're repaired or ensure that the older person doesn't use them. (You'll have to make other arrangements for getting the person to different levels of the house.)

● Is the floor free of cords and wires and small objects that the older person could trip over? (Pets and small children should also be kept out of the way when older people are moving about.)

● Is furniture arranged so that the older person can see it clearly, and is it then left in place? If a piece of furniture is hard to distinguish from its surroundings, place an item of contrasting color on it — for example, a colorful throw over the back of a chair that blends into the wallpaper.

In the hospital and nursing home, take the following steps:

● Keep rooms as free of clutter as possible, and see that frequently used items are kept within functional reach.

● Place call bells within reach, on a surface of contrasting color, with a brightly colored dot on the button. (Too often, a white call bell is placed on a white sheet, making it difficult for the patient to find.)

● Arrange telephone wires, call bell cords, tubing, poles, and other equipment so they're not in the patient's way when he's getting out of bed.

● Keep beds in the lowest position, with the wheels locked or removed.

● Keep bathroom lights on at night to help the patient find his way there in a hurry.

● Orient new patients to their surroundings thoroughly and repeatedly if necessary. Older people take longer to process information and may have a hard time absorbing a lot of information at one time. Write down information or make signs or draw pictures as reminders, if necessary.

● Advise the patient not to wear loose or long clothing that could catch on his heels or on doors or other objects.

● Make sure footwear fits properly, fully surrounds the foot (no open-back shoes or slippers), and has slip-resistant soles. Suggest sneakers, crepe-soled shoes, or slippers with nonskid treads for walking on tile floors or similar surfaces. For people whose step height is poor or who have a shuffling gait, leather-soled shoes are more suitable because they allow some gliding across floor surfaces. A physical or occupational therapist can suggest proper footwear if necessary.

● Inspect assistive devices to ensure that they're in good working order and that no parts, such as rubber tips, are missing. Make sure that each device is the proper size for the patient and that the patient is using it correctly. A physical or occupational therapist can help make these determinations.

Dealing with alcohol abuse

Confronting a person who abuses alcohol is a difficult task that requires all available resources. The elderly person or the family may deny that he has a problem or maintain that drinking is not important in an older person. Remember to address underlying issues, such as loneliness, in drawing up the plan of care.

Be alert for signs and symptoms of alcohol withdrawal, and be supportive and nonjudgmental in caring for the patient. Inform the patient and his family about available support services. Monitor medication use carefully for adverse effects. (Alcoholism may have caused decreased hepatic function, which impairs drug metabolism.)

Reducing iatrogenic risk factors

If you detect a change in a patient's mental status, review his medications at once. Be aware of drugs that have a high incidence of adverse effects or drug interactions in the elderly, and become familiar with suggested dosages and common adverse effects.

Make sure invasive treatments and devices are discontinued as soon as possible, and begin ambulation early to help reduce the incidence of delirium and deconditioning. If the patient becomes agitated or restless, look for causes before attempting to treat these symptoms with either drugs or physical restraints. First address the patient's basic needs: pain relief, toileting, food and fluids, warmth and comfort, activity (such as walking), increased or decreased stimulation, and reorientation. Watch closely for signs of pain, even if the patient denies having it; a delirious or demented person can't always verbalize his needs. If you can determine what's causing the patient's delirium, you can treat it and thus reduce the risk of falls as well.

Handling restraints

If a person's condition requires the use of restraints, use a device that provides the desired effect with the least restriction. Four-point restraints are painful, demoralizing, and likely to cause injuries, so try every alternative before using them. A rollbelt is a good choice for someone who must remain in bed, but it must be applied correctly to be effective. This device allows the person to roll freely from side to side but prevents him from climbing out of bed. By allowing some degree of movement, it decreases agitation, the adverse effects of immobility, and the risk of falls.

Monitor patients in restraints carefully and frequently. Perform toileting, turning, and other routine care as you did before. For example, if you took a patient to the bathroom every 90 minutes before he was restrained, continue that schedule. Because a restrained person often feels that he's being punished and abandoned, offer frequent reassurances, encouragement, and explanations.

Patient teaching

Preventing falls is everyone's business. If you care for elderly people in the community, teach the patients and their families how to perform routine safety checks and how to monitor for risk factors. Then review this information with them routinely. If you're a visiting nurse, make risk assessment a regular part of home visits.

If you work in a nursing home or in a subacute or acute care facility, make sure all staff members know how to identify risk factors and how to intervene appropriately. Develop and implement protocols for preventing falls, and be creative in formulating interventions.

Evaluation

You'll be able to determine the effectiveness of your fall prevention program primarily by monitoring the incidence of falls and noting trends and patterns through a review of incident reports. The reports will reveal areas that need to be reviewed or improved. Also encourage primary caregivers to evaluate the effectiveness of prevention measures and to continually look for ways to further reduce or eliminate risks.

Keep in mind that the benefits of prevention — for patients, family, staff members, and the health care system as a whole — far outweigh the costs in money, time, and effort.

6

Managing ear and eye problems

As a person ages, sensory capabilities — hearing, vision, touch, taste, and smell — deteriorate. Hearing and vision losses are most upsetting, because they directly affect the ability to perform activities of daily living (ADLs), threaten bodily safety, and distort communication.

The major forms of hearing loss are classified as *conductive loss* (interrupted passage of sound from the external ear to the junction of the stapes and oval windows) and *sensorineural loss* (impaired cochlear or acoustic [eighth cranial] nerve dysfunction, causing failure of sound impulse transmission within the inner ear or brain). Common age-related conductive losses include external blockage resulting from cerumen (wax) accumulation and otosclerosis, a slow stiffening of the tiny bones (ossicles) in the inner ear.

The most common sensorineural loss, *presbycusis,* affects the inner ear and retrocochlear area. It begins with the loss of high-frequency sounds and may progress to middle and low frequencies; degeneration of vestibular structures and atrophy of the cochlea and organ of Corti also occur.

Age-related vision changes are first noticed in the fifth decade of life. During the early to mid-forties, presbyopia, the inability to focus properly, causes most middle-aged adults to need corrective eyeglasses. The visual field narrows, reducing peripheral vision. The iris loses elasticity and responds less efficiently to light and dark. The lens yellows, making it difficult for the older adult to distinguish low tones of blue, green, and violet. Floaters (bits of debris or condensation) accumulate in the vitreous humor and float across the visual field. Intraocular fluid reabsorption loses efficiency, increasing intraocular pressure and the risk of glaucoma. A white circle (arcus senilus) may develop around the periphery of the cornea.

Common vision problems discussed in this chapter include *cataracts,* opacities that develop in the lens and further cloud the vision; *dry eyes,* which result from diminished lacrimal gland secretions; *entropion* and *ectropion,* or inversion and eversion of the eyelids, which cause irritation and poor drainage of tears through the nasolacrimal system; *glaucoma,* marked by high intraocular pressure (IOP) that damages the optic nerve; and *macular degeneration,* which results from hardening of retinal arteries.

Because hearing and vision loss in an older person can interfere significantly with individual pursuits and social interactions, you must periodically assess each older patient thoroughly to rule out conditions that can be treated by surgery or medication. In this chapter you'll also learn appropriate interventions to mitigate or restore these deficits.

CERUMEN IMPACTION

A frequently overlooked cause of hearing loss in older people, cerumen impaction is easily treatable.

However, most older adults who have the condition don't realize that their hearing is reduced and don't seek treatment. Such persons may be inappropriately labeled as "confused" or "uncooperative" when they misinterpret spoken instructions or respond improperly. In some cases, the cerumen causes sudden tinnitus and hearing loss. Impacted cerumen may be rock hard; in men, it also may contain a generous amount of exfoliated hair.

Causes

Cerumen is produced by the ceruminous glands that line the outer two-thirds of the external ear canal. Cerumen functions to intercept small particles that find their way into the ear canal and to prevent them from reaching the tympanic membrane, where they might cause irritation. In older people, the keratin component of cerumen is increased, making it thicker and liable to form a blockage.

Assessment findings

The patient may complain of hearing loss or a feeling of fullness in the ear. The blockage is usually visible on inspection of the ear canal. If the blockage occurs in the medial portion of the canal, the doctor may insert instruments, such as cotton-tipped applicators, into the canal to try to dislodge it.

Treatment

Gentle removal of the blockage is usually all that's required. The doctor may use a cerumen spoon and aural speculum for good visualization. Because the skin of the external canal is easily traumatized and sensitive to manipulation, the doctor may instead order application of a cerumen-softening agent for several days to a week, followed by irrigation. If an infection is suspected, the softening agent may contain an antibiotic solution. Irrigation is contraindicated if the tympanic membrane is perforated, because it may cause an infection.

Complications

As with other forms of hearing loss, blockage-related loss can lead to social isolation, depression, inappropriate acting out, and paranoia. Older adults with hearing loss may think that people around them are mumbling or deliberately excluding them from conversations. The hearing impairment may cause older adults to become labeled as confused.

Nursing interventions

● Inspect the older person's ear canals during initial physical examination and periodically thereafter.
● Administer eardrops to soften the blockage as ordered, and tell the patient to lie on his side for 5 to 10 minutes after instillation to allow the medication to travel down into the ear canal.
● Perform irrigation as ordered, taking care not to direct the stream of liquid directly at the canal.

Patient teaching

● Warn your patient not to insert anything into the ear to avoid the risk of perforating the eardrum and subsequent infection.
● Encourage regular ear examinations, and tell the patient to report any changes in hearing acuity.
● Explain that although loss of hearing often occurs with advancing age, it is often treatable and not something to be ashamed of.

OTOSCLEROSIS

The most common cause of conductive hearing loss among older adults, otosclerosis is the slow formation of spongy bone in the otic capsule, particularly at the oval window. This otosclerotic bone growth eventually causes the footplate of the stapes to become fixed in position, disrupting the conduction of vibrations from the tympanic membrane to the cochlea. Otosclerosis occurs in at least 10% of whites, is twice as common in women as in men, and usually begins between ages 15 and 50. With surgery, the prognosis is good.

Causes

Otosclerosis may result from a genetic factor transmitted as an autosomal dominant trait. Many people who have this disorder report a family history of hearing loss (excluding presbycusis).

Assessment findings

Carefully assess and document your patient's ability to hear (see *Assessing hearing loss*). The patient may report a history of gradual hearing loss in one ear, which may have progressed to both ears, without middle ear infection. He may also describe tinnitus and the ability to hear a conversation better in a noisy environment than in a quiet one (paracusis of Willis).

Otoscopic examination usually reveals a tympanic membrane that appears normal. Occasionally, however, a faint pink blush may be seen through the membrane from the vascularity of the active otosclerotic bone.

Diagnostic tests

In otosclerosis, the Rinne test demonstrates that a bone-conducted tone is heard longer than an air-conducted tone (normally, the reverse is true). As otosclerosis progresses, bone conduction also deteriorates. Weber's test detects sound lateralizing to the more damaged ear. Audiometric testing reveals hearing loss, ranging from 60 dB in early stages to total loss as the disease advances. (See *Reviewing Weber's and Rinne tests,* page 108.)

Treatment

In most cases, treatment consists of stapedectomy (removal of the stapes) and insertion of a prosthesis to restore partial or total hearing. This procedure is performed on one ear at a time, beginning with the ear that has sustained greater damage. Postoperative treatment includes hospitalization for 2 to 3 days and antibiotics to prevent infection. Other surgical procedures include fenestration and stapes mobilization; all require normal cochlear function.

Sometimes further hearing loss can be prevented by giving the patient sodium fluoride and calcium supplements to promote recalcification and arrest spongy bone formation. Hearing aids may be an acceptable alternative and enable the patient to hear conversation in normal surroundings.

Complications

Unilateral at first, this disorder may advance to bilateral conductive hearing loss.

Assessing hearing loss

Your general observations of your patient's ability to hear form an important part of your initial assessment. Be sure to watch for and document these specific characteristics.
● Hears well enough to respond to questions
● Hard of hearing; wears hearing aid; speaker must speak loudly into left or right ear
● Deaf; reads lips or uses sign language.

Nursing interventions

● Address your patient's questions, encourage him to discuss his concerns about hearing loss, and offer reassurance when appropriate.
● If the patient has trouble understanding procedures and treatments because of hearing loss, give clear, concise explanations. Provide written materials, if possible. Face the patient when speaking; enunciate clearly, slowly, and in a normal tone; give the patient time to grasp what you've said. Supply a pencil and paper to aid communication, and alert the staff to the communication problem.
● Follow the doctor's orders regarding specific postoperative positioning of the patient on the unaffected side to prevent graft displacement or on the affected side to facilitate drainage. Some doctors allow any position that doesn't cause vertigo.
● After surgery, keep the bed's side rails raised and help the patient walk. Administer prescribed medication for pain and assess the patient's response. Meperidine may be given at first, followed by milder analgesics.

Patient teaching

For a patient undergoing surgery, provide preoperative and postoperative teaching.
● After surgery, advise the patient to move slowly to prevent vertigo.
● Advise the patient to avoid any activities that provoke dizziness, such as straining, bending, or heavy lifting, and to avoid contact with anyone who has an upper respiratory tract infection.

Reviewing Weber's and Rinne tests

Tell your patient that the two most common tests used to detect hearing loss and provide preliminary information about its type are Weber's test and the Rinne test. Explain that you'll be performing these tests, using a tuning fork.

Weber's test

Inform your patient that this test determines whether he hears the tone of the tuning fork in only one ear. In this test you'll place the base of a vibrating tuning fork at the vertex of his head or midline on his forehead (as shown below). Alternative sites include the bridge of the nose, the central incisors, or the mandibular symphysis.

TUNING FORK POSITION FOR WEBER'S TEST

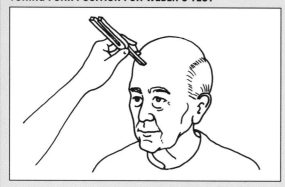

Does the patient hear the tone equally well in both ears? If he does, he has normal hearing. But if the tone is louder in one ear, he may have conductive hearing loss in that ear. This is because the tone lateralizes to the affected ear through bone conduction, while background noise prevents similar detection by the unaffected ear.

Although this test is inconclusive for sensorineural hearing loss, tell the patient that if he has one normal ear, and he hears the tone equally or more loudly in that ear, he may have sensorineural hearing loss in the other ear.

The Rinne test

Inform your patient that this test evaluates his ability to hear sounds through bone conduction and air conduction. This time, you'll place the vibrating tuning fork against his mastoid process and hold it there until he no longer hears the tone (shown at top of next column).

FIRST TUNING FORK POSITION FOR THE RINNE TEST

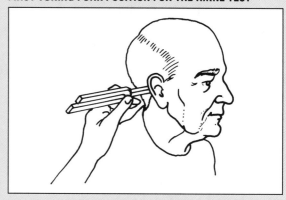

This tests bone conduction. Next, you'll quickly move the vibrating tuning fork to a position in front of his ear canal, but not touching his auricle (as shown below) until he no longer hears the tone. This tests air conduction. Then you'll repeat the test on his other ear.

SECOND TUNING FORK POSITION FOR THE RINNE TEST

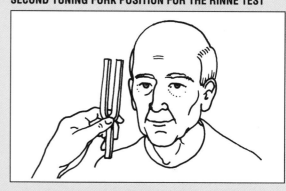

Explain that if his hearing is normal, he'll hear the air-conducted tone twice as long as the bone-conducted tone. But if he hears the bone-conducted tone for as long as he hears the air-conducted tone or longer, he may have conductive hearing loss. Explain that a positive test result can also indicate sensorineural hearing loss because the inner ear's perception of sound waves by air or bone conduction is compromised.

- Teach the patient and a family member how to change the external ear dressing (eye or gauze pad) and care for the incision. Stress the importance of protecting the ears against cold.
- Emphasize the need to complete the prescribed antibiotic regimen and to return for scheduled follow-up care, which includes removing the packing. Point out that hearing may be masked by packing and dressing as well as by swelling from the operation. Inform the patient that hearing may not be noticeably improved until 1 to 4 weeks after surgery.
- Before discharge, instruct the patient to avoid loud noises and sudden pressure changes, such as those that occur while diving or flying, until healing is complete (usually within 6 months). Advise him against blowing his nose for at least 1 week to prevent bacteria-contaminated air from entering the eustachian tubes.
- Advise the patient not to wet his head while showering, and to avoid washing his hair for 2 weeks. (If this is unacceptable, suggest that dry shampoo can be used as long as none is allowed to enter the ears.) Then, for the next 4 weeks, he should avoid getting water in his ears when washing his hair. Tell him not to swim for 6 weeks.
- Instruct the patient not to strain while defecating, and to avoid constipation.

PRESBYCUSIS

Also known as sensorineural, senile, or progressive hearing loss, presbycusis is marked by bilateral, symmetrical dysfunction of the sensory elements (hair cells) or neural structures (cochlear nerve fibers). The most common type of hearing loss in older people, it affects both men and women (men are usually more impaired than women of the same age). Sensorineural loss usually affects high-frequency sounds, but this in itself doesn't interfere with understanding speech until the disorder affects those high frequencies involved in consonant discrimination.

Four types of presbycusis are known: sensory, neural, metabolic, and cochlear. *Sensory presbycusis* begins in middle age and progresses slowly. A loss of cochlear neurons occurs, which parallels loss in the organ of Corti.

In *neural presbycusis,* which develops later in life, loss of cochlear neurons occurs without loss in the organ of Corti. Neural presbycusis progresses rapidly and may be accompanied by other signs of central nervous system decline, including intellectual deterioration, memory loss, and loss of motor coordination. *Metabolic presbycusis* tends to run in families, usually begins in middle age, and progresses slowly. *Cochlear conductive presbycusis* also starts in middle age and is related to alterations in the motion mechanism of the cochlear duct.

Causes

Although the exact cause is unknown, the incidence of sensorineural hearing loss rises with age. Noise exposure, high-cholesterol diet, hypertension, metabolic factors, and heredity are contributing factors. Vascular lesions resulting in hypoperfusion may aggravate age-related changes in the ear and central nervous system.

Assessment findings

The patient complains of difficulty in understanding people with high-pitched voices, such as women and young children. He also complains of difficulty in hearing conversations in large groups or in locations where there is a lot of background noise.

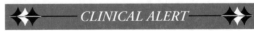

CLINICAL ALERT

Instead of recognizing and acknowledging his hearing loss, the person with sensorineural hearing loss often feels that people are mumbling.

Diagnostic tests

The definitive test for sensorineural hearing loss is pure tone audiometry, sometimes called an audiogram. The audiogram can help identify the type of sensorineural hearing loss.

Sensory presbycusis produces an abrupt loss of high-frequency sound, but preserves good word discrimination. Neural presbycusis produces a loss of high-frequency sound and poor word discrimination. Metabolic presbycusis produces a flat threshold of audibility with normal speech discrimination until speech volume falls below 50 dB. Cochlear conductive presbycusis produces a bilaterally symmetrical, descending threshold of audibility; speech discrimination is better at steeper thresholds.

Treatment

Treatment for sensorineural hearing loss usually involves a hearing aid. Hearing aids are available in different forms: behind-the-ear aid, in-the-ear aid, eyeglass hearing aid, and body hearing aid.

The behind-the-ear aid, used for mild to moderate hearing loss, is easy to conceal, comfortable to wear, and has no long wires. It's also durable, and some models are equipped with a telephone pickup device. Disadvantages include the close proximity of the microphone to the receiver, which causes feedback and limits the amount of amplification.

The in-the-ear aid fits directly into the ear canal and is supported by the outer ear. It's lightweight, easy to conceal, and lacks external wires. But it's suitable only for mild hearing loss because it provides less amplification than other aids. It also allows some sound distortion and is less durable. Its small size may make it difficult to operate for someone who has stiff fingers or arms.

The eyeglass aid also is used for mild to moderate hearing loss. It's similar to a behind-the-ear aid, except that the hearing unit is built into the arm of an eyeglass frame. The frame can carry a signal from one ear to the other, so it's good for amplification in both ears. Bone-conduction hearing aids are also available in the eyeglass style. However, this type of hearing aid requires eyeglasses with bulky, often unattractive, frames. If the aid or frame breaks, the wearer may be without both hearing aid and glasses, unless he keeps a second pair of glasses for such emergencies.

In the body aid, the microphone, amplifier, and battery lie in a single case, which attaches to clothing or is carried in a pocket. The external receiver attaches directly to the earmold and connects to the amplifier by a long wire. The most powerful type, this aid is usually used for severe hearing loss. It allows the wearer to hear wide ranges of amplification, and the controls are easier to adjust than those of other aids. Since the receiver and microphone are separated, there's little or no acoustical feedback. Some models also have variable tone control. This type of aid is usually less expensive than others.

People who have become profoundly deaf but have no associated medical problems may benefit from a cochlear implant, a surgically inserted device that stimulates the auditory nerve. The device consists of an external microphone, a transmitter, and an implanted receiver. The transmitter receives signals from the microphone, then sends them to the receiver located near the auditory nerve. The signals travel along an implanted wire to the nerve.

Complications

As with other forms of hearing loss, sensorineural hearing loss can cause embarrassment and may lead to withdrawal from social activities. Profound isolation can have both psychological and physical effects.

Nursing interventions

● When speaking to a patient with hearing loss, stand directly in front of him, with the light on your face, and speak slowly and distinctly in a low tone. Avoid shouting. When approaching the patient, move to within his visual range and elicit his attention by raising your arm or waving; touching him may be unnecessarily startling.
● Carefully explain all diagnostic tests and hospital procedures. The patient may depend totally on visual clues, so make sure he's in an area where he can observe unit activities and see people approaching.
● Provide emotional support and encouragement if the patient is learning how to use a hearing aid. Be sure other caregivers are aware of the patient's handicap and his established method of communication (such as writing on a pad, or signing).

Patient teaching

● Teach the patient how to care for his hearing aid and give him the handout, *Using and caring for your hearing aid,* pages 111 to 113.

(Text continued on page 114.)

TEACHING AID

Using and caring for your hearing aid

Dear Patient:

Adjusting to your hearing aid takes patience, practice, and hours of wear. Several weeks or even several months may pass before you feel completely comfortable. But don't be discouraged. Once you learn how, inserting, removing, and caring for your hearing aid will become just another daily routine, like brushing your teeth. And you'll be glad that you made the effort when you notice how much your hearing improves.

The guidelines below will help you learn to use and care for your hearing aid, as well as ease the period of adjustment.

Inserting your hearing aid

First, wash your hands. Make sure that the hearing aid is turned off and the volume is turned all the way down.

Next, examine the earmold to determine whether it's for the right or left ear. Now look in the mirror and line up the parts of the earmold with the corresponding parts of your external ear. Then, rotate the earmold slightly forward, and insert the canal portion.

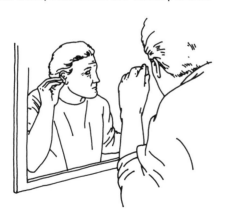

Gently push the earmold into the ear while rotating it backward. Adjust the folds of your ear over the earmold, if necessary. The earmold should fit snugly and comfortably.

After inserting the earmold, adjust other parts of the hearing aid as needed. For example, place a behind-the-ear hearing aid over your ear and clip a body aid to your shirt pocket, undergarment, or hearing-aid harness carrier.

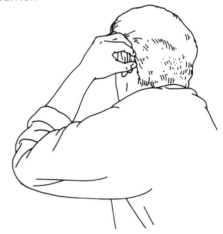

Finally, set the switch to the *on* position and slowly turn the volume halfway up. Adjust the volume as necessary.

Removing your hearing aid

First, set the switch to the *off* position and lower the volume. Then, looking in the mirror, remove the earmold by rotating it forward and pulling outward. Next, remove or unclip the hearing-aid case. After removal, store the hearing aid in a safe place. If possible, use the same place each time.

(continued)

Using and caring for your hearing aid (continued)

Adjusting to your hearing aid
To help ease your period of adjustment, follow the guidelines below:
● Wear your hearing aid only for short periods at first. For example, wear it for 15 minutes the first 2 days, then increase your time 30 minutes each day until you feel completely comfortable. If you get nervous or tired, turn off the aid and rest for awhile.
● Once you're comfortable wearing the aid, wear it as much as possible.
● Don't turn the volume up too high. This distorts sound and also may cause feedback, a whistling or squealing noise. (These sounds may also signal a loose-fitting earmold.)
● Try to block out background sounds when listening to conversations. This takes practice. If the background noise gets too annoying, turn down the volume on your hearing aid and watch the speaker's face closely.
● Talk to only one person at a time until you get used to the hearing aid. Experiment to see if you can hold a conversation in difficult situations—for example, with loud music in the background.
● When you're in a large group, sit as close to the speaker as possible.

Cleaning the earmold
Keep the earmold of your hearing aid clean and free of excess wax to prevent infection and keep the aid working efficiently.
● To clean a body aid, first detach the earmold from the receiver. For a behind-the-ear or eyeglass aid, first detach the earmold where its tubing meets the hook of the

hearing-aid case, if possible. Don't remove the earmold if glue or a small metal split ring secures the earmold tubing to the hearing-aid case.
● After detaching the earmold, soak it in a mild soapy solution, then rinse and dry it well. Blow out excess moisture through the earmold opening.
● If the opening is clogged with wax or debris, use a pipe cleaner or toothpick to remove it, but avoid pushing debris into the opening.
● Store the dry, clean earmold in the hearing-aid case.
● If you wear an in-the-ear aid with an unremovable earmold, wipe the earmold with a damp cloth.

Maintaining your hearing aid
● Your hearing aid is a delicate electronic instrument, so avoid wearing it outside for long periods in very hot, humid, or cold weather.
● Never store it near a stove, heater, or on a sunny windowsill.
● Don't wear it in the rain, in the bathtub or shower, during activities that cause excessive perspiration, when using a blow-dryer or hairspray, or when using a vaporizer.
● Never clean or immerse any part except the earmold in water. Don't insert sharp objects into the microphone or receiver opening — only an audiologist or hearing-aid dealer should clean these parts.
● Take care not to drop your hearing aid on a hard surface. Work over a bed or similar soft area when changing batteries or removing the aid from your ear.
● Replace dead batteries with new ones of the

EACHING AID

Using and caring for your hearing aid (continued)

same type. When inserting a battery, first turn off the hearing aid, then match the negative (–) and positive (+) signs. If you use your hearing aid 10 to 12 hours a day, you'll probably need to replace the battery weekly.

● If you won't be using the hearing aid for several days, remove the battery to prevent it from leaking and causing corrosion. Leave the battery case open, storing your hearing aid in an airtight container with a silica-gel packet, especially in humid climates.

● To clean the battery, gently rub it with a sharpened pencil eraser to remove corrosion. If the battery gets damp, dry the contacts with a cotton swab. Store extra batteries in the freezer to lengthen shelf life.

When you have problems

● If you have pain or drainage in your ear — a sign of a skin or cartilage infection, a middle-ear infection, a tumor, or an improperly fitted earmold — call your doctor.

● If you have any questions about wearing, caring for, or maintaining your hearing aid, call your doctor or audiologist.

● If the hearing aid fails to operate, first review instructions in the operator's manual. Or consult the checklist below.

PROBLEM AND POSSIBLE CAUSE	POSSIBLE SOLUTIONS
No sound or weak sound	
● Incorrect battery insertion	● Reinsert battery.
● Dead battery	● Try a new battery.
● Clogged earmold opening	● Unclog the earmold opening.
● Twisted plastic tubing	● Untwist plastic tubing.
● Switch is *off* or on *T* for use with telephone	● Switch to *on* or *M* position.
● Volume not turned high enough	● Turn volume control at least one-half rotation.
Whistling or squealing sound	
● Incorrect earmold insertion	● Reinsert earmold.
● Volume turned too high	● Turn down volume.
● Earmold not securely snapped to a receiver of a body hearing aid. (A whistling sound is normal when the earmold isn't inserted and the hearing aid is turned on. Such whistling indicates that the aid is working and that the battery is inserted correctly.)	● Secure earmold to receiver.

- Teach the family how to improve the patient's understanding of what they're saying.
- Teach the patient the importance of regular hearing evaluations. Stress that hearing loss, although an inconvenience, is often treatable.
- Instruct the patient to maintain a low-cholesterol diet and to avoid loud noises.

CATARACTS

A common cause of gradual vision loss, a cataract is an opacity of the lens or the lens capsule of the eye. Light shining through the cornea is blocked by this opacity, and a blurred image is cast onto the retina. As a result, the brain interprets a hazy image. Cataracts commonly affect both eyes, but each cataract progresses independently. Cataracts are most prevalent in people over age 70. Surgical removal of the cataracts restores vision in about 95% of patients.

Causes
Cataracts are classified by their causes. *Senile cataracts* are believed to develop as a result of chemical changes in lens proteins. *Complicated cataracts* occur secondary to uveitis, glaucoma, retinitis pigmentosa, or retinal detachment, or in the course of a systemic disease, such as diabetes, hypocalcemia, myotonic dystrophy, and exposure to ionizing radiation or infrared rays. Toxic cataracts occur as a result of toxicity from drugs or chemicals such as systemic corticosteroids, phenothiazines, ergot, dinitrophenol, and naphthalene.

Assessment findings
Typically, the person complains of painless, gradual vision loss. He may also report a blinding glare from headlights when driving at night, poor reading vision, and an annoying glare and poor vision in bright sunlight. If he has a central opacity, he may report seeing better in dim light than in bright light. That's because this cataract is nuclear, and as the pupil dilates, the person can see around the opacity.

Inspection with a penlight may reveal a milky white pupil and, with an advanced cataract, a grayish white area behind the pupil.

Diagnostic tests
Indirect ophthalmoscopy reveals a dark area in the normally homogeneous red reflex. Slit-lamp examination confirms the diagnosis of lens opacity. A visual acuity test confirms the degree of vision loss.

Treatment
Cataracts are treated surgically by extracting the opacified lens and implanting an intraocular lens (IOL) to correct the visual deficit. The surgery is usually performed as a same-day or outpatient procedure. *Extracapsular cataract extraction,* the most common procedure, involves removing the anterior lens capsule and cortex and leaving the posterior capsule intact. In this procedure, the surgeon implants a posterior chamber where the patient's own lens has been. *Intracapsular cataract extraction* involves removing the entire lens within the intact capsule by cryoextraction — the moist lens sticks to an extremely cold metal probe for easy and safe removal with gentle traction. After the surgeon removes the lens, he implants an IOL in either the anterior or posterior chamber. Another procedure, called *phacoemulsification,* uses ultrasonic vibrations to disintegrate the opaque lens, which is then aspirated from the capsule.

A patient with an IOL implant may experience improved vision almost immediately. However, the IOL corrects distance vision only; the patient will also need either corrective reading glasses or a corrective contact lens, which can be fitted 4 to 8 weeks after surgery. If the patient did not receive an IOL, he may be given temporary corrective cataract glasses or contact lenses. Then, sometime between 4 and 8 weeks after surgery, he'll have a refraction examination for permanent glasses.

Some patients who have an extracapsular cataract extraction develop a secondary membrane that causes decreased visual acuity in the posterior lens capsule (which has been left intact). This membrane can be removed by the Nd:YAG laser, which cuts an area from the membrane's center, thus restoring vision.

Complications

Without surgery, a cataract eventually involves the entire lens, causing blindness. Possible complications of surgery include loss of vitreous humor (during the procedure), wound dehiscence from loosening sutures, "flattening" of the anterior chamber, iris prolapse into the wound, hyphema, glaucoma, retinal detachment, and infection.

Nursing interventions

Preoperatively, provide a safe environment with bright lighting. Explain all procedures and tests, and encourage your patient to ask questions. Postoperatively, monitor vital signs until the patient recovers from the effects of the anesthetic. Keep the bed's side rails raised, and assist the patient with early ambulation. Apply an eye shield or an eye patch, as ordered.

Patient teaching

Because your patient will be discharged after he recovers from the anesthetic, remind him to return for a checkup the next day. Caution him to avoid activities that increase intraocular pressure, such as straining with coughing, bowel movements, or lifting.

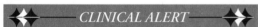

CLINICAL ALERT

Explain to your patient that wearing an eye patch may cause a change in his depth perception.

Review safety precautions with your patient. Advise him to abstain from sex until he receives his doctor's approval. Teach the patient or a family member how to instill ophthalmic ointment or drops. Alert the patient to notify his doctor immediately if he experiences increased eye discharge, sharp eye pain (unrelieved by analgesics), or a deterioration in vision.

DRY EYES

Dry eyes is one of the most common complaints of older adults. The problem can result from a decrease in function of lacrimal glands, which normally produce the tears that lubricate the eyes. Other causes include drugs such as antihypertensives, antihistamines, anticholinergics, and sympatholytics.

The doctor may prescribe artificial tears to lubricate the eyes. Untreated, dry eyes can lead to infection.

Teach the patient or a family member how to instill the eyedrops. (For more information about instilling eye medications, see Chapter 16, *Administering and Monitoring Medications*.) Instruct the patient never to rub his eyes, because this may damage the cornea. Instruct him to report to the doctor any signs of infection or drainage.

ECTROPION AND ENTROPION

The eyes in an older adult sometimes appear to be sunken, and the eyelid turned inward (entropion). In other persons, the eyelid sometimes falls away, taking on the appearance of turning outward (ectropion). Although these conditions are seen in many elderly patients, they are not problematic unless they cause eye irritation.

Causes

Entropion results from a spasm in the lower orbicular muscle of the eyelid margin. This occurs more often in the lower lid, causing the lid to turn inward and abrade its margin against the eyeball. The lashes rub against the cornea with each blink and can cause chronic irritation.

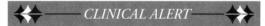

CLINICAL ALERT

In entropion, the fat cushion behind the eye shrinks, causing the eyes to recess into the sockets. Thus, in an elderly patient, sunken eyes may not always indicate dehydration.

Ectropion results from loss of strength of the orbicular muscle — the muscle that squeezes the eyelids shut. When the margin of the lower lid no longer touches the eye, the punctum of the medial lower lid doesn't touch it either, and tears can't drain from the conjunctival sac into the lacrimal sac.

Assessment findings

The patient with *entropion* will complain of a constant sensation that something is lodged in his eye. Inspection reveals the margin of the eyelid turning inward. As the patient blinks, the lashes can be seen stroking the eyeball.

The patient with *ectropion* may complain of excessive tears and of tears draining down his face. His lids may not close when he sleeps, and he may complain of awakening with dry eyes. Inspection reveals eyes that appear sunken, with the lid hanging down from the margin of the eye (that is, where the pink conjunctiva meets the white).

Treatment

Entropion is usually treated surgically. The treatment for ectropion usually focuses on relieving symptoms. If the cornea becomes dry, surgical intervention may be indicated.

Complications

Entropion can result in corneal and conjunctival scarring if not treated. With ectropion, the lid often doesn't close completely during sleep; this can cause corneal drying, secondary abrasions, redness, and irritation.

Nursing interventions

Instruct the patient not to rub his eyes. Use warm compresses to relieve irritation.

Patient teaching

Instruct the patient on the importance of having regular eye checkups. Advise the patient who has excessive tears to carry tissues and blot his eyes, not rub them. Instruct him to report any persistent dryness or itching of the eyes to the doctor.

GLAUCOMA

A group of disorders, glaucoma is characterized by high IOP that damages the optic nerve. Glaucoma may occur as a primary or congenital disease, or it may be secondary to other diseases or conditions.

Primary glaucoma has two forms: open-angle (also known as chronic, simple, or wide-angle) glaucoma and angle-closure (also known as acute or narrow-angle) glaucoma. Open-angle glaucoma is the most common type of glaucoma affecting older adults.

Secondary glaucoma can develop from such conditions as infections, uveitis, injury, surgery, prolonged drug use (such as with corticosteroids), venous occlusion, and diabetes. Sometimes, new blood vessels may form (neovascularization) and block the drainage of aqueous humor.

One of the leading causes of blindness in the United States, glaucoma accounts for about 12% of newly diagnosed cases of blindness. It affects about 2% of Americans over age 40; the incidence is highest among African-Americans. However, early detection and effective treatment contribute to a good prognosis for preserving vision.

Causes

Open-angle glaucoma results from degenerative changes in the trabecular meshwork. These changes block the flow of aqueous humor from the eye, which causes IOP to rise. The result is optic nerve damage. Open-angle glaucoma accounts for about 90% of all cases of glaucoma, and commonly occurs in families.

Angle-closure glaucoma results from reduced outflow of aqueous humor caused by an anatomically narrow angle between the iris and the cornea. This causes IOP to increase suddenly. Attacks of angle-closure glaucoma may be triggered by trauma, pupillary dilation, stress, or any ocular change that pushes the iris forward (a hemorrhage or a swollen lens, for example).

Assessment findings

Because open-angle glaucoma begins insidiously and progresses slowly, the patient may have no symptoms. Later he may complain of a dull headache in the morning, mild aching in the eyes, loss of peripheral vision, the appearance of halos around lights, and reduced visual acuity (especially at night) that's uncorrected by glasses.

Inspection may reveal unilateral eye inflammation, a cloudy cornea, and a moderately dilated pupil that's nonreactive to light. Increased IOP may be discovered by applying gentle fingertip pressure to the patient's closed eyelids; the eyeball resists such pressure.

Diagnostic tests

Tonometry (with an applanation, Schiotz, or pneumatic tonometer) measures IOP and provides a baseline for reference. Normal IOP ranges from 8 to 21 mm Hg. However, patients whose pressure falls within the normal range can develop signs and symptoms of glaucoma, and patients who have abnormally high pressure may have no clinical effects. Slit-lamp examination reveals the effects of glaucoma on the anterior eye structures, including the cornea, iris, and lens. Gonioscopy determines the angle of the eye's anterior chamber, enabling the examiner to distinguish between open-angle and angle-closure glaucoma. The angle is normal in open-angle glaucoma, abnormal in angle-closure glaucoma. In older patients, however, partial closure of the angle may occur, allowing the two forms of glaucoma to coexist.

Ophthalmoscopy facilitates visualization of the fundus. In open-angle glaucoma, cupping of the optic disk may be seen earlier than in angle-closure glaucoma. Perimetry or visual field tests determine the extent of peripheral vision loss, which helps evaluate deterioration in open-angle glaucoma. Fundus photography monitors and records optic disk changes.

Treatment

For open-angle glaucoma, initial drug treatment aims to reduce pressure by decreasing aqueous humor production. The drugs include beta blockers such as timolol (used cautiously in patients with asthma and those with bradycardia) and betaxolol. Other drug treatments include epinephrine to dilate the pupil (contraindicated in angle-closure glaucoma) and miotic eyedrops, such as pilocarpine, to promote aqueous humor outflow.

Patients who don't respond to drug therapy may benefit from argon laser trabeculoplasty or from a surgical filtering procedure called trabeculectomy. To perform argon laser trabeculoplasty, the ophthal-mologist focuses an argon laser beam on the trabecular meshwork of an open angle. This produces a thermal burn that changes the meshwork surface and facilitates the outflow of aqueous humor.

To perform a trabeculectomy, the surgeon dissects a flap of sclera to expose the trabecular meshwork. He removes a small tissue block and performs a peripheral iridectomy, which creates an opening (fistula) for the outflow of aqueous humor under the conjunctiva and produces a filtering bleb. Postoperatively, subconjunctival injections of fluorouracil may be given to maintain the fistula's patency. The iridectomy relieves pressure by excising part of the iris to reestablish the outflow of aqueous humor. A few days later, the surgeon performs a prophylactic iridectomy on the other (normal) eye to prevent an episode of acute glaucoma in that eye.

If the patient has severe pain, treatment may include narcotic analgesics. After peripheral iridectomy, treatment includes cycloplegic eyedrops to relax the ciliary muscle and to decrease inflammation, thereby preventing adhesions.

Complications

Untreated glaucoma can progress to total blindness.

Nursing interventions

● After trabeculectomy, give medications as ordered to dilate the pupil. Also apply topical corticosteroids as ordered to rest the pupil.
● Protect the affected eye by applying an eye patch and shield, positioning the patient on his back or unaffected side, and following general safety measures.
● Administer pain medication as ordered.
● Encourage ambulation immediately after surgery to help prevent secondary complications. Also encourage the patient to express his concerns related to having a chronic condition.

Patient teaching

● Stress to your patient the importance of meticulous compliance with his prescribed drug therapy to maintain low IOP and prevent optic disk changes that can cause vision loss. Teach the patient or a family member how to instill the eye medications.

• Explain all procedures and treatments, especially surgery, to help reduce the patient's anxiety. Inform the patient that lost vision cannot be restored, but that treatment can usually prevent further vision loss.
• Instruct the family in ways to modify the patient's environment for safety. For example, suggest keeping pathways clear and reorienting the patient to room layouts, if necessary.
• Emphasize to the patient the signs and symptoms that require immediate medical attention, such as sudden vision change and eye pain. Discuss with family members the importance of glaucoma screening for early detection and prevention. Point out that all persons over age 35 should have an annual tonometric examination.

MACULAR DEGENERATION

Commonly affecting both eyes, this disorder is a leading cause of blindness among all age-groups in the United States. Two primary forms are the atrophic (also called the involutional or dry) form, which accounts for about 70% of cases, and the exudative (also called the hemorrhagic or wet) form.

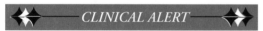

CLINICAL ALERT

At least 10% of older Americans have irreversible central vision loss from age-related macular degeneration.

Causes

Age-related macular degeneration results from hardening and obstruction of the retinal arteries, usually associated with age-related degenerative changes. Thus, formation of new blood vessels (neovascularization) in the macular area obscures central vision. The disorder can also be genetic or the result of an injury, inflammation, or infection.

Assessment findings

The history should include questions about your patient's ability to see and read. The patient may complain of seeing a blank spot (scotoma) in the center of a page while reading. He may tell you that his central vision blurs intermittently and has gradually worsened. He may also report that straight lines appear distorted.

Diagnostic tests

Indirect ophthalmoscopy through a dilated pupil discloses changes in the macular region of the fundus. Fluorescein angiography may identify (in sequential photographs) leaking vessels in the subretinal neovascular net. Amsler grid tests can detect visual distortion (metamorphopsia) on a daily basis, if appropriate.

Treatment

No cure currently exists for the atrophic form of macular degeneration. In 5% to 10% of patients with the exudative form, argon laser photocoagulation may slow the progression of severe vision loss.

Complications

Age-related macular degeneration may result in blindness. Bilateral lesions may lead to nystagmus.

Nursing interventions

Help the patient obtain vision aids, such as magnifiers and special lamps. Offer emotional support, and encourage the patient to express any concerns.

Patient teaching

Point out ways the patient can modify his home for safety. Explain that macular degeneration usually doesn't affect peripheral vision, which should be adequate for performing routine activities. If the patient likes to read, refer him to an agency such as the American Foundation for the Blind.

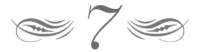

Managing cardiovascular problems

No body system wears out, breaks down, or otherwise malfunctions as often as the cardiovascular (CV) system. Heart disease affects people of all ages and takes many forms, but it's especially prevalent among older adults.

As the body ages, changes occur that reduce functional status and compromise CV health. The walls of the ventricle and the aorta become stiffer, decreasing the heart's pumping efficiency. Atherosclerotic lesions develop in the coronary and peripheral arteries, compromising the heart's blood supply. Also, the vasculature's ability to react to oxygen demand declines, which may increase the risk of ischemia. Delayed ventricular filling, valvular disease, stiffening of the myocardium, and decreased heart rate responses that prolong the relaxation phase contribute to impaired diastolic performance. However, these changes don't occur all at once, and they vary from person to person.

The risk of heart failure is highest in people over age 65. Half of those who develop heart failure die within 5 years of being diagnosed. The incidence of hypertension also increases with age; its presence represents a key risk factor for CV disorders, such as coronary artery disease (CAD) and cerebrovascular accident (CVA), as well as for renal disorders. CAD, one of the primary causes of impaired function among older people, is found on autopsy in over half the men in North America over age 60 and causes more than two-thirds of deaths in older adults.

Myocardial infarction (MI), one of the most common causes of death in developed nations, has a mortality rate of about 25%. Studies have shown that up to 68% of adults over age 64 have had an unrecognized MI. Most adults with peripheral vascular disease are over age 55. Although peripheral vascular disease usually occurs more frequently in men, after the eighth decade of life it affects women more often. Ischemic heart disease, heart failure, and hypertension all can precipitate atrial fibrillation.

You need to be familiar with the causes and treatments of these problems in older people. You also need good assessment skills, adapted to older adults, to guide your interventions. And your teaching is critical in helping older adults learn how to live with CV problems.

This chapter focuses on CV problems that commonly affect older people. The high incidence of these problems and the seriousness of their complications continually reaffirm your need to know how to assess the complex CV system and intervene appropriately.

HEART FAILURE

In this condition, the heart fails to pump enough blood to meet the body's metabolic needs. Pump failure usually occurs in a damaged left ventricle (left ventricular failure). However, it may occur in the right ventricle, either as primary failure or a secondary failure brought on by left ventricular dysfunction. Left and right ventricular failure may also develop simultaneously.

Heart failure is usually classified by the site of the failure (left or right ventricle, or both), but it may also be classified by level of cardiac output (high or low), stage (acute or chronic), and direction (forward or backward). These classifications represent different aspects of heart failure, not distinct diseases.

For many older adults with heart failure, the disorder's symptoms restrict the ability to perform activities of daily living, severely affecting quality of life. Advances in diagnostic and therapeutic techniques have greatly improved the outlook for these people, but the prognosis still depends on the underlying cause and its response to treatment.

Causes

Heart failure in older adults can be precipitated by CAD, hypertensive heart disease, cor pulmonale, mitral stenosis, subacute bacterial endocarditis, bronchitis, pneumonia, or myxedema. Among the age-related changes that cause heart failure are reduced elasticity and lumen size of the vessels and rises in blood pressure that interfere with the heart's blood supply.

Most older people with chronic heart failure have CAD. Another cause is mechanical disturbances in ventricular filling during diastole, with impaired ability of the ventricle to accept blood. Systolic hemodynamic disturbances that increase cardiac work load and limit the heart's pumping ability are also found in older people. Such disturbances include aortic stenosis and systemic hypertension, which increase resistance to ventricular emptying, and mitral or aortic insufficiency, which causes high blood volume. In older people with underlying heart disease, arrhythmias also can cause heart failure — for example, tachyarrhythmias reduce ventricular filling time, bradycardia reduces cardiac output, and other arrhythmias disrupt the synchrony of normal atrial and ventricular filling, leading to heart failure.

Assessment findings

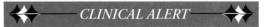
— CLINICAL ALERT —

Overwhelming fatigue may be the first symptom of heart failure in an older person, so be sure to assess carefully a patient with this complaint. Other assessment findings commonly include nighttime wandering, depression, dyspnea, orthopnea, weight gain, and bilateral ankle edema.

Your patient may complain of shortness of breath during exertion. He may also report having difficulty breathing when lying flat. He may have to prop up his head with several pillows or sit in a chair to sleep comfortably. His family may report episodes of confusion, agitation, or being "out of sorts." If heart failure has progressed, he may complain of awakening shortly after falling asleep with a need to sit bolt upright to catch his breath.

In chronic heart failure, shortness of breath develops gradually over weeks or months and may be accompanied by a persistent cough. Because of the insidious onset, patients may not realize there has been a change unless questioned carefully. In acute heart failure, the patient may experience shortness of breath at rest. Peripheral edema may cause shoes and rings to fit tightly. Ask the patient what medications he's taking (over-the-counter and prescription). If he takes medication for chronic heart failure, find out if he has stopped taking the medication or altered the prescribed dosage.

During the initial examination, check for signs that reveal the duration and severity of heart failure. Patients with heart failure of recent onset appear acutely ill but are usually well nourished, whereas those with chronic heart failure often appear malnourished, even cachectic. Observation may reveal dyspnea, anxiety, and respiratory distress. In mild heart failure, dyspnea may occur while the patient is lying down or active; in acute heart failure, it won't be affected by position or activity. If the patient has pulmonary edema, his cough will produce pink, frothy sputum.

Inspection may reveal cyanosis of the lips and nail beds, pale skin, dependent peripheral and sacral edema, and jugular venous distention. Ascites may be present, especially in patients with right ventricular failure. Palpation may reveal a rapid pulse and pulsus alternans. The skin may feel cool and clammy. Palpation and percussion of the abdomen may reveal hepatomegaly and splenomegaly. Percussion over the lung bases may reveal dullness if the lungs are filled with fluid.

Auscultation of blood pressure may reveal decreased pulse pressure, indicating reduced stroke volume. Auscultation may also disclose an S_3 gallop and a systolic murmur of mitral or tricuspid insufficiency. Auscultation of the lungs may reveal moist, bibasilar crackles. If pulmonary edema is present, typically you'll hear crackles accompanied by rhonchi and expiratory wheezing. However, if the person has severe pulmonary edema, you may not be able to hear crackles, even if the lungs are filled with fluid, because air may not have sufficient space in which to move and thereby produce sounds.

Diagnostic tests

Tests that help identify heart failure include electrocardiography (ECG), chest X-ray, pulmonary artery pressure monitoring, echocardiography, and arterial blood gas measurements (ABGs). ECG may show patterns of ventricular hypertrophy and myocardial ischemia, injury, or infarction. It may also reveal atrial enlargement and arrhyth-mias, especially atrial fibrillation and premature ventricular contractions. Chest X-rays may confirm the presence or absence of cardiomegaly and may show increased pulmonary vascular markings, interstitial edema, or pleural effusion.

Pulmonary artery monitoring may indicate elevated pulmonary artery diastolic pressure, pulmonary artery systolic pressure, and pulmonary artery wedge pressure (PAWP). Echocardiography may show ventricular hypertrophy, decreased contractility, and decreased ejection fraction and may identify valvular and other disorders causing heart failure.

ABG values may show low partial pressure of oxygen in arterial blood (PaO_2) and low pH in persons with pulmonary edema. Because of decreased peripheral circulation, persons with pulmonary edema experience an accumulation of lactic acid and a corresponding decrease in pH and bicarbonate values (metabolic acidosis). Severely ill people often show increased partial pressure of carbon dioxide in arterial blood ($PaCO_2$). However, with tachypnea, rapid breathing may cause a low $PaCO_2$.

Treatment

People experiencing heart failure require immediate care to stabilize their condition, followed by measures to relieve symptoms. Treatment in older adults mirrors treatment for the middle-aged population. It seeks to minimize discomfort and prolong life and includes medical interventions, such as drug therapy, and lifestyle changes, such as modifications in diet, fluid intake, exercise, and sleep habits.

Supplemental oxygen and intravenous (I.V.) diuretics are central to treatment. The doctor will order an I.V. line for the administration of medications. A central line may be used to monitor cardiac status. An indwelling urinary catheter is inserted if the person is in acute heart failure or if aggressive diuresis is necessary.

If the person develops cardiogenic shock or responds poorly to treatment or if the cause of pulmonary edema is unclear, hemodynamic monitoring will be needed. The doctor may insert a pulmonary artery catheter to monitor cardiac output and PAWP. A cardiac index of 2.2 L/min/m^2 or higher and a PAWP below 18 mm Hg are the desired targets.

Record the patient's response to prescribed medications. For example, 15 to 20 minutes after an I.V. bolus injection of furosemide (given over 1 to 2 minutes), tachypnea should decrease, and PaO_2 and urine output should increase. If, after aggressive therapy, the patient's PaO_2 falls below 50 mm Hg and his $PaCO_2$ rises above 50 mm Hg, intubation and mechanical ventilation may be necessary.

Morphine is commonly used, especially in acute heart failure, to stimulate vasodilation, decrease preload, and reduce anxiety. If the patient receives morphine, monitor for hypoventilation. Some doctors reserve morphine for intubated patients. If the patient doesn't respond well to oxygen and the first dose of diuretic agents, and his systolic pressure exceeds 100 mm Hg, a vasodilator will be ordered. Monitor his pulse rate, respiratory rate, and blood pressure closely.

If the patient's systolic pressure falls below 90 mm Hg, he may require inotropic drugs. In severe hypotension, expect to administer dobutamine and dopamine. Both of these drugs, however, can cause arrhythmias, so you'll need to monitor the patient closely. Correlate arterial blood pressure and other hemodynamic indices with assessment findings and titration of medications.

Alternatively, you may administer amrinone, possibly along with dopamine or dobutamine. If you do, watch for hypotension, arrhythmias, and thrombocytopenia.

If you're giving digoxin, monitor its level and observe for signs of toxicity. Collect a blood sample for determining the drug's level 12 hours after an oral dose; note both the time the blood was obtained and the time the dose was given on the laboratory slip. Also monitor serum potassium and magnesium levels because people with hypokalemia and hypomagnesemia are more likely to develop digoxin toxicity. Once the crisis is over, digoxin may be used for long-term therapy.

If the patient is receiving nitroprusside, monitor his serum lactate and thiocyanate levels.

Assess the person's ECG, serum electrolyte level, and digoxin level. Also monitor his blood urea nitrogen (BUN) and creatinine levels. Impending renal shutdown may require emergency dialysis. Administer medications as prescribed and enforce fluid restrictions.

Complications
Chronic heart failure may worsen as a result of respiratory tract infections, pulmonary embolism, stress, increased sodium or water intake, or failure to comply with the prescribed treatment regimen.

Nursing interventions
Nursing interventions focus on relieving symptoms and incorporating the medical treatment regimen into the person's routine.
- Place the person in Fowler's position and give him supplemental oxygen to help him breathe more easily. Organize all activity to provide maximum rest periods.
- Obtain a baseline weight. Check for peripheral edema and areas of skin breakdown. Also, monitor I.V. intake and urine output (especially if the patient is receiving diuretics). Weigh the person daily, preferably before breakfast, to determine fluid retention. Measure the circumference of his feet and ankles. To assess changes accurately, mark the area you measure with a permanent marker so the same spot can be measured each day. Assess skin turgor.
- Assess vital signs (for increased respiratory and heart rates and for narrowing pulse pressure) and mental status. If possible, apply an automatic cuff to monitor blood pressure closely. For certain patients, the doctor may insert a catheter into the radial or femoral artery for continuous blood pressure monitoring and convenient blood sampling. Auscultate for abnormal heart and breath sounds. Report any changes immediately.
- Frequently monitor BUN and serum creatinine, potassium, sodium, chloride, and magnesium levels. Provide continuous cardiac monitoring during acute and advanced stages to identify and treat arrhythmias promptly.
- To prevent deep vein thrombosis resulting from vascular congestion, assist the person with range-of-motion exercises. Enforce bed rest, and apply antiembolism stockings. Watch for calf pain and tenderness.
- If a person has multiple I.V. and pressure-monitoring lines, color-code each one. For instance, label arterial lines with a piece of red tape, pulmonary artery catheter lines with green tape, and central venous catheter lines with yellow tape.
- Monitor for pulmonary edema, poor response to therapy, increasing acidosis, confusion, and a decreasing level of consciousness. Be prepared to assist with intubation and mechanical ventilation. Resuscitate the person as needed.
- Monitor the patient's ABG levels. Maintain his PaO$_2$ at 80 mm Hg and PaCO$_2$ at 30 to 40 mm Hg with a normal pH. Once the patient's condition has stabilized, monitor cardiopulmonary status at least every 4 hours. Assess blood pressure, apical and radial pulse rates and rhythm, respiratory rate, heart

and breath sounds, and skin color. Keep in mind that arrhythmias, MI, and hypertensive crisis may accompany acute heart failure.

● Organize all activity to provide long rest periods. Assist the patient with gradual increases in activity as his condition warrants. Report changes in the patient's condition immediately.

Patient teaching

Explain the disorder, its treatment, and any ordered tests to the patient. Discuss the need for diet and lifestyle modifications. Stress the importance of regular checkups.

Many older adults don't understand the concept of a chronic illness that can't be cured. As a result, they continually search for a method to "fix" the problem. Explain that congestive heart failure is a chronic disorder, and that continued treatment and lifestyle modifications are needed to keep him functional.

● Teach the patient to manage the disorder at home. Advise him to avoid foods high in sodium content, such as canned or commercially prepared foods and dairy products, to curb fluid overload. Instruct him to limit his fluid intake.

● Teach your patient how to take his pulse.

● Advise him to weigh himself daily, and explain why this is important.

● Suggest ways that the person can stay active without exhausting himself. Encourage him to walk and to increase his distance gradually. Suggest that he plan most activities for the morning and rest periodically during the day. Discuss ways to simplify his routine and conserve energy. Help the person delegate tasks.

● Stress the importance of taking medications as prescribed. Help the person simplify his drug regimen and set up a medication schedule. Suggest organizing a week's worth of medication in a pillbox or empty egg carton and using an alarm clock to remind him when to take medication.

● Provide the person with a wallet-size card listing medications and emergency phone numbers.

● If the person is taking digoxin, teach him the signs of toxicity: anorexia, vomiting, confusion, a slow or irregular pulse rate, and blurred vision or visible

yellow-green halos. An older adult may also experience flulike symptoms. Tell him to report any signs of toxicity immediately.

● If the person is also taking cholestyramine (a lipid-lowering drug), tell him to take digoxin 2 to 3 hours before cholestyramine. That's because cholestyramine decreases digoxin levels and its bioavailability.

● Tell your patient to take digoxin at least 1 to 2 hours before taking antacids or eating high-bran foods. They can decrease drug bioavailability.

● Explain the importance of follow-up blood tests. Discuss any sleep pattern disturbances. If nocturia is a problem, help the person adjust his diuretic schedule. For example, if he's taking a diuretic twice a day, advise him to take the second dose in the late afternoon or early evening. Otherwise, the drug's peak action will occur in the middle of the night.

If orthopnea is a problem, suggest that the person elevate the head of his bed on blocks or sleep in a recliner. Raising the bed is more effective than piling up pillows.

✦✦ — CLINICAL ALERT — ✦✦

If dyspnea awakens the person shortly after he goes to bed, encourage him to elevate his feet for an hour before lying down. Explain that fluid that has pooled in his legs suddenly returns to circulation when he lies down; this excess fluid then floods the lungs, causing shortness of breath. By elevating his feet before retiring, he can reduce pooling in the legs and allow his kidneys to clear excess fluid before he lies down. (During an episode of acute dyspnea, however, he should dangle his legs over the side of the bed to help drain fluid from his lungs.)

● Instruct him to inform the doctor if he experiences dizziness, palpitations, blurred vision, an unusually irregular pulse rate, a pulse rate below 60 beats/minute, increased shortness of breath or fatigue during regular activities, a persistent dry cough, swelling in the legs or ankles that doesn't go away with elevation, decreased urine output, or a weight gain of 2 lb (about 0.9 kg) or more in 2 days.

● Because the person may be more susceptible to respiratory infections, suggest that he ask the doctor

about pneumonia and influenza vaccinations.
• Teach relaxation techniques to reduce anxiety.

HYPERTENSION

This disorder is marked by an intermittent or sustained elevation of diastolic or systolic blood pressure. Generally, a sustained systolic pressure of 160 mm Hg or more or a diastolic pressure of 90 mm Hg or more qualifies as hypertension. The incidence rises with age. In older adults, hypertension often results from vasoconstriction associated with aging, which produces peripheral resistance. Other causes include hyperthyroidism, parkinsonism, Paget's disease, anemia, and thiamine deficiency. Hypertension affects more than 60 million adults in the United States. Blacks are twice as likely as whites to be affected, and they're four times as likely to die of the disorder.

Aside from characteristic high blood pressure, hypertension is classified according to its cause, severity, and type. The two major types are *essential* (also called *primary* or *idiopathic*) *hypertension,* which comprises 90% to 95% of cases, and *secondary hypertension,* which results from renal disease or another identifiable cause. *Malignant hypertension* is a severe, fulminant form of hypertension that commonly arises from both types.

Causes

Along with the normal physiologic changes of aging, other risk factors for hypertension include diabetes, obesity, and nonhealthy habits.

The exact cause of essential hypertension is unknown. Family history, race, stress, obesity, a diet high in sodium or saturated fat, use of tobacco or oral contraceptives, sedentary lifestyle, and aging have all been studied to determine their role in the development of hypertension. Secondary hypertension may result from renovascular disease, renal parenchymal disease, pheochromocytoma, primary hyperaldosteronism, Cushing's syndrome, diabetes mellitus, coarctation of the aorta, neurologic

disorders, and dysfunction of the thyroid, pituitary, or parathyroid glands.

Assessment findings

In many cases, the hypertensive person has no symptoms, and the disorder is revealed incidentally during evaluation for another disorder or during a routine blood pressure screening program. When symptoms do occur, they reflect the effect of hypertension on the organ systems.

The person may report awakening with a headache in the occipital region, which subsides spontaneously after a few hours. This symptom usually is associated with severe hypertension. He may also complain of dizziness, memory loss, palpitations, fatigue, and impotence. With vascular involvement, the person may complain of nosebleeds, bloody urine, weakness, and blurred vision. Complaints of chest pain and dyspnea may indicate cardiac involvement. Slow tremors, nausea, and vomiting may also occur.

◆◆ CLINICAL ALERT ◆◆

Blood pressure measurement is a critical element of the physical examination. Take special care to ensure an accurate reading in an older adult.

Make sure the person has rested before you take the measurement. Even the activity of walking into the room and sitting down can cause blood pressure to rise.

To obtain an immediate blood pressure reading on a person whose upper arm is too large for the available cuff, wrap the cuff around the forearm and auscultate Korotkoff sounds over the radial artery. Verify this measurement as soon as possible by using a proper size cuff on the upper arm.

A rise in the diastolic blood pressure when the person changes from a sitting to a standing position suggests essential hypertension, whereas a fall in blood pressure with a change from the sitting to the standing position indicates secondary hypertension.

Inspection may reveal peripheral edema in late stages when heart failure is present. Ophthalmoscopic evaluation may reveal hemorrhages, exudates, and papilledema in late stages if hypertensive retinopathy is present.

Palpation of the carotid artery may disclose stenosis or occlusion. Palpation of the abdomen may reveal a pulsating mass, suggesting an abdominal aneurysm. Enlarged kidneys may point to polycystic disease, a cause of secondary hypertension.

An abdominal bruit may be heard just to the right or left of the umbilicus midline, or in the flanks if renal artery stenosis is present. Bruits may also be heard over the abdominal aorta and femoral arteries.

Diagnostic tests

Several tests may elicit predisposing factors and help identify the cause of hypertension: A urinalysis may show protein, red blood cells, or white blood cells, suggesting renal disease, or glucose, suggesting diabetes mellitus. Excretory urography may reveal renal atrophy, indicating chronic renal disease. One kidney that is more than $\frac{5}{8}$" (1.6 cm) shorter than the other suggests unilateral renal disease. Serum potassium levels less than 3.5 mEq/L may indicate adrenal dysfunction (primary hyperaldosteronism). BUN levels that are normal or elevated to more than 20 mg/dl and serum creatinine levels that are normal or elevated to more than 1.5 mg/dl suggest renal disease.

Other tests that help detect CV damage and other complications include ECG, which may show left ventricular hypertrophy or ischemia, and chest X-rays, which may demonstrate cardiomegaly.

Treatment

Although essential hypertension has no cure, drugs and modifications in diet and lifestyle can control it. Generally, nondrug treatment, such as lifestyle modification, is tried first, especially in early, mild cases. If this is ineffective, treatment progresses in steps to include various types of antihypertensives. Many older adults with hypertension can be treated with diuretics alone.

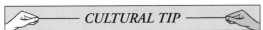

CULTURAL TIP

Most blacks respond poorly to beta-adrenergic blocking agents; however, for unclear reasons, they respond well to a combination of a diuretic and an angiotensin-converting enzyme inhibitor.

Treatment of secondary hypertension includes correcting the underlying cause and controlling hypertensive effects.

Complications

Hypertension is a major cause of CVA, cardiac disease, and renal failure. Complications occur late in the disease and can attack any organ system. Cardiac complications may include CAD, angina, MI, heart failure, arrhythmias, and sudden death. Neurologic complications include cerebral infarctions and hypertensive encephalopathy. Hypertensive retinopathy can cause blindness. Renovascular hypertension can lead to renal failure. Severely elevated blood pressure (hypertensive crisis) may be refractory to medications and may be fatal.

Nursing interventions

● If a person is hospitalized with hypertension, find out if he was taking his prescribed antihypertensive. If he wasn't, ask why. The most common reason that people stop taking their medication or alter the dose is unpleasant adverse effects, such as constipation, drowsiness, depression, and dizziness. If that's the case with your patient, his medication regimen may need to be modified. Also, many older adults may not be able to afford the medication and may need a referral to an appropriate social service department.
● When routine blood pressure screening reveals elevated pressure, make sure the sphygmomanometer cuff size is appropriate for the patient's upper arm circumference. Take the pressure in both arms in lying, sitting, and standing positions. Ask the patient if he smoked, drank a beverage containing caffeine, or was emotionally upset before the test. Advise him to return for blood pressure testing at frequent and regular intervals.
● To help identify hypertension and prevent untreated hypertension, participate in public education programs dealing with hypertension and ways to reduce risk factors. Encourage public participation in blood pressure screening programs. Routinely

screen all patients, especially those at risk (blacks and people with family histories of hypertension, CVA, or heart attack).

Patient teaching

Focus your teaching on helping the person learn to live with and control his hypertension. Emphasize that lifelong therapy is needed, even when overt signs and symptoms of ill health are absent.
• Teach the person to use a self-monitoring blood pressure cuff and to record the reading at least twice weekly in a journal for review by the doctor at every office appointment. Tell him to take his blood pressure at the same hour each time with relatively the same type of activity preceding the measurement.
• To encourage compliance with antihypertensive therapy, suggest establishing a daily routine for taking medication. Warn the person that uncontrolled hypertension may cause stroke and heart attack. Tell him to keep a record of the drugs he takes and the effectiveness of each, and to discuss this information with the doctor during follow-up visits. Explain that suddenly stopping drug therapy is dangerous. Instruct him to report any adverse effects to the doctor immediately.
• Advise the person to avoid high-sodium antacids and over-the-counter cold and sinus medications containing harmful vasoconstrictors.
• For people who smoke tobacco, describe the effects of smoking and the importance of quitting smoking, or refer the person to a smoking cessation program. Explain the proper use of nicotine-containing patches, chewing gum, or nasal spray.
• Advise the person to limit daily consumption of alcohol to 1 oz.
• Help the person examine and modify his lifestyle. Suggest stress-reduction groups, dietary changes, and an exercise program (such as aerobic walking), to improve cardiac status and reduce obesity and serum cholesterol levels. Encourage a change in dietary habits. Help the obese patient plan a weight-loss diet. Tell him to avoid high-sodium foods (pickles, potato chips, canned soups, cold cuts), table salt, and foods high in cholesterol and saturated fat.

• Continue to monitor the patient's blood pressure and compliance with treatment. Provide positive reinforcement and psychosocial support, as needed.

CORONARY ARTERY DISEASE

In CAD, fatty fibrous plaques or calcium-plaque deposits, or combinations of both, narrow the lumens of coronary arteries, reducing the volume of blood that can flow through them. The diminished coronary blood flow leads to a loss of oxygen and nutrients to myocardial tissue.

This disease is nearly epidemic in the Western world. CAD is more prevalent in men, whites, and middle-aged and older people than in women or in people of other races and ages.

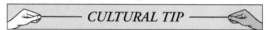
CULTURAL TIP

CAD is a leading health problem among Japanese and native Hawaiians.

Causes

Atherosclerosis, the most common cause of CAD, has been linked to many risk factors. This condition and some risk factors, such as advanced age, male or postmenopausal female gender, and heredity, can't be controlled. A positive family history of CAD and a nonwhite racial origin also increase the risk. However, the patient can modify other risk factors, such as blood pressure, cholesterol level, cigarette smoking, obesity, exercise, and stress, with good medical care and appropriate lifestyle changes.

Uncommon causes of reduced coronary artery blood flow include dissecting aneurysms, infectious vasculitis, and syphilis. Coronary artery spasms may also impede blood flow. Because CAD is so widespread, prevention is crucial.

Assessment findings

The classic symptom of CAD is angina, the direct result of inadequate flow of oxygen to the myocardium. The person usually describes it as a burning, squeezing, or crushing tightness in the substernal or precordial area of the chest that may radiate to the left arm, neck, jaw, or shoulder blade. Typically, the person clenches his fist over his chest or rubs his left arm when describing the pain. Nausea, vomiting, fainting, sweating, and cool extremities may accompany the feeling of tightness.

Angina commonly occurs after physical exertion but may also follow emotional excitement, exposure to cold, or a large meal. It may also develop during sleep, and symptoms may awaken the patient.

When assessing for anginal pain, remember that older adults often have an increased tolerance and won't complain as much of pain as younger people will. Instead, they may compensate by slowing their activity levels.

The person's health history may suggest a pattern to the type and onset of pain. If the pain is predictable and relieved by rest or nitrates, it's called *stable angina*. If it increases in frequency and duration and is more easily induced, it's referred to as *unstable angina* or *unpredictable angina*. Unstable angina generally indicates extensive or worsening disease and may progress to MI. An effort-induced pain that occurs with increasing frequency and with decreasing provocation is referred to as *crescendo angina*. If severe pain occurs at rest without provocation, it's called *variant angina* or *Prinzmetal's angina*.

Inspection may reveal evidence of atherosclerotic disease, such as xanthelasma (a yellowish, slightly raised tumor that's usually found on the eyelids). Ophthalmoscopic inspection may show increased light reflexes and arteriovenous nicking, suggesting hypertension, an important risk factor for CAD. Palpation can uncover thickened or absent peripheral arteries, signs of cardiac enlargement, and abnormal contraction of the cardiac impulse, such as left ventricular akinesia or dyskinesia. Auscultation may detect bruits, an S_3, an S_4, or a late systolic murmur (if mitral insufficiency is present).

Diagnostic tests

ECG serves as the chief diagnostic test. During an angina attack, the ECG shows ischemia as demonstrated by T-wave inversion or ST-segment depression and, possibly, arrhythmias, such as premature ventricular contractions. ECG results may or may not be normal during pain-free periods.

Arrhythmias may occur without infarction, secondary to ischemia. A treadmill or bicycle exercise test may provoke chest pain and ECG signs of myocardial ischemia in response to physical exertion. Monitoring electrical rhythm may demonstrate T-wave inversion or ST-segment depression in the ischemic areas.

Coronary angiography reveals coronary artery stenosis or obstruction, collateral circulation, and the arteries' condition beyond the narrowing. Myocardial perfusion imaging with thallium-201 during treadmill exercise detects ischemic areas of the myocardium, visualized as "cold spots."

Treatment

The goal of treatment in patients with angina is to reduce myocardial oxygen demand or increase the oxygen supply and reduce pain. Activity restrictions may be required to prevent onset of pain. Rather than eliminating activities, performing them more slowly often averts pain. Stress reduction techniques are also essential, especially if known stressors precipitate pain.

Pharmacologic therapy consists primarily of nitrates, such as nitroglycerin or isosorbide dinitrate, or beta-adrenergic blockers. Long-acting nitrates are not usually prescribed for older adults.

Obstructive lesions may necessitate atherectomy or coronary artery bypass graft surgery (CABG) using vein grafts. Percutaneous transluminal coronary angioplasty (PTCA) may be performed during cardiac catheterization to compress fatty deposits and relieve occlusion. In patients with calcification, PTCA may reduce the obstruction by fracturing the plaque.

PTCA carries certain risks but causes fewer complications than surgery. Complications after PTCA can include circulatory insufficiency, MI, restenosis of the vessels, retroperitoneal bleeding, sudden coronary occlusions, vasovagal response and arrhythmias, and death (rarely). PTCA is a viable alternative to grafting in older adults or in those who otherwise cannot tolerate cardiac surgery. However, persons with a left main coronary artery occlusion, lesions in extremely tortuous vessels, or occlusions older than 3 months are usually not candidates for PTCA.

Laser angioplasty corrects occlusion by vaporizing fatty deposits with an excimer or hot-tip laser device. Rotational ablation (or rotational atherectomy) removes atheromatous plaque with a high-speed, rotating burr covered with diamond crystals.

Complications

When a coronary artery goes into spasm or is occluded by plaque, blood flow to the myocardium supplied by that vessel decreases, causing angina. Failure to remedy the occlusion causes ischemia and, eventually, myocardial tissue infarction.

Nursing interventions

● During anginal episodes, monitor blood pressure and heart rate. Take a 12-lead ECG before administering nitroglycerin or other nitrates.
● Record the duration of pain, the amount of medication required to relieve it, and accompanying symptoms. Ask the patient to grade the severity of his pain on a scale of 1 to 10. This allows him to assess his own pain as well as the effectiveness of pain-relieving medications. Keep nitroglycerin available for immediate use. Instruct the patient to call immediately whenever he feels chest, arm, or neck pain and before taking nitroglycerin.
● During cardiac catheterization, monitor the patient for adverse reactions to the dye. If he has such symptoms as falling blood pressure, bradycardia, diaphoresis, and light-headedness, increase parenteral fluids as ordered, administer nasal oxygen, place the patient in Trendelenburg's position, and administer I.V. atropine if necessary.
● After catheterization, review the expected course of treatment with the patient and his family. Monitor the catheter site for bleeding. Also check for distal pulses. To counter the diuretic effect of the dye, increase I.V. fluids and make sure the patient drinks plenty of fluids. Assess potassium levels, and add potassium to the I.V. fluid, if necessary.
● After PTCA, maintain heparinization, observe for bleeding systemically and at the site, and keep the affected leg immobile. After rotational ablation,

monitor the patient for chest pain, hypotension, coronary artery spasm, and bleeding from the catheter site. Provide heparin and antibiotic therapy for 24 to 48 hours, as ordered.
● After bypass surgery, provide care for the I.V. site, pulmonary artery catheter, and endotracheal tube. Monitor blood pressure, intake and output, breath sounds, chest tube drainage, and cardiac rhythm, watching for signs of ischemia and arrhythmias. I.V. administration of epinephrine, nitroprusside, dopamine, albumin, potassium, and blood products may be necessary. The patient may also need temporary epicardial pacing, especially if the surgery included replacement of the aortic valve.
● Insertion of an intra-aortic balloon pump may be necessary until the patient's condition stabilizes. Also observe for and treat chest pain. Perform vigorous chest physiotherapy and guide the person in pulmonary toilet.

Patient teaching

Teach the person what he needs to know about CAD, its treatment, and any prescribed lifestyle and diet modifications.
● Before cardiac catheterization, explain the procedure to the patient. Make sure he knows why it's necessary, understands the risks, and realizes that it may indicate a need for interventional therapies such as PTCA, CABG, atherectomy, and laser angioplasty. If the patient is scheduled for surgery, explain the procedure, provide a tour of the intensive care unit, introduce him to the staff, and discuss postoperative care.
● Help the patient determine which activities precipitate episodes of pain. Help him identify and select more effective coping mechanisms to deal with stress.
● Emphasize the need to follow the prescribed drug regimen. Teach the patient how to use nitroglycerin.
● Encourage the patient to maintain the prescribed low-sodium diet and to start a low-calorie, low-cholesterol diet as well.
● If the patient smokes, refer him to a program to stop smoking. Acknowledge that this will be difficult but that he should make every attempt to stop smoking immediately and never restart.

• Encourage regular, moderate exercise. Teach your patient how to exercise safely and how to personalize his exercise program. Help him find his personal target heart rate and heart rate range for aerobic exercise (see Chapter 3). Urge other family members or a friend to join in the physical activity to encourage the patient's commitment to the exercise program.

• Reassure the patient that he can resume sexual activity and that modifications can allow for sexual fulfillment without fear of overexertion, pain, or reocclusion.

• Explain that recurrent angina symptoms after PTCA or rotational ablation may signal reobstruction, and the patient should call the doctor immediately.

MYOCARDIAL INFARCTION

MI results from reduced blood flow through a coronary artery. This, in turn, results in myocardial ischemia and necrosis.

The infarction site depends on the vessels involved. For instance, occlusion of the circumflex coronary artery causes a lateral wall infarction; occlusion of the left anterior coronary artery causes an anterior wall infarction. True posterior and inferior wall infarctions result from occlusion of the right coronary artery or one of its branches. Right ventricular infarction also can result from right coronary artery occlusion, can accompany inferior infarctions, and may cause right ventricular failure. In transmural (Q wave) MI, tissue damage extends through all myocardial layers; in subendocardial (non–Q wave) MI, usually only the innermost layer is damaged.

The incidence of MI in men resembles that in postmenopausal women. In North America and Western Europe, MI is one of the most common causes of death, which usually results from cardiac damage or complications. The mortality rate for persons over age 70 is twice that for younger persons.

Age-related changes in the CV system, along with other risk factors, predispose the older person to MI. Additional risk factors for this age-group include eating a large meal or physical exertion. The older population is also at greater risk for silent MI, which often results in sudden death from arrhythmias. Because of the high incidence and mortality of MI, teaching about prevention is a critical aspect of nursing care for the older adult (see *Preventing MI,* page 130).

Causes
MI results from occlusion of one of the coronary arteries. Such occlusion can stem from atherosclerosis, thrombosis, platelet aggregation, or coronary artery stenosis or spasm. Predisposing factors include aging; diabetes mellitus; elevated serum, triglyceride, low-density lipoprotein, and cholesterol levels; and decreased serum high-density lipoprotein levels.

Other risk factors include excessive intake of saturated fats, carbohydrates, or salt; hypertension; obesity; positive family history of CAD; sedentary lifestyle; smoking; and stress or type A personality (aggressive, competitive attitude, addiction to work, chronic impatience).

Assessment findings
Older adults with MI often don't report its usual symptom: persistent, crushing substernal pain that may radiate to the left arm, jaw, neck, and shoulder blades. Instead, an older adult may not have pain, or it may be mild and confused with indigestion. In people over age 85, dyspnea is a more common presenting symptom.

The patient with CAD may report increasing anginal frequency, severity, or duration (especially when an angina attack not precipitated by exertion, a heavy meal, or exposure to cold and wind). The patient may also report a feeling of impending doom, fatigue, nausea, vomiting, and shortness of breath. Sudden death, however, may be the first and only indication of MI.

Inspection may reveal an anxious or confused patient with dyspnea. If right ventricular failure is present, you may note jugular venous distention.

Preventing MI

All of your older patients should be instructed in ways to prevent a myocardial infarction (MI). This instruction can be incorporated into any routine history or cardiovascular assessment.

Teaching about diet and alcohol
● Teach the patient risk-reducing dietary modifications, such as reducing cholesterol, saturated fat, sodium, and if needed, caloric intake. Instruct him to limit his cholesterol intake to less than 300 mg/day and limit his fat intake to less than 30% of total calories. Explain the benefits of adding fiber, fish, and olive oil to the diet. A dietitian's input can be invaluable in helping the person make dietary changes.
● If the patient drinks alcoholic beverages, advise him to limit daily intake to no more than 1 oz of ethanol daily (equivalent to 2 oz of 100-proof whiskey, 8 oz of wine, or 24 oz of beer). Explain that alcohol can raise blood pressure and adversely affect his heart. Make sure the patient understands how his medications interact with alcohol.

Teaching about smoking cessation
● If the patient smokes, stress the need to stop smoking. Explain that smoking reduces serum high-density lipoproteins, constricts arteries, and reduces the blood's ability to carry oxygen. Provide repetitive counseling and refer the patient to an effective smoking cessation program.
● Explain the use of the nicotine patch, nicotine gum, or nicotine nasal spray.
● Refer the patient to local support and information groups, such as local branches of the American Cancer Society, American Heart Association, and American Lung Association.

Teaching about warning signs and symptoms
● Teach your patient how to respond to symptoms. Tell him to notify the doctor if he experiences chest pain, dizziness, excessive shortness of breath, rapid or irregular pulse rate, or prolonged recovery time after exercise or sexual activity.

Palpitations, worsening heart failure, stroke, syncope, dizziness, and acute renal failure are other symptoms seen in the older adult. Subtle changes, such as excessive fatigue, altered mental status, unusual behaviors, and changes in eating patterns should be carefully assessed, because they may be the result of MI.

Within the first hour after an anterior MI, about 25% of patients exhibit sympathetic nervous system hyperactivity, such as tachycardia and hypertension. Up to 50% of patients with an inferior MI exhibit parasympathetic nervous system hyperactivity, such as bradycardia and hypotension.

In patients who develop ventricular dysfunction, auscultation may disclose S_4, S_3, paradoxical splitting of S_2, and decreased heart sounds. A systolic murmur of mitral insufficiency may be heard with papillary muscle dysfunction secondary to infarction. A pericardial friction rub may also be heard, especially in patients who have a transmural MI or have developed pericarditis.

Fever is unusual at the onset of an MI, but a low-grade fever may develop during the next few days.

Diagnostic tests
Serial 12-lead ECG readings may be normal or inconclusive during the first few hours after an MI and difficult to interpret in the older patient with preexisting heart disease. Characteristic abnormalities include serial ST-segment depression in subendocardial MI and ST-segment elevation and Q waves, representing scarring and necrosis, in transmural MI.

The serum creatine kinase (CK) level is usually elevated, especially the CK-MB isoenzyme, the cardiac muscle fraction of CK.

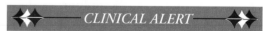

In older adults, laboratory test results, especially the CK, can be confusing because of the person's lean body mass.
Echocardiography shows ventricular wall dyski-

nesia with a transmural MI and helps evaluate the ejection fraction.

Scans, using I.V. technetium-99m pertechnetate, can identify acutely damaged muscle by picking up accumulations of radioactive nucleotide, which appears as a "hot spot" on the film. Myocardial perfusion imaging with thallium-201 reveals a "cold spot" in most patients during the first few hours after a transmural MI.

Treatment

The goals of treatment are to relieve chest pain, to stabilize heart rhythm, and to reduce cardiac work load. Treatment includes revascularization to preserve myocardial tissue. Arrhythmias, the most common problem during the first 48 hours after MI, may require antiarrhythmics and possibly a pacemaker. On rare occasions, they may also require cardioversion.

Morphine I.V. is the drug of choice for pain and sedation. Meperidine or hydromorphone may be used alternatively. Inotropic drugs that increase contractility or blood pressure, such as dobutamine and amrinone, are used to treat reduced myocardial contractility. Beta-adrenergic blockers, such as propranolol and timolol, may be used after acute MI to help prevent reinfarction.

Drug therapy usually includes nitroglycerin (sublingual, topical, transdermal, or I.V.); calcium channel blockers, such as nifedipine, verapamil, or diltiazem (sublingual, oral, or I.V.); or isosorbide dinitrate (sublingual, oral, or I.V.) to relieve pain by redistributing blood to ischemic areas of the myocardium, increasing cardiac output, and reducing myocardial work load. Lidocaine may be used for ventricular arrhythmias. If lidocaine is ineffective, procainamide, quinidine sulfate, bretylium, or disopyramide can be used. Atropine I.V. or a temporary pacemaker is used for heart block or bradycardia.

Oxygen is usually administered (by face mask or nasal cannula) at a modest flow rate for 24 to 48 hours; a lower concentration is necessary if the patient has chronic obstructive pulmonary disease. Bed rest with a bedside commode is enforced to decrease the cardiac work load. Pulmonary artery

catheterization may be performed to detect left or right ventricular failure and to monitor response to treatment, but it's not routinely done. An intra-aortic balloon pump may be inserted for cardiogenic shock.

Revascularization therapy is used more often for patients under age 70 who don't have a history of CVA, bleeding, GI ulcers, marked hypertension, recent surgery, or chest pain lasting longer than 6 hours. Thrombolytic therapy must begin within 6 hours of the onset of symptoms, using intracoronary or systemic (I.V.) streptokinase or tissue plasminogen activator (t-PA). The best response occurs when treatment begins within the first hour after onset of symptoms. Cardiac catheterization, PTCA, and CABG may also be performed.

Complications

Typically, older patients are more prone to complications and death after an acute MI. Cardiac complications may include arrhythmias, cardiogenic shock, pericarditis, and heart failure causing pulmonary edema. Other complications include rupture of the atrial or ventricular septum, ventricular wall, or valves; ventricular aneurysms; mural thrombi causing cerebral or pulmonary emboli; and extensions of the original infarction. Dressler's syndrome (post-MI pericarditis) can occur days to weeks after an MI and cause residual pain, malaise, and fever. Psychological problems can also occur, either from the person's fear of another MI or from an organic brain disorder caused by tissue hypoxia. Some older adults may have a personality change following MI.

Nursing interventions

• When the patient is admitted to the intensive care unit, monitor and record his ECG readings, blood pressure, temperature, and heart and breath sounds. Assess pain and give analgesics, as ordered. Record the severity, location, type, and duration of pain. Don't give the patient I.M. injections because absorption from the muscle is unpredictable and I.V. administration gives more rapid relief of signs and symptoms.

• Check the patient's blood pressure after giving nitroglycerin, especially after the first dose. Frequently monitor ECG readings to detect rate changes and arrhythmias. Analyze rhythm strips and place a representative strip in the patient's chart if any new arrhythmias are documented, if chest pain occurs, or at least every shift or according to your facility's protocol.

• During episodes of chest pain, obtain ECG readings and blood pressure and pulmonary artery catheter measurements (if applicable) to determine changes.

• Watch for crackles, cough, tachypnea, and edema, which may indicate impending left ventricular failure. Carefully monitor daily weight, intake and output, respiratory rate, serum enzyme levels, ECG readings, and blood pressure.

• Auscultate for adventitious breath sounds periodically (patients on bed rest frequently have atelectatic crackles, which may disappear after coughing) and for S_3 or S_4 gallops.

• Organize patient care and activities to maximize uninterrupted rest periods. Ask the dietitian to provide a clear liquid diet until nausea subsides. A low-cholesterol, low-sodium diet, without beverages that contain caffeine, may be ordered.

• Provide a stool softener to prevent straining at stool, which causes vagal stimulation and may slow heart rate. Allow the patient to use a bedside commode, and provide as much privacy as possible.

• Assist with range-of-motion exercises. If the patient is immobilized by a severe MI, turn him often. Antiembolism stockings help prevent venostasis and thrombophlebitis.

• Provide emotional support, and help reduce stress and anxiety; administer tranquilizers, as needed.

• If the patient has undergone PTCA, sheath care is necessary. Keep the sheath line open with a heparin drip. Observe for generalized and site bleeding. Keep the leg with the sheath insertion site immobile. Maintain strict bed rest. Check peripheral pulses in the affected leg frequently. Provide analgesics for back pain, if needed.

• After thrombolytic therapy, administer continuous heparin, as ordered. Measure the partial thromboplastin time every 6 hours, and monitor the patient for evidence of bleeding. Check ECG rhythm strips for reperfusion arrhythmias and treat them accord-

ing to your facility's protocol. If the artery reoccludes, the patient will experience the same symptoms as before. If this occurs, prepare the patient for return to the cardiac catheterization laboratory.

Patient teaching

Focus your teaching on helping the person and his family understand and cope with MI. Explain all procedures and answer any questions. Describe the intensive care unit environment and routine. Remember that you may need to repeat explanations during the emergency situation and again after it has resolved.

• To promote compliance with the prescribed medication regimen and other treatment measures, thoroughly explain dosages and therapy. Inform the patient of the drug's adverse effects, and advise him to watch for and report signs of toxicity (for example, anorexia, nausea, vomiting, mental depression, vertigo, blurred vision, and yellow vision, if the patient is receiving digitalis).

• Review dietary restrictions with the patient. If he must follow a low-sodium or low-fat and low-cholesterol diet, provide a list of foods to avoid. Ask the dietitian to speak to the patient and his family.

• Encourage the patient to participate in a cardiac rehabilitation exercise program. The doctor and the exercise physiologist should determine the appropriate level of exercise and then discuss it with the patient and secure his agreement to a stepped-care program.

• Counsel the patient to resume sexual activity progressively. Don't overlook this aspect of care with older adults. Most older adults are sexually active and may not feel comfortable asking about this topic. The patient may need to take nitroglycerin before sexual intercourse to prevent chest pain from the increased activity. Give him the teaching handout, *Resuming sex after a heart attack.*

• Instruct the patient to report any typical or atypical chest pain. Post-MI syndrome may develop, producing chest pain that must be differentiated from recurrent MI, pulmonary infarction, and heart failure. If appropriate, stress the need to stop smoking. If necessary, refer the person to a support group.

EACHING AID

Resuming sex after a heart attack

Dear Patient:

After you're discharged from the hospital, you can expect to gradually resume most, if not all, of your usual activities, including sex. Most patients, in fact, can resume having sex 3 to 4 weeks after a heart attack. As far as physical demands, sex is a moderate form of exercise, no more stressful than a brisk walk. However, keep in mind that sex can place a strain on your heart if it's accompanied by emotional stress.

Read over the following guidelines. They can help you have a satisfying sex life. And be sure to discuss any concerns with your doctor or nurse.

The setting

Choose a quiet, familiar setting for sex. A strange environment may cause stress. Make sure the room temperature is comfortable for you. Excessive heat or cold makes your heart work harder.

When to have sex

Have sex when you are rested and relaxed. A good time is in the morning, after you've had a good night's sleep.

When not to have sex

Don't have sex when you're tired or upset. Also avoid having sex after drinking a lot of alcohol. Alcohol expands your blood vessels, which makes your heart work harder. And don't have sex after a big meal; wait a few hours.

Positioning for comfort

Choose positions that are relaxing and permit unrestricted breathing. Any position that's comfortable for you is okay. Don't be afraid to experiment. At first, you may be more comfortable if your partner assumes a dominant role. You may also want to avoid positions that require you to use your arms to support yourself or your partner.

A few precautions

Ask your doctor if you should take nitroglycerin before having sex. This medication can prevent angina attacks during or after sex.

Remember, it's normal for your pulse and breathing rates to rise during sex. But they should return to normal within 15 minutes. Call your doctor at once if you have any of these symptoms after sex:
- sweating or palpitations for 15 minutes or longer
- breathlessness or increased heart rate for 15 minutes or longer
- chest pain that's not relieved by two or three nitroglycerin tablets (taken 5 minutes apart) or a rest period, or both
- sleeplessness after sex or extreme fatigue the next day.

PERIPHERAL VASCULAR DISEASE

Peripheral vascular disease can occur in the arterial or venous system. In older adults, it typically occurs as aneurysms, arteriosclerosis obliterans, varicose veins, and deep vein thrombi. Aneurysms are abnormal dilatations of an arterial wall. The weakened wall can rupture, become occluded, or be the source of emboli. Arteriosclerosis obliterans is the most common type of peripheral vascular disease in the geriatric population. Varicose veins are tortuous vessels engorged with blood. They may eventually cause venous insufficiency or venous stasis ulcers, especially around the ankles. A deep vein thrombosis is a clot that forms in one of the large veins, most commonly in the legs.

Aneurysms occur most commonly in men over age 50. Age-related changes in the vessels contribute to the occurrence of peripheral arterial disease. Calcium and cholesterol and other lipids accumulate in the arteries, and increased amounts of connective tissue and mucopolysaccharides are found in the intima. The resulting loss of elasticity causes the vessels to dilate and elongate.

Primary varicose veins tend to run in families, affect both legs, and are twice as common in women as in men. Usually, secondary varicose veins occur in only one leg. Both types most commonly begin in middle adulthood.

Superficial vein thrombophlebitis is usually self-limiting. It's also less likely to cause complications, because superficial veins have fewer valves than deep veins. Deep vein thrombophlebitis (DVT) affects small vessels, such as the lesser saphenous vein, and large veins, such as the vena cava and the iliac, femoral, and popliteal veins. Because it affects the veins that carry 90% of the venous outflow from the legs, DVT is more serious than superficial vein thrombophlebitis. Studies indicate that up to 35% of hospitalized patients develop this disorder, which occurs more commonly in people with a sedentary lifestyle or those who have limited mobility because of an acute or chronic illness. The incidence of deep subclavian vein thrombophlebitis is increasing as the use of subclavian vein catheters becomes more common.

Causes

Peripheral vascular disease results from a reduced blood supply to the tissues. The onset can be gradual or sudden. Buildup of atherosclerotic plaque in the vessels or changes in the vessels resulting from diabetes will cause a gradual onset. A sudden onset occurs when the vessel suddenly becomes occluded, such as by a thrombus, embolus, or trauma.

The most common cause of aneurysms of the leg vessels in older adults is progressive atherosclerotic changes in the medial layer of the arterial wall. The weakened area of the wall balloons outward with the pressure in the CV system.

In arteriosclerosis obliterans, the vessels become stiff and lose their elasticity because of the buildup of arteriosclerotic plaque. When the person exercises, the tissues require a larger oxygen supply and the sclerotic vessels are unable to dilate to increase the supply. Symptoms also occur with postural changes and extreme changes in temperature.

Primary varicose veins can result from congenital weakness of the valves or venous wall; from conditions that produce prolonged venous stasis, such as wearing tight clothing; or from occupations that necessitate standing for an extended period. Secondary varicose veins result from disorders of the venous system, such as DVT, trauma, and occlusion. With venous compromise, blood and fluid pool in dependent extremities. The resultant edema causes increased pressure in the tissues, further compromising the ability of blood to get to the tissues.

Three factors — hypercoagulability, venous stasis, and endothelial damage — together cause thrombophlebitis. These factors are known as Virchow's triad. Movement of blood through the veins is dependent on the pumping of the skeletal muscles through one-way valves. Any condition that results in a decreased use of the skeletal muscles or that compromises the valves can lead to DVT. Risk factors include immobilization, decreased physical activity, venous damage, obesity, heart failure, polycythemia, thrombocytosis, dehydration, malignancy, hip fracture, and estrogen use. Once in place, the DVT will further compromise the valves, contributing to the recurrent nature of this condition.

Although peripheral vascular disease can't be prevented, people can take steps to decrease the risk.

Assessment findings

As part of your assessment, review the person's medical history for possible causes of peripheral vascular disease. A person with peripheral vascular disease usually reports pain, but he may be asymptomatic. Varicose veins usually run in families, so check for a family history. Also document the presence and character of peripheral pulses and skin temperature for all extremities.

Aneurysm

If the aneurysm is large enough to compress a nerve, the person may report pain in the area of the compression. If the artery is thrombosed, the person may report feeling a nonpulsating mass.

With a femoral aneurysm, the person may report feeling a pulsating mass in the upper thigh. Later on, thrombosis or embolism may produce symptoms of ischemia.

Arteriosclerosis obliterans

The person will report intermittent claudication — pain with activity that subsides with rest. Document the amount of exercise the person can tolerate before pain occurs. Inspect the extremities for cold feet and legs, edema, and trophic changes, such as hair loss on the affected limb; thick toenails; dry, shiny or atrophic skin; or possible ischemic ulcers on the toes and heels. You also may see deep purple pregangrenous lesions or gangrenous lesions that are black, shriveled, and hard.

Test for postural color changes, indicating moderate to severe arterial occlusive disease. Ask the person to elevate his feet for 1 minute. With elevation, the feet will turn pale. When returned to a dependent position, the feet develop a dusky color.

Use a Doppler device to probe for pulses that are difficult to detect. Grade pulses from 0 to +4 (0 = absent, +1 = weak, +2 or +3 = normal, +4 = bounding). Absence of a posterior tibial pulse is the most reliable sign of arterial occlusive disease of the legs.

Varicose veins

A person with varicose veins may be asymptomatic or may complain of mild to severe leg symptoms, including a heavy feeling that worsens in the evening and in warm weather; cramps at night; diffuse, dull aching after prolonged standing or walking; aching during menses; and fatigue. Exercise may relieve symptoms because venous return improves.

Inspection of the affected leg reveals dilated, purplish, ropelike veins, particularly in the calf. Deep vein incompetence causes orthostatic edema and stasis of the calves and ankles. Palpation may reveal nodules along affected veins and valve incompetence, which can be checked by the manual compression test and Trendelenburg's test (see *Testing for varicose veins*, page 136).

Deep vein thrombophlebitis

The classic sign of DVT is new, rapidly occurring swelling of one limb with dependent edema. The person usually discovers the swelling on awakening. If pain is present, it's usually not severe. The person may report painful tenderness or a heavy, dull achiness in the involved extremity, commonly the calf. Exercise doesn't affect the level of pain. The person also may complain of fever, chills, and malaise.

The circumference measurement of the affected extremity will be larger than the unaffected one, especially just above the ankle. Inspection may reveal redness or swelling of the affected leg or arm. Gentle dorsiflexion of the foot may disclose a positive Homans' sign (pain in the affected calf). However, this sign's reliability as an indicator of DVT is questionable. Pitting edema is present on assessment, along with a mild to moderate temperature increase.

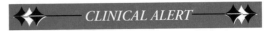

CLINICAL ALERT

There is always a gap between the level of thrombosis and the location of edema. For example, edema of the lower calf and ankle usually indicates a thrombus in the popliteal or lower femoral vein.

Testing for varicose veins

Two simple tests for varicose veins can be done as part of the assessment if this condition is suspected.

Manual compression test

The manual compression test is used to detect competent saphenous valves. Start by palpating the dilated vein with the fingertips of one hand. With the other hand, firmly compress the vein at a point at least 8"(20 cm) higher. Feel for an impulse transmitted to your lower hand. With competent saphenous valves, you won't detect any impulse. A palpable impulse indicates incompetent valves in a vein segment between your hands.

Trendelenburg's test

To do Trendelenburg's test (retrograde filling test), mark the distended veins with a pen while the patient stands. Then have him lie on the examination table and elevate his leg for about a minute to drain the veins. Next, have him stand while you measure venous filling time. Competent valves take at least 30 seconds to fill. If the veins fill in less than 30 seconds, have the patient lie on the examination table again and elevate his leg for 1 minute. Then apply a tourniquet around his upper thigh. Next, have him stand. If leg veins still fill in less than 30 seconds, suspect incompetent perforating veins and deep vein valves (functioning valves block retrograde flow). Now remove the tourniquet. If the veins fill again in less than 30 seconds, suspect incompetent superficial vein valves that allow backward blood flow.

Diagnostic tests

Arteriography helps confirm the diagnosis and can disclose the type, location, and degree of an obstruction or aneurysm and the status of any collateral circulation. Ultrasonography determines the size of femoral and popliteal arteries and shows aneurysmal dilation, decreased blood flow distal to an arterial occlusion, or the presence or absence of venous backflow in deep or superficial veins. It is also the current diagnostic test of choice for DVT. A computed tomography scan confirms the size and location of the aneurysm. Segmental limb pressures and pulse volume measurements help evaluate the location and extent of an occlusion.

Photoplethysmography, a noninvasive test used for venous disease, characterizes venous blood flow by noting changes in the skin's circulation. Venous outflow and reflux plethysmography can detect deep venous occlusion. Ascending and descending venography can demonstrate venous occlusion and patterns of collateral flow. Although it's the gold standard for diagnosing DVT, it's an invasive test and not routinely used.

Treatment

Medical treatment varies with the type and severity of disease, and may include surgery, drug therapy, or supportive measures.

Aneurysm

Aneurysms are usually repaired surgically. Depending on the size and location of the aneurysm, the doctor may monitor the extremity before surgically intervening.

Arteriosclerosis obliterans

In mild, chronic occlusive disease, treatment usually consists of supportive measures. The doctor may encourage the person to quit smoking, to control hypertension, to reduce dietary cholesterol and saturated fats, to exercise mildly, and to provide foot and leg care. In more severe cases, drug therapy, surgery, or both may be necessary.

For persons with intermittent claudication caused by chronic arterial occlusive disease, pentoxifylline may be prescribed to improve blood flow through the capillaries. This drug is particularly useful for poor surgical candidates. Other prescribed drugs may include heparin to prevent emboli and dextran to reduce platelet adhesion and clot formation. Thrombolytics, such as urokinase, streptokinase, and alteplase, can dissolve clots and relieve the obstruction caused by a thrombus.

Acute arterial occlusive disease usually requires surgery — typically, embolectomy, thromboendartectomy, or PTCA.

In embolectomy, a balloon-tipped, indwelling urinary catheter is used to remove thrombotic material from the artery. Embolectomy is used mainly for mesenteric, femoral, or popliteal artery occlusion. Thromboendarterectomy involves opening the artery and removing the obstructing thrombus and the medial layer of the arterial wall. Plaque deposits remain intact. Thromboendarterectomy is usually performed after angiography and is often used in conjunction with autogenous vein or Dacron bypass surgery (femoropopliteal or aortofemoral). PTCA uses fluoroscopy and a special balloon catheter to dilate the stenotic or occluded artery to a predetermined diameter without overdistending it.

In laser surgery, an excimer, or a hot-tipped laser, vaporizes the clot and plaque. Patch grafting involves removing the thrombosed arterial segment and replacing it with an autogenous vein or Dacron graft. In bypass grafting, blood flow is diverted through an anastomosed autogenous or woven Dacron graft to bypass the thrombosed arterial segment. Depending on the condition of the sympathetic nervous system, lumbar sympathectomy may be an adjunct to reconstructive surgery. If arterial reconstructive surgery fails or if gangrene, uncontrollable infection, or intractable pain develops, amputation may be necessary.

Varicose veins

Treatment for varicose veins depends on the severity of the disorder. In mild or moderate forms of the disorder, treatment may focus on self-care measures, such as wearing elastic stockings; avoiding tight clothing and prolonged standing; walking or other exercise that promotes muscle contraction, minimizes venous pooling, and forces blood through the veins; or elevating the legs.

For severe cases, the doctor may order custom-fitted, surgical-weight stockings with graduated pressure (pressure is highest at the ankle, lowest at the top). Stripping and ligation may be performed if the patient fatigues easily and has pain, heaviness, recurrent superficial thrombophlebitis, and external bleeding. Surgery may also be performed for cosmetic reasons. For persons who are poor surgical risks, the doctor may inject a sclerosing agent into small segments of affected veins.

Thrombophlebitis

Therapy for severe superficial vein thrombophlebitis may include use of an anti-inflammatory drug (such as indomethacin), antiembolism stockings, warm compresses, and leg elevation. For DVT, the doctor may prescribe activity restrictions, drug therapy, and in rare cases, surgery. Initial treatment usually includes anticoagulants (initially heparin, later Warfarin). Activity restrictions include bed rest with elevation of the affected arm or leg; application of warm, moist compresses to the affected area; and analgesics. After the acute episode subsides, the person may begin to walk while wearing antiembolism stockings that are applied before he gets out of bed. For lysis of acute, extensive DVT, treatment may include streptokinase or urokinase, provided the risk of bleeding does not outweigh the potential benefits of thrombolytic treatment.

In rare cases, DVT may cause complete venous occlusion. This complication necessitates venous interruption by simple ligation, vein plication, or clipping. Embolectomy may be indicated if clots are shed to the pulmonary and systemic vasculature and other treatment is unsuccessful. Caval interruption with an umbrella filter placed transvenously can trap emboli, preventing them from traveling to the pulmonary vasculature.

Complications

Peripheral vascular disease can lead to complete disruption of the circulation. Stasis ulcers, gangrene, and necrosis can result. Ulcers associated with peripheral vascular disease are usually difficult to heal. If they become infected, the diminished blood flow inhibits the ability of antibiotics to reach the tissues. Aneurysms can rupture or can form thrombi, which may embolize, causing ischemia and necrosis. Necrosis or gangrene in an extremity may require amputation. The major complications of thrombophlebitis are pulmonary embolism and chronic venous insufficiency.

Nursing interventions

Managing the care of an older person with peripheral vascular disease involves a wide range of tasks. Among other duties, you'll need to assess your patient's circulatory status and skin condition, administer drugs, and monitor coagulation times. If surgery is ordered, you'll need to prepare him for the procedure and monitor for complications afterward. You'll also need to provide emotional support as he learns to cope with his disorder.

- Assess and record your patient's circulatory status, noting the location and quality of peripheral pulses in the affected leg.
- Administer prophylactic antibiotics, anticoagulants, and analgesics, as prescribed.
- If the person is receiving anticoagulants, monitor coagulation times: activate partial thromboplastin time (APTT) for heparin therapy and prothrombin time (PT) and international normalized ratio (INR) for warfarin therapy. Therapeutic values for APTT and PT are $1\frac{1}{2}$ times the control; for the INR, a result between 2 and 3 is considered therapeutic. Watch for signs and symptoms of bleeding, such as tarry stools, coffee-ground vomitus, and ecchymoses. Monitor the person for bleeding at I.V. sites, and check gums for bleeding.
- Remind the person not to rub or massage the extremity. Place a cradle over the foot of the bed to keep the weight of the linens off the legs if needed.
- Measure and record the circumference of the affected arm or leg daily and compare it to measurements of the unaffected arm or leg. To ensure consistency, mark the skin where the measurement is taken.
- Assess the extremity daily for redness, tenderness, and signs of breakdown. Check the presence and status of peripheral pulses every 2 to 4 hours or as dictated by the person's signs and symptoms.
- During an acute episode of DVT, enforce bed rest and elevate the affected limb until the episode has passed. When you use pillows, position them to support the entire leg and prevent compression of the popliteal space. After an acute episode, increase the person's activity level according to his tolerance level, and apply antiembolism stockings. Apply warm compresses or a covered aquathermia pad to increase circulation to the affected area and to relieve pain and inflammation.

◆◆ — CLINICAL ALERT — ◆◆

To relieve limb pain caused by arterial occlusion, place the foot in a dependent position; elevation aggravates the pain. To ease pain caused by venous occlusion, elevate the limb.

- Provide clear and concise information about any impending surgery. Allow the person to express fears and anxieties about the disorder and about surgery. Encourage discussion about the impact the disorder will have on his life.
- Ask the person to describe activities that increase comfort. Encourage him to perform these activities so that he feels a sense of control. Encourage family members and friends to provide emotional support.
- Following surgery, carefully monitor the person for early signs of thrombosis or graft occlusion, including severe pain, loss of pulse, or decreased skin temperature, sensation, and motor function. Monitor for signs of infection, such as fever. Palpate distal pulses hourly for the first 24 hours and as ordered thereafter. Correlate your findings with those from the preoperative assessment. Mark the pulse sites on the person's skin for future reference.
- Encourage walking to prevent venous stasis and thrombus formation. Administer a plasma volume expander, such as dextran, as prescribed, to decrease platelet adhesion and to prevent early graft closure.
- Observe the person's behavior for nonverbal signs of pain. Administer analgesics, as prescribed, to alleviate pain.

Patient teaching

You'll need to teach the person with peripheral vascular disease what to expect during surgery and what to watch for after surgery. Also discuss drug therapy and activity restrictions.

• Before surgery, teach the person about surgical bypass and reconstruction of the artery. A person with an aneurysm may not be scheduled for surgery right away. Review expected postoperative procedures and answer any questions directly and honestly.

• After surgery, instruct the person to report any indications of failure of the saphenous vein or prosthetic graft replacement, such as a faint or absent pulse, a pale or blue color in the leg or foot, or coldness to the touch in the leg or foot. If the person has atherosclerosis, explain the risk for further arterial occlusions. Tell the person to report the return of any preoperative symptoms, such as decreased motor function, evidence of leg ulcer or injury, pain in the extremity, or evidence of decreased blood flow to the affected area.

• Teach the person how to care for his incision properly. Tell him to monitor the incision and report any drainage, redness, swelling, or tenderness near the incision. Explain that persistent swelling may occur after popliteal artery resection. If antiembolism stockings are ordered, make sure they fit properly and demonstrate how to put them on. Emphasize the need to avoid constrictive clothing.

• If the person is taking anticoagulants, emphasize the need to prevent bleeding. Instruct him to use an electric razor for shaving. Explain the importance of follow-up blood studies to monitor anticoagulant therapy. Caution against the use of tobacco and aspirin, and urge him to report evidence of bleeding, including bleeding gums, tarry stools, or bruising. Give him the teaching aid *Do's and don'ts of anticoagulant therapy,* page 140.

• If the person is taking pentoxifylline, teach him the use and adverse effects of this medication. Excretion is slower in an older person, so stress the importance of reporting any adverse effects.

• Discuss the activity level recommended by the doctor. The person may be allowed to go on daily walks. Describe the benefits of wearing a medical identification bracelet. Discuss the benefits of participating in a rehabilitation program to promote reconditioning.

ATRIAL FIBRILLATION

The most common arrhythmia in the older population, atrial fibrillation is characterized by a lack of organized atrial activity and irregular timing of the ventricular response. If the ventricular response is too fast, the ventricle will not have a chance to fill, compromising the cardiac output.

In older adults, atrial fibrillation is more likely to be chronic than acute and usually signifies organic heart disease. As the body ages, the number of pacemaker cells decreases and myocardial fat, collagen, and elastin fibers increase. The sinus node, which is responsible for initiating atrial contraction, has 90% fewer cells at age 75 than at age 20.

Causes

Atrial fibrillation results from impulses in many circus reentry pathways in the atria. In atrial fibrillation, these impulses usually fire at a rate of 400 to 600 per minute, causing the atria to quiver rather than contract regularly. The most common predisposing factors in older people are hypertension, CAD, and mitral valve disease. Stimulants such as nicotine and caffeine as well as amyloidosis, sick sinus syndrome, and thyrotoxicosis may also trigger atrial fibrillation.

Assessment findings

With rapid atrial fibrillation, the ventricle does not have time to fill, and the person may complain of his heart racing or of feeling faint. The heart rate will be irregularly irregular, meaning that there is no pattern to the irregularity of the pulse. Many people, especially those who have a ventricular rate less than 100 beats/minute, won't have any symptoms.

An ECG reveals an irregular tracing. The atrial rhythm is grossly irregular, with a rate of more than 400 beats/minute. The QRS complexes, depicting ventricular response, have a uniform configuration and duration but occur erratically. There are no discernible P waves, which depict atrial contraction in a normal heart rhythm, and no discernible PR

*T*EACHING AID

Do's and don'ts of anticoagulant therapy

Dear Patient:

To hinder your blood's ability to clot, your doctor has prescribed an anticoagulant drug. Follow this list of do's and don'ts when taking this drug.

Do's

● Carry medical identification stating that you're taking an anticoagulant.
● Use an electric razor to shave or a depilatory to remove unwanted hair.
● Place a rubber mat and safety rails in your bathtub to prevent falls.
● Wear gloves while gardening.

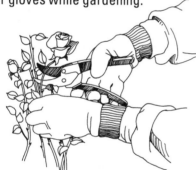

● Use a soft-bristled toothbrush.
● Ensure adequate intake of foods high in vitamin K: green leafy vegetables, tomatoes, bananas, and fish.
● Avoid sharp objects and roughhousing. Report abdominal or joint pain or swelling to your doctor.
● Draw a line around the margins of new bruises. If the bruises extend outside the line, notify your doctor.
● Maintain pressure on all cuts for 10 minutes. If you cut your arm or leg, also elevate it above

heart level. If the bleeding doesn't stop, call for help. Then call your doctor immediately.
● Check your urine and stool for any signs of blood.
● Notify your doctor of bleeding gums, nosebleeds, bleeding hemorrhoids, reddish or purplish skin spots, or excessive menses. Also report vomiting, diarrhea, or fever that lasts longer than 24 hours.
● Keep all appointments for blood tests.
● Refill your prescription at least 1 week before your supply runs out.
● Take your medication at the same time each day, as prescribed. Change your dosage only as directed by your doctor.
● Store your medication away from extreme heat or cold.

Don'ts

● Avoid taking aspirin, drugs containing aspirin, or any other drug (including nonprescription cough and cold remedies and vitamins) without checking with your doctor or pharmacist.
● Don't take an extra dose of your anticoagulant. If you forget to take a dose, just take your next dose at the scheduled time. If you miss two doses, call your doctor.
● Never put toothpicks or sharp objects into your mouth.
● Avoid walking barefoot.
● Don't trim calluses and corns yourself; instead, consult a podiatrist.
● Never use power tools.
● Avoid heavy alcohol consumption.

interval. Instead, a wavy baseline, indicating quivering of the atria, is present between the QRS complexes.

Treatment

Atrial fibrillation in older people is treated the same as in younger people. The goal of treatment is to decrease the ventricular rate to 60 to 100 beats/minute. Digoxin and verapamil are the most common agents used for chemical conversion.

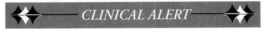

CLINICAL ALERT

Digoxin and verapamil are contraindicated in Wolff-Parkinson-White syndrome, which is rare in older adults. Quinidine may also be added; however, recent studies suggest that people receiving long-term quinidine therapy have an increased mortality rate.

Approximately one-third of older adults with atrial fibrillation have a controlled ventricular response and require no therapy.

If drug therapy is not successful, or if the arrhythmia is newly diagnosed (within a few weeks of onset), the doctor may perform cardioversion. Because of the risks involved, careful consideration is given to the cause and duration of the rhythm, the size of the atria, and the risks of alternative therapy.

Older adults have an increased risk of cerebral embolism. Anticoagulation therapy is usually initiated with heparin, followed by warfarin.

Complications

Complications usually arise from clots forming in the poorly functioning atria. Studies have shown that established atrial fibrillation in an otherwise healthy man substantially increases the risk of CV mortality to twice that of men with a normal rhythm. The incidence of CVA increases 13 times. Pulmonary embolism and acute arterial occlusion may also occur. Compromised cardiac output may result in hypotension or decreased urine output.

Nursing interventions

● Place the person on a continuous heart monitor and check his vital signs frequently (see *Cardiac monitoring,* page 142). Document any arrhythmias

and assess for hypotension or decreased urine output.

● Administer cardiac medications as ordered. Monitor digoxin or quinidine levels. If the person is receiving quinidine, document the QT interval before starting therapy and daily thereafter. A prolonged QT interval could lead to ventricular arrhythmias. Assist with cardioversion if ordered.

Patient teaching

Teach the person about atrial fibrillation, its treatment, and any necessary lifestyle modifications.

● Explain that atrial fibrillation, if managed properly, usually won't interfere with normal activities. Encourage the person to establish a regular exercise routine, under his doctor's supervision, to improve his overall CV fitness. Remind him to avoid overexertion, and warn him to stop exercising immediately if he experiences dizziness, light-headedness, dyspnea, or chest pain. Also warn against driving or operating heavy machinery if the atrial fibrillation causes periodic dizziness or syncope.

● Emphasize the importance of taking medications as prescribed. Point out that medication can only control, not cure, the arrhythmia. Tell the person to continue taking antiarrhythmics and other prescribed drugs according to schedule, even if he's free of symptoms. Advise him to call his doctor if he experiences adverse reactions. Tell him not to stop any medication until he contacts his doctor.

● If the person is taking digoxin, emphasize the importance of reporting any adverse effects and keeping follow-up appointments with his doctor and appointments for blood testing.

● Teach him how to take his pulse, making sure he is counting the beats for a full 60 seconds. Instruct him to call the doctor if his heart rate is greater than 100 or less than 50. Instruct him to report any episodes of dizziness, syncope, or palpitations.

● Explain that caffeine and nicotine are stimulants, and can increase the heart rate. Explain the dangers of "holiday heart syndrome" — the combination of increased food and alcohol consumption, smoking, and emotional excitement associated with holiday get-togethers can trigger or worsen arrhythmia.

● If the person will be undergoing cardioversion,

CHARTING GUIDE

Cardiac monitoring

In your notes, document the date and time that monitoring begins and the monitoring leads used. Commit all rhythm strip readings to the record. Be sure to label the rhythm strip with the patient's name, his room number, and the date and time. Also document any changes in the patient's condition.

7/8/96	07:20	Pt. on 5-lead electrode system. ECG strip shows Afib @ a ventricular rate of 96-120, QRS .08, ventricular rate up to 130 @ 0710 hr. Dr. Solon notified. Pt. asymptomatic. Peripheral pulses irregular; no edema noted. Heart irregular. No murmurs, gallops or rubs. Pt. denied chest pain/discomfort. J. Steele, RN

Atrial fibrillation

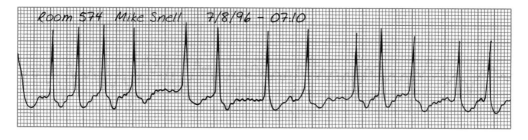

Room 574   Mike Snell   7/8/96 - 07:10

inform him that this procedure uses an electric current to restore the normal heart rate and relieve symptoms. Instruct him to abstain from food and fluids for at least 8 hours before the procedure. Explain that he'll be given an I.V. sedative to induce sleep and that while he's asleep, an electric current will be delivered to his heart through paddles placed on his chest. Reassure him that he'll feel no pain or discomfort from the procedure and that he'll be able to eat and move about once the sedative has worn off. Inform him that he may notice a reddened area of skin where the paddles were placed. The area may feel tender and itchy for a day or two.

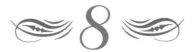

Managing respiratory problems

The aging process degrades the structure and function of the respiratory system, putting older adults at greater risk for respiratory disorders and diseases. Age-related anatomic changes include increased anteroposterior diameter of the chest wall, which causes reduced rib mobility and partial contraction of intercostal muscles, and elevated ribs and flattened diaphragm, which cause decreased chest expansion. Also, because of such factors as osteoporosis and vertebral collapse, kyphosis (spinal curvature) advances with age. Mobility and physical activity also decline. Stress, often well tolerated in the younger adult, causes fatigue and dyspnea in an older person.

As aging progresses, degenerative changes in lung tissue include loss of collagen (the elastic fibers within the alveolar walls that provide elastic recoil) and reduced ciliary activity in the tracheobronchial tree. Smaller airways collapse, producing poor ventilation of some basal areas. Forced vital capacity (the amount of air that can be expired after a maximal inspiration) decreases, and the residual volume of the lung increases. As a result, the lung surface area available for gas exchange decreases, reducing diffusion capacity.

Decreased ciliary activity and a diminished cough reflex impair clearing of mucus and foreign material from airways. Coupled with a decreased immune response, these conditions predispose older people to pneumonia, chronic obstructive pulmonary disease (COPD), tuberculosis, influenza, and adult respiratory distress syndrome (ARDS).

Because older people are particularly susceptible to respiratory disease, you'll need to perform respiratory assessment frequently. You'll probably be the first person the older patient meets who can detect early changes in his pulmonary function, thus ensuring prompt treatment. However, accurate respiratory assessment can be a challenge; changes in lung structure and mobility lead to increased dead space, which mimics COPD. What's more, the signs of infection in an older person are often misleading, placing him at risk for a late diagnosis and a more complicated course of illness.

PNEUMONIA

An acute infection of the lung parenchyma that often impairs gas exchange, pneumonia can be classified in several ways. Based on microbiologic etiology, it may be viral, bacterial, fungal, protozoal, mycobacterial, mycoplasmal, or rickettsial in origin. Based on location, pneumonia may be classified as bronchopneumonia, lobular pneumonia, or lobar pneumonia. Bronchopneumonia involves distal airways and alveoli; lobular pneumonia, part of a lobe; and lobar pneumonia, an entire lobe.

As well, the infection can be classified as one of three types: primary, secondary, or aspiration pneumonia. Primary pneumonia results directly from inhalation or aspiration of a pathogen, such as bacteria or a virus; it includes pneumococcal and viral pneumonia. Secondary pneumonia may follow initial lung damage from a noxious chemical or other insult (superinfection) or may result from hematogenous spread of bacteria from a distant area. Aspiration pneumonia results from inhalation of foreign matter, such as vomitus or food particles, into the bronchi.

Pneumonia occurs in both sexes and at all ages. Older adults run a greater risk of developing it because their weakened chest musculature reduces their ability to clear secretions. Those in long-term care facilities are particularly susceptible. The infection carries a good prognosis for patients with normal lungs and an adequate immune system. In debilitated patients and those over age 100, however, bacterial pneumonia ranks as the leading cause of death. Pneumonia is also the leading cause of death from infectious disease in the United States.

Bacterial pneumonia is the most common type of pneumonia found in older adults; viral pneumonia is the second most common type. Aspiration pneumonia occurs in older adults from impaired swallowing ability and a diminished gag reflex. These changes can occur after a cerebrovascular accident or any prolonged illness.

Causes

The decreased immune response of older people, along with decreased mobility, increases the likelihood of developing pneumonia. Other predisposing factors include chronic illness and debilitation, cancer (particularly lung cancer), abdominal and thoracic surgery, atelectasis, common colds or other viral respiratory infections, chronic respiratory disease, influenza, smoking, malnutrition, alcoholism, tracheostomy, exposure to noxious gases, aspiration, and immunosuppressive therapy. Aspiration pneumonia occurs in older or debilitated people, those receiving nasogastric (NG) tube feedings, and those with an impaired gag reflex, poor oral hygiene, or a decreased level of consciousness.

In bacterial pneumonia, which can occur in any part of the lungs, an infection initially triggers alveolar inflammation and edema. Capillaries become engorged with blood, causing stasis. As the alveolocapillary membrane breaks down, alveoli fill with blood and exudate, resulting in atelectasis. In severe bacterial infections and in ARDS, the lungs assume a heavy, liverlike appearance.

Viral infection, which typically causes diffuse pneumonia, first attacks bronchiolar epithelial cells, causing interstitial inflammation and desquamation. It then spreads to the alveoli, which fill with blood and fluid. In advanced infection, a hyaline membrane may form. As with bacterial infection, severe viral infection may clinically resemble ARDS.

In aspiration pneumonia, aspiration of gastric juices or food triggers similar inflammatory changes and also inactivates surfactant over a large area. Decreased surfactant leads to alveolar collapse. Acidic gastric juices may directly damage the airways and alveoli. Particles with the aspirated material may obstruct the airways and reduce airflow, which in turn leads to secondary bacterial pneumonia.

Assessment findings

An older adult with pneumonia may report fatigue and a slight cough. Pleuritic pain, if present, may not be as severe as that described in a younger person. Cerebral hypoxia may cause confusion, restlessness, and behavioral changes.

On assessment, you may note that the patient has a rapid respiratory rate and a fever. A decline in functional status often indicates an infectious process.

❖❖ ─── CLINICAL ALERT ─── ❖❖

Absence of a fever does not mean absence of infection in an older adult. Many adults develop a subnormal temperature in response to infection.

During inspection, you may observe that the person is shaking and coughing up sputum. Creamy yellow sputum suggests staphylococcal pneumonia, green sputum denotes pneumonia caused by *Pseudomonas* organisms, and sputum that looks like currant jelly indicates pneumonia caused by *Klebsiella*. Clear sputum usually indicates that the person doesn't have an infective process.

In advanced cases of all types of pneumonia,

you'll hear dullness when you percuss. Auscultation may disclose crackles, wheezing, or rhonchi over the affected lung area, as well as decreased breath sounds and decreased vocal fremitus.

Because older adults can tire easily when asked to take deep breaths, begin auscultation at the base of the lungs, and work toward the apex, alternating left to right. Normal breath sounds for the older adult often include diminished breath sounds and some chronic, mild adventitious sounds.

Be sure to respect the older adult's feelings of modesty and desire for privacy during your assessment, and assure him that the hospital gown sufficiently covers his body.

Diagnostic tests

A chest X-ray will disclose infiltrates, confirming the diagnosis. A sputum specimen for Gram stain and culture and sensitivity tests will show the bacterial cause of an infection. Because of age-related changes in the respiratory system, obtaining an adequate sputum specimen from an older adult is often more difficult.

Blood cultures will detect bacteremia and help determine the causative organism. An elevated white blood cell (WBC) count may be found in bacterial pneumonia; a normal or low WBC count in viral or mycoplasmal pneumonia.

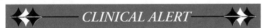

CLINICAL ALERT

In some older adults, the WBC count may be in the normal range, even with bacterial pneumonia. Look for an elevated band count in the differential for a better indicator of bacterial infection.

Arterial blood gas (ABG) levels vary, depending on the severity of the pneumonia and the underlying lung state. Bronchoscopy or transtracheal aspiration allows the collection of material for culture. Invasive procedures, however, afford a greater risk for the older adult, especially if he is frail or unable to cooperate. Pleural fluid cultures may also be obtained. Pulse oximetry may show a reduced arterial oxygen saturation (SaO_2) level.

Treatment

Antimicrobial therapy is based on the causative agent. The doctor will choose the initial antimicrobial agent, depending on whether or not he believes the pneumonia to be community acquired or nosocomial. Once culture results are available, he may change the drug to match the sensitivity reports. Therapy should also be evaluated by looking at the patient's temperature, respiratory comfort, sputum production, and results of the WBC count and differential.

Supportive measures include humidified oxygen therapy for hypoxia, bronchodilator therapy, antitussives, mechanical ventilation for respiratory failure, a high-calorie diet and adequate fluid intake, bed rest, and an analgesic to relieve pleuritic chest pain. A patient with severe pneumonia who is receiving mechanical ventilation may need positive end-expiratory pressure (PEEP) treatment to maintain adequate oxygenation.

Complications

Without proper treatment, pneumonia can lead to such life-threatening complications as septic shock, hypoxemia, respiratory failure, and ARDS. The infection can also spread within the patient's lungs, causing empyema or lung abscess. Or it may spread by way of the bloodstream or by cross-contamination to other parts of the body, causing bacteremia, endocarditis, pericarditis, or meningitis.

Nursing interventions

Focus your efforts on providing supportive care and assisting with implementation or monitoring of medical therapy.
● Maintain a patent airway and adequate oxygenation. Measure the patient's ABG or SaO_2 levels, especially if he's hypoxic. Administer supplemental oxygen if his partial pressure of arterial oxygen (PaO_2) falls below 60 mmHg. If he has an underlying chronic lung disease, give oxygen cautiously (usually limited to 2 to 3 L/minute).
● In severe pneumonia that requires endotracheal intubation or a tracheostomy with or without mechanical ventilation, provide thorough respiratory care and suction often, using sterile technique,

to remove secretions.

● Obtain sputum specimens as needed. Use suction if the patient can't produce a specimen. Collect the specimens in a sterile container and deliver them promptly to the microbiology laboratory. Administer antibiotics, as ordered, and pain medication, as needed. Administer I.V. fluids and electrolyte replacements, if needed, for fever and dehydration. Adequate hydration loosens secretions and makes them easier to expectorate.

● Provide a high-calorie, high-protein diet of soft foods to offset the calories the patient uses to fight the infection. To improve intake, offer nutritional supplements, such as Ensure or Pulmocare, between meals.

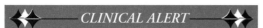
CLINICAL ALERT

Small, frequent meals are recommended for older adults because abdominal congestion due to a flattened diaphragm causes satiety after consuming just a small amount of food.

● If the patient is extremely debilitated, supplement oral feedings with NG tube feedings or parenteral nutrition. To prevent aspiration during NG tube feedings, elevate the patient's head, check the tube position, and administer the feeding slowly. Don't give large volumes at one time because this could cause vomiting. If the patient has an endotracheal tube, inflate the tube cuff before feeding. Keep his head elevated for at least a half hour after feeding. Monitor fluid intake and output.

● To control the spread of infection, dispose of secretions properly. Tell the patient to sneeze and cough into a disposable tissue, and tape a waxed bag to the side of the bed for used tissues.

● Provide a quiet, calm environment, with frequent rest periods. Make sure the patient has appropriate diversionary activities. Listen to the patient's fears and concerns, and remain with him during periods of severe stress and anxiety. Encourage him to identify actions and care measures that promote comfort and relaxation.

● Whenever possible, include the patient in decisions about care. Include the family in all phases of the patient's care, and encourage them to visit.

Patient teaching

Explain all procedures (especially intubation and suctioning) to the patient and family. Also discuss treatment, home care measures, and steps to avoid infection.

● Emphasize the importance of adequate rest to promote full recovery and prevent a relapse. Explain to the patient that the doctor will advise him when he can resume full activity or return to work.

● Review the medication regimen. Tell the patient to take the entire course of medication, even if he feels better, to prevent a relapse.

● Teach procedures to clear lung secretions, such as deep-breathing and coughing exercises, as well as home oxygen therapy. Explain deep breathing and pursed-lip breathing.

● Urge the patient to drink 2 to 3 qt (2 to 3 L) of fluid a day to maintain adequate hydration and keep mucus secretions thin for easier removal.

● Teach the patient and family how to perform chest physiotherapy. Explain that postural drainage, percussion, and vibration help to mobilize and remove mucus from the lungs. Urge a bedridden or postoperative patient to perform deep-breathing and coughing exercises frequently. Reposition the patient at least every 2 hours, and get him out of bed as much as possible.

● If appropriate, teach the patient how to use oxygen therapy safely at home.

● Advise the patient to avoid using antibiotics indiscriminately for minor infections. Doing so could result in upper airway colonization with antibiotic-resistant bacteria. If pneumonia develops, the organisms that produce the pneumonia may require treatment with more toxic antibiotics.

● Encourage the older adult to ask his doctor about an annual influenza vaccination and the pneumococcal pneumonia vaccination, which he would receive only once. Urge him to avoid irritants that stimulate secretions, such as cigarette smoke, dust, and significant environmental pollution. Advise the patient to avoid crowds during the influenza season as well as people with active upper respiratory infections. If necessary, refer him to community programs or agencies that can help him stop smoking, or suggest that he talk with his doctor.

● Discuss ways to avoid spreading the infection to others. Remind the patient to sneeze and cough into tissues and to dispose of the tissues in a waxed or plastic bag. Advise him to wash his hands thoroughly after handling contaminated tissues.

CHRONIC OBSTRUCTIVE PULMONARY DISEASE

Also called chronic airflow limitation disease, COPD is characterized by a reduced airway lumen from mucosal thickening and increased airway compliance from destruction of the lumen. In older adults, this disease most commonly takes two forms: emphysema and chronic bronchitis. Emphysema distends or ruptures the terminal alveoli, causing a loss of elasticity. These changes in the lung tissue interfere with expiration.

Chronic bronchitis is marked by excessive production of tracheobronchial mucus sufficient to cause a cough for at least 3 months each year for 2 consecutive years. It results in hypertrophy and hyperplasia of the bronchial mucous glands, increased goblet cells, ciliary damage, squamous metaplasia of the columnar epithelium, and chronic leukocytic and lymphocytic infiltration of bronchial walls. Additional effects include widespread inflammation, airway narrowing, and mucus within the airways, all producing resistance in the small airways and, in turn, a severe ventilation-perfusion mismatch. The severity of the disease is linked to the amount of cigarette smoke or other pollutants inhaled and the duration of the inhalation. A respiratory tract infection typically exacerbates the cough and related symptoms.

Emphysema appears to be more prevalent in men than in women; about 65% of people with well-defined emphysema are men; about 35% are women. Postmortem findings reveal few adult lungs without some degree of emphysema. Many older adults have persistent productive cough, wheezing, recurrent respiratory infections, and shortness of

breath associated with chronic bronchitis. The symptoms usually develop gradually, and are often first noticed when the patient has difficulty breathing in cold or damp weather. Older adults with a combination of chronic bronchitis and emphysema usually have a long history of smoking.

Causes
Emphysema may be caused by cigarette smoking or a deficiency of alpha$_1$-antitrypsin, although this is usually seen in younger people. Recurrent inflammation associated with the release of proteolytic enzymes from lung cells causes abnormal, irreversible enlargement of the air spaces distal to the terminal bronchioles. This leads to the destruction of alveolar walls, which results in a breakdown of elasticity.

The most common cause of chronic bronchitis is cigarette smoking, although some studies suggest a genetic predisposition to the disease as well. The disease is directly correlated with heavy pollution and is more prevalent in people exposed to organic or inorganic dusts and noxious gases.

Assessment findings
Usually, a person with emphysema or chronic bronchitis seeks medical treatment for a productive cough and exertional dyspnea. Typically, the dyspnea worsens and takes increasingly longer to subside. With chronic bronchitis, the cough may be described as initially prevalent in the winter months but gradually becomes a year-round problem with increasingly severe episodes.

The person may have a history of longtime cigarette smoking or, with chronic bronchitis, frequent respiratory tract infections. The history may also reveal anorexia with resultant weight loss and a general feeling of malaise. If weight gain occurs, it may be due to congestive heart failure.

Inspection may reveal a barrel chest, pursed-lip breathing, and use of accessory muscles for breathing. You may notice peripheral cyanosis, clubbed fingers and toes, and tachypnea. The characteristic cough produces copious gray, white, or yellow sputum.

Palpation may reveal decreased tactile fremitus,

decreased chest expansion, pedal edema, and neck vein distention. Percussion may detect hyperresonance. On auscultation, you may hear decreased breath sounds, rhonchi, crackles, and wheezing during inspiration; a prolonged expiratory phase with grunting respirations; and distant heart sounds.

Diagnostic tests

In advanced disease, the chest X-ray may show a flattened diaphragm, reduced vascular markings at the lung periphery, overaeration of the lungs, a vertical heart, enlarged anteroposterior chest diameter, and large retrosternal air space.

Pulmonary function tests typically indicate increased residual volume and total lung capacity, and reduced diffusing capacity. In emphysema, the inspiratory flow is increased and the diffusing capacity is decreased. In chronic bronchitis, the static compliance is normal, the diffusion capacity is normal, and the expiratory flow is decreased. ABG analysis usually shows reduced PaO_2 and normal partial pressure of arterial carbon dioxide ($PaCO_2$) until late in the disease.

Electrocardiography may reveal tall, symmetrical P waves in leads II, III, and aV_F; vertical QRS axis; and signs of right ventricular hypertrophy late in the disease.

A red blood cell count usually demonstrates an increased hemoglobin level late in the disease when the patient has persistent severe hypoxia. Sputum culture may reveal many microorganisms and neutrophils with chronic bronchitis.

Treatment

The most effective treatment is for the person to stop smoking and to avoid air pollutants as much as possible. The doctor may order antibiotics to treat recurrent infections, and bronchodilators to relieve bronchospasm and facilitate mucus clearance. Corticosteroids also may be used for their anti-inflammatory effects, although the risks for older adults may outweigh the benefits.

Some older patients may require oxygen therapy (limited to 2 to 3 L/minute) to correct hypoxia.

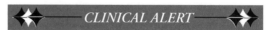

CLINICAL ALERT

Remember, respirations in people with severe COPD are stimulated by low oxygen levels, not high carbon dioxide levels. These patients may also require transtracheal catheterization to receive oxygen at home. And they'll need counseling about avoiding smoking, air pollutants, and sources of infection.

Adequate fluid intake (up to 2 to 3 L/day) is essential, and chest physiotherapy may be needed to mobilize secretions. Ultrasonic or mechanical nebulizer treatments may help to loosen and mobilize secretions. Diuretics may be used to treat edema.

Most older adults should be immunized to prevent influenza and pneumococcal pneumonia.

Complications

In COPD, complications may include recurrent respiratory tract infections, cor pulmonale, right ventricular hypertrophy, and respiratory failure. Peptic ulcer disease strikes between 20% and 25% of people with this disease. Additionally, alveolar blebs and bullae may rupture, leading to spontaneous pneumothorax or pneumomediastinum.

Nursing interventions

Provide supportive care and help the older adult adjust to lifestyle changes necessitated by a chronic illness. Answer any questions, and encourage him and his family to express their concerns about the illness. Include the patient and his family in care decisions. Remain with him during periods of extreme stress and anxiety. Refer him to appropriate support services as needed.

● Assess the patient for changes in baseline respiratory function. Evaluate sputum quality and quantity, restlessness, increased tachypnea, and altered breath sounds.
● Weigh the patient three times weekly, and assess for edema. Report changes immediately.
● Perform chest physiotherapy, if ordered, including postural drainage and chest percussion and vibra-

CHARTING GUIDE

Documenting chest physiotherapy

Whenever you perform chest physiotherapy, document the date and time of your interventions, the patient's positions for secretion drainage, the length of time the patient remains in each position, the chest segments percussed or vibrated, and the characteristics of the secretion expelled (include color, amount, odor, viscosity, and the presence of blood). Also record the indications of complications, the nursing actions taken, and the patient's tolerance of the treatment.

11/20/96	14:15	Pt. placed on ① side c̄ foot
		of bed elevated. Chest PT
		and postural drainage per-
		formed for 10 min. from
		upper to middle then upper
		lobes as ordered. Pt. had
		productive cough and ex-
		pelled large amt. of thick
		yellow sputum. Lungs clear p̄
		chest PT. Procedure toler-
		ated w/o difficulty. ———
		Colleen Durkin, RN

tion, several times daily. Document the date and time, as well as the specific interventions and results. (See *Documenting chest physiotherapy.*)

- Provide the patient with a high-calorie, protein-rich diet to promote health and healing. Give small, frequent meals to conserve energy and prevent fatigue.
- Schedule respiratory treatments at least 1 hour before or after meals. Provide mouth care after bronchodilator therapy. Make sure the patient receives adequate fluids (at least 3 L/day) to loosen secretions.
- Administer medications, as ordered, and record the person's response.
- Encourage daily activity, and provide diversionary activities as appropriate. To conserve energy and prevent fatigue, have the patient plan alternate periods of rest and activity.
- Assess the oral cavity.

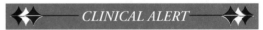
CLINICAL ALERT

Infections of the oral cavity can lead to respiratory infections or decreased appetite and contribute to poor general health. Teeth that are loose or brittle can dislodge or break, leading to lung abscesses and infections. The patient may have fewer respiratory infections when loose or diseased teeth are removed.

- Watch for complications, such as respiratory tract infections, cor pulmonale, spontaneous pneumothorax, respiratory failure, and peptic ulcer disease.

Patient teaching

Teaching people with obstructive lung disease how to manage the disorder is crucial, because self-care measures play a large role in treatment. Pertinent teaching topics include infection control, breathing techniques, chest physiotherapy, oxygen safety in the home, drug therapy, diet and activity regimens, and when to seek medical help.

● Advise the patient to avoid crowds and people with known infections, and to talk with his doctor about obtaining influenza and pneumococcal immunizations. Encourage him to have regular dental examinations.

● Teach the patient abdominal breathing and pursed-lip breathing techniques to use when he feels short of breath. Give the patient the teaching handout *How to overcome shortness of breath.*

● If the patient will be receiving home oxygen therapy, explain the rationale for oxygen therapy and proper use of equipment. If he requires a transtracheal catheter, instruct him about catheter care, precautions, and follow-up.

● Teach the patient and his family how to perform postural drainage and chest percussion. Instruct them to maintain each position for about 10 minutes and then perform percussion and cough. Give them the teaching handout *How to perform chest physiotherapy,* pages 152 and 153. Also, teach the patient coughing and deep-breathing techniques to promote good ventilation and mobilize secretions.

● Review the medication regimen and explain the rationale, dosage, and adverse effects of the prescribed drug. Stress the importance of not taking more than the prescribed amount of medication, even if symptoms are worsening. Advise the patient to report adverse reactions to the doctor immediately.

● If appropriate, show the patient how to use an inhaler correctly. Remember, because of age-related arthritic changes, an older adult may have more difficulty manipulating the equipment and, therefore, may need more practice.

● If the patient takes theophylline, warn him that cigarette smoking causes the drug to be metabolized faster. Instruct him to notify his doctor if he quits smoking, because he may experience adverse reactions associated with higher blood levels of theophylline.

● Encourage the patient to eat high-calorie, protein-rich foods. Urge him to drink plenty of fluids to prevent dehydration and to help loosen secretions.

● If he smokes, encourage him to stop. Provide him with smoking cessation resources or counseling, if necessary.

● Advise the patient to avoid respiratory irritants, such as automobile exhaust fumes, aerosol sprays, and industrial pollutants. Warn him that exposure to blasts of cold air may precipitate bronchospasm. Suggest that he avoid going out in cold, windy weather or that he cover his mouth and nose with a scarf or mask if he must go outside.

● Encourage daily exercise, and help the patient develop a regimen. Explain that conditioned muscles use oxygen more efficiently, so his exercise tolerance should improve.

● Advise the patient that sexual activity may be more comfortable earlier in the day while using oxygen and after taking bronchodilators.

● If appropriate, describe signs and symptoms of peptic ulcer disease. Instruct the patient to check his stools every day for blood and to notify the doctor if he has persistent nausea, vomiting, heartburn, indigestion, constipation, diarrhea, or bloody stools.

● Teach the patient the signs and symptoms that suggest ruptured alveolar blebs and bullae. Explain the seriousness of possible spontaneous pneumothorax. Urge him to notify the doctor if he feels sudden, sharp pleuritic pain that's exacerbated by chest movement, breathing, or coughing.

TUBERCULOSIS

An acute or chronic infection, tuberculosis (TB) is characterized by pulmonary infiltrates and by formation of granulomas with caseation, fibrosis, and cavitation. The American Lung Association estimates that active disease afflicts nearly 14 of every 100,000 people, and the incidence is on the rise.

TB is twice as common in men as in women and four times as common in nonwhites as in whites. But incidence is highest in people who live in crowded, poorly ventilated, unsanitary conditions, such as those in some tenement houses and home-

(Text continues on page 154.)

T EACHING AID

How to overcome shortness of breath

Dear Patient:

When you're having trouble breathing, performing special exercises will help you feel better. Practice these exercises twice a day for 5 to 10 minutes until you get used to doing them.

Abdominal breathing

1. Lie comfortably on your back and place a pillow beneath your head. Bend your knees to relax your stomach.
2. Press one hand on your stomach lightly but with enough force to create slight pressure. Rest the other hand on your chest.
3. Now breathe slowly through your nose, using your stomach muscles. The hand on your stomach should rise when you breathe in and fall when you breathe out. The hand on your chest should remain almost still.

Pursed-lip breathing

1. Breathe in slowly through your nose to avoid gulping air. Hold your breath as you count to yourself: one-1,000; two-1,000; three-1,000.
2. Purse your lips as if you're going to whistle.
3. Now, breathe out slowly through pursed lips as you count to yourself: one-1,000; two-1,000; three-1,000; four-1,000; five-1,000, six-1,000.

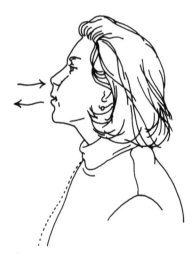

You should make a soft whistling sound while you breathe out. Exhaling through pursed lips slows down your breathing and helps get rid of the stale air trapped in your lungs.

When performing pursed-lip breathing during activity, inhale before exerting yourself; exhale while performing the activity.

If the recommended counting rhythm feels awkward, find one that feels more comfortable. Keep in mind that you must breathe out longer than you breathe in.

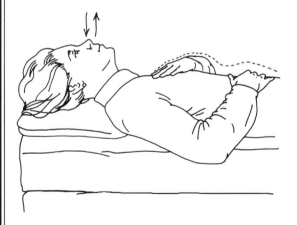

TEACHING AID

How to perform chest physiotherapy

Dear Patient:

The doctor wants you to perform chest physio-therapy to help make your breathing easier. This treatment has three parts: postural drainage, percussion, and coughing. You'll be able to perform postural drainage and cough-ing yourself, but you'll need a family member's or friend's help to percuss your back.

Postural drainage lets the force of gravity drain mucus from the bottom of your lungs. Then percussion helps move thick, sticky mucus from the smaller airways of your lungs into the larger airways. Coughing — the last and most important step — clears mucus from your lungs.

Follow the instructions for each step.

When to perform chest physiotherapy

Unless the doctor tells you differently, perform chest physiotherapy when you get up in the morning and before you have dinner or go to bed. When you have more mucus than usual (for example, during a respiratory infection), increase the number of treatments.

Getting ready

Don't eat for 1 hour before chest physiotherapy to avoid abdominal bloating and the risk of choking on vomited food. If ordered, use your inhaler 10 to 15 minutes before percussion to improve effectiveness.

Avoid wearing tight or restrictive clothing around your chest, neck, or stomach. Wear a light shirt or gown to avoid friction from percussion.

Postural drainage

1. Place a box of tissues within easy reach. Also stack pillows on the floor next to your bed or couch.
2. Next, lie on your stomach over the side of your bed. Support your head, chest, and arms with the pillows you've placed on the floor. Stay in this position for 10 to 20 minutes, as tolerated.

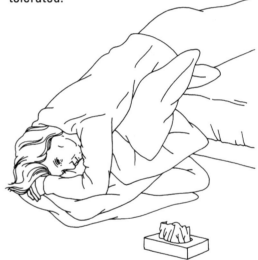

(This is the usual position for postural drainage. If it is difficult for you, use the following posi-tion: Stack two or three pillows on the bed and lay face down across them so that the pillows are under your hips and pelvis.)

Percussion

1. Remain in the postural drainage position. Have a family member or friend position his hands in a cupped shape, with his fingers

TEACHING AID

How to perform chest physiotherapy (continued)

flexed and thumbs pressed tightly against the side of his index fingers.

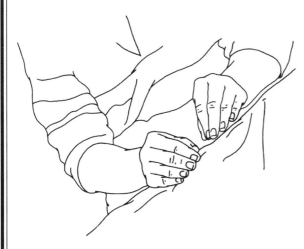

2. Next, have him rhythmically pat your back for 3 to 5 minutes, alternating his cupped hands. He can start on one side of the back, just above

the waist, and percuss upward, changing sides as he continues. Percussion will feel firm but shouldn't hurt. You should hear a hollow sound like a horse galloping.

Coughing

1. While remaining in the postural drainage position, take a slow deep breath through your nose. Hold the breath as you count to yourself: one-1,000; two-1,000; three-1,000.
2. Briefly cough three times through a slightly open mouth as you breathe out. An effective cough sounds deep, low, and hollow; an ineffective one sounds high-pitched.
3. Next, take a slow deep breath through your nose and breathe normally for several minutes. Repeat this coughing procedure, as tolerated.
4. After chest physiotherapy, return to an upright position slowly to prevent light-headedness and possible fainting.

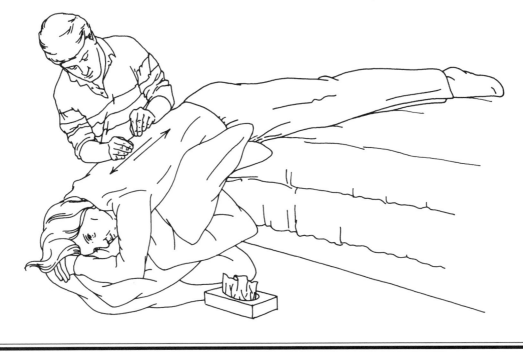

less shelters and those who live in institutional settings. Nursing home patients are 10 times as likely to contract TB as the general population.

Diagnosis is often delayed in older adults because the typical presenting symptoms, fever and night sweats, are often not seen. With age, diaphoresis decreases and alterations in body temperature commonly occur. These factors highlight the importance of periodic screening for older adults. All older patients entering a hospital and any group of older people, such as in a senior center, should be tested with a two-step Mantoux test.

Causes

TB results from exposure to *Mycobacterium tuberculosis* and sometimes other strains of mycobacteria. Transmission occurs when an infected person coughs or sneezes, spreading infected droplets.

When a person inhales these droplets, the bacilli lodge in the alveoli, causing irritation. The immune system responds by sending leukocytes, lymphocytes, and macrophages to surround the bacilli, and the local lymph nodes swell and become inflamed. If the encapsulated bacilli (tubercles) and the inflamed nodes rupture (as in an immunocompromised person), the infection contaminates the surrounding tissue and may spread through the blood and lymphatic circulation to distant sites.

After exposure to *M. tuberculosis*, roughly 5% of infected people develop active TB within 1 year; in the remainder, microorganisms cause a latent infection. The host's immunologic defense system usually destroys the bacillus or walls it up in a tubercle. But the live, encapsulated bacilli may lie dormant within the tubercle for years, reactivating later during the aging process to cause active infection.

The risk for TB is higher in older people who have close contact with a newly diagnosed TB patient, those who have had TB before, gastrectomy patients, and those affected with silicosis, diabetes, malnutrition, cancer, Hodgkin's disease, or leukemia. Drug and alcohol abusers, patients in mental institutions, and nursing home residents also have a higher incidence. The aging process weakens the immune system, further increasing the likelihood of

tubercular infection in older people. The incidence is higher in people receiving treatment with immunosuppressants or corticosteroids and in those who have diseases that affect the immune system.

Assessment findings

An older person with TB may complain of weakness and fatigue, anorexia, and weight loss. A cough that produces blood-tinged sputum is a less common initial sign in this population.

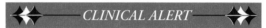

Fever and night sweats, the typical hallmarks of TB, may not be present in an older adult who exhibits a change in activity level or weight; assess the patient carefully.

When you percuss, you may note dullness over the affected area, a sign of consolidation or the presence of pleural fluid. On auscultation, you may hear crepitant crackles, bronchial breath sounds, wheezes, and whispered pectoriloquy.

Diagnostic tests

Chest X-rays show nodular lesions, patchy infiltrates (mainly in upper lobes), cavity formation, scar tissue, and calcium deposits. However, they may not help distinguish between active and inactive TB.

A tuberculin skin test reveals that the person has been infected with TB at some point, but it doesn't indicate active disease. In this test, 5 tuberculin units (0.1 ml) of intermediate-strength purified protein derivative are injected intradermally on the forearm, with results read in 48 to 72 hours. A positive reaction (equal to or more than a 10-mm induration) develops within 2 to 10 weeks after infection with the tubercle bacillus in both active and inactive TB.

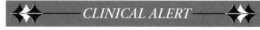

In older people, a two-step test should be performed. If the initial test is negative, it should be repeated in 1 week. If the response has waned, the second test will cause a conversion.

The most definitive test is isolation of *M. tuberculosis* in the sputum, cerebrospinal fluid, urine, abscess drainage, or pleural fluid using stains and cultures that show heat-sensitive, nonmotile, aerobic, acid-fast bacilli. Bronchoscopy may be performed if the person can't produce an adequate sputum specimen. Several specimens may need to be tested to distinguish TB from other diseases that may mimic it (such as lung carcinoma, lung abscess, pneumoconiosis, and bronchiectasis). Computed tomography or magnetic resonance imaging scans allow the evaluation of lung damage or confirm a difficult diagnosis.

Treatment

Antitubercular therapy with daily oral doses of isoniazid or rifampin (with ethambutol added in some cases) for at least 6 to 9 months usually cures TB. After 2 to 4 weeks, the disease is no longer infectious, and the patient can resume his normal activities while continuing to take medication.

A person with atypical mycobacterial disease or drug-resistant TB may require second-line drugs, such as capreomycin, streptomycin, para-aminosalicylic acid, pyrazinamide, and cycloserine. The adverse effects of these medications can be particularly hazardous to older adults. Para-aminosalicylic acid can cause GI tract irritation, anorexia, nausea, vomiting, and diarrhea, which can lead to malnutrition. Streptomycin can damage the peripheral and central nervous systems, resulting in disequilibrium and hearing loss, which can compromise the person's safety.

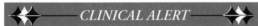

CLINICAL ALERT

Changes in gastric secretions can cause the medications to be passed through the intestinal tract without being absorbed. Check the stools of older people for undissolved tablets.

Complications

TB can cause massive pulmonary tissue damage, with inflammation and tissue necrosis eventually leading to respiratory failure. Bronchopleural fistulas can develop from lung tissue damage, resulting in pneumothorax. The disease can also lead to hemorrhage, pleural effusion, and pneumonia. Small mycobacterial foci can infect other body organs,

including the kidneys and the central nervous and skeletal systems.

Nursing interventions

Most of your interventions will focus on providing supportive care and administering prescribed medications. You'll also need to help the older adult with TB adjust to his diagnosis and learn to adapt his lifestyle accordingly.

● Until he's no longer contagious, isolate the infectious patient in a private room with an airflow control that prevents the circulation of air to other parts of the facility. Provide diversional activities and check on him frequently. Make sure the call button is nearby.

● Place a covered trash can nearby, or tape a waxed bag to the bedside for used tissues. Tell the patient to wear a mask when outside his room. Visitors should also wear masks in the patient's room. The Occupational Safety and Health Administration requires staff to wear a HEPA-filtered respirator when caring for a person with TB.

● Make sure the patient gets plenty of rest. Provide for periods of rest and activity to promote health, conserve energy, and reduce oxygen demand.

● Provide the patient with well-balanced, high-calorie foods, preferably in small, frequent meals to conserve energy. (Small, frequent meals may also encourage the anorexic patient to eat more.) Record the patient's weight weekly. If he needs oral supplements, consult with the dietitian.

● Administer prescribed antibiotics and antitubercular agents.

● Watch for adverse reactions to the medications. Administer isoniazid with food. This drug can cause hepatitis or peripheral neuritis, so monitor levels of aspartate aminotransferase and alanine aminotransferase. To prevent or treat peripheral neuritis, give pyridoxine (vitamin B_6) as ordered. If the patient receives ethambutol, watch for signs of optic neuritis; report them to the doctor, who will probably discontinue the drug. Check the patient's vision monthly and give this medication with food. If he is receiving rifampin, watch for signs of hepatitis, purpura, and a flulike syndrome, as well as other complications, such as hemoptysis. Monitor

liver and kidney function tests throughout therapy.
● Perform chest physiotherapy, including postural drainage and chest percussion, several times a day. Give the patient supportive care, and help him adjust to the changes he may have to make during his illness. Include the patient in care decisions, and let the family take part in his care whenever possible.
● An older person can have a very difficult time accepting the diagnosis of TB. Most older adults remember living in a time when people with TB were sent away to sanitariums for long periods of time. They may be unaware of new treatment methods and fearful of being institutionalized. Provide education on the treatment plan, and emphasize that treatment can be provided in the person's current living environment, once the initial infectious period has passed.

Patient teaching
The following teaching topics commonly apply to older adults with TB.
● Show the patient and his family how to perform postural drainage and chest percussion. Also, teach coughing and deep-breathing techniques. Instruct him to maintain each position for 10 minutes and then to perform percussion and cough.
● Explain the medication regimen, including therapeutic and adverse effects. Tell the patient to report adverse effects immediately. Warn the patient taking rifampin that the drug will temporarily make his body secretions appear orange; reassure him that this effect is harmless.
● Emphasize the importance of regular follow-up examinations, and teach the patient and his family to recognize the signs and symptoms of recurring TB. Stress the importance of complying with long-term treatment. Advise anyone exposed to an infected person to receive tuberculin tests and, if ordered, chest X-rays and prophylactic isoniazid.
● Teach the patient to report increased cough, hemoptysis, unexplained weight loss, fever, and night sweats. Stress the importance of eating high-calorie, high-protein, balanced meals.
● Explain respiratory and universal precautions to the hospitalized patient. Before discharge, tell him

that he must take precautions to prevent spreading the disease, such as wearing a mask around others, until his doctor tells him he's no longer contagious. He should tell all health care practitioners with whom he is in contact, including his dentist and eye doctor, that he has TB so that they can institute infection-control precautions.
● Teach the patient other specific precautions to avoid spreading the infection. Tell him to cough and sneeze into tissues and to dispose of the tissues properly. Stress the importance of washing his hands thoroughly in hot, soapy water after handling his own secretions. Also, instruct him to wash his eating utensils separately in hot, soapy water.
● Refer the patient to support groups such as the American Lung Association.

INFLUENZA

Also called the grippe or the flu, influenza is an acute, highly contagious infection of the respiratory tract. Although it affects all age-groups, influenza is more serious in older people and people with chronic diseases. In these groups, it can sometimes lead to death.

Causes
Influenza results from three types of viruses. Type A, the most prevalent form, strikes every year, with new serotypes causing epidemics every 3 years. Type B also strikes annually but only causes epidemics every 4 to 6 years. Type C is endemic and causes only sporadic cases.

The infection is transmitted by inhaling a respiratory droplet from an infected person or by indirect contact, such as drinking from a contaminated glass. The virus then invades the epithelium of the respiratory tract, causing inflammation and desquamation.

A remarkable feature of the influenza virus is its ability to mutate into different strains so that those at high risk have no immunologic resistance.

Assessment findings

The patient's history usually reveals recent exposure to a person with influenza. Most patients report that they didn't receive an influenza vaccine in the past flu season.

Flu symptoms appear after an incubation period of 24 to 48 hours. The patient typically reports sudden onset of chills, fever (101° to 104° F [38.3° to 40° C]), headache, malaise, myalgia, a nonproductive cough and, occasionally, laryngitis, hoarseness, rhinitis, and rhinorrhea. These signs usually subside within 3 to 5 days, but older people may feel tired and listless for several weeks.

Inspection may reveal red watery eyes, clear nasal discharge, and erythema of the nose and throat without exudate.

As the infection progresses, respiratory findings become more apparent. The patient coughs frequently and looks tired. If pulmonary complications occur, he may exhibit tachypnea, cyanosis, and shortness of breath. With bacterial pneumonia, you'll see purulent or bloody sputum.

Palpation may reveal cervical adenopathy and tenderness. Auscultation may disclose transient gurgles or crackles. With pneumonia, breath sounds may be diminished in areas of consolidation.

Diagnostic tests

Isolation of the influenza virus is essential at the first sign of an epidemic. Nose and throat cultures and increased serum antibody titers can help confirm the diagnosis. Once an epidemic has been confirmed, diagnosis requires only observation of clinical signs and symptoms. Uncomplicated cases show a decreased WBC count and an increased lymphocyte count.

Treatment

The patient with uncomplicated influenza needs bed rest, adequate fluids, acetaminophen or aspirin to relieve fever and muscle pain, and expectorant to relieve nonproductive coughing. Antibiotics have no effect on the influenza virus.

The antiviral drug amantadine has effectively reduced the duration of type A infection. In influenza complicated by pneumonia, the patient needs supportive care (fluid and electrolyte replacement, oxygen, and assisted ventilation) and appropriate antibiotics for bacterial superinfection.

Complications

The most common complication of influenza is pneumonia, which can be primary viral pneumonia or secondary to bacterial infection. Influenza also may cause myositis, exacerbation of COPD, Reye's syndrome and, rarely, myocarditis, pericarditis, transverse myelitis, and encephalitis.

Nursing interventions

● Administer analgesics, antipyretics, and decongestants, as ordered.
● Watch for signs and symptoms of developing pneumonia, such as crackles, increased fever, chest pain, dyspnea, and coughing accompanied by bloody or purulent sputum.
● Follow respiratory and blood and body fluid precautions.
● Provide cool, humidified air, but change the water daily to prevent *Pseudomonas* superinfection.
● Encourage the patient to rest in bed and drink plenty of fluids. Administer I.V. fluids if ordered.
● Administer oxygen if warranted.
● Help the patient to gradually resume his normal activities.

Patient teaching

● If the patient doesn't need to be hospitalized, teach him supportive care measures and signs and symptoms of serious complications.
● Teach him the importance of drinking plenty of fluids to prevent dehydration.
● Suggest a warm bath or a heating pad to relieve myalgia.
● Advise the patient to use a vaporizer to provide cool, moist air and to clean the reservoir and change the water every 8 hours.
● Tell the patient to get an annual influenza vaccine at the start of flu season (late autumn) unless he's allergic to eggs or chickens (the vaccine is made from chicken embryos). Inform the patient about possible adverse effects (discomfort at the vaccination site, fever, malaise and, rarely, Guillain-Barré syndrome).

ADULT RESPIRATORY DISTRESS SYNDROME

A form of pulmonary edema that causes acute life-threatening respiratory failure, ARDS is associated with various acute pulmonary injuries. It begins with increased permeability of the alveolo capillary membrane. Fluid accumulates in the lung interstitium, alveolar spaces, and small airways, causing the lung to stiffen. Ventilation becomes impaired, prohibiting adequate oxygenation of pulmonary capillary blood. Severe ARDS can cause intractable and fatal hypoxemia; however, people who recover may have little or no permanent lung damage.

Older adults, who have decreased lung elasticity and fewer functioning capillaries because of aging, are more likely to develop ARDS after a pulmonary incident.

Causes

In older people, ARDS usually arises from a variety of respiratory and nonrespiratory insults, including aspiration of gastric contents, sepsis (usually gram-negative), trauma, oxygen toxicity, and shock. It can also occur with pneumonia, microemboli, and disseminated intravascular coagulation. Drug overdose, blood transfusion, inhalation of smoke or chemicals, ingestion of hydrocarbons, pancreatitis, and near-drowning are less common causative factors.

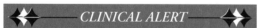
CLINICAL ALERT

The older person may appear to be doing well following an initial ARDS episode. Symptoms often appear 2 or 3 days later.

Once the syndrome is triggered, altered permeability of the alveolo capillary membranes causes fluid to accumulate in the interstitial space. If the pulmonary lymphatics can't remove this fluid, interstitial edema develops. The fluid collects in the peribronchial and peribronchiolar spaces, producing bronchiolar narrowing. Hypoxemia occurs as a result of fluid accumulation in alveoli and subsequent alveolar collapse, causing the shunting of blood through nonventilated lung regions. As well, regional differences in compliance and airway narrowing cause regions of low ventilation and inadequate perfusion, which also contribute to hypoxemia.

Assessment findings

In the early stages, the person will exhibit signs of respiratory distress, rapid respiratory rate, use of accessory muscles, apprehension, and restlessness. He will usually be cyanotic and may grunt with respiratory effort. As the hypoxemia worsens, mental sluggishness, motor dysfunction, and tachycardia (possibly with transient increased arterial blood pressure) will occur.

Auscultation of the lungs will reveal crackles and rhonchi from fluid accumulation.

Diagnostic tests

Serial chest X-rays may initially be normal or may show bilateral infiltrates. In later stages, a ground glass appearance is present and eventually (as hypoxemia becomes irreversible), "whiteouts" of both lung fields occur.

On room air, ABG analysis initially shows a decreased PaO_2 (less than 60 mm Hg) and $PaCO_2$ (less than 35 mm Hg). The resulting pH usually reflects respiratory alkalosis. As ARDS becomes more severe, ABGs show respiratory acidosis ($PaCO_2$ more than 45 mm Hg) and metabolic acidosis (bicarbonate less than 22 mEq/L) and a decreasing PaO_2 despite oxygen therapy.

Pulmonary artery catheterization helps identify the cause of pulmonary edema by evaluating pulmonary artery wedge pressure (PAWP); allows collection of pulmonary artery blood, which shows decreased oxygen saturation, reflecting tissue hypoxia; measures pulmonary artery pressure; and measures cardiac output by thermodilution techniques.

Treatment

When possible, treatment is designed to correct the underlying cause of ARDS and to prevent progression and potentially fatal complications of hypoxemia and respiratory acidosis. Supportive medical care consists of administering humidified oxygen by a tight-fitting mask, which allows for use of continuous positive airway pressure. Hypoxemia that doesn't respond adequately to these measures requires ventilatory support with intubation, volume ventilation, and PEEP. Other measures include correction of electrolyte and acid-base abnormalities.

When ARDS requires mechanical ventilation, sedatives, narcotics, or neuromuscular blocking agents, such as tubocurarine or pancuronium bromide, may be ordered to minimize restlessness (which in turn minimizes oxygen consumption and carbon dioxide production) and to facilitate ventilation. When ARDS results from fat emboli or chemical injuries to the lungs, a short course of high-dose steroids may help if given early. Treatment to reverse severe metabolic acidosis with sodium bicarbonate may be necessary, and use of fluids and vasopressors may be required to maintain blood pressure. Infections require antimicrobial drugs, if treatable.

Complications
Severe ARDS causes overwhelming hypoxemia that, if uncorrected, results in hypotension, decreasing urine output, respiratory and metabolic acidosis, and eventually, ventricular fibrillation or standstill.

Nursing interventions
Most of your interventions will focus on monitoring respiratory and neurologic status, serum electrolyte levels, and ABG studies. You'll also need to provide supportive care and emotional support as the patient learns to cope with ARDS.
- Frequently assess the patient's respiratory status. Be alert for retractions on inspiration. Note rate, rhythm, and depth of respirations, and watch for dyspnea and the use of accessory muscles for respiration. On auscultation, listen for adventitious or diminished breath sounds. Check for clear, frothy sputum that may indicate pulmonary edema. Document the date and time mechanical ventilation begins and any changes in the settings or the patient's response. (See *Documenting mechanical ventilation,* page 160.)

- Observe and document the hypoxemic patient's neurologic status (level of consciousness, mental sluggishness). Maintain a patent airway by suctioning, using sterile, nontraumatic technique. Ensure adequate humidification to help liquefy tenacious secretions. Closely monitor heart rate and blood pressure. Watch for arrhythmias that may result from hypoxia, acid-base disturbances, or electrolyte imbalance. With pulmonary artery catheterization readings, know the desired PAWP level; check readings often and watch for decreasing mixed venous oxygen saturation.
- Monitor serum electrolyte levels and correct imbalances. Measure intake and output, and weigh the patient daily. Check ventilator settings frequently, and empty condensation from tubing promptly to ensure maximum oxygen delivery. Monitor ABG studies; check for metabolic and respiratory acidosis and PaO_2 changes. The patient with severe hypoxemia may need controlled mechanical ventilation with positive pressure. Give sedatives, as needed, to reduce restlessness.
- Because PEEP may decrease cardiac output, check for hypotension, tachycardia, and decreased urine output. Suction only as needed so that PEEP is maintained, or use an in-line suctioning apparatus. Reposition the patient often, and record any increase in secretions or temperature or hypotension that may indicate a deteriorating condition.
- Monitor nutrition, maintain joint mobility, and prevent skin breakdown. Accurately record caloric intake. Give tube feedings and parenteral nutrition, as ordered. Perform passive range-of-motion exercises or help the patient perform active exercise, if possible. Provide meticulous skin care. Plan care sessions to allow periods of uninterrupted sleep.
- Provide emotional support. Warn the patient who is recovering from ARDS that recovery will take some time and that he will feel weak for a while.

Patient teaching
Prepare the patient and his family for treatment, and teach them what to expect.
- Explain all procedures and care routines to the patient and his family. Also explain the workings of the intensive care unit, and the roles of the different

Documenting mechanical ventilation

Document the date and time that mechanical ventilation began. Note the type of ventilator used for the patient and its settings. Describe the patient's subjective and objective responses to mechanical ventilation (including vital signs, breath sounds, use of accessory muscles, intake and output, and weight).

Throughout mechanical ventilation, list any complications and subsequent interventions. Record all pertinent laboratory data, including results of any arterial blood gas (ABG) analyses and oxygen saturation findings.

If the patient is receiving pressure support ventilation or using a T-piece or tracheostomy collar, note the duration of spontaneous breathing and the patient's ability to maintain the weaning schedule. If the patient is receiving intermittent mandatory ventilation, with or without pressure-support ventilation, record the control breath rate, the time of each breath reduction, and the rate of spontaneous respirations.

Record any adjustments made in ventilator settings as a result of ABG levels, and document any adjustments of ventilator components, such as draining condensation into a collection trap and changing, cleaning, or discarding the tubing.

12/6/95	10:15	Pt. on Servo ventilator set at TV 750, FIO2 45%, 5 cm PEEP; AC of 12, RR 20 nonlabored. #8 ETT in Ⓡ corner of mouth taped securely at 22-cm mark. Suctioned via ETT for large amt. of thick white secretions. Pulse oximeter reading 98%. Ⓛ lung clear, Ⓡ lung with basilar crackles and expiratory wheezes. No SOB noted. ——— Maria Duarte, RN

people who will be participating in the patient's care. Explain the ventilator and the different sounds the patient will hear. If he's intubated, provide a pen and paper for him to write down questions and allow him to communicate. Reassure him that he will be able to talk once the tube is removed.

• Emphasize the importance of suctioning and positioning, to encourage the patient's participation in his care.

• Provide emotional support. If possible, teach the family basic mouth care and provide the necessary supplies, so they can feel as if they are participating in the patient's care.

Managing neurologic problems

The neurologic system is the body's communications network. It regulates every mental and physical function during a person's lifetime, from birth to death. This dynamic control system coordinates and organizes all body systems. Therefore, changes in the neurologic system affect every body system.

As the body ages, the neurologic system changes. The number of neurons in the brain and spinal cord decreases, and the overall weight of the brain drops by 5% to 17%. Synthesis and metabolism of neurotransmitters diminish, slowing impulses that travel along neural pathways and decreasing response and reaction times. Kinetic sensing decreases, leading to impaired balance and reaction time. The sleep cycle is altered, with increased insomnia and night wakening and less deep sleep and REM sleep. Also, the sensory organs lose efficiency.

Keep these age-related changes in mind when caring for patients who are even further compromised by neurologic disorders such as those discussed below.

HERPES ZOSTER

Also known as shingles, herpes zoster is a virus that causes acute inflammation of the nerves of the skin, eyes, and ears. Each nerve emanates from the spine, banding and branching around the body to inner-vate a skin area called a dermatome. The virus produces vesicular skin lesions confined to a dermatome. The herpes zoster rash erupts along the course of the affected nerve fibers, covering the skin in one or several of the dermatomes. The thoracic and lumbar dermatomes are the most commonly affected, but others, such as those covering the cervical and sacral areas, can also be affected. Affected dermatomes can vary and overlap.

Exposure to the virus begins at birth and is cumulative with age. The infection, found primarily in adults over age 50, seldom recurs. Weakening of the immune system, which comes with age, is believed to contribute to the increased incidence of herpes zoster in older people. Other factors that compromise the immune system, such as chemotherapy and radiation, can cause herpes zoster. This virus is more severe in the immunocompromised patient but is seldom fatal.

The prognosis for people with herpes zoster is good, and most patients recover completely unless the infection spreads to the brain. Researchers are attempting to develop attenuated live-virus vaccines for susceptible populations.

Causes
The varicella-zoster virus, a herpes virus, causes herpes zoster. For unknown reasons and by an unidentified process, the disease erupts when the virus reactivates after dormancy in the cerebral ganglia (extramedullary ganglia of the cranial nerves) or the ganglia of posterior nerve roots.

Although the process is unclear, the virus may multiply as it reactivates, and antibodies remaining from the initial infection may neutralize it. Without opposition from effective antibodies, the virus continues to multiply in the ganglia, destroys neurons, and spreads along the sensory nerves to the skin.

Herpes zoster may be more prevalent in people who had chickenpox at a very young age, especially before age 1, but this is still a hypothesis.

Assessment findings

The typical patient reports no history of exposure to others with the varicella-zoster virus. He may complain of fever, malaise, pain that mimics appendicitis, pleurisy, musculoskeletal pain, or other conditions. In 2 to 4 days, he may report severe, deep pain; pruritus; and paresthesia or hyperesthesia (usually affecting the trunk and occasionally the arms and legs). Pain, described as intermittent, continuous, or debilitating, usually lasts from 1 to 4 weeks and occurs in areas bordering the inflamed nerve root ganglia.

During examination of a patient within 2 weeks after the initial symptoms, you might observe small, red, nodular skin lesions that spread unilaterally around the thorax or vertically over the arms or legs. Instead of nodules, you may see vesicles filled with clear fluid or pus. About 10 days after they appear, these vesicles dry, forming scabs. The lesions are most vulnerable to infection after rupture; some may become gangrenous. During palpation, you may detect enlarged regional lymph nodes.

Herpes zoster can involve the cranial nerves (especially the trigeminal and geniculate ganglia or the oculomotor nerve). With geniculate involvement, you might observe vesicle formation in the external auditory canal and ipsilateral facial palsy. The patient might complain of hearing loss, dizziness, and reduced sense of taste. With trigeminal involvement, the patient might complain of eye pain. He also might have corneal and scleral damage and impaired vision. Rarely, oculomotor involvement causes conjunctivitis, extraocular weakness, ptosis, and paralytic mydriasis.

In an elderly patient, recurrent infection or widespread dissemination calls for an evaluation for underlying lymphoma or other immune deficiency conditions.

Diagnostic tests

Vesicular fluid and infected tissue analyses typically show eosinophilic intranuclear inclusions and varicella virus. Differentiation of herpes zoster from localized herpes simplex requires staining vesicular fluid and identifying antibodies under fluorescent light. Usually, though, the locations of herpes simplex and herpes zoster lesions are distinctly different. Herpes simplex lesions commonly are found on the tongue, gingivae, cheeks, or genital area. Herpes zoster lesions typically appear in a unilateral distribution around the thorax or vertically over the arms or legs.

With central nervous system (CNS) involvement, results of a lumbar puncture indicate increased intracranial pressure (ICP). Cerebrospinal fluid (CSF) analysis demonstrates increased protein levels and possibly pleocytosis.

Treatment

Primary therapeutic goals include relief of itching with antipruritics (such as calamine lotion) and relieving neuralgic pain with analgesics (such as aspirin, acetaminophen, or possibly codeine). Tricyclic antidepressants help relieve neuritic pain.

Secondary infection may be prevented by applying a demulcent and skin protectant (such as collodion or tincture of benzoin) to unbroken lesions. If bacteria infect ruptured vesicles, treatment consists of an appropriate systemic antibiotic. Herpes zoster affecting trigeminal and corneal structures calls for instilling idoxuridine ointment or another antiviral agent.

Older adults are most likely to experience postherpetic neuralgia. To help patients cope with this intractable pain, a systemic corticosteroid, such as cortisone or corticotropin, may be ordered to reduce inflammation. The doctor also may prescribe tranquilizers, sedatives, or tricyclic antidepressants with phenothiazines.

Acyclovir may be prescribed for immunocompromised patients at high risk for complications and for patients with infections of the ophthalmic branch of the trigeminal nerve. This drug halts the progressing rash, reduces the duration of viral shedding and acute pain, and prevents visceral complications.

As a last resort for pain relief, transcutaneous peripheral nerve stimulation, patient-controlled analgesia, or a small dose of radiotherapy may be considered.

Complications

Herpes zoster ophthalmicus might result in vision loss. Complications of generalized infection might involve acute urine retention and unilateral paralysis of the diaphragm. In postherpetic neuralgia, intractable neuritic pain can persist for years, and scars may be permanent. In rare cases, herpes zoster may be complicated by generalized CNS infection, muscle atrophy, motor paralysis (usually transient), acute transverse myelitis, and ascending myelitis.

Nursing interventions

● Administer topical treatments as directed. If the doctor orders calamine, apply it liberally to your patient's lesions. Avoid blotting contaminated swabs on unaffected skin areas.
● Be prepared to administer drying therapies, such as oxygen, if the patient has severe disseminated lesions. Use silver sulfadiazine, as ordered, to soften and debride infected lesions.
● Give analgesics exactly as scheduled to minimize severe neuralgic pain. For a patient with postherpetic neuralgia, follow a pain specialist's recommendations to maximize pain relief without risking tolerance to the analgesic.
● Maintain meticulous patient hygiene to prevent spreading the infection to other parts of the body. If the patient has open lesions, follow contact isolation precautions to prevent the spread of infection to immunocompromised patients.

Patient teaching

● Inform your patient that treatment consists primarily of drug therapy to relieve pain and promote healing of the skin lesions. Reassure him that herpetic pain eventually subsides.
● Teach the patient how to apply the prescribed topical medication to the skin.

● Teach him how to apply cool compresses for additional relief from pain and itching.
● Suggest diversionary or relaxation activities to take the patient's mind off the pain and pruritus.
● To decrease discomfort from oral lesions, tell the patient to use a soft toothbrush, eat soft foods, and use a saline- or bicarbonate-based mouthwash and oral anesthetics.
● Stress the need for rest during the acute phase.
● Explain that herpes zoster isn't contagious (except to immunocompromised patients), but stress the need for meticulous hygiene to prevent spreading infection to other parts of the body.

SUBDURAL HEMATOMA

A subdural hematoma results from blood leaking into the subdural space. It can occur days or weeks after an injury, and the onset is usually insidious. Because the presenting symptoms can mimic cerebrovascular accident (CVA) or dementia, careful assessment is necessary.

There are three types of subdural hematomas, classified by their onset. An *acute subdural hematoma* involves rapid onset of neurologic deterioration, occurring 3 to 6 hours after the injury. The mortality rate is usually greater than 50%, and survivors may have neurologic deficits. A *subacute subdural hematoma* has a slower course, with a more gradual neurologic descent occurring 24 to 36 hours after the initial injury. The outcome for people with subacute hematoma is more favorable than for those with an acute hematoma. A *chronic subdural hematoma* produces neurologic symptoms up to 6 weeks after the causative injury, which the patient usually forgets or deems insignificant. Without cerebral herniation, the outcome for chronic subdural hematoma is good, with a mortality rate below 10%.

A high incidence of subdural hematomas is found in elderly patients with gait or balance problems or anyone at risk for falls. Chronic subdural hematomas commonly occur in alcoholics, patients with seizure disorders, and patients with prolonged coagulation.

Causes

Most subdural hematomas are caused by the head hitting a broad, hard object. Bleeding into the subdural space is either arterial or venous. Bleeding from an arterial source is usually severe and occurs with an acute trauma or, rarely, an aneurysm. Bleeding from large veins can also cause an acute hematoma. Subacute hematomas are more often associated with slow venous bleeding.

The initial injury in a chronic hematoma is small and usually doesn't produce any signs. As the hematoma develops, new capillaries form, which leak red blood cells and proteins. Local fibrinolysis prevents any further clot formation, and there is a cycle of clot lysis and reabsorption and minor bleeding. If bleeding occurs faster than reabsorption, a chronic subdural hematoma forms. This hematoma can grow quite large without causing any symptoms.

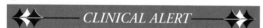

CLINICAL ALERT

An older person with cerebral atrophy can tolerate a larger subdural hematoma for a longer period of time than a younger person can before the hematoma causes neurologic changes. So a hematoma in an older patient can be very large before any symptoms are seen, even in an acute condition.

Assessment findings

Your patient may report a fall or injury to the head occurring anytime from hours to 3 days before the start of his symptoms, or he may not be able to recall any injury. He may complain of weakness in one or more extremities. Caregivers may report confusion and memory loss. Depending on the location of the hematoma, the patient may have difficulty speaking, ambulating, or balancing.

The patient with an acute subdural hematoma may report intense headache, vomiting, and visual deterioration from papilledema. The patient with a chronic subdural hematoma may complain of a recurring headache.

Inspection may reveal an old bruise or scab over the site of a head injury, but you may find no sign of injury at all. Early neurologic signs depend on the location of the hematoma. Assessment of strength and motor control may reveal weakness in one or more of the extremities. Assessment of pupils may demonstrate unequal size and reactions. Aphasia may be present.

The patient with an acute subdural hematoma displays a rapid decline in level of consciousness (LOC) and may present in a coma. The patient with a subacute subdural hematoma is initially lucid, with a slower deterioration in LOC. In a patient with a chronic subdural hematoma, LOC fluctuates; periods of coherence and alertness alternate with periods of confusion and lethargy.

Diagnostic tests

Computed tomography (CT) scanning is usually performed to visualize the collection of blood below the dura. Magnetic resonance imaging (MRI) yields the same image as a CT scan but may also allow visualization of the dura. Angiography is rarely used but may be indicated if the source of bleeding is suspected to be an aneurysm.

Treatment

The treatment in most cases is surgical evacuation. A craniotomy is usually performed for acute and subacute subdural hematomas to evacuate the hematoma and identify and treat the cause of bleeding. Surgery for a chronic hematoma most often involves the creation of burr holes under local anesthesia. The hematoma is evacuated, and the area irrigated. In 25% of cases, blood collection recurs.

An elderly patient with a small chronic subdural hematoma may be monitored with frequent CT scans to check on resolution or expansion. If no expansion is seen, the hematoma is allowed to remain. Evacuation of the chronic hematoma in an older adult may be further complicated by decreased elasticity of the brain. In this case, if the fluid is present for any length of time, drainage leaves a space and the fluid reaccumulates.

HARTING GUIDE

Using the Glasgow coma scale

The Glasgow coma scale is used to assess a patient's level of consciousness (LOC). It was designed to help predict a patient's survival and recovery after a head injury. This scale minimizes subjective impressions in evaluating LOC. The scale scores three observations: eye response, motor response, and response to verbal stimuli. Each response receives a point value. If the patient is alert, can follow simple commands, and is completely oriented to person, place, and time, his score will total 15 points. If the patient is comatose, his score will total 7 or less. A score of 3, the lowest possible score, indicates deep coma and a poor prognosis. Many facilities display the Glasgow coma scale on neurologic flowsheets to show changes in the patient's LOC over time.

OBSERVATION	RESPONSE	SCORE
Eye response	Opens spontaneously	4
	Opens to verbal command	3
	Opens to pain	2
	No response	1
Motor response	Reacts to verbal command	6
	Reacts to painful stimulus:	
	• Identifies localized pain	5
	• Flexes and withdraws	4
	• Assumes flexor position	3
	• Assumes extensor posture	2
	No response	1
Verbal response	Is oriented and converses	5
	Is disoriented, but converses	4
	Uses inappropriate words	3
	Makes incomprehensible sounds	2
	No response	1
TOTAL SCORE		3 to 15

Complications

The outcome for a patient with a subdural hematoma depends on the length of time between injury and surgery, how quickly ICP increases, and any associated intracranial damage. Complications include seizures and cerebral atrophy, which can lead to permanent neurologic deficits. In rapidly accumulating hematomas, brain stem herniation and death can occur as increased pressure and volume force the brain stem down into the base of the skull.

Nursing interventions

• Prepare the patient for ordered diagnostic tests. Perform frequent neurologic assessments to detect changes in LOC, which may indicate expansion of the hematoma. Document LOC using the Glasgow coma scale to minimize the subjective impressions in your evaluation. (See *Using the Glasgow coma scale.*)
• Keep the call button within the patient's reach, and instruct him to use it if headache symptoms begin or increase. Keep the bed's side rails raised at

night, as appropriate, and at other times if warranted. Keep the room free of clutter.
• If surgery is required, prepare the patient physically and emotionally.
• Following surgery, assess the patient's neurologic status to detect early signs of complications, especially increased ICP and cerebral ischemia. Also check vital signs. Assess for changes in respiratory patterns, which may be related to cerebral swelling or hematoma reaccumulation, and evaluate the patient for signs of infection.

Patient teaching

• Explain the nature of the disorder and the need for prompt treatment to help prevent complications. Also explain the purpose of diagnostic tests.
• Tell the patient to be sure to notify the doctor if he develops a headache. Explain the importance of keeping follow-up appointments with the doctor.
• Inform the patient about planned surgery. Clarify his risks and explain preoperative, postoperative, and follow-up home care.
• To prevent falls, instruct the patient to sit down and rest immediately if he experiences dizziness, disturbed balance, or weakness. To help prevent falls at home, advise the patient on making minor changes, such as installing a grab bar in the tub area.

ALZHEIMER'S DISEASE

A chronic condition characterized by declining intellectual capacity, Alzheimer's disease (AD) is the most common form of dementia. This progressive degenerative disorder of the cerebral cortex (especially the frontal lobe) causes gradual loss of memory with loss of at least one other cognitive function, such as language, abstraction, or spatial orientation.

An estimated 5% of people over age 65 have a severe form of this disease, and 12% suffer from mild to moderate dementia. Because this is a primary progressive dementia, the prognosis for a person with AD is poor. Typically, patients die of

debilitating brain disease 2 to 15 years after the onset of symptoms. The average duration of the illness before death is 8 years.

Causes

The cause of AD is unknown. However, several factors are thought to be closely connected to this disease. They include neurochemical factors, such as deficiencies of the neurotransmitters acetylcholine, somatostatin, substance P, and norepinephrine; viral factors such as slow-growing central nervous system viruses; trauma; and genetic factors.

Some researchers believe that up to two-thirds of AD cases may stem from genetic abnormalities that in some way interact with other factors to cause the disorder. Age also has been identified as a possible factor. Between ages 65 and 75, 3% to 5% of people are likely to develop AD; between ages 75 and 85, 18% are at risk; and over age 85, 48% to 50% may develop AD.

Assessment findings

As you assess your patient, keep in mind that the onset of AD is insidious and that initial changes are almost imperceptible but gradually progress to serious problems. The patient history is almost always obtained from a family member or caregiver.

Typically, the patient's history shows initial onset of very small changes, such as forgetfulness and subtle memory loss without loss of social skills and behavior patterns. It also reveals that over time, the patient began experiencing recent memory loss and had difficulty learning and remembering new information. The history also may reveal a general deterioration in personal hygiene and appearance and an inability to concentrate.

Depending on the severity of the disease, the patient history may reveal that this person experiences several of the following problems: difficulty with abstract thinking and activities that require judgment; progressive difficulty in communicating; and a severe deterioration of memory, language, and motor function that in the more severe cases finally results in loss of coordination and an inability to speak or write. He may also perform repetitive actions and experience restlessness; exhibit negative personality changes, such as irritability, depression, paranoia, hostility, and combativeness; experience sleep disturbances; and become disoriented.

The person giving you the patient's history may explain that the patient is suspicious and fearful of imaginary people and situations, misperceives his environment, misidentifies objects and people, and complains of stolen or misplaced objects.

He also may report that the patient seems overdependent on caregivers and has difficulty in using correct words, often substituting meaningless words. He may report that conversations with the patient drift off into nonsensical phrases. The patient's emotions may be described as labile; he may laugh or cry inappropriately, and have mood swings and sudden angry outbursts.

Neurologic examination confirms many of the problems revealed during the history. In addition, it often reveals an impaired sense of smell (usually an early symptom), impaired stereognosis (inability to recognize and understand the form and nature of objects by touching them), gait disorders, tremors, and loss of recent memory. In the final stages, the patient typically has urinary or fecal incontinence and may twitch and have seizures.

◆◆— CLINICAL ALERT —◆◆

The patient with AD has a positive snout reflex. The test involves tapping or stroking the patient's lips or the area just under the nose. Grimacing or puckering the lips is a positive sign for AD in an adult. (A positive result in early infancy is normal.)

Diagnostic tests
AD is diagnosed by exclusion. Various tests, such as those described below, are performed to rule out other disorders. However, the diagnosis cannot be confirmed until death, when pathologic findings come to light at autopsy.

EEG allows evaluation of the brain's electrical activity and may show slowing of the brain waves in the late stages of the disease. This diagnostic test also helps identify tumors, abscesses, and other intracranial lesions that might cause the patient's symptoms.

CSF analysis may help determine if the patient's signs and symptoms stem from a chronic neurologic infection. Cerebral blood flow studies may reveal abnormalities in blood flow to the brain.

Treatment
No cure or definitive treatment exists for AD. Tacrine is the only drug currently approved by the Food and Drug Administration for AD treatment. It has been used successfully in approximately 10% of cases to delay onset of AD by about 6 to 12 months when used in the beginning of the disease process.

Other treatments include cerebral vasodilators, such as ergoloid mesylates, isoxsuprine, and cyclandelate, to enhance the brain's circulation; hyperbaric oxygen to increase oxygenation to the brain; psychostimulators, such as methylphenidate, to enhance the patient's mood; and antidepressants if depression seems to exacerbate the dementia. Most other drug therapies are experimental. These include choline salts, lecithin, physostigmine, enkephalins, and naloxone, which may slow the disease process.

Complications
In this disorder, complications include injury from the patient's own violent behavior or from wandering or unsupervised activity; pneumonia and other infections, especially if the person doesn't exercise enough; malnutrition and dehydration, especially if the patient refuses or forgets to eat; and aspiration.

Nursing interventions
● Expect the patient's symptoms to get worse, at least temporarily, when he enters a facility. Away from the familiar home environment, he may become more disoriented and confused.
● To decrease the patient's adjustment time, ask the caregiver to describe the patient's usual routine at home. Use this information to plan a schedule of daily activities for his hospital stay.
● Use a soft tone, simple sentences, and a slow, calm manner when speaking to a person with AD. If he doesn't understand you, repeat yourself using the same words. Your nonverbal communication is more important than the words you use. The patient will respond to your tone of voice and gestures more than your actual spoken message. Don't use a

hurried tone, which will make the patient feel stressed. Move slowly and maintain eye contact.

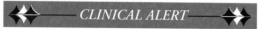

CLINICAL ALERT

Watch for loss of eye contact, a fearful look, wringing of the hands, and other signs of anxiety. When a person with AD is overwhelmed with anxiety, he'll become dysfunctional and acutely confused, agitated, compulsive, or fearful. Intervene by validating his fear and helping him focus on another activity, such as helping you set the table for a meal.

• Because the patient's thought processes are slow, allow him sufficient time to answer questions.
• Be supportive and acknowledge his feelings when he expresses them.
• Prevent excessive stimulation, and keep familiar objects and pictures at the patient's bedside.
• If the patient can still follow directions and read, leave memory aids, such as notes or pictures.
• Allow choices, even in small areas such as food or clothing. The perception of control decreases his anxiety and maximizes his ability to participate in his care.
• Administer ordered medications and note their effects. If the patient has trouble swallowing, crush tablets and open capsules and mix them with a semisoft food. (Always check with the pharmacist first; some drugs shouldn't be altered.)
• Protect the patient from injury by providing a safe, structured environment.

CLINICAL ALERT

Because most falls occur during the daytime, try bringing high-risk patients to one central location, such as the unit lounge. There, one staff member can supervise several patients, freeing the rest of the staff for other duties.

• Because the patient has a short attention span, provide task-oriented activities based on things the patient is familiar with. For instance, ask a housewife to fold hand towels or washcloths.
• Break tasks into parts. For instance, tell the patient to pick up the toothbrush, then to put toothpaste on it, then to brush, and then to rinse.
• Provide rest periods between activities because AD patients tire easily. But discourage frequent daytime naps, which may alter nighttime sleeping patterns.
• Encourage the patient to exercise, as ordered, to help maintain mobility, keep joints and muscles healthy, and promote better sleep cycles.
• Assist the patient with hygiene and dressing, as necessary. Many patients with advanced AD become incapable of performing these tasks.
• Encourage sufficient fluid intake and adequate nutrition. Provide assistance with menu selection, and allow the patient to feed himself as much as possible. Offer finger foods to patients who have short attention spans and frequently move from place to place. This allows them to walk as they eat, increasing their independence and caloric intake.
• Provide a well-balanced diet with adequate fiber. Avoid stimulants, such as coffee, tea, cola, and chocolate. Give the patient semisolid foods if he has dysphagia. Insert and care for a nasogastric (NG) tube or a gastrostomy tube for feeding, as ordered.
• Because the patient may be disoriented or have impaired neuromuscular function, take him to the bathroom at least every 2 hours, and make sure he knows its location. Paste a picture of a toilet on the door to help him remember where it is.
• Provide emotional support to the patient and his family. Encourage them to discuss their concerns. Answer their questions honestly and completely. Establish an effective communication system with the patient and his family to help them adjust to the patient's altered cognitive abilities.

Patient teaching

• Give the family the teaching handout *Planning home care*, pages 169 to 171. Tell them to create a routine for all the patient's activities, which will reduce confusion. If the patient becomes upset, tell the family to remain calm and to try redirecting him after validating his feelings.
• Give caregivers the teaching handout *Avoiding caregiver burnout*, pages 172 and 173. Advise them to get plenty of sleep, exercise, and support from others. Also, help them contact support services as appropriate.
• Provide the teaching handout *Promoting patient safety*, pages 174 and 175. Encourage family mem-

(Text continues on page 176.)

TEACHING AID

Planning home care

Dear Caregiver:

Taking care of a person with Alzheimer's disease requires a great deal of patience and understanding. It also requires you to look at the person's typical daily routine and his environment with new eyes, and make necessary changes to help him function at the highest possible level. The following tips can help you plan your daily care.

Reduce stress

Too much stress can worsen the patient's symptoms. Try to protect him from the following potential sources of stress:
● a change in routine, caregiver, or environment
● fatigue
● excessive demands
● overwhelming, misleading, or competing stimuli
● illness and pain
● over-the-counter (nonprescription) medications.

Establish a routine

Keep the patient's daily routine stable so he can respond automatically. Adapting to change may require more thought than he can handle. Even eating a different food or going to a strange grocery store may overwhelm him. Ask yourself: What are the patient's daily activities? Then make a schedule:
● List the activities necessary for his daily care and include ones that he especially enjoys, such as weeding in the garden. Designate a time frame for each activity.

● Establish bedtime rituals — especially important to promote relaxation and a restful night's sleep for both of you.
● Stick to your schedule as closely as possible (for example, breakfast first, then dressing) so the patient won't be surprised or need to make decisions.

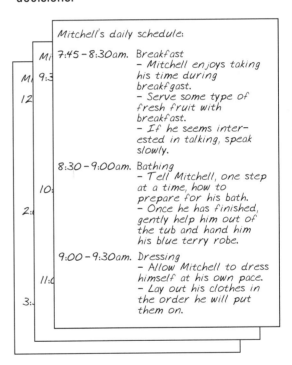

Mitchell's daily schedule:

7:45 – 8:30am. Breakfast
 – Mitchell enjoys taking his time during breakfast.
 – Serve some type of fresh fruit with breakfast.
 – If he seems interested in talking, speak slowly.

8:30 – 9:00am. Bathing
 – Tell Mitchell, one step at a time, how to prepare for his bath.
 – Once he has finished, gently help him out of the tub and hand him his blue terry robe.

9:00 – 9:30am. Dressing
 – Allow Mitchell to dress himself at his own pace.
 – Lay out his clothes in the order he will put them on.

● Keep a copy of the patient's schedule to give to other caregivers. To help them give better care, include notes and suggestions about techniques that work for you; for instance, "Speak in a quiet voice" or "When helping Mitchell dress or take a bath, take things one step at a time and wait for him to respond."

(continued)

TEACHING AID

Planning home care (continued)

Practice reality orientation

In your conversations with the patient, orient him to the day and the activity he'll perform. For instance, say "Today is Tuesday, and we're going to have breakfast now." Do this every day. This keeps the patient aware of his immediate environment and tells him what to expect without challenging him to remember events.

Simplify the surroundings

The patient will eventually lose the ability to interpret correctly what he sees and hears. Protect him by trying to decrease the noise level in his environment and by avoiding busy areas, such as shopping malls and restaurants. Does the patient mistake pictures or images in the mirror for real people? If so, remove the photos and mirrors. Also avoid rooms with busy patterns on wallpaper and carpets, because they can overtax his senses.

To avoid confusion and encourage the patient's independence, provide cues. For example, hang a picture of a toilet on the bathroom door.

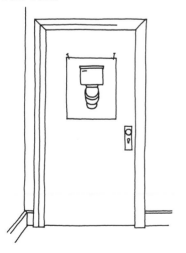

Avoid fatigue

The patient will tire easily, so plan important activities for the morning when he's functioning best. Save less demanding ones for later in the day. Remember to schedule breaks — one in the morning and one in the afternoon. About 15 to 30 minutes of listening to music or just relaxing is sufficient in the early stages of Alzheimer's disease. As the disease progresses, schedule longer, more frequent breaks (perhaps 40 to 90 minutes). If the patient naps during the day, have him sleep in a reclining chair rather than in a bed to prevent him from confusing day and night.

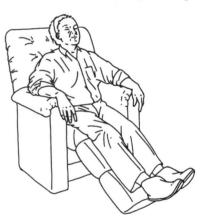

Don't expect too much

Accept the patient's limitations. Don't demand too much from him — this forces him to think about a task and causes frustration. Instead, offer help when needed, and distract him if he's trying too hard. You'll feel less stressed, too.

Prepare for illness

If the patient becomes ill, expect his behavior to deteriorate and plan accordingly. He'll have a low tolerance for pain and discomfort.

*T*EACHING AID

Planning home care *(continued)*

Never rely on the patient to take his own medicine. He may forget to take it or miscount what he has taken. Always supervise him.

Use the sense of touch

Because the patient's visual and auditory perceptions are distorted, he has an increased need for closeness and touching. Remember to approach the patient from the front. You don't want to frighten him or provoke him into becoming belligerent or aggressive.

Respect the patient's need for personal space. Limit physical contact to his hands and arms at first; then move to more central parts of his body, such as his shoulders or head.

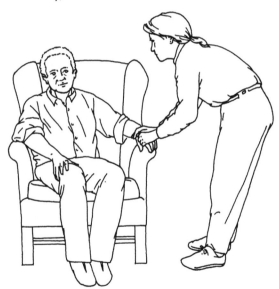

Using long or circular motions, lightly stroke the patient to help relieve muscle tension and give him a sense of his physical self. Physical contact also expresses your feelings of intimacy and caring.

Allowing the patient to touch objects in the environment can help relieve stress by providing information. Let him handle, poke, pull, or shake objects — for example, a handbag, a brush, or a comb. Make sure they're unbreakable and can't harm him.

Handle problem behavior

If the patient becomes restless or agitated, divert his attention with an appropriate activity. Good choices include walking, rocking in a rocking chair, sanding wood, folding laundry, or hoeing the garden.

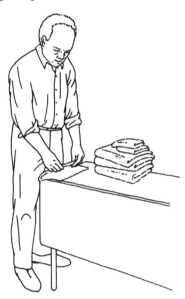

These repetitive activities don't require any particular sequence or planning. A warm bath, a drink of warm milk, or a back massage can also be calming.

Although problem behavior can be taxing for you, try to remember that the patient can't help himself. Your understanding and compassion can increase his sense of security.

Avoiding caregiver burnout

Dear Caregiver:

Caring for a person who needs full-time supervision and care makes you a prime candidate for burnout. Seemingly endless responsibilities can leave you feeling emotionally and physically drained, with virtually no time for yourself. If you feel inadequate to handle an unexpected crisis, both you and the patient suffer.

How can you cope? Start by learning the warning signs of burnout so you'll know if you're reaching your physical and emotional limits. Ask yourself the following questions:
● Do I have trouble getting organized?
● Do I cry for no reason?
● Am I short-tempered?
● Do I feel numb and emotionless?
● Are everyday tasks getting harder to accomplish?
● Do I feel constantly pressed for time?
● Do I feel that I just can't do anything right?
● Do I feel that I have no time for myself?

If you answered "yes" to any of the above questions, you're probably suffering from burnout or heading toward it. If so, the tips below will help you meet your own needs so you can give better patient care.

Get enough rest

Exhaustion magnifies pressures and reduces your ability to cope. So the first step in combatting burnout is getting a good night's sleep every night, if possible. Here's how:

First, decide how much sleep you usually need — say 7 hours — and set aside this much time. Then, when you go to bed, try not to replay the day in your mind. This isn't the time to solve problems.

To help control disturbing thoughts, practice relaxation techniques, such as deep breathing, reading, or listening to soft music. Or try dimming the bathroom lights and taking a warm bath or shower to relieve muscle tension and help you wind down.

Strenuous activity earlier in the day (not near bedtime) can promote sleep by tiring you physically. It also increases your physical stamina, improves your self-image, brightens your outlook, and gets you out of the house.

If possible, hire a relief caretaker so you can attend aerobics classes, go for a brisk walk, or get some kind of exercise for at least 1 hour three times a week.

In addition, try to schedule three or four short breaks during the day. Resting for 10 minutes with your feet up and your eyes closed can rejuvenate you and counteract the cycle of frantic activity that's probably keeping you up at night.

Use sleeping pills or tranquilizers only as a last resort, and only temporarily. Both types of drugs have side effects that can cause more problems for you in the long run. Instead, to induce drowsiness, try drinking a glass of warm milk.

Eat well

Eating regular, well-balanced meals helps you keep up your energy and increases your resistance to illness. Skipping meals or eating on the run can cause vitamin and mineral

Avoiding caregiver burnout (continued)

deficiencies — such as anemia (a shortage of iron in the blood) — that deplete your strength and make you feel exhausted.

Choose foods from the five food groups every day, avoid empty calories, and — unless you're overweight and your doctor advises it — don't diet. You need increased calories to fuel your increased activity.

Don't try to be superhuman

After you've been giving home care for several weeks, reappraise your earlier plans. How much can you really do? How much time do you need for yourself?

Now delegate tasks. If possible, hire extra caretakers or someone to help with housework and shopping. Contact local support agencies for help. Send your laundry out. Remember, you don't have to do it all today, or accomplish everything on your list. Do only what's absolutely necessary, and learn to set priorities.

Remember to save some time for pleasant activities. If you have 15 minutes of free time, listen to music or take a walk. If you want to have friends over for dinner, go ahead; just ask everyone to bring a course.

Confide in someone

A family member or close friend can help you resolve conflicts, be a sounding board for your anger and frustration, and offer emotional support. A support group can accomplish this too, as well as offer practical hints for patient care.

Schedule some quality time alone

Free time won't happen automatically; you have to schedule it. In fact, your patient also needs time for himself. So allow yourself and him some personal space and private time. If you don't, you'll become too dependent on each other.

Try to keep your life as normal as possible. Continue to do things that you enjoy, either by yourself or with your friends. Remember: Meeting your own needs isn't selfish, even if the patient is homebound. If you continue to feel guilty about taking some time for yourself, go for counseling.

How much time alone is necessary? The answer depends on you. At the very least, you need to take the time to attend to your important personal needs, such as bathing, washing your hair, and dressing. Or, you might want or need to have a part-time or full-time job. If so, arrange for a caregiver to take care of the patient while you're working away from home. Make sure this arrangement fits your needs and your relationship with the patient.

Your goal is to provide the best quality of life for the patient without sacrificing your own. How you accomplish this is up to you. But if you feel happy with the arrangement and the patient seems to be reasonably content, it's working.

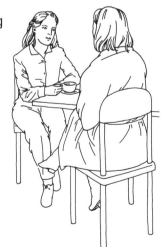

*T*EACHING AID

Promoting patient safety

Dear Caregiver:

A person with Alzheimer's disease requires intensive physical care as well as almost constant supervision to keep him from hurting himself. This means removing potential safety hazards from his environment and installing assistive devices where needed.

You can purchase many of these devices from large pharmacies or medical supply stores. You can also use childproofing devices, such as safety caps for electrical outlets, soft plastic corners for furniture, and doorknob covers. They're available from catalogs and where baby products are sold.

Use the following guidelines to help you provide a safe environment for the person in your care.

Remove potential safety hazards
● Move knives, forks, scissors, and other sharp objects beyond the patient's reach.
● Remove the knobs from the stove and other potentially hazardous kitchen appliances. Put dangerous small appliances, such as food processors and irons, out of reach.
● Taste the patient's food before serving it, so he won't burn his mouth or skin if he accidentally spills it.
● Serve the patient's food on unbreakable dishes.
● Adjust your water heater to a lower temperature (no higher than 120° F [48.8° C]) to prevent accidental burns.
● Cover unused electrical outlets, especially

those above waist level, with masking tape or safety caps.

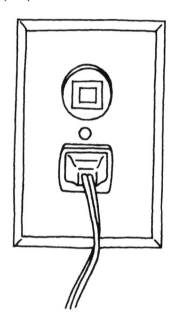

● Remove mirrors or install ones with safety glass in rooms the patient uses.
● Remove all breakable wall hangings and pictures, and attach curtains to the wall with Velcro.
● Get rid of throw rugs and cover slippery floors with large area rugs. Place pads under the rugs, and secure them so they don't slide.
● Keep traffic patterns open by moving unsafe furniture to the walls.
● Keep floors and stairways clear of toys, shoes, and other objects that can trip the patient.

Promoting patient safety *(continued)*

- Barricade stairways with high gates.

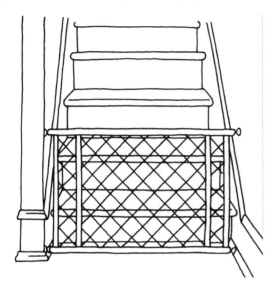

- Lock doors or camouflage them with murals or posters so they don't look like exits. Install locks at the bases of doors as an extra security measure, or install childproofing devices over the knobs.
- Store all medications out of the patient's reach, preferably in a locked container.

Install assistive devices

- Pad sharp furniture corners with masking tape or plastic corners.
- Provide a low bed for the patient.
- Keep the house well illuminated during waking hours. Keep a night-light in the bathroom.
- If the patient uses the stairs, mark the edges with strips of yellow or orange tape to compensate for poor depth perception.
- Encourage the patient to use the bathroom by making a "path" of colored tape leading in that direction.
- Attach safety rails in the bathtub, near the toilet, and on stairways.

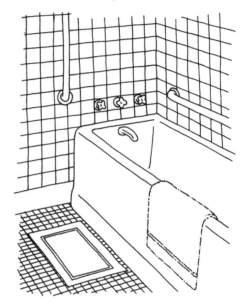

- Glue nonskid strips in the bathtub and by the toilet.
- Provide an identification bracelet for the patient, listing his name, address, phone number, and medical problems.

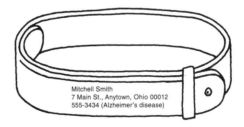

Mitchell Smith
7 Main St., Anytown, Ohio 00012
555-3434 (Alzheimer's disease)

- Give the local police a photograph and description of the patient, in case he's found wandering in the streets.

bers to allow the patient as much independence as possible while ensuring his and others' safety.

• Teach the patient's family about AD. Explain that the cause of the disease is unknown. Review the signs and symptoms of the disease with them, and advise them to expect deterioration. To help them plan future care, discuss the stages of this inevitably progressive disease. Be sure to explain that the disease progresses at an unpredictable rate and that the patient will eventually suffer complete memory loss and total physical deterioration. Bear in mind that family members may refuse to believe that the disease is advancing. So be sensitive to their concerns and, if necessary, review the information again when they're more receptive.

• Review the diagnostic tests that will be performed and the treatment the patient will require.

• Advise the family to provide the patient with exercise. Suggest physical activities that he enjoys, such as walking or light housework.

• Stress the importance of diet. Instruct the family to limit the number of foods on the patient's plate so he won't have to make decisions. If the patient has coordination problems, tell family members to cut his food and to provide finger foods, such as fruit and sandwiches. Suggest using plates with rim guards, built-up utensils, and cups with lids and spouts.

TRANSIENT ISCHEMIC ATTACKS

Transient ischemic attacks (TIAs) are sudden, brief episodes of neurologic deficit caused by focal cerebral ischemia. They usually last 5 to 20 minutes and are followed by rapid clearing of neurologic deficits (typically within 24 hours).

There are two types of TIAs: vertebrobasilar and carotid. Vertebrobasilar TIAs result from inadequate blood flow from the vertebral arteries. The two vertebral arteries (on either side of the head) extend from the subclavian artery, through the upper six cervical vertebrae, then enter the skull through the foramen magnum and join to form the basilar

artery. A vertebrobasilar TIA may occur secondary to occluded blood flow from the subclavian artery, which supplies blood to the vertebrobasilar arterial pathway.

Carotid TIAs result from inadequate blood flow from the carotid artery. Inadequate blood flow may be due to a narrowing or partial occlusion at the bifurcation of the common carotid artery where it branches into the internal and external carotid arteries.

TIAs occur most often in people over age 50. They affect men more commonly than women, and blacks have a higher risk than whites. TIAs may warn of an impending CVA. About 50% to 80% of patients who experience a thrombotic CVA have previously suffered a TIA. Accurately predicting when a CVA will occur after a TIA is difficult. One patient may suffer a single TIA followed by a CVA only hours later, whereas another patient, who may have had 50 TIAs, might not have a CVA for years.

Causes

TIAs may be caused by vascular disorders, such as extensive extracranial atherosclerosis, arteritis, and fibromuscular dysplasia, or blood disorders, such as hypercoagulability, polycythemia, and recurrent embolism. Any condition that lowers cerebrovascular blood flow, such as diminished cardiac output or subclavian steal syndrome (decreased supply of blood to the subclavian artery), can cause a TIA. Sometimes, a TIA can result from hyperextension and flexion of the head, for example, when a person falls asleep in a chair, impairing cerebral blood flow.

Assessment findings

Because a TIA usually resolves itself by the time the patient reaches the hospital, focus your assessment on obtaining a thorough health history, including previous medical conditions.

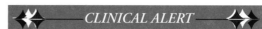

CLINICAL ALERT

To get the best assessment results, ask the patient about recent falls, especially frequent falls. This is important because an older patient is less likely to forget about or minimize frequent falls than other signs of a TIA.

If the patient experienced a vertebrobasilar TIA, he may complain of dizziness, diplopia, dark or blurred vision, visual field deficits, ptosis, difficulty in speaking, or difficulty in swallowing. He may report unilateral or bilateral weakness and numbness in the fingers, arms, or legs (or all three sites), a staggering gait, or veering to one side.

If the patient experienced a carotid TIA, he may complain of transient blindness in one eye, altered LOC, numbness of the tongue, seizures, or unilateral or bilateral weakness or numbness in the fingers, arms, or legs (or in all three sites).

A neurologic examination usually discloses varied deficits, which are transient and brief. A cardiac examination may reveal heart or vascular disease. For example, auscultation of the carotid artery may reveal bruits. Palpation may disclose faint peripheral pulses. A blood pressure check may reveal hypertension.

Diagnostic tests

Oculoplethysmography may indicate carotid occlusive disease by revealing delayed pulse arrival in one eye. A carotid Doppler or transcranial Doppler study may disclose blood flow disturbances. Cerebral angiography may be needed to confirm carotid stenosis or occlusion.

Digital subtraction angiography may reveal carotid occlusion or severe carotid stenosis. MRI and magnetic resonance arteriography may provide additional information.

Treatment

Aspirin is the preferred drug for treating a TIA and is probably most helpful when the TIA is caused by emboli due to atherosclerotic plaque. Warfarin may be prescribed, but prolonged therapy increases the risk of hemorrhagic complications. Short-term I.V. heparin may be ordered for patients suspected of having carotid or vertebrobasilar stenosis from thrombus formation. Dipyridamole and sulfinpyrazone are now only occasionally prescribed.

If the patient doesn't respond to drug therapy and is at high risk for a CVA, surgery may be considered. However, surgery is used primarily to treat carotid artery obstruction resulting from atherosclerosis or stenosis. With vertebrobasilar TIAs (which usually don't lead to CVA), surgery is rarely performed because only the proximal vertebrobasilar arteries are surgically accessible. Surgical procedures include carotid endarterectomy and extracranial-intracranial bypass; however, the latter is controversial.

Recommended lifestyle changes to reduce risk factors may include weight loss, smoking cessation, hypertension and diabetes management, and daily exercise.

Complications

TIAs significantly increase a person's risk of CVA.

Nursing interventions

● Prepare the patient for ordered diagnostic tests. After invasive procedures, monitor him for complications.

● Monitor neurologic status and vital signs to detect TIA recurrence or progression to CVA.

● Administer ordered medications, and assess for bleeding.

● Monitor the results of laboratory tests, including prothrombin time in patients receiving oral anticoagulants and partial thromboplastin time in patients receiving heparin. Also monitor the patient's hemoglobin level, hematocrit, and platelet count.

● Keep the call button near the patient, and instruct him to use it if he experiences any symptoms.

● Keep the bed's side rails raised at night and at other times, if warranted. Keep the patient's room free of clutter.

● If the patient fears a CVA, offer emotional support. Allow him to express his fears and concerns. Explain clearly the goals of treatment.

● If the patient requires surgery, prepare him physically and emotionally.

● Following surgery, assess the patient's neurologic status to detect early signs of complications, especially increased intracranial pressure and cerebral ischemia. Also assess his vital signs. Expect to maintain his systolic blood pressure at 120 to 170 mm Hg to ensure cerebral perfusion. Also assess for airway obstruction, which may be related to excessive swelling in the neck, hematoma formation, or faulty head positioning.

- Ask the doctor if the patient can drive or operate dangerous equipment.

Patient teaching

- Explain the nature of the disorder and the need for prompt treatment to help prevent a CVA. Also explain the purpose of diagnostic tests and the importance of keeping follow-up laboratory appointments.
- Inform the patient about prescribed drugs, including their purpose, action, dosage, route, possible adverse effects, and precautions. Tell the patient to be sure to notify the doctor if bleeding occurs.
- To prevent falls, instruct the patient to sit down and rest immediately if dizziness, disturbed balance, or weakness occurs. To help prevent falls at home, suggest making minor changes, such as installing a grab bar in the tub area.
- Inform the patient about planned surgery. Clarify the risks, and explain preoperative, postoperative, and follow-up home care.
- Help the patient plan to reduce TIA risk. Work with him on a program of moderate exercise. Refer him to a smoking cessation or weight loss program, if needed. Discuss the need to comply with all treatments, which may include taking prescribed medications to control blood pressure or diabetes mellitus.
- Tell the patient to immediately report any neurologic symptoms, especially those lasting longer than 24 hours. Stress the need for keeping follow-up appointments.

CEREBROVASCULAR ACCIDENT

Also called a stroke, a cerebrovascular accident (CVA) occurs when impaired circulation in the brain disrupts the supply of oxygen. Recovery from a CVA depends on how quickly and completely circulation is restored. However, almost half of all patients who survive a CVA are permanently disabled and suffer a recurrent attack.

CVA is the third leading cause of death and the most common cause of neurologic disability in North America. It strikes more than 500,000 people each year, killing more than 250,000. Though CVA can strike people of any age, it affects mostly men over age 65. Blacks face an especially high risk. Improved control of hypertension, the main risk factor for CVA, and improved treatment for TIAs have helped reduce the incidence of CVA over the past 30 years.

Causes

A CVA results from impaired circulation in one or more blood vessels of the brain, usually due to thrombosis, embolism, or hemorrhage. The most common cause of CVA is thrombosis, which is usually related to atherosclerosis. Plaque and atheromatous deposits gradually occlude the artery. Occlusion leads to ischemia and infarction of brain tissue, followed by edema and necrosis. Thrombosis usually occurs in the extracerebral vessels, but sometimes occurs in the intracerebral vessels.

With embolism, fragments usually break off from a mural thrombus in the left atrium or ventricle or from bacterial vegetations affecting heart valves. These emboli travel through the carotid artery and typically lodge in the smaller cerebral vessels, most often the left middle cerebral artery. Ischemia may occur suddenly, often followed by necrosis and edema. However, if the embolus breaks apart, then enters and is absorbed by a smaller vessel, the person's symptoms may subside.

CVA due to hemorrhage occurs when a cerebral vessel ruptures and blood flows into brain tissue or the subarachnoid space. Hemorrhagic CVAs are usually caused by rupture of an arteriosclerotic vessel due to prolonged hypertension, a cerebral aneurysm, or an arteriovenous malformation. Effects may be severe. More than 50% of patients die of brain herniation within the first 3 days.

Risk factors for CVA include head injury, atherosclerosis, hypertension, arrhythmias, myocardial infarction, rheumatic heart disease, postural hypotension, cardiac hypertrophy, previous heart surgery, emboli, diabetes mellitus, and gout. Other risk factors include obesity; high serum cholesterol, lipoprotein, or triglyceride levels; lack of exercise;

smoking; and a family history of cerebrovascular disease.

Assessment findings

If you suspect that a person is having or has had a CVA, contact the doctor immediately. Make certain that the patient has an unobstructed airway and is adequately ventilated. Assess his vital signs and perform as complete a neurologic examination as the situation allows (see *Understanding neurologic deficits,* page 180).

If the patient isn't in immediate danger, obtain a health history. As you speak with him, you may observe an altered LOC and cognitive or emotional problems. Note any communication problems, such as dysarthria or aphasia.

The patient or members of his family may report recent complaints of headache, vomiting, seizures, confusion, or changes in sensation or motor function. The patient may also have memory loss, mood swings, problems with vision, or bowel or bladder incontinence. Use a standard tool such as the Glasgow Coma scale to assess LOC and cognition.

Physical effects of a CVA vary with the part of the brain affected, the severity of the episode, and the extent that collateral circulation develops to help the brain compensate for its decreased blood supply.

A large hemorrhagic CVA usually causes sudden unconsciousness. In smaller hemorrhagic CVAs, unconsciousness may be preceded by disorientation, restlessness, decreased attention span, difficulties with comprehension, forgetfulness, impaired judgment, lack of motivation, and emotional difficulties, such as anxiety or mood swings.

Impairment of cranial nerves that control swallowing, gagging, and coughing may cause aspiration and inadequate nutrition. Damage to other cranial nerves may cause visual field deficits and loss of the pupillary reflex or loss of the corneal reflex.

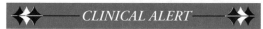

CLINICAL ALERT

Failure of the patient's pupils to react to light or a unilateral and sluggish pupillary response may indicate increased ICP, which requires immediate intervention.

Assessment of the patient's cerebellar and motor functions helps determine which cerebral hemisphere is affected. Left hemiparesis or hemiplegia means the right hemisphere is affected; right hemiparesis or hemiplegia means the left hemisphere is affected. If the patient can stand, he may exhibit problems with balance (ataxia) or gait.

Assessment of the patient's sensations may reveal losses ranging from slight impairment of touch to an inability to perceive the position and motion of body parts. The patient may be unaware of one side of his body (neglect syndrome) because the nondominant (usually right) cerebral hemisphere has been disrupted. If paralyzed, he may actually deny any motor impairment. Visual-spatial problems may also exist.

The patient may have difficulty interpreting visual, tactile, and auditory stimuli. A visual examination may reveal diplopia or visual field deficits — for example, hemianopia (blindness in half the visual field) caused by damage to the optic tract or the occipital lobe.

Assessment of muscle tone may initially reveal flaccid paralysis with decreased deep tendon reflexes. Later, these reflexes usually return to normal, whereas muscle tone, and sometimes spasticity, increases. Bowel and bladder incontinence may result from impaired muscle control and altered LOC and cognition. Cardiovascular signs, such as murmurs or bruits, may indicate a cause of the CVA.

Diagnostic tests

Cerebral angiography is used to detect disruption or displacement of cerebral circulation by occlusion or hemorrhage. Digital subtraction angiography allows evaluation of the patency of cerebral vessels and shows their position. It also aids detection and evaluation of lesions and other vascular abnormalities. A CT scan, commonly used for patients with TIAs, reveals structural abnormalities, edema, and lesions, such as nonhemorrhagic infarction and aneurysms.

Positron emission tomography is used to evaluate cerebral metabolism and cerebral blood flow changes, especially in an ischemic CVA. Single-photon emission tomography is used to identify cerebral blood flow and cerebral infarction. MRI

Understanding neurologic deficits

A cerebrovascular accident (CVA) can cause neurologic deficits ranging from mild hand weakness to complete unilateral paralysis. Such functional loss results from damaged brain tissue normally perfused by the occluded or ruptured artery. Most CVAs affect anterior cerebral circulation and damage the middle cerebral artery, internal carotid artery, or anterior cerebral artery. The list below correlates CVA symptoms with damage sites.

Middle cerebral artery

When a CVA occurs in the middle cerebral artery, the patient may experience:
- aphasia
- dysphasia
- reading difficulty (dyslexia)
- writing inability (dysgraphia)
- visual field deficits
- contralateral hemiparesis (more severe in the face and arm than in the leg)
- altered level of consciousness (LOC)
- contralateral sensory deficit.

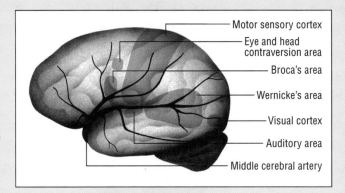

Motor sensory cortex
Eye and head contraversion area
Broca's area
Wernicke's area
Visual cortex
Auditory area
Middle cerebral artery

Internal carotid artery

When a CVA occurs in the internal carotid artery, the patient may experience:
- headaches
- weakness, paralysis, numbness, sensory changes, and visual deficits, such as blurring, on the affected side
- altered LOC
- bruits over the carotid artery
- aphasia
- dysphasia
- ptosis.

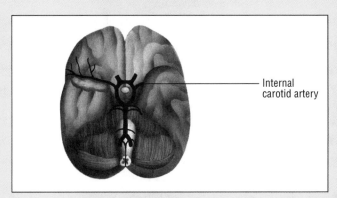

Internal carotid artery

Anterior cerebral artery

When a CVA occurs in the anterior cerebral artery, the patient may experience:
- confusion, weakness, and numbness on the affected side
- paralysis of the contralateral foot and leg
- footdrop
- incontinence
- loss of coordination
- impaired sensory functions
- personality changes.

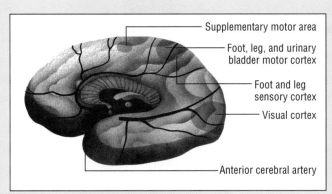

Supplementary motor area
Foot, leg, and urinary bladder motor cortex
Foot and leg sensory cortex
Visual cortex
Anterior cerebral artery

reveals the location and size of lesions. Although not as useful as a CT scan for distinguishing among hemorrhage, tumor, and infarction, MRI is more useful for examining the cerebellum and brain stem.

Transcranial Doppler studies are used to evaluate the size of intracranial vessels and the direction and velocity of cerebral blood flow. Cerebral blood flow studies are used to measure blood flow to the brain and help detect abnormalities. Ophthalmoscopic examination reveals hypertension and atherosclerotic changes in retinal arteries.

Electroencephalography is used to detect reduced electrical activity in an area of cortical infarction. It's especially useful when the CT scan is inconclusive, and can be used to differentiate seizure activity from a CVA. Neuropsychological tests are used to evaluate mental and verbal abilities and sometimes personality traits. Electrocardiography reveals abnormalities caused by a cardiac-induced CVA.

Treatment

Acute care for a patient with a CVA may include antithrombolytic therapy, mechanical ventilation, ICP and cardiac monitoring, administration of I.V. fluids and electrolytes, and NG intubation. Tissue-plasminogen activator, if given within 3 hours of the onset of symptoms, works to improve blood flow and can result in better recovery of function.

The need for and type of surgery required for a CVA depend on its cause and extent and may include a craniotomy to remove a hematoma, an endarterectomy to remove atherosclerotic plaque from the inner arterial wall, or a bypass to circumvent an artery blocked by occlusion or stenosis. Ventricular shunts may be needed to drain CSF.

Drug therapy for a CVA may include anticonvulsants, such as phenytoin or phenobarbital, to treat or prevent seizures; stool softeners to prevent straining, which increases ICP; corticosteroids to reduce associated cerebral edema; antihypertensives to treat high blood pressure; vasodilators to treat ischemia; and analgesics to relieve headache. Anticoagulants are usually ordered to prevent thrombotic or embolic CVAs and to treat a thrombotic CVA in progress.

Physical rehabilitation and a special diet help

decrease a person's risk factors. Other care measures may help him adapt to specific deficits, such as speech impairment and paralysis.

Complications of a CVA include unstable blood pressure from loss of vasomotor control, fluid imbalances, malnutrition, depression, contractures, pulmonary emboli, and infections, such as encephalitis, brain abscess, and pneumonia.

Nursing interventions

● Before surgery, monitor the patient's vital signs, fluid and electrolyte balance, and intake and output.
● After surgery, dress the incision area, provide analgesics, and monitor for surgical complications, including further neurologic deficits, infection, hemorrhage, and fluid and electrolyte imbalance. Maintain an open airway, ventilate adequately, and administer supplementary oxygen. Assist with endotracheal intubation and mechanical ventilation if necessary. Continue monitoring the patient's airway, breathing, and circulation (ABCs). Remember, if the patient's LOC deteriorates, his respirations may deteriorate as well.
● Monitor vital and neurologic signs as needed. Compare the results with baseline findings. Report any deterioration immediately. During the first 72 hours, watch for signs of increased ICP, especially altered LOC. Also look for delayed response to verbal suggestions, slowed speech, and increasing restlessness and confusion. If the patient's LOC deteriorates significantly, assist the doctor with ICP monitoring.
● Continue to assess sensory function, speech, skin color, and temperature. Note the presence of nuchal rigidity or headache.

◆◆ ━━━ *CLINICAL ALERT* ━━━ ◆◆

An impending CVA causes a sudden increase in blood pressure and a rapid, bounding pulse; the patient may complain of a headache. When increasing ICP accompanies a CVA, blood pressure increases but pulse rate decreases.

● To prevent increases in ICP, elevate the head of the bed 30 to 45 degrees and maintain the patient's head in a midline neutral position to encourage venous return. Avoid extreme hip flexion and, if the patient is alert, instruct him to avoid isometric muscle contractions and Valsalva's maneuver.

● Hyperoxygenate and hyperventilate the patient receiving mechanical ventilation. Remove secretions by continual suctioning for no more than 10 seconds at a time. Allow the patient time to rest between interventions.

● Consult with the doctor concerning the desired blood pressure range. Give medications such as vasopressors and antihypertensives, if prescribed.

● Maintain fluid and electrolyte balance. If the patient can take liquids orally, offer them as often as fluid limitations permit. Administer I.V. fluids as ordered, but never give too much too fast because this can increase ICP. Monitor the patient's fluid intake and output.

● Repeatedly explain to the patient what is happening and why.

● Offer the urinal or bedpan every 2 hours. If the patient is incontinent, consider using an indwelling urinary catheter, but remember that this device increases the risk of infection.

● Establish a bowel training program if needed. Watch for signs that the patient is straining during defecation, which can increase ICP.

● Provide a high-fiber diet, and administer stool softeners as ordered. Offer prune juice or apple juice. Give laxatives only if necessary.

● Consult with the dietitian about proper nutrition and with the speech pathologist about managing the impaired swallowing and gag reflex.

● When feeding the patient, place the food tray within his sight. Have him sit upright, and tilt his head slightly forward to eat. If the patient has dysphagia or one-sided facial weakness, give him semisoft foods and tell him to chew on the unaffected side of his mouth. Stay with a patient who may aspirate food. If oral feedings aren't possible, insert a NG feeding tube as ordered.

● Carefully clean and irrigate the patient's mouth, and care for his dentures as needed.

● Remove secretions from the patient's eyes with a cotton ball moistened with 0.9% sodium chloride solution. For loss of corneal reflex, apply eyedrops or ointment as ordered.

● Give medications as ordered. Watch for and report any adverse reactions.

● Report signs of deep vein thrombosis, such as calf pain, or signs of pulmonary emboli, such as chest pain, dyspnea, dusky color, tachycardia, fever, and changed sensorium. To prevent thrombosis and emboli, apply antiembolism stockings, frequently change the patient's position, and help him ambulate. For the immobile patient, use continuous pneumatic compression sleeves.

● Align the patient appropriately. Prevent footdrop and contractures by using such devices as cradle boots, footboards, or high-topped sneakers.

● Prevent pressure ulcers by turning or repositioning the patient frequently and by using a convoluted foam mattress, flotation pads, or pulsating mattress.

● Prevent pneumonia by turning the patient at least every 2 hours.

● Control dependent edema by elevating the affected hand and arm and placing the hand in a functional position.

● Protect the patient from injury by keeping the bed's side rails raised, if appropriate, and padding them as needed. Place the call button on his unaffected side, and have him call you before he gets out of bed. When he's out of bed, supervise his activities, including the use of ambulation aids.

● After consulting with the physical therapist, plan a rehabilitation schedule with the patient and his family. Coordinate the rehabilitation plan with the nursing staff.

● Assist the patient with passive range-of-motion (ROM) exercises for both the affected and unaffected sides at least four times a day while he's unconscious or immobilized. Encourage the conscious or mobile patient to participate in his own rehabilitation, while ensuring that his efforts don't cause recurrence of hemorrhage. Teach him to use his unaffected side to exercise his affected side. Encourage him to raise his hands over his head by clasping them together in front and then raising his arms.

● Apply pressure splints to the arms or legs with sensory loss. Alternate inflation and deflation to help restimulate sensory function.

● If the patient has a limited field of vision, encourage him to turn his head and look in the affected direction. If unilateral neglect occurs, encourage him to look at the affected side and to exercise it with his unaffected hand.

• With the patient, family, and speech therapist, help the patient develop an effective means of communicating. Make sure that the nursing staff knows of any communication problem the patient may have. Post a sign above the patient's bed to inform the health care team and visitors of alternative communication methods.

• If the patient has receptive (Wernicke's) aphasia, speak slowly, using simple sentences. Use gestures or pictures when necessary. If the patient has expressive (Broca's) aphasia or dysarthria with difficulty speaking, give him enough time to speak. To help this patient, create a communication board displaying pictures of common needs, such as a bedpan or a glass of water. Or create conversation cards by printing simple messages on index cards, such as "I am thirsty" or "Please raise my bed." Punch holes in the cards, and attach them to a large key ring. The patient can express his needs by showing you the appropriate card.

• Encourage the patient to express himself, but remember that mood changes from brain damage and resentment over dependence may make establishing rapport difficult.

• Discuss realistic, short-term goals with the patient and his family, and involve them in his care. Help the patient and his family find effective means to cope with his condition and care. If necessary, refer them for counseling.

• Encourage your patient to be as independent as possible. Consult with an occupational therapist for help with teaching self-care techniques. Develop a consistent daily routine for performing activities of daily living (ADLs), allowing sufficient time for completion.

Patient teaching

• Teach the patient and his family about CVA. Explain diagnostic tests, treatments, and the rehabilitation program. If surgery is scheduled, make sure that the patient and his family understand the procedure and any associated consequences.

• After consulting an occupational therapist and a physical therapist, teach the patient self-care skills. When describing self-care skills to patients with sensory or cognitive impairment, demonstrate each step of the activity. Then re-demonstrate the complete skill. Be sure to give the patient time to understand.

• If speech therapy is necessary, encourage him to begin as soon as possible.

• If a special diet or food is required, have the dietitian explain it to the patient. If appropriate, explain the danger of aspiration to the patient's family, and teach preventive measures. Make sure that family members are skilled in the abdominal thrust maneuver.

• Inform the patient and family members about special glasses, cups, plates, and utensils that can make eating easier and more enjoyable for the patient and his family.

• Explain to the patient and his family the importance of following the prescribed exercise program, and make sure they can perform the exercises.

• Emphasize the importance of wearing slings, splints, or other prescribed devices to prevent complications.

• Make sure the patient and his family understand transfer techniques and the use of ambulatory aids. If the patient is going home with a walker, give him the teaching handout *Using a walker to sit and stand,* page 184.

• Devise a discharge plan with the patient and his family. Suggest appropriate home safety equipment, such as ramps and grab bars for the toilet and bathtub. Teach them about the importance of home safety measures, such as removing throw rugs and securing carpets to the floor.

• Urge the patient and his family to report any signs of an impending CVA, such as a severe headache, drowsiness, confusion, and dizziness. Emphasize the importance of regular follow-up doctor's visits.

• Teach the patient and, if necessary, a family member about the purpose, dosage, and possible adverse effects of all prescribed medications. Make sure that the patient taking aspirin realizes that he mustn't substitute acetaminophen.

• Counsel the patient and his family about lifestyle

Using a walker to sit and stand

Dear Patient:

Follow these directions to help you sit down in a chair and then stand up.

Sitting down

1. Begin by choosing a sturdy armchair. Stand with your back to the chair and with the walker directly in front of you.

2. Place the back of your stronger leg against the seat of the chair. Carefully lift your weaker leg slightly off the floor. Now grasp the chair's arm with the hand on your weak side. Shift your weight to your stronger leg and the hand grasping the armrest. Then grasp the other armrest with your free hand.

3. Balancing yourself between both arms, gently lower yourself into the chair and slide backward. After you're seated, place the walker beside your chair.

Getting up

1. Pull the walker in front of you. Slide forward in the chair.

2. Place the back of your stronger leg against the seat. Then move your weaker leg forward. Now, placing both hands on the armrests, push yourself to a standing position. Support your weight with your stronger leg and the opposite hand. Then grasp the walker's handgrip with your free hand.

3. Grasp the free handgrip with your other hand. Now, distribute your weight evenly between your hands and your stronger leg. Take a moment to get your balance. Steady yourself, take a deep breath, and you're off.

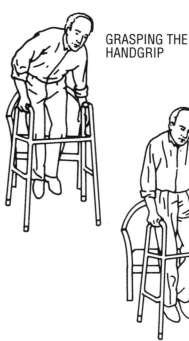

GRASPING THE
HANDGRIP

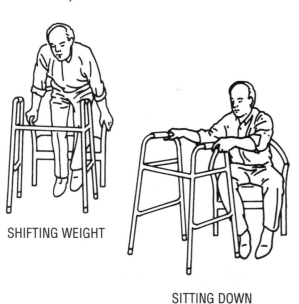

SHIFTING WEIGHT

SITTING DOWN
AND PLACING WALKER

SECURING GRIP

changes that may reduce the risk of another CVA, such as smoking cessation and measures to control diabetes or hypertension, if applicable. Explain the importance of increasing activity, avoiding prolonged bed rest, minimizing stress, and following a low-cholesterol, low-salt diet.

● Encourage the patient and his family to contact a local support group and to obtain information from the National Institute of Neurological Disorders and Stroke. Refer them to a local home health care agency, if necessary.

PARKINSON'S DISEASE

One of the most common cripplers, Parkinson's disease is a slowly progressive, chronic, degenerative condition. It characteristically causes progressive muscle rigidity, postural instability, bradykinesia, and resting tremors. As the person loses mobility, he may experience injury from falls and skin breakdown. Deterioration progresses for an average of 10 years, culminating in death, which usually results from aspiration pneumonia or another infection.

Parkinson's disease occurs throughout the world in all racial and ethnic groups. It strikes 1 in every 100 people over age 60 — men more than women — although it occasionally occurs before age 40. As the general population ages, the incidence of Parkinson's disease is growing. Roughly 60,000 new cases are diagnosed annually in the United States.

Causes
Parkinson's disease results from a deficiency of the neurotransmitter dopamine. Neurons in the brain's substantia nigra that project into the corpus striatum degenerate, causing a dopamine deficiency in the basal ganglia. As a result, the excitative effect of acetylcholine is unchecked, causing symptoms of cholinergic excess, such as rigidity, tremors, bradykinesia, and postural instability.

Parkinson's disease may occur after epidemic encephalitis. Trauma or ischemia may produce parkinsonian symptoms, as may long-term adminis-

tration of certain drugs, such as phenothiazines and reserpine. Rarely, parkinsonian symptoms stem from exposure to toxins, such as manganese dust or carbon monoxide.

Assessment findings
Symptoms are often subtle and occur in varying combinations. They also change as the disease progresses. Early symptoms, such as fatigue and generalized slowness, may be mistaken for normal aging. Therefore, assessment requires a health history, physical examination findings, and diagnostic test results. Inquire about past medical conditions and obtain a thorough medication history to uncover possible causes of parkinsonian symptoms.

Initially, the patient may complain of fatigue when performing ADLs. He also may report muscle cramps in his legs, neck, and trunk. Constipation, urine retention, and dysphagia may eventually occur.

The patient or members of his family may report gait, balance, and posture disturbances. They may also mention slow movements or difficulty in initiating movements. Ask when symptoms began and if they've gotten progressively worse.

The patient may report tremors, which typically begin in the fingers. Although he may not be able to pinpoint when the tremors began, he may report that they increase with stress or anxiety and decrease with purposeful movement and sleep.

He may also report secondary symptoms from autonomic nervous system involvement, including oily skin, increased perspiration, lacrimation, heat sensitivity, and postural hypotension. Family members may report that the patient has rapid mood swings or experiences depression.

Rigidity is a cardinal sign of parkinsonism and can involve any or all of the striated muscles. Inspection may reveal a masklike facial expression, with fixed, wide-open eyes. Drooling may be apparent. Vocal cord rigidity may lead to dysarthria and hypophonia. Passive movement of the extremities may reveal "cogwheel" or "lead-pipe" rigidity.

You may also note that the patient takes a long time to perform a purposeful action, such as sitting down, standing, or walking to the door. This symptom is called bradykinesia, another classic sign of Parkinson's disease. To easily assess the patient for bradykinesia, ask him to quickly alternate his hands from a palms-up to a palms-down position. If he has bradykinesia, he won't be able to do this. You may also observe akinesia, an inability to initiate and carry out simple motor movements — such as standing up when you ask him to do so.

The person with Parkinson's disease may exhibit a stooped posture. His gait will lack normal parallel motion and may be propulsive (the tendency to take rapid steps forward) following slow initiation of movement. At times, he may take rapid steps backward instead of going forward, which places him in danger of falling. You may also note that he has difficulty pivoting and seems to lose his balance if he moves suddenly.

In some people, the combined effects of rigidity, bradykinesia, and postural instability result in the characteristic slow, shuffling gait of Parkinson's disease, including short steps and the absence of coordinated swinging of the arms.

Observe the patient's fingers while his hands are at rest. Look for the classic "pill-rolling" tremor, in which the thumb moves against the distal second and third fingers of the hand.

Parkinson's disease doesn't usually affect the intellect. However, you may note cognitive disturbances, such as memory deficits or confusion in the patient with severe Parkinson's disease. Usually, these symptoms result from drug toxicity or a form of dementia. Rarely, oculogyric crisis (eyes fixed upward, with involuntary tonic movements) or blepharospasm (contraction of the orbicular muscle) occurs.

Diagnostic tests
CT scan or MRI may be performed to rule out other disorders, such as intracranial tumors. Although urinalysis may reveal reduced dopamine levels, it usually has little value in identifying Parkinson's disease; only autopsy reveals a dopamine deficiency.

Treatment
Parkinson's disease has no cure, so the goal of treatment is to relieve symptoms and keep the patient mobile and functioning independently as long as possible.

Levodopa, a dopamine replacement, is most effective during the first few years it's prescribed. The drug is given in increasing doses until signs and symptoms are relieved or adverse reactions appear. Because adverse effects can be serious, levodopa is frequently given in combination with carbidopa (a dopa-decarboxylase inhibitor) to halt peripheral dopamine synthesis. The patient may also receive bromocriptine to reduce the levodopa dose.

Selegiline may be administered with carbidopa and levodopa, especially when their combined effectiveness decreases. Some neurologists now initiate selegiline therapy as a first-line therapy in early-stage Parkinson's disease because evidence suggests that this drug slows the destruction of dopaminergic neurons in the substantia nigra.

Anticholinergics, such as trihexyphenidyl or benztropine, and antihistamines, such as diphenhydramine, are alternative therapies. These drugs may be prescribed when levodopa proves ineffective or too toxic. Anticholinergics may be used to control tremors and rigidity. They may also be used in combination with levodopa. Antihistamines may help decrease tremors because of their central anticholinergic and sedative effects. Amantadine, an antiviral agent, is used early in treatment to reduce rigidity, tremors, and akinesia. Tricyclic antidepressants may be given to decrease the depression that often accompanies the disease.

Physical therapy helps the patient maintain normal muscle tone and function. Appropriate physical therapy includes both active and passive ROM exercises, routine daily activities, walking, and baths and massage to help relax muscles.

Stereotaxic surgery to reduce tremors and rigidity is rarely performed today because of the advent of more effective drug therapy. However, with new advances in equipment, neurosurgeons are revisiting this technique. Experimental attempts at surgical implantation of the patient's own adrenal medulla cells into the corpus striatum have been made; however, these attempts have generally not been successful. Other experimental surgeries involve transplantation of fetal substantia nigra tissue.

Complications

The patient with Parkinson's disease is at risk for pressure ulcers, depression, and contractions. Because no cure exists, the disease eventually progresses to death.

Nursing interventions

• Provide emotional and psychological support to your patient and his family. Listen to their specific concerns and answer their questions. Encourage the patient to use coping skills. Help him identify social activities that he can continue to participate in; then encourage him to participate to help bolster self-esteem and prevent depression.

• Encourage independence by asking the patient to participate in care-related decisions. Help him identify ADLs that he can perform, and teach him necessary self-care skills. Counsel the patient to help himself as much as possible, and provide positive reinforcement. Make certain that all caregivers are aware of the patient's capabilities. Allow sufficient time for the patient to complete his care. Assist him with self-care in later stages of illness when disability is more profound.

• Provide assistive devices as appropriate. For example, to help the patient turn himself in bed, tie a rope to the foot of the bed and extend it to the patient so that he can grasp it and pull himself to a sitting position. Make sure that the patient and caregiver demonstrate proper use of any assistive devices, such as a walker or cane.

• Monitor drug treatment and report any adverse reactions or failure to relieve symptoms.

• Because fatigue may make the patient more dependent on others, provide rest periods between activities.

• If the patient's speech is affected, consult with the speech therapist.

• Assess the patient's nutritional status, and monitor his body weight. Observe for conditions that can hinder adequate nutritional intake, such as difficulty swallowing because of tremors or depression. Consult with the dietitian, physical therapist, doctor, and occupational therapist, as needed, to plan an effective nutritional program.

◆◆——— CLINICAL ALERT ———◆◆

To decrease the risk of aspiration, instruct the patient to sit upright when eating. Keep suction equipment available. Offer semisolid foods if he has difficulty in swallowing. Provide supplementary feedings or small, frequent meals to increase caloric intake, if needed.

• Help establish a regular bowel elimination routine by encouraging the patient to drink at least 2 liters of liquids daily (unless contraindicated), eat high-fiber foods, exercise daily, and establish a regular time for elimination. Also make sure he has an elevated toilet seat to ease sitting.

• Work with the physical therapist to develop a program of daily exercises to increase muscle strength, decrease muscle rigidity, prevent contractures, and improve coordination. The program should include stretching and postural exercises, swimming, and stationary bicycling.

• If the patient experiences depression that isn't easily resolved without drug therapy, discuss the problem with the doctor, who may prescribe antidepressants.

• Provide frequent warm baths and massage to help relax muscles and relieve cramps.

• Protect the patient from injury by raising the bed's side rails, as appropriate, and assisting him as necessary when he walks. Keep his environment free of clutter that could result in falls. Make certain he sits in chairs with armrests and back supports.

Patient teaching

• Teach the patient and his family about the disorder, its progressive nature, and all prescribed treatments.

• Encourage the patient to exercise daily and to follow the planned physical therapy program. Teach him simple stretching exercises to promote flexibility. Give him the teaching handout *How to do stretching exercises,* pages 188 and 189.

• Explain the purpose, dosage, possible adverse effects, and precautions for all prescribed drugs. Tell the patient to notify the doctor if any drugs lose

(Text continues on page 190.)

How to do stretching exercises

Dear Patient:

Your doctor has prescribed exercises to help you maintain flexibility and muscle strength. At first, do each exercise 1 to 5 times daily. Then, gradually increase to 10 to 20 times daily. If you're unable to do these exercises standing up, you can do most of them sitting down.

Facial muscle exercises

Raise your eyebrows and then lower and squeeze them together. Next, open your eyes wide; then close them tight.

Now wrinkle your nose. Follow this by opening your mouth wide in a big "O" and then closing it tight. Shift your jaw from side to side. Finally, give a big smile; then purse your lips, as though trying to whistle. Repeat the exercises.

Neck exercises

Begin by turning your head from side to side. Next, bend your head down and back. Repeat the exercises.

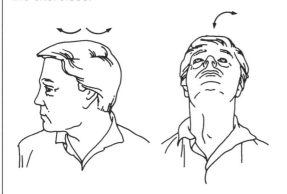

Shoulder exercises

Raise your shoulders toward your ears as high as you can. Then lower them. Repeat a few more times.

Arm and shoulder exercises

Raise your arms over your head. Then, swing them down, extending them behind your back. Repeat.

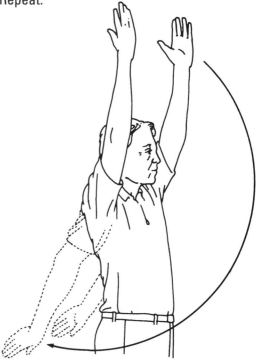

Trunk exercises

With your hands on your hips, twist your body at the waist from side to side, keeping your hips and legs in place. Repeat.

How to do stretching exercises (continued)

Hip and knee exercises

While holding on to a counter or sturdy piece of furniture, raise your right knee toward your right shoulder. Lower it and then raise your left knee toward your left shoulder. Lower the knee and repeat these movements.

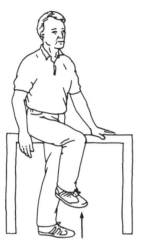

Stand facing a wall, about 8" (20 cm) away. Place your hands on the wall until they're above your head. Then raise your right leg up behind you, keeping your knee straight. Do the same with the left leg. Repeat.

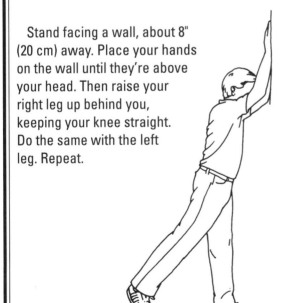

Knee exercises

While sitting down, straighten your right knee, extending your right leg out in front of you. Then bend your right leg back under the chair as far as you can. (Keep your ankle flexed to avoid a muscle spasm.) Repeat with your left leg. Perform this exercise several times.

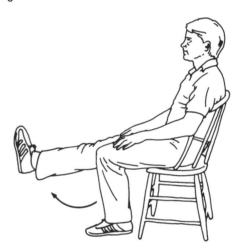

Ankle and foot exercises

While sitting down, make circles with your right foot, first in one direction and then in the other. Repeat with your left foot. Do this a few more times.

Ankle and toe exercises

While sitting down, extend your leg and point your toes toward the floor. Then point them up toward your nose. Try this several more times.

their effectiveness or cause adverse reactions. Explain that the doctor may need to adjust the dosage or change medications.

• If appropriate, show the family how to prevent pressure ulcers and contractures by proper positioning.

• Explain household safety measures to the patient and caregiver. For example, suggest installing hand rails in bathrooms, halls, and stairs. Instruct them to remove throw rugs to prevent falls.

• Teach the patient to ambulate with a wide-based gait to improve his balance and prevent falls. Also instruct him to rise slowly to a sitting position and to change positions slowly.

• Explain the importance of daily bathing to the patient with oily skin and increased perspiration.

• Consult with the occupational therapy department regarding the use of dressing aids. Clothing with zippers or Velcro fasteners can make dressing easier.

• If appropriate, advise the patient how to eat. Teach him to place food on the tongue, close the lips, chew first on one side and then the other, then lift the tongue up and back and make a conscious effort to swallow. Tell family members to allow plenty of time for meals.

• Refer the patient and his family to the National Parkinson Foundation, the American Parkinson Disease Association, or the United Parkinson Foundation.

10

Managing musculoskeletal problems

*A*ge changes the musculoskeletal system in many ways. The number of muscle fibers decreases and muscles become smaller and weaker. Muscle tone, strength, and endurance decline. Stiffening ligaments and tendons reduce joint mobility, especially in the knees, hips, and spine. Wear and tear on the auricular surfaces of the joints increases with loss of synovial elasticity. Bone density decreases, weakening the bones. The intervertebral disks thin, causing older adults to lose 1.2 cm of height every 20 years. Pronounced curvature of the thoracic and cervical curves of the spine causes a stooped posture, with the head and neck thrust forward and the hips and stance widened. The older person's movement becomes cautious and deliberate, making it harder to walk and maintain balance.

OSTEOARTHRITIS

Osteoarthritis — the most common arthritis — causes deterioration of joint cartilage and formation of new bone at the margins and subchondral areas of the joints. The chronic degeneration of osteoarthritis results from a breakdown of chondrocytes. It occurs most often in weight-bearing joints, especially in the hips and knees.

Osteoarthritis occurs equally in both sexes and affects 83% to 87% of people between ages 55 and 64. More than half of all people over age 30 have some features of primary osteoarthritis. And nearly all people over age 60, when examined radiographically, exhibit evidence of the disorder, although fewer than half experience symptoms.

In osteoarthritis, the breakdown of cartilage begins long before symptoms appear. As the disease progresses, whole sections of cartilage may disintegrate, osteophytes (bony spurs) form, and fragments of cartilage and bone float freely in the joint. Progression rates vary; joints may remain stable for years in the early stage of deterioration.

Depending on the site and severity of joint involvement, disability can range from minor limitation of the fingers to near immobility in some people with hip or knee disease. Some joints, such as hips and knees, can be replaced to improve mobility and function.

Causes

Primary osteoarthritis may be related to aging. Although researchers don't understand exactly why, wear and tear on the joints as a person ages is thought to play a major role in its development. Other factors that may lead to primary osteoarthritis are obesity and repetitive overuse of a joint. For example, a baseball player may develop osteoarthritis of the shoulder. In some older adults, however, it may be hereditary.

Secondary osteoarthritis usually follows a specific event or circumstance; most commonly a traumatic injury or a congenital abnormality, such as hip dysplasia. Endocrine disorders (such as diabetes mellitus), metabolic disorders (such as chondrocalcinosis), and other types of arthritis also can lead to secondary osteoarthritis.

Assessment findings

The aging adult usually complains of gradually increasing signs and symptoms of osteoarthritis and may report a predisposing incident, such as a traumatic injury. In early osteoarthritis, the geriatric patient has no symptoms or has a mild, dull ache when the joint is used. Rest relieves the discomfort. In more advanced disease, pain becomes more common and may be present even during rest, typically worsening as the day progresses. He commonly describes a deep, aching joint pain after exercising or bearing weight on the affected joint. Rest may relieve the pain.

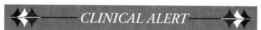
CLINICAL ALERT

Don't assume that an older person's complaints of pain and mobility problems are inevitable signs of age. Investigate them as possible signs of disease.

Additional complaints include stiffness in the morning and after exercise, aching during changes in weather, contractures, limited movement, and a "grating" feeling when the joint moves. These symptoms tend to be worse in older people with poor posture, obesity, or occupational stress.

Inspection may reveal joint swelling, muscle atrophy, deformity of the involved areas, and gait abnormalities (when arthritis affects hips or knees). Osteoarthritis of the interphalangeal joints produces hard nodes on the distal and proximal joints. Painless at first, these nodes eventually become red, swollen, and tender. The most common of these nodes, Heberden's nodes, occur on the dorsolateral aspect of the distal interphalangeal joint. Bouchard's nodes, which occur less often, appear on the proximal interphalangeal joint. The fingers may become numb and lose dexterity.

Palpation may reveal joint tenderness and warmth without redness, grating with movement, joint instability, muscle spasms, and limited movement.

Diagnostic tests

X-rays of the affected joint may help confirm the diagnosis; however, findings may be normal in the early stages. X-ray studies may require many views and typically show a narrowing of the joint space or margin, cystlike bony deposits in the joint space and margins, sclerosis of the subchondral space, joint deformity caused by degeneration or articular damage, bony growths at weight-bearing areas, and joint fusion in people with erosive, inflammatory osteoarthritis.

Synovial fluid analysis can be used to rule out inflammatory arthritis. Radionuclide bone scans also can be used to rule out inflammatory arthritis by showing normal uptake of the radionuclide.

Arthroscopy identifies soft-tissue swelling by showing internal joint structures. Magnetic resonance imaging produces clear cross-sectional images of the affected joint and adjacent bones and can illustrate disease progression. Neuromuscular tests may disclose reduced muscle strength (reduced grip strength, for example).

Treatment

The goal of treatment is pain relief, improved mobility, and minimized disability. Treatment options include medications, rest, physical therapy, assistive mobility devices and, possibly, surgery.

Aspirin, nonsteroidal anti-inflammatory drugs, and salicylates are the most commonly used medications. In some older adults, intra-articular injections of corticosteroids may be necessary. Such injections, given every 4 to 6 months, may delay nodal development in the hands.

Adequate rest is essential and should be balanced with activity. Physical therapy methods include massage, moist heat, paraffin dips for the hands, supervised exercise to maintain muscle tone and posture and to decrease muscle spasms and atrophy, and protective techniques for preventing undue joint stress. Some people may reduce stress and increase stability by using crutches, braces, a cane, a walker, a cervical collar, or traction. Weight reduction may help an obese patient.

In some instances, older adults with severe disability or uncontrollable pain may undergo surgery. Partial or total arthroplasty — replacement of a deteriorated part of the joint with a prosthetic appliance — is common with severe hip and knee disease. Arthrodesis — surgical fusion of the bones — is used primarily in the spine. Osteoplasty involves scraping and lavaging deteriorated bone from the joint. Osteotomy — removing a wedge of bone (usually in the lower leg) — is performed to change alignment and relieve stress.

Complications

Osteoarthritis may cause flexion contractures, subluxation and deformity, ankylosis, bony cysts, gross bony overgrowth, central cord syndrome (with cervical spine osteoarthritis), nerve root compression, and *cauda equina* syndrome.

Nursing interventions

- Provide emotional support and reassurance to help your patient cope with limited mobility. Give him opportunities to voice his feelings about immobility and nodular joints.
- Include the patient and his family members in all phases of care. Answer their questions as honestly as you can.
- Encourage the geriatric patient to perform as much self-care as mobility and pain levels allow. Give him adequate time to perform activities at his own pace.
- Administer anti-inflammatory medication and other drugs, as ordered. Watch for and document adverse reactions; tell the doctor if any occur.
- Assess the patient's pain pattern. Give analgesics as needed, and monitor and document his response.
- To help the older person sleep, adjust pain medications to allow maximum rest. Provide normal sleep aids, such as a pillow, bath, or a back rub.
- Help the geriatric patient identify techniques and activities that promote rest and relaxation and encourage him to perform them regularly.
- For joints in the hand, provide hot soaks and paraffin dips to relieve pain, as ordered.
- For lumbosacral spinal joints, provide a firm mattress (or bed board) to decrease morning pain.
- For cervical spinal joints, adjust the patient's cervical collar to prevent constriction; watch for

irritated skin with prolonged use.
- For the hip, use moist heat pads to relieve pain. Administer antispasmodic drugs, as ordered.
- For the knee, assist the patient with prescribed range-of-motion (ROM) exercises twice daily to maintain muscle tone, and progressive resistance exercises to increase muscle strength.
- Provide elastic supports or braces if needed. Check the crutches, cane, braces, or walker for a proper fit.

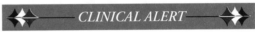
CLINICAL ALERT

An older person with unilateral joint involvement should use an orthopedic appliance (such as a cane or walker) on the normal side.

Patient teaching

- Instruct your patient to take medications exactly as prescribed. Tell him which adverse reactions to report immediately.
- Teach him to plan for adequate rest during the day, after exertion, and at night.
- Encourage the patient to learn and use energy conservation methods, such as pacing and simplifying work procedures. For example, a wheeled cart is an inexpensive work-saving device to move objects from one place to another while giving him some support.
- Teach the patient joint-protecting methods. Instruct him to stand and walk correctly, to minimize weight-bearing activities, and to be especially careful when stooping or picking up objects. Tell him to wear well-fitting, supportive shoes and to repair worn heels.
- Advise an older adult to maintain proper body weight to minimize strain on the joints.
- Recommend sitting on cushions and using an elevated toilet seat. These measures reduce stress when rising from a seated position.
- Advise your patient to have safety devices installed at home, such as grab bars in the bathroom.
- Instruct him to do ROM and isometric exercises, performing them as gently as possible.

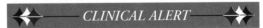
CLINICAL ALERT

The benefits of isometric and mild exercise for osteoarthritis are well known. Excessive exercise, however, can cause more pain and degeneration. So advise against overexertion. Give the patient the teaching handouts *Performing active range-of-motion exercises,* pages 195 to 197, and *Performing isometric exercises,* pages 198 and 199.

• Teach the older patient how to use crutches or other orthopedic devices. Stress the importance of proper fit and regular, professional readjustment of the aids. Warn him that impaired sensation might allow tissue damage from these devices without signs of discomfort.

• Use positive reinforcement to acknowledge your patient's efforts to adapt. Point out improved or stabilized physical functions.

• As necessary, provide referrals to occupational therapists or a home health nurse to help the older adult cope with activities of daily living (ADLs). Although not covered by most insurance policies (except in conjunction with a skilled home care provider), homemaker services may relieve him of strenuous activities.

OSTEOPOROSIS

In this metabolic bone disorder, the rate of bone resorption accelerates, and the rate of bone formation decelerates, resulting in decreased bone mass. The bones lose calcium and phosphate, becoming porous, brittle, and abnormally vulnerable to fracture. The immobility that follows a fracture can exacerbate osteoporosis.

Osteoporosis may be primary or secondary to an underlying disease. Primary osteoporosis may be classified as idiopathic, type I, or type II. Idiopathic osteoporosis affects children and adults. Type I (or postmenopausal) osteoporosis usually affects women ages 51 to 75. Type I osteoporosis — related to the loss of estrogen's protective effect on bone — results in trabecular bone loss and some cortical bone loss. In type I osteoporosis, vertebral and wrist fractures are common. Type II (or senile) osteoporosis occurs most commonly between ages 70 and 85. Trabecular and cortical bone loss and consequent fractures of the proximal humerus, proximal tibia, femoral neck, and pelvis characterize type II osteoporosis.

Causes

The cause of primary osteoporosis is unknown. However, clinicians suspect several contributing factors: mild but prolonged negative calcium balance, which can occur from inadequate dietary calcium intake; declining gonadal adrenal gland function and estrogen deficiency, which causes faulty protein metabolism; and a sedentary lifestyle are believed to contribute to primary osteoporosis.

Secondary osteoporosis may result from prolonged therapy with steroids or heparin, bone immobilization or disuse (as occurs with hemiplegia), alcoholism, malnutrition, rheumatoid arthritis, liver disease, malabsorption, scurvy, lactose intolerance, hyperthyroidism, osteogenesis imperfecta, and Sudeck's atrophy (localized in hands and feet, with recurring attacks).

Assessment findings

The medical history typically discloses a postmenopausal woman or one with a condition known to cause secondary osteoporosis. She may report that she bent down to lift something, heard a snapping sound, and felt a sudden pain in her lower back. Or she may say that the pain developed slowly over several years. If the older woman has vertebral collapse, she may describe a backache and pain radiating around the trunk. Any movement or jarring aggravates the pain.

◆◆ *CLINICAL ALERT* ◆◆

A dowager's hump is the clinical hallmark of osteoporosis. This malformation is caused by increased spinal curvature from repeated vertebral fractures.

Inspection may reveal that the aging woman has a humped back and a markedly aged appearance. She may report a loss of height. Assess height loss by having your patient stand with her arms raised laterally and parallel to the floor. A measured

(Text continues on page 200.)

T EACHING AID

Performing active range-of-motion exercises

Dear Patient:

Review the following guidelines before you begin active range-of-motion exercises:
- Do your exercises daily to get the most benefit.
- Repeat each exercise three to five times or as often as your doctor recommends. (As you get stronger, the doctor may tell you to increase your activity.)
- Perform the exercises top to bottom. When exercising all your major joints, begin at your neck and work toward your toes.
- Move slowly and gently, so you don't injure yourself. If an exercise is painful, *stop doing it*. Then ask your doctor if you should keep doing that particular exercise.
- Take a break and rest after an exercise that's especially tiring.
- Divide your exercise routine into several sessions throughout the day, if you prefer this to a single session.

Neck exercise

Slowly tilt your head as far back as possible. Next, move it to the right, toward your shoulder.

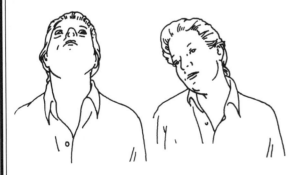

Still with your head to the right, lower your chin as far as it will go toward your chest. Then move your head toward your left shoulder. Complete a full circle by moving your head back to its usual upright position. Complete the recommended number of counterclockwise circles. Then reverse the exercise, doing an equal number of clockwise circles.

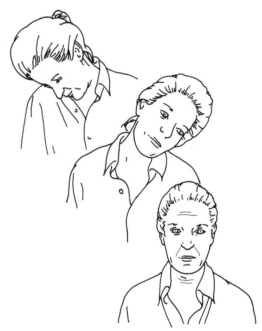

Shoulder exercises

Raise your shoulders as if to shrug. Then move them forward, down, then up, in a circular motion. Now move them backward, down, then

(continued)

Performing active range-of-motion exercises (continued)

up again in a circular motion. Alternate forward and backward shoulder circles for the recommended repetitions.

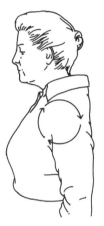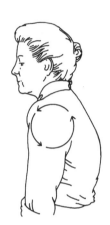

Elbow exercise

Extend your arm straight out to the side. Open your hand, palm up, as if to catch a raindrop. Now slowly reach back with your forearm so that you touch your shoulder with your fingers. Then slowly return your arm to its straight

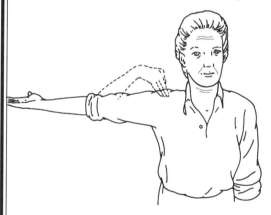

position. Repeat with your other arm. Alternate arms while completing the recommended repetitions.

Wrist and hand exercise

Extend your arms in front of you, palms down and fingers straight. Keeping your palms flat, slowly raise your fingers and point them back

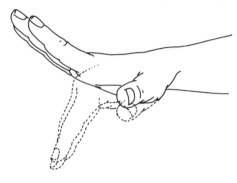

toward you. Then, slowly lower your fingers and point them as far downward as you comfortably can.

Finger exercise

Spread the fingers and thumb on each hand as

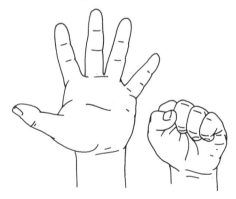

far as possible without causing discomfort. Then bring the fingers back together into a fist.

Leg and knee exercise

Lie on a bed or the floor. Bend one leg so the knee is up and the foot is flat.

*T*EACHING AID

Performing active range-of-motion exercises (continued)

Now bend the other leg and slowly bring your knee as close to your chest as you can without discomfort. Then straighten the leg slowly as you lower it to the floor. Repeat the exercise with your other leg.

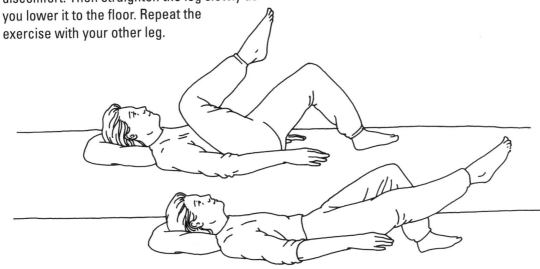

Ankle and foot exercise

Raise one foot and point your toes away from you. Move the foot in a circular motion, first to the right, then to the left. Next, point your toes back toward you. With your foot in this position, make a circle with it, first to the right, then to the left.

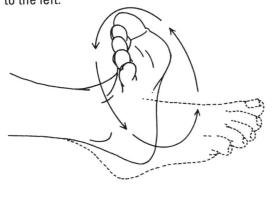

Toe exercise

Sit in a chair or lie on your bed. Stretch your legs out in front of you, with your heels resting on the floor. Slowly bend your toes down and away from you. Next, bend your toes up and back toward you. Finally, spread out your toes so that they're totally separated. Then squeeze your toes together.

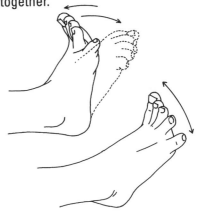

*T*EACHING AID

Performing isometric exercises

Dear Patient:

When performed correctly, isometric exercises increase muscle strength. Repeat each exercise as many times (typically three) as your doctor directs.

Some guidelines

In isometric exercise, you contract your muscles against the resistance of a stationary object, such as a bed, a wall, or another body part. This is a basic isometric exercise: Press your palms together (pushing with one, resisting with the other) until you feel a tightness in your chest and upper arm muscles.

   You don't have to be in any special position for most isometric exercises, so you can do them anytime and anywhere. Hold each contraction for 3 to 5 seconds. Repeat the entire series at least five times a day.

   For the first week, don't contract your muscles fully to give them a chance to adjust to the exercise. After that, contract them fully.

Neck exercises

● Place the heel of your right hand above your right ear. Without moving your head, neck, or arm, push your head toward your hand. Repeat the exercise with your left hand above your left ear.

● Clasp your fingers behind your head. Without moving your neck or hands, push your head back against your hands.

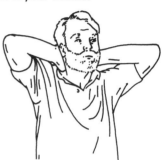

Shoulder and chest exercise

First, hold your right arm straight down at your side. Grasp your right wrist with your left hand. Then try to shrug your right shoulder, but prevent this by keeping a firm grip on your right wrist.

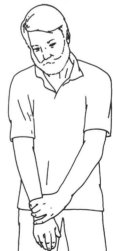

Repeat the exercise with your left arm and shoulder.

EACHING AID

Performing isometric exercises *(continued)*

Arm exercises

With your right arm at your side, bend your elbow at a 90-degree angle. Turn your right palm up and place your left fist in it. Then try to bend your right arm upward while resisting this force with your left fist.

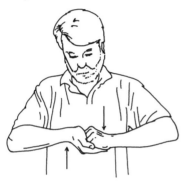

Repeat the exercise with your left arm and right fist.

Abdominal exercise

Begin by sitting on the floor or on a bed with your legs out in front of you. Then bend forward and place your hands palm down on the midfront of your thighs. Try to bend farther forward, but resist this movement by pressing your palms against your thighs.

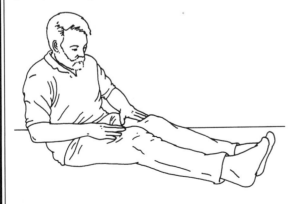

Buttocks exercise

While standing, squeeze your inner thighs and buttocks together as tightly as possible. When doing this exercise in bed, place a pillow between your knees to make the exercise more effective.

Thigh exercise

Sit on the floor or on a bed. With your legs completely straight, vigorously tighten the muscles above your knees so that your knee-caps move upward.

Calf exercise

While sitting up in bed, bend forward and grasp your toes. Then pull gently backward, and hold this position briefly.

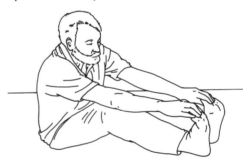

Still touching your toes, push them forward and down as far as possible, and hold this position briefly.

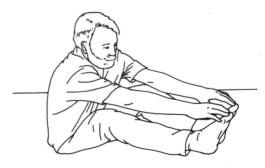

difference exceeding 1½" (3.8 cm) between her height and the distance across the outstretched arms (from longest fingertip to longest fingertip) suggests height loss.

Palpation may reveal muscle spasm, especially in the lumbar region. The older woman may also have decreased spinal movement with flexion more limited than extension.

Diagnostic tests

Differential diagnosis must exclude other causes of rarefying bone disease, especially those that affect the spine, such as metastatic carcinoma and advanced multiple myeloma. X-ray studies show characteristic degeneration in the lower thoracolumbar vertebrae. The vertebral bodies may appear flatter and denser than usual. Loss of bone mineral appears in later disease.

Serum calcium, phosphorus, and alkaline phosphatase levels remain within normal limits. Parathyroid hormone levels may be elevated.

Transiliac bone biopsy may be performed to directly examine osteoporotic changes in bone cells. Computed tomography (CT) scan allows accurate assessment of spinal bone loss. Bone scans that use a radionuclide agent display injured or diseased areas as darker portions.

Treatment

To control bone loss, prevent additional fractures, and control pain, treatment focuses on a physical therapy program of gentle exercise and activity and drug therapy to slow disease progress. Other treatment measures include supportive devices and, possibly, surgery.

Estrogen may be prescribed within 3 years after menopause to decrease the rate of bone resorption. Sodium fluoride may be given to stimulate bone formation. Calcium and vitamin D supplements may help to support normal bone metabolism. Calcitonin may be used to reduce bone resorption and slow the decline in bone mass. Etidronate is the first agent approved to restore lost bone. Studies show that etidronate, used for 2 weeks every 4 months, increases bone mass.

Weakened vertebrae should be supported, usually with a back brace. Surgery (open reduction and internal fixation) can correct pathologic fractures of the femur. Colles' fracture requires reduction and immobilization (with a cast) for 4 to 10 weeks.

Complications

Bone fractures are the major complication of osteoporosis. They occur most commonly in the vertebrae, the femoral neck, and the distal radius.

Nursing interventions

• Design your care plan with the patient's fragility in mind. Focus on careful positioning, proper body mechanics, ambulation, and prescribed exercises.
• Provide emotional support and reassurance to help her cope with limited mobility. Give her opportunities to voice her feelings. If possible, arrange for her to interact with others who have similar problems.
• Include the patient and her family in all phases of care. Answer their questions as honestly as you can.
• Encourage the older woman to perform as much self-care as her mobility and pain levels allow. Allow her adequate time to perform these activities at her own pace.
• Encourage activities that involve mild exercise. For example, help her walk several times daily.
• As appropriate, have your patient perform passive ROM exercises, or encourage active exercises. Also, make sure she attends scheduled physical therapy sessions.
• Check a geriatric patient's skin daily for redness, warmth, and new sites of pain, which may indicate new fractures.
• Impose safety precautions. For example, keep side rails up on the bed and insist she use any prescribed assistive device.
• Move the older woman gently and carefully at all times and discuss with ancillary facility personnel how easily an osteoporotic patient's bones can fracture.
• Provide a balanced diet rich in nutrients that support skeletal metabolism: vitamin D, calcium, and protein.
• Administer analgesics and heat to relieve pain, as prescribed, and assess and document your patient's response.

Patient teaching

- Explain all treatments, tests, and procedures. Make sure the older woman and her family members clearly understand the prescribed drug regimen. Tell them how to recognize significant adverse reactions and to report them immediately.
- Thoroughly explain osteoporosis to the patient and her family members. If they don't understand the disease process, they may feel needless guilt, thinking that they could have acted to prevent bone fractures.
- If your patient takes a calcium supplement, encourage liberal fluid intake to help maintain adequate urine output and avoid renal calculi, hypercalcemia, and hypercalciuria.
- Teach the patient taking estrogen to perform breast self-examination. Tell her to perform this examination at least once a month and to report any lumps right away. Emphasize the need for regular gynecologic examinations and tell the older woman to report abnormal vaginal bleeding promptly.
- Tell her to report any new pain sites immediately, especially after trauma. Teach her how to use a back brace properly, if appropriate.
- Advise your patient to sleep on a firm mattress and to avoid excessive bed rest. Placing a board between the mattress and the box spring will make the mattress firmer and may reduce the older woman's morning stiffness.
- Demonstrate proper body mechanics. Show her how to stoop before lifting anything and how to avoid twisting movements and prolonged bending. Also, encourage the patient to install safety devices, such as grab bars and railings, at home.
- Advise the older woman to eat a diet rich in calcium, and give her a list of calcium-rich foods. Explain that type II osteoporosis may be prevented by adequate dietary calcium and regular exercise. Hormonal and fluoride treatments also may help prevent osteoporosis.
- Explain that secondary osteoporosis may be prevented by effectively treating underlying disease, mobilizing soon after surgery or trauma, decreasing alcohol consumption, carefully observing for signs of malabsorption, and promptly treating hyperthyroidism.
- Provide positive reinforcement for the aging adult's efforts to adapt, and show her how her condition is improving or stabilizing.
- As necessary, refer her to an occupational therapist or a home health nurse to help her cope with ADLs. A physical therapist who can institute a home exercise program may be indicated to promote the patient's optimum flexibility and functioning.

HIP FRACTURE

Hip fractures — the most frequent fall-related injuries resulting in hospitalization — are a leading cause of disability among older adults. They are one of many events that may permanently change your patient's level of functioning and independence. Many who survive a hip fracture never return to their pre-fracture ambulatory status.

Fractures in the older person are related to falls, cancer metastasis, osteoporosis, and other skeletal diseases. The most common site of fracture is the head of the femur, with women having a higher incidence than men. Older adults' bones fracture more easily because they are more brittle. They also heal more slowly, increasing the risk of immobility complications.

Causes

Falls are the most common cause of hip fracture in older adults. Poor footing, uneven surfaces, or slippery conditions can cause falls. People who are confused and restrained with side rails or body vests can sometimes experience hip fractures while attempting to get out of bed. The aging adult with bony metastasis or severe osteoporosis can fracture his hip by twisting in bed.

Assessment findings

Suspect a hip fracture whenever an older person falls or has any trauma to the bones. The person with a hip fracture typically reports pain in the affected hip and leg. The pain is exacerbated by any movement.

With the patient lying flat, examine the legs. The fractured leg is usually rotated outward and may appear shorter than the other leg. The fractured limb also has limited or abnormal ROM. Edema and discoloration of the surrounding tissue may also be present. In an open fracture, the bone protrudes through the skin.

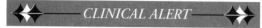

CLINICAL ALERT

A shortened leg and outward rotation are the classic signs of a fractured hip.

Diagnostic tests

X-rays are used to diagnose most fractures. Pictures are usually taken from two angles. CT scans may be ordered for complicated fractures to pinpoint the abnormalities.

Treatment

Treatment for the patient with a hip fracture focuses on restoring function and motion to the injured leg. Activity and weight bearing are limited to allow the fracture to mend properly. Depending on the location, the fracture is treated with immobilization or joint replacement. Skin traction may be ordered preoperatively to decrease muscle spasms. Bedrest with immobility is ordered initially for the older adult who is not going to be surgically treated. Narcotic or nonnarcotic analgesics are ordered to treat pain. Physical therapy is used to teach the patient non-weight-bearing transfers and a therapist works with the patient as his weight-bearing status changes.

Complications

Complications of a hip fracture can be devastating to the older adult. They include pneumonia, venous thrombosis, pressure sores, and voiding dysfunction. These complications can delay or prevent rehabilitation, and may require his admission to a nursing home.

Nursing interventions

- If the bone is protruding from the skin, immediately apply a sterile dressing to cover the bone and open wound, stabilize the leg, and notify the doctor.
- Offer your patient opportunities to express fears and concerns. Answer all questions honestly.
- If the patient has skin traction, remove it daily to check the skin for redness or other signs of breakdown. Maintain alignment of the traction, and check the setup to assure that the weights are hanging freely, not touching the bottom of the bed or the floor.
- Maintain proper body alignment, and use an abductor splint or trochanter roll between the older person's legs to prevent loss of alignment. A foot board and sandbags can also be used to maintain proper positioning. Use log-rolling techniques to turn your patient in bed.
- Have someone assist you when transferring the patient, to maintain non-weight-bearing status.
- Increase his activity level as prescribed. Assist with active ROM exercises to the unaffected limbs to maintain function.
- Encourage the older person to perform coughing and deep-breathing exercises.
- Keep his skin clean and dry.

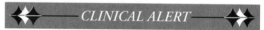

CLINICAL ALERT

Do not massage the patient's extremities in an effort to promote circulation. Massage could increase the risk of thromboembolus.

- Turn your patient often, and consider using a sheepskin or alternating pressure mattress to prevent skin breakdown.
- Good nutrition promotes healing and increases resistance. Encourage the older person to eat as much of his meals as possible. Offer high-protein, high-calorie snacks.
- As soon as the doctor permits, help the patient to mobilize. Reassure him that the healed limb is safe to use. Plan progress in small steps. Start by helping him stand at the bedside. At the next session, have him walk to a nearby chair, as prescribed. Your patient's early involvement in physical therapy is vital to his successful recovery.

Patient teaching

- Instruct the patient to use a splint to maintain body alignment while he sleeps.
- Teach him ROM exercises and the importance of good skin care.

• Emphasize the need for coughing and deep-breathing exercises and incentive spirometry to prevent pulmonary complications.

• Advise the patient to obtain a raised toilet seat and to ask the doctor about a raised chair seat, also called a hip chair.

• Explain the physiology of healing bones to help the patient understand the importance of activity restrictions and lifestyle changes.

• Encourage your patient to use safe ambulation practices. Advise him to wear properly fitting shoes with low, broad heels. Teach him to place both feet near the edge of a curb or stairs before stepping down or up, rather than stepping with the legs stretched and poorly balanced.

• Tell the patient to consider wearing sunglasses outside to improve vision on bright days. Advise him to use a night-light in the hall and bathroom to avoid falls during night visits, and tell him to remove loose rugs and clutter from the floors and stairs.

• Stress the importance of following a nutritious diet to promote bone healing. Encourage the patient to eat foods rich in vitamin C (such as citrus fruits and tomatoes) and calcium (such as dairy products, salmon, and broccoli). Advise him to get enough vitamin D (found in fortified milk and produced by sun-exposed skin), to promote calcium absorption and bone repair, and to eat adequate amounts of protein and foods with vitamin A for proper wound healing.

• If the patient is taking a narcotic analgesic, such as codeine, advise him to avoid activities that require alertness. Also, tell him to report a rash, itching, or gastrointestinal (GI) upset. Because older people are more prone to constipation, a direct side effect of narcotic use, have him talk to his doctor about using a stool softener.

• Tell the patient who is taking a nonsteroidal anti-inflammatory drug that the drug may cause GI upset and bleeding. Instruct him to report loss of appetite, nausea, vomiting, diarrhea, or other GI symptoms. Tell him to call his doctor immediately if he has black, tarry stools, bloody vomit, or other signs of GI bleeding.

HIP REPLACEMENT

Total or partial replacement of the hip joint with a synthetic prosthesis restores mobility and stability and relieves pain. Recent improvements in surgical techniques and prosthetic devices have made joint replacement an increasingly common treatment. More than 500,000 total hip replacements are performed worldwide every year. The benefits of a hip replacement include not only improved, pain-free mobility but also an increased sense of independence and self worth.

The earliest workable hip prosthesis, introduced in 1939, was a metal cup that fit between the acetabulum and the squared-off head of the femur. Metal-on-metal prostheses followed in 1958, with limited success. Most were removed due to wear of the components that left metal particles in the joint. In the 1960s, plastic-to-metal prostheses were tried along with a plastic femoral head. Most femoral prostheses today are made from titanium, vanadium, and nickel-cobalt with various polymers or plastics used for the acetabular cap. Originally, a methyl methacrylate "cement" was used to hold the prostheses in place. Porous-coated prostheses were introduced in the 1980s, making the cement unnecessary.

Today, there are at least 100 different varieties on the market. The acetabular cups are metal cups with or without screws, plastic, or ceramic. The majority of the femoral components are made of metal, although some are ceramic. There is an equal distribution of porous and nonporous prostheses.

Causes

The most common indication for total hip replacement is primary degenerative arthritis. The replacement is also performed for patients with other forms of severe chronic arthritis, extensive joint trauma, and hip fractures. A protruding acetabulum associated with rheumatoid arthritis, osteomalacia, or Paget's disease are less common indications.

Assessment findings

Because the joint replacement is complex, patient assessment begins long before the day of surgery.

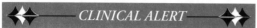
CLINICAL ALERT

The patient's home should be assessed for safety and functionality. Available seating, bathroom setup, location of bedrooms and bathrooms (first or second floor), and number of steps to enter the house are all evaluated to ensure the necessary postoperative preparations.

Treatment

During the procedure, the surgeon must remove the head of the femur, exposing the marrow cavity of the femoral shaft. The femoral component of the prosthesis is inserted into the cavity, at an angle that allows it to articulate with the acetabular cup. The acetabular cup is attached to the pelvic bones.

Hip replacements are performed using either a cemented or uncemented technique. With a cemented prosthesis, the surgeon cements the femoral head of the prosthesis in a position that allows articulation with a studded cup, which he then cements into the deepened acetabulum. Because of the many complications associated with the methyl methacrylate cement, porous-coated prostheses were developed.

In a porous-coated prosthesis, the smooth metal surface is studded with metal beads and sprayed with a bone-stimulating material. Ceramic and hydroxyapatite, a biochemical substance, are the most common materials used. The coated beads are designed to stimulate bone growth in between the beads to hold the prosthesis in place. The incidence of loosening with this technique is no higher than that found with the cemented technique.

Complications

Infection and fractures are two common complications of hip replacement. Fractures can occur if the prosthesis is too large for the marrow cavity or if an incorrect angle is used. Dislocation, usually caused by excess forward or backward motion of the hip or loosening of the prosthesis, may require a second

surgery. Fat embolism can develop within 72 hours after surgery. Hypovolemic shock from blood loss during surgery is a rare complication of this procedure. Among older adults, cerebrovascular accidents and myocardial infarction may also result.

If removal of a septic prosthesis is necessary, a Girdlestone procedure may be performed. The Girdlestone procedure, performed often before the advent of joint replacement, involves removing the femoral head and neck as well as the adjacent synovium. The top of the femoral shaft migrates up between the posterior aspect of the iliac crest and the gluteal muscles, forming a pseudo-acetabulum. The patient will have a shorter leg following this procedure, but will usually be pain free, because the nerve endings involved in arthritis pain were in the removed synovium of the femoral head.

If methyl methacrylate cement is used, pulmonary edema may result. Other complications associated with the cement include arterial thrombosis, pseudoaneurysms, hematomas, cardiac arrest, hypertension, and fracture of the cement with the possibility of a loose piece of cement in the joint, displacing the femoral head.

Nursing interventions

● After surgery, assess the older adult's vital signs frequently and report any hypotension; narrowed pulse pressure; tachycardia; decreased level of consciousness; rapid, shallow respirations; or cold, pale, clammy skin. Maintain bedrest for the prescribed period. Maintain the hip in proper alignment. If traction is used, periodically check the weights and other equipment.

● Assess the patient's level of pain and provide analgesics, as ordered. Be alert for signs of toxicity or oversedation.

● Monitor the older person for signs of fat embolism, including apprehension, diaphoresis, fever, dyspnea, pulmonary effusion, tachycardia, cyanosis, seizures, and petechial rash on the chest and shoulders.

● Inspect the incision site and dressing frequently for signs of infection. Change the dressing as necessary, maintaining strict aseptic technique. Document the appearance of the incision and the

CHARTING GUIDE

Documenting surgical incision care

In addition to documenting vital signs and level of consciousness when the patient returns from surgery, keep careful records of the appearance of the surgical incision and the care provided.

4/10/96	08:30 Dressing removed from left hip incision; no drainage on dressing. Incision well approximated and intact with staples. Margins ecchymotic; small amt. of serosanguineous drainage from distal portion of wound. Dry 5″ x 9″ sterile gauze pad applied.
	Renata Connor, RN

Also, read the records that came with the patient from the postanesthesia care unit. Look for a doctor's order directing whether you or the doctor will perform the first dressing change. Document the following features of surgical wound care:

- the date, time, and type of wound care performed
- the wound's appearance (size, condition of margins, necrotic tissue if any), odor (if any), location of any drainage, and drainage characteristics (type, color, consistency, and amount)
- dressing information, such as type and amount of new dressing applied
- the patient's tolerance of the procedure.

Record special or detailed wound care instructions and pain management measures on the nursing plan of care. Document the color and amount of measurable drainage on the intake and output form.

If the patient is expected to need wound care after discharge, provide and document appropriate instructions. This record documents that you explained aseptic technique and the signs of infection and other complications, that you demonstrated how to change the dressing, and that you provided written instructions for home care.

care given (see *Documenting surgical incision care*).
- Periodically assess neurovascular and motor status distal to the site of joint replacement. Immediately report any abnormalities.
- Check for signs of dislocation, such as sudden severe pain, shortening of the involved leg, or external rotation of the leg.
- Reposition your patient often to enhance his comfort and prevent pressure ulcers. Encourage frequent coughing and deep breathing exercises to prevent pulmonary complications, and promote adequate fluid intake to prevent urinary stasis and constipation.
- Help him begin exercising the affected leg soon after surgery. Some doctors routinely order physical therapy to begin on the day of surgery.
- Before the patient leaves the hospital, provide referrals for home physical therapy and any needed

equipment, including a hip chair and toilet seat with a high seat and arm rests.

Patient teaching
- Reinforce the doctor's and physical therapist's instructions for an exercise regimen. Remind the patient to closely adhere to the prescribed schedule and not to rush rehabilitation, no matter how good he feels.
- Review prescribed limits of activity. Caution the older adult against extensive stair climbing, prolonged sitting, and overuse of the hip.
- Give him the teaching handout, *Adjusting to a total hip replacement*, pages 206 and 207. To reduce the risk of dislocating the prosthesis, tell your patient to keep his hips abducted, to never cross his legs when sitting, and to avoid sleeping on his side

(Text continues on page 208.)

Adjusting to a total hip replacement

Dear Patient:

Your new artificial hip should eliminate hip pain and help you get around better. But go easy at first.

   To give your hip time to heal and to avoid placing too much stress on it, follow these do's and don'ts for the next 3 months, or for as long as your doctor orders.

Do's

● Sit only in chairs with arms that you can lean on for support when you get up. Before standing, ease to the edge of your chair. Then, place your affected leg in front of the unaffected one, which should be well under your chair. Now,

grip the chair's arms firmly, and push up with your arms, *not with your legs.* Support most of your weight with your arms and your unaffected leg.

● Wear support stockings except when you're in bed.

● Turn in bed only as directed by your doctor.

● Place a pillow between your legs when you lie on your side and when you go to bed at

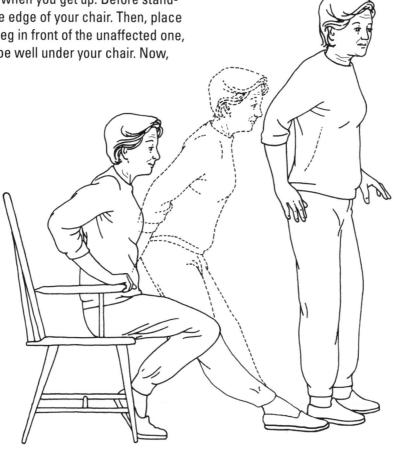

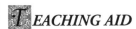

Adjusting to a total hip replacement (continued)

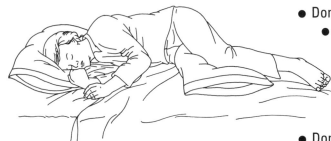

night. This keeps your leg from twisting and dislodging your new hip.

● Always keep your affected leg facing forward when sitting, lying down, or walking.

● Exercise regularly, as ordered. Stop exercising immediately, though, if you feel severe hip pain.

● Lie down and elevate your feet and legs, if they swell after walking.

● Rent or purchase a raised toilet seat to use at home and use public toilets that are designated for the disabled.

● Sit on a firm pillow when riding in a car and keep your affected leg extended (if your knee suddenly hits the dashboard, your hip prosthesis could be dislodged).

● To pick up dropped objects, position yourself as your therapist teaches you.

Don'ts

● Don't lean far forward to stand up.

● Don't sit on low chairs or couches.

● Don't bend too far over when picking up objects or tying your shoes.

● Don't cross your legs or turn your hip or knee inward or outward, which can dislodge your hip.

● Don't scrub your hip incision.

  ● Don't take tub baths.

    ● Don't lift heavy items.

      ● Don't have sexual intercourse until your doctor says it's okay to do so.

      ● Don't play tennis, run, jog, or do other strenuous activities.

● Don't drive a car.

● Don't reach to the end of your bed to pull up blankets.

When to call your doctor

Call your doctor if you have:

● redness, swelling, or warmth around your incision

● drainage from your incision

● fever or chills

● severe hip pain uncontrolled by prescribed medicine

● sudden sharp pain and a clicking or popping sound in your joint

● leg shortening, with your foot turning outward

● loss of control over leg motion or complete loss of leg motion.

An important precaution

Your doctor or dentist will prescribe an antibiotic for you to take before and after tooth extractions, dental procedures other than routine fillings, any other surgery, and some diagnostic tests and procedures.

or rolling to his side when getting up. Remind him to keep his toes and kneecap pointing forward. Tell him to avoid flexing his hips more than 90 degrees when arising from a bed or chair. Encourage him to sit in chairs with arms and a firm, high seat and to sleep only on a firm mattress.

● Caution your patient to promptly report any signs of possible infection, such as persistent fever and increased pain, tenderness, or stiffness in the joint and surrounding area. Explain that infection may develop even several months after joint replacement.

● Tell him to report a sudden increase in pain, which may indicate dislodgment of the prosthesis.

● Provide him with written instructions for incision care. Stress the importance of keeping follow-up appointments and ensure that he knows when his sutures or staples are to be removed.

11

Managing urinary tract problems

*A*s the body ages, the urinary system changes in several ways. Bladder muscles become weaker and bladder capacity decreases. The older adult has more difficulty emptying his bladder, leaving more residual volume. The micturition reflex is delayed. The pelvic diaphragm weakens, especially in women who've had twins or triplets. In aging men, an enlarged prostate gland often leads to urinary tract problems.

URINARY INCONTINENCE

Urinary incontinence is never a normal sign of aging. It is always a symptom of an underlying problem. Millions of older adults suffer from some loss of voluntary control.

Problems with urinary continence are called acute or persistent and can range from mild loss of bladder control to total incontinence. Acute incontinence occurs suddenly and is usually related to an acute illness. Common in hospitalized people, it usually ends once the illness is resolved. Acute incontinence can also be associated with medications, treatments, and other environmental factors.

Persistent incontinence is classified as urge incontinence, stress incontinence, overflow incontinence, and functional incontinence. Urge incontinence is a sudden strong desire to void accompanied by a leakage of urine. Stress incontinence is a

sudden leakage of urine associated with activity such as laughing, sneezing, coughing, lifting, jumping, or bending. Overflow incontinence is a frequent, sometimes constant leakage of urine from a too-full bladder. Functional incontinence occurs with an intact lower urinary tract, as the result of immobility or cognitive impairment. Several types of incontinence may co-exist.

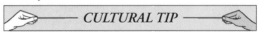
CULTURAL TIP

Many older adults accept incontinence as a part of the aging process, and do not report problems. Women who have had children often accept stress incontinence as a normal consequence of aging and childbirth. Incontinence can be embarrassing or frustrating, making some older adults reluctant to discuss it. They may fear surgery or be unaware that treatment options exist. Also, older adults often feel that health care professionals are not interested in the problem.

Advertising is in part responsible for perpetuating the idea that incontinence is an acceptable, normal part of aging, as noted in commercials that use active, youthful-looking people to sell incontinence products. The ads fail to mention that all incontinence should be investigated by a health care provider, who may be able to eliminate the cause. The media present a misleading message of hopelessness to the older person.

Incontinence is a leading cause of nursing home

placement. The costs of incontinence care, supplies, laundry, and nursing care, are extremely high. Continence is a learned ability, requiring an intact genitourinary tract, competent sphincters, adequate cognitive and physical function, motivation, and an appropriate environment for toileting.

Causes

Causes of acute incontinence include confusion, dehydration, medications, urethritis, and atrophic vaginitis. Infection, especially a symptomatic urinary tract infection (UTI), can also cause incontinence. Urinary incontinence can result from some endocrine imbalances, such as hypercalcemia and hyperglycemia. Restricted mobility or conditions that cause urinary retention can precipitate urinary incontinence. Or it may result from depression in the older adult.

Urge incontinence is the result of involuntary bladder contractions. Irritation of the detrusor muscle (the external muscle coating the bladder) caused by local irritating factors such as infection, stones, tumor, or obstruction can lead to urge incontinence, as can hyperactivity of the detrusor associated with cerebrovascular accident, suprasacral spinal disease, Parkinson's disease, dementia, and demyelinating disease.

Stress incontinence is caused by weakened anatomic support in the pelvic floor. Perinatal trauma, tissue weakening associated with aging, estrogen deficiency, pudendal nerve damage, and gynecologic trauma from surgery can cause weakening of the pelvic floor. Medications such as alpha-adrenergic blockers, analgesics, sedatives, and hypnotics can cause bladder outlet relaxation and incontinence.

Overflow incontinence occurs when the bladder becomes over-distended, due to incomplete emptying. The aging adult often is unable to feel the full bladder. More common in men, overflow incontinence can be caused by an atonic or underactive detrusor muscle or obstruction. Diabetes and medications that lead to urine retention — such as analgesics, psychotropics, alpha-adrenergic agonists, calcium channel blockers, and anticholinergic agents — can decrease activity of the detrusor.

Anatomic obstruction can include prostatic hypertrophy, pelvic prolapse, stricture, tumor, or neurogenic conditions such as multiple sclerosis or suprasacral lesions.

Functional incontinence is caused by disruption of a person's continence routine. Immobility and cognitive impairment are two common causes. The use of physical or chemical restraints or environmental barriers, such as side rails, can lead to functional incontinence in an older adult. Psychological issues, such as depression, regression, or bipolar disorders, are other causes.

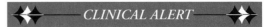

CLINICAL ALERT

Not every patient with cognitive impairment is incontinent, so incontinence should not be automatically expected or accepted in these individuals.

Assessment findings

Use nonthreatening questions when asking about incontinence. Questions like "Do you sometimes have to rush to the bathroom?" will get more responses than "Do you have a problem with incontinence?" The patient needs to be questioned carefully about his symptoms to ascertain the type of incontinence and identify the cause and possible treatment. Whenever possible, document the patient's response in his own words.

The patient with urge incontinence reports feeling the urge to void, but is not able to hold it until he reaches the bathroom. This patient's report indicates urgency, frequency, and nocturia. The patient with stress incontinence reports leaking small amounts of urine when laughing, sneezing, jumping, coughing or bending. These symptoms usually occur only in the daytime.

The patient with overflow incontinence reports a poor or slow stream, and the feeling of hesitancy or straining. He complains of having to void frequently in small amounts and periodic or continuous dribbling of urine.

The patient with functional incontinence reports adequate urine volume and stream.

Observations of how the patient ambulates, rises, and sits provide clues to their ability to get to the toilet. Look at the way they undress and refasten clothing to determine how well they are able to disrobe for toileting and how long the process takes.

Inspection of the perineal area may reveal poor hygiene or signs of infection. A rectal examination of the male patient may reveal prostate enlargement or pain, possibly indicating benign prostatic hypertrophy or infection.

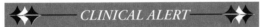

The absence of an enlarged prostate does not exclude an obstructive process.

Vaginal examination may reveal vaginal dryness or atrophic vaginitis, indicating estrogen deficiency. Asking the female patient to bear down during the exam may reveal pelvic laxity, a cystocele, urethrocele, or rectocele. Asking the patient to cough during the exam may reveal leaking urine with increased intra-abdominal pressure.

On palpation, the bladder of the patient with overflow incontinence is above the symphysis pubis.

Diagnostic tests

Postvoid residual catheterization is used to determine the extent of bladder emptying and the amount of urine left in the bladder after the patient has voided. For accurate results, catheterization should be done within 15 minutes of voiding. A hand-held bladder scanner can be used to determine bladder residual urine when an invasive procedure is contraindicated.

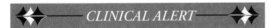

Always check to ensure that the patient is not constipated when performing this test. Constipation interferes with bladder emptying and will increase the amount of residual urine in the bladder.

Urinalysis is used to look for bacteria, blood, and glucose in urine. A cloudy appearance or foul odor may indicate infection. Urine cultures are sent to a laboratory to identify bacteria in the urine.

Uroflowmetry is used to evaluate voiding pattern and to demonstrate bladder outlet obstruction by measuring the flow rate of the stream as the patient voids. Cystometry is used to assess the bladder's neuromuscular function by measuring the efficiency of the detrusor muscle reflex, intravesical pressure and capacity, and the bladder's reaction to thermal stimulation. The results of cystometry can be ambiguous, and are usually supported by the results of excretory urography and voiding cystourethrography.

Excretory urography, also called intravenous pyelography, is used to evaluate the structure and function of the kidneys, ureter and bladder. It involves I.V. administration of a contrast medium. Voiding cystourethrography is used to detect abnormalities of the bladder and urethra and to assess hypertrophy of the prostate lobes, urethral stricture, and the degree of compromise of a stenotic prostatic urethra (in men).

Retrograde urethrography, used almost exclusively in men, aids diagnosis of urethral stricture and outlet obstruction. External sphincter electromyography measures electrical activity of the external urinary sphincter. Needle electrodes are inserted in the perineal or periurethral tissues, in an anal plug, or in skin electrodes. Skin electrodes are most commonly used.

Treatment

Treatment for urinary incontinence involves exercises to strengthen the pelvic muscles, dietary modifications and fluid restrictions, medications to treat underlying conditions, and procedures and devices such as behavioral therapies, habit training, bladder retraining, pessaries, condom catheters, artificial sphincter implantation, and intermittent self-catheterization. Occasionally, the treatment may include surgery.

If urinary incontinence results from inflammation caused by bacterial infection, an antibiotic is prescribed. If detrusor muscle instability is suspected, anticholinergic drugs are ordered to improve bladder function and treat bladder spasms. Antispasmodic drugs are prescribed for detrusor hyperreflexia to suppress the bladder's smooth muscle activity. Estrogen, in either oral, topical or suppository form, is used if atrophic vaginitis is present.

Stress incontinence can sometimes be treated with antidepressant drugs.

Behavioral therapies include bladder training, habit and clock training, prompted voiding, and pelvic muscle exercises (Kegel exercises). The approach is selected to suit the patient's underlying problem. Habit and bladder training are well suited to the patient with urge incontinence. Pelvic floor exercises can be well utilized by the cognitively intact patient with stress incontinence. Behavioral interventions are generally not selected for patients with incontinence secondary to overflow.

Behavioral therapies have no reported side effects and involve the patient in the treatment process. When the patient is motivated and properly taught, treatment results with these therapies are reported in ranges from significant reduction of wetness to complete dryness. Outcomes of behavioral techniques were reported as "percent cured" and "percent improved" in the clinical practice guidelines published by the U.S. Department of Health and Human Services (1992). Pelvic muscle exercise reportedly improved outcomes in 75% of cases and cures in 12%. Bladder training improved 54% and cured 16%, with no adverse effects or complications from either modality.

Additional techniques, such as biofeedback and electrical stimulation, serve as adjuncts to behavioral therapy. (For more information about these techniques, see Chapter 17.)

Habit training, helpful for patients with dementia or cognitive impairment, involves maintaining a rigid voiding schedule, usually every 2 to 4 hours. The patient's objective is to void before an accident occurs. Bladder retraining may be useful for the patient who has full cognitive function. It teaches the patient to resist the urge to void, gradually increasing bladder capacity and the intervals between voiding. As capacity increases, urgency and frequency decrease.

A pessary may be prescribed for the female patient with an anatomic abnormality, such as severe uterine prolapse or pelvic relaxation. The pessary is worn internally, like a contraceptive diaphragm, and stabilizes the bladder's base and the urethra, preventing incontinence during physical strain. Short-term use of a condom catheter may be prescribed for the male patient to effectively help him avoid accidents.

Long-term use should be avoided, as it can lead to UTI and skin irritation.

An artificial sphincter — consisting of a silicone cuffed sphincter with a pressure-regulating balloon and a bulb pump — may be inserted in the male patient after radical prostatectomy or in the female patient with stress incontinence that is unresponsive to other treatment. The cuff is placed around the bladder neck. The balloon holds the fluid that is used to inflate the cuff. The bulb pump is implanted in the scrotum or labia. As the bladder fills with urine, the pressure-sensitive cuff inflates to prevent urine from leaking around the bladder neck. The patient squeezes the pump to move fluid from the cuff into the pressurized balloon, allowing urination.

Surgical repair of the anterior vaginal wall or retropubic suspension of the bladder and urethra may be options for treatment of women with stress incontinence. Retropubic suspension restores the bladder and urethra to their proper intra-abdominal positions. In men with urge incontinence resulting from prostatic hypertrophy, treatment may include transurethral resection of the prostate or open prostatectomy. Surgery may be used to remove obstructive lesions that cause urge or overflow incontinence.

Patients with overflow incontinence from urine retention may benefit from intermittent catheterization. Removal of barriers, adequate lighting, and frequent orientation will help the patient with functional incontinence.

Complications

Complications from urinary incontinence include UTI and skin irritation and breakdown. These conditions, if not treated quickly or completely, can lead to sepsis. Incontinence in the geriatric patient also has severe psychological consequences, such as depression, loss of self esteem, isolation, frustration, and feelings of hopelessness.

Nursing interventions

● Explain all tests and procedures to your patient. Allow him to ask questions, and answer them honestly. Provide privacy for any discussions.
● Administer antibiotics and other medications, as ordered.

• Orient the patient to the location of the bathroom and any call devices. Provide adequate lighting in the bathroom to help him avoid mishaps during the night. If he needs help to get to the bathroom, offer it every 2 hours or when he awakens.

• Explain bladder training routines and post the schedule. Assist the patient receiving bladder training in deep breathing exercises to delay the urge to void. Give ample, positive reinforcement for all efforts toward continence.

• Provide frequent perineal care and watch the aging adult for skin breakdown. Wash with mild soap and water, and pat the skin to dry it. Wash from the front to the back to avoid spreading contamination.

• Help the patient insert a pessary, as ordered. If intermittent catheterization is ordered, perform it on time and document the amount of urine returned.

• For the postoperative patient, record accurate intake and output measurements. Provide catheter care and ambulate him as soon as permitted.

Patient teaching

• Tell the aging adult that strong pelvic muscles can help prevent incontinence. Teach the female patient how to do Kegel exercises to strengthen muscles that control urine flow.

• Instruct the older person to limit or eliminate foods that irritate the bladder and cause urinary frequency, such as foods and beverages with caffeine (coffee, tea, cola, dark chocolate), alcohol, and the artificial sweetener aspartame (Nutrasweet). Explain that many prescription and nonprescription drugs contain caffeine. Urge your patient to check food and drug labels carefully.

• If the doctor asks the patient to keep a record of fluid intake and voiding and incontinence episodes, advise him to review the record daily to make sure he's taking in at least eight 8-oz glasses (2,000 ml) of fluid daily. Explain that many incontinent patients consciously or unintentionally restrict fluids, which isn't the aim of treatment. Teach patients that a reduction in daytime fluid intake will not cure incontinence or the need to get up and void at night. If the patient is concerned about nocturia, suggest that he consume most fluids in the daytime and limit

evening intake to small sips after 6 p.m.

• Because urinary incontinence may stem from pressure on the bladder and urethra due to constipation or fecal impaction, recommend a fiber-rich diet to help counter these conditions.

• Teach the older person the actions and adverse effects of any medications that are prescribed. If an antibiotic is ordered, stress the importance of taking all of the pills in the prescription.

• Describe all procedures and devices used to improve or manage urinary incontinence. If habit training is in the treatment plan, make sure to include the patient's family members and other caregivers in your teaching. Stress the importance of keeping accurate records to help the doctor monitor progress and adjust treatment. Direct the patient to urinate at the specified times, whether or not he feels the urge. If he needs to urinate at additional times, instruct him to do so immediately. Also advise him to urinate just before going to bed.

• If the patient is undergoing bladder retraining, demonstrate how to suppress the urge to void by breathing slowly and deeply. Encourage him to practice this procedure.

• Teach the patient with a pessary the correct technique for inserting and positioning the device. Also teach her to remove and clean it according to the doctor's directions. Stress infection prevention methods.

• Teach the male patient how to apply and wear a condom catheter, and point out ways to avoid complications such as contact dermatitis and penile maceration, ischemia, and obstruction.

• Review preoperative and postoperative instructions for the patient undergoing artificial sphincter implantation, including complications that may necessitate implant repair or removal. For example, the cuff or balloon can leak (uncommon) or trapped blood or other fluid contaminants can disable the bulb pump, impairing fluid passage to and from the cuff. Other complications include tissue erosion around the bulb or in the bladder neck or urethra, infection, inadequate occlusion pressure, and kinked tubing.

• Teach the patient and caregivers the correct technique for intermittent catheterization. Reassure them that although this procedure may seem difficult at first, practice makes it easier. Stress the importance of clean technique and tell them to report any signs of infection to the doctor.

• For the woman undergoing surgical repair, explain that retropubic suspension restores the bladder and urethra to their proper intra-abdominal positions. Explain that the operation may be effective for only a short time in some women.

• For the male patient undergoing prostatic resection, explain the procedure and the preoperative and postoperative care.

• Discuss wearing protective pads and garments to augment habit training and bladder retraining. Mention that these absorbent devices boost comfort and confidence and allow the patient more mobility during treatment for urinary incontinence. Describe the different types available.

• Teach the patient how to prevent skin irritation and breakdown. After each incontinence episode, direct the patient to wash skin that's exposed to urine with mild soap and water. Instruct him to pat the area dry and then to apply a protective barrier cream.

BENIGN PROSTATIC HYPERPLASIA

Most men over age 50 have some prostatic enlargement. In most cases, prostatic enlargement is benign, but it does increase the risk of malignancy and requires regular evaluation.

In benign prostatic hyperplasia (BPH), the prostate gland enlarges enough to compress the urethra and cause urinary obstruction. It's the most common cause of bladder outlet obstruction in men. BPH begins with changes in periurethral glandular tissue. As the prostate enlarges, it may extend into the bladder and obstruct urine outflow by compressing or distorting the prostatic urethra. BPH may also cause a diverticulum musculature that retains urine when the rest of the bladder empties.

Symptoms of BPH progress slowly but continuously. Many men, embarrassed by the symptoms, avoid seeking medical attention.

Causes

The exact cause of BPH is unknown, but its appearance in older men strongly suggests a link to changes associated with aging. Recent evidence implicates hormonal activity as a causative factor. As men age, androgenic hormone production decreases, causing an imbalance in androgen and estrogen levels and high levels of dihydrotestosterone, the main prostatic intracellular androgen. Other theoretical causes include neoplasm, arteriosclerosis, inflammation, and metabolic or nutritional disturbances.

Assessment findings

Clinical features of BPH depend on the extent of prostatic enlargement and on the lobes affected. Characteristically, the patient complains of a group of symptoms known as prostatism: decreased urine stream caliber and force, an interrupted stream, urinary hesitancy, and difficulty starting urination, which results in straining and a feeling of incomplete voiding. As the obstruction increases, the patient may report frequent urination with nocturia, dribbling, urine retention, incontinence and, possibly, hematuria. Prostatism affects 75% of men age 65 and older.

Physical examination reveals a visible midline mass above the symphysis pubis, which represents an incompletely emptied bladder. Palpation of the abdomen discloses a distended bladder. An enlarged prostate is felt during the rectal examination.

Diagnostic tests

Excretory urography is used to identify urinary tract obstruction, hydronephrosis, calculi or tumors, and filling and emptying defects in the bladder. Elevated blood urea nitrogen and serum creatinine levels suggest impaired renal function. Urinalysis and urine culture show hematuria, pyuria and, when the bacterial count exceeds 100,000/mm³, UTI.

When symptoms are severe, cystourethroscopy is the definitive diagnostic measure and is used to determine the best surgical procedure. It can show prostate enlargement, bladder wall changes, calculi, and a raised bladder. A prostate-specific antigen test may be performed to rule out prostatic cancer.

Treatment

Depending on the size of the enlarged prostate, the age and health of the patient, and the extent of the obstruction, BPH may be treated surgically or symptomatically. Conservative therapy includes prostatic massages, sitz baths, short-term fluid restriction (to prevent bladder distention) and, if infection develops, antimicrobials. Regular sexual intercourse may help relieve prostatic congestion.

Treatment with terazosin and finasteride is also effective. Two investigational drugs, leuprolide acetate (Lupron) and nafarelin acetate hold promise for older men who aren't candidates for surgery. Leuprolide acetate reduces prostate volume and improves signs and symptoms such as urinary frequency and urgency and diminished urinary stream. Researchers believe nafarelin acetate helps BPH by blocking testosterone production. It can cause impotence, which persists until the drug is discontinued.

Surgery is the only effective therapy for relieving acute urine retention, hydronephrosis, severe hematuria, and recurrent UTI, and for palliative relief of intolerable symptoms. A transurethral resection may be performed if the prostate weighs less than 2 oz (57 g). In this procedure, a resectoscope is used to remove tissue with a wire loop and an electric current. For high-risk patients, continuous drainage with an indwelling urinary catheter alleviates urine retention. Other transurethral procedures include vaporization of the prostate or a prostate incision with a scalpel or laser.

Other procedures involve open surgical removal of the prostate. Suprapubic (transvesical) prostatectomy is the most common and is especially useful when prostatic enlargement remains within the bladder area. Perineal prostatectomy is usually performed for a large gland in an older patient. The operation commonly causes impotence and incontinence. Retropubic (extravesical) prostatectomy allows direct visualization; potency and continence usually are maintained.

Less frequently performed procedures include balloon dilatation, ultrasound needle ablation, and use of stents.

Complications

Because BPH causes urinary obstruction, a patient may have urinary stasis, UTI, or calculi. Bladder wall trabeculation, detrusor muscle hypertrophy, bladder diverticuli and saccules also may occur. Other complications include urethral stenosis, hydronephrosis, paradoxical (overflow) incontinence, acute or chronic renal failure and acute postobstructive diuresis.

Nursing interventions

- Prepare the patient for diagnostic tests and surgery.
- Monitor and record his vital signs, intake and output, and daily weight. Watch closely for signs of postobstructive diuresis (such as increased urine output and hypotension), which may lead to serious dehydration, lowered blood volume, shock, electrolyte losses, and anuria.
- Administer antibiotics, as ordered, for UTI, urethral procedures that involve instruments, and cystoscopy. If he retains urine, try to insert an indwelling urinary catheter. If the catheter can't be passed transurethrally, assist with suprapubic cystostomy. Watch for rapid bladder decompression.

◆◆ —— CLINICAL ALERT —— ◆◆

Avoid giving an older person with BPH decongestants, tranquilizers, alcohol, antidepressants, or anticholinergics because these drugs can worsen the obstruction.

- After prostatic surgery, maintain his comfort, and watch for and prevent postoperative complications. Observe for signs of shock and hemorrhage. Check your patient's catheter frequently (every 15 minutes for the first 2 to 3 hours) for patency and urine color and check the dressings for bleeding.
- Postoperatively, many urologists insert a three-way catheter and establish continuous bladder irrigation. Keep the solution flowing at a rate sufficient to maintain patency and ensure that returns are clear

Speeding your recovery after prostate surgery

Dear Patient:

Here's what you can expect after prostate surgery, along with directions for caring for yourself.

Expect trouble urinating

At first, you may have a feeling of heaviness in the pelvic area, burning during urination, a frequent need to urinate, and loss of some control over urination. Don't worry, these symptoms will disappear with time.

If you notice blood in your urine during the first 2 weeks after surgery, drink some fluids and lie down to rest. The next time you urinate, the bleeding should decrease.

Let your doctor know right away if you continue to see blood in your urine, you can't urinate at all, or you develop a fever.

Prevent constipation

Eat a well-balanced diet and drink 12 glasses of fluid daily, unless the doctor prescribes otherwise. Don't strain to have a bowel movement. If you do become constipated, take a mild laxative.

Don't use an enema or place anything, such as a suppository, into your rectum for at least 4 weeks after surgery.

Cut back on activities

Take only short walks, and avoid climbing stairs as much as possible. Don't lift heavy objects. Also, don't exercise strenuously for at least 3 weeks.

Strengthen your perineal muscles

Perform this simple exercise to strengthen your perineal muscles after surgery: Press your buttocks together, hold this position for a few seconds, and then relax. Repeat this 10 times.

Perform this exercise as many times daily as your doctor orders.

Don't have sex just yet

Don't have sex for at least 4 weeks after surgery, because sexual activity can cause bleeding.

When you do have sex, most of the semen (the fluid that contains sperm) will pass into your bladder rather than out through your urethra. This won't affect your ability to have an erection or an orgasm. However, it will decrease your fertility.

Don't be alarmed if the semen in your bladder causes cloudy urine the first time you urinate after intercourse.

Ask about resuming activity

At your next doctor's appointment, ask when you can return to your usual activities. The timing will vary by the type of surgery you had, your usual kind of activities, and your general health.

Schedule an annual checkup

Continue to have an annual examination, so your doctor can check the prostate area that wasn't removed during surgery.

and light pink. Watch for fluid overload from absorption of the irrigating fluid into the systemic circulation. If a regular catheter is used, observe it closely. If drainage stops because of clots, irrigate the catheter, as ordered, usually with 80 to 100 ml of normal saline solution, while maintaining strict aseptic technique.

● Watch for septic shock, the most serious complication of prostatic surgery. Immediately report severe chills, sudden fever, tachycardia, hypotension, or other signs of shock. Start rapid infusion of intravenous antibiotics, as ordered. Watch for signs of pulmonary embolism, congestive heart failure, and acute renal failure.

● Monitor vital signs, central venous pressure, and arterial pressure. Administer belladonna and opium suppositories or other anticholinergics, as ordered, to relieve bladder spasms that may occur after transurethral resection.

● Continue infusing I.V. fluids until the patient can drink enough on his own (2,000 to 3,000 ml daily) to maintain adequate hydration.

● Administer stool softeners and laxatives, as ordered, to prevent straining.

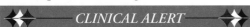
CLINICAL ALERT

Don't check for fecal impaction because a rectal examination may cause bleeding.

Patient teaching

● Tell the patient having a prostatectomy to expect blood in his urine for several days. Inform him that the catheter will remain in place until the bleeding subsides. Warn that he may have bladder spasms, but that medication can be given to provide relief.

● After the catheter is removed, the patient may experience urinary frequency, dribbling and, occasionally, hematuria. Reassure him that he'll gradually regain urinary control. Reinforce your teaching by providing a copy of the teaching handout *Speeding your recovery after prostate surgery.*

● If the patient is to go home with an indwelling catheter, teach him how to care for the catheter.

● Reinforce prescribed activity limits. Warn against lifting, strenuous exercise, and long car rides for at least 1 month after surgery because these activities

can cause bleeding. Also caution him not to have sexual intercourse for at least several weeks after discharge.

● Teach your patient to recognize the signs of UTI and report them immediately to the doctor, because infection can worsen the obstruction. Instruct the patient to follow the prescribed oral antibiotic regimen, and tell him the indications for using gentle laxatives. Urge him to seek medical care immediately if he can't void at all, passes bloody urine, or develops a fever.

● Rarely, an older man experiences temporary or permanent impotence after surgery. More commonly, he may be able to have an erection but will become sterile because his semen is expelled backward into the bladder instead of being ejaculated. Reassure him that seminal fluid in the bladder does no harm; it is simply eliminated in the urine. If your patient has problems adjusting sexually, refer him and his partner to a counselor.

LOWER URINARY TRACT INFECTION

Lower urinary tract infections (UTIs) are the most common cause of bacterial sepsis in older adults. Although these infections are nearly 10 times more common in women — affecting 10% to 20% of all females at least once — their incidence also increases in men over age 65.

The two forms of lower UTI are cystitis (infection of the bladder) and urethritis (infection of the urethra). In adult males, lower UTIs typically are associated with anatomic or physiologic abnormalities and therefore need close evaluation. Most UTIs respond readily to treatment, but recurrence and resistant bacterial flare-ups during therapy are possible.

Weakened bladder muscles in women and enlarged prostates in men — changes associated with aging — can contribute to incomplete emptying of the bladder. Incontinence and decreased ability of aging people to provide proper hygiene for themselves also increase the incidence of UTI by giving bacteria an entry route to the bladder. Older adults with chronic indwelling catheters are also at higher risk because the catheter provides an entry port for bacteria.

Causes

Most lower UTIs are caused by ascending infection by a gram-negative, enteric bacterium, such as *Escherichia coli, Klebsiella, Proteus, Enterobacter, Pseudomonas,* and *Serratia.* In a person with neurogenic bladder, an indwelling urinary catheter, or a fistula between the intestine and bladder, a lower UTI may result from simultaneous infection with multiple pathogens.

Studies suggest that infection results from a breakdown in local defense mechanisms in the bladder, which allows bacteria to invade the bladder mucosa and multiply. These bacteria can't be eliminated readily by normal urination.

Bacterial flare-up during treatment usually is caused by the pathogen's resistance to the prescribed antimicrobial therapy. Even a small number of bacteria (fewer than 10,000/ml) in a midstream urine specimen obtained during treatment casts doubt on the effectiveness of treatment.

In almost all patients, recurrent lower UTIs result from reinfection by the same organism or by some new pathogen. In the remaining patients, recurrence is associated with renal calculi, chronic bacterial prostatitis, or a structural anomaly that's a source of persistent infection.

The high incidence of lower UTI among females probably occurs because natural anatomic features facilitate infection. The female urethra is shorter than the male urethra (about 1" to 2" [2.5 to 5 cm] compared with 7" to 8" [18 to 20 cm]). It's also closer to the anus, allowing bacterial entry into the urethra from the vagina, perineum, or rectum, or from a sexual partner. In young men, release of prostatic fluid serves as an antibacterial shield. Men lose this protection around age 50 when the prostate gland begins to enlarge, resulting in a higher incidence of infection in older men.

Fecal matter, sexual intercourse, and instruments such as catheters and cystoscopes can introduce bac-

teria into the urinary tract and trigger infection. A narrowed ureter or calculi lodged in the ureter or bladder can obstruct urine flow. Slowed urine flow allows bacteria to remain and multiply, posing a risk of damage to the kidneys. Urinary stasis can promote infection, which, if undetected, can spread to the entire urinary system. In addition, because urinary tract bacteria thrive on sugars, diabetes also is a risk factor.

Vesicourethral reflux results when pressure inside the bladder (caused by coughing or sneezing) pushes a small amount of urine from the bladder into the urethra. When the pressure returns to normal, the urine flows back into the bladder, bringing bacteria from the urethra with it. In vesicoureteral reflux, urine flows from the bladder back into one or both ureters. The vesicoureteral valve normally shuts off reflux, but a damaged valve may not do its job.

Assessment findings

Symptoms of lower UTI in an older adult are often nonspecific. The older person may not consider urinary urgency, urinary frequency, and nocturia unusual.

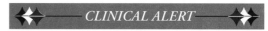

Often the first sign of lower UTI in an older adult is decreased alertness.

In other cases, the patient may report nausea, vomiting, loss of appetite, bladder cramps or spasms, itching, a feeling of warmth during urination, low back pain, chills, and flank pain. The urine may smell bad. Low-grade fever is also a symptom, but not usually in older people. A male patient may have a urethral discharge.

Diagnostic tests

Microscopic urinalysis showing red blood cell and white blood cell counts greater than 10 per high-power field suggests lower UTI.

Clean-catch urinalysis revealing a bacterial count of more than 100,000/mm³, confirms UTI. Lower counts don't necessarily rule out infection, especially if the patient urinates frequently, because bacteria require 30 to 45 minutes to reproduce in urine. Clean-catch collection is preferred to catheterization, which can reinfect the bladder with urethral bacteria. However, catheterization may be the only option in an older patient.

Sensitivity testing is used to select the appropriate antimicrobial drug. Voiding cystourethrography or excretory urography may disclose congenital anomalies that predispose to recurrent UTI.

Treatment

Appropriate antimicrobials are the treatment of choice for most initial lower UTIs.

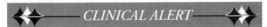
CLINICAL ALERT

A 7- to 10-day course of antibiotics is standard treatment for lower UTI. Although studies suggest that a single dose or a 3- to 5-day regimen may be sufficient to render urine sterile, older patients may still need 7 to 10 days of antibiotics to fully benefit from treatment.

A repeat culture is done to rule out resistance. If the culture shows that urine isn't sterile after 3 days of antibiotic therapy, bacterial resistance probably has occurred, requiring a different antimicrobial.

A single dose of amoxicillin or co-trimoxazole may be effective for females with an acute, uncomplicated lower UTI. A urine culture taken 1 to 2 weeks later indicates whether the infection has been eradicated. Recurrent infections due to infected renal calculi, chronic prostatitis, or structural abnormalities may require surgery. Prostatitis also requires long-term antibiotic therapy. In older adults without these predisposing conditions, long-term, low-dose antibiotic therapy is preferred.

Complications

If untreated, chronic UTIs can seriously damage the urinary tract lining. Infection of adjacent organs and structures (for example, pyelonephritis and renal failure) also may occur. When this happens, the prognosis is poor.

Nursing interventions

- Watch for GI disturbances from antimicrobial therapy. If ordered, give nitrofurantoin macrocrystals with milk or meals to prevent GI distress.
- If sitz baths don't relieve perineal discomfort, apply warm compresses sparingly to the perineum, but be careful not to burn the patient.
- Apply topical antiseptics on the urethral meatus, as necessary.
- Collect all urine specimens for culture and sensitivity testing carefully and promptly.

Patient teaching

- Provide copies of the teaching handout *Self-care tips for urinary tract infections,* page 220, to reinforce your instructions to both men and women.
- Explain the nature and purpose of antimicrobial therapy. Emphasize the importance of completing the prescribed course of therapy and strictly adhering to the ordered dosage.
- Familiarize the patient with prescribed medications and their possible adverse effects. Suggest taking nitrofurantoin macrocrystals with milk or a meal to prevent GI distress. Warn the patient that phenazopyridine turns urine red-orange and stains clothing.
- Explain that an uncontaminated midstream urine specimen is essential for accurate diagnosis. Before collection, teach an older woman to clean the perineum properly and to keep the labia separated during urination.
- Suggest warm sitz baths for relief of perineal discomfort.
- Explain that fruit juices, especially cranberry juice, and oral doses of vitamin C may help acidify urine and enhance the action of some drugs. Urge the older person to drink at least eight 8-oz glasses (2,000 ml) of fluids a day during treatment. More or less than this amount may alter the drug's effect. Be aware that the aging adult may resist this suggestion because it causes him to make frequent trips, possibly up and down stairs, to urinate.
- To prevent recurrent lower UTIs, teach an older woman to carefully wipe the perineum from front to back and to thoroughly clean it with soap and water after bowel movements. If she is infection-prone, she should urinate immediately after sexual intercourse. Tell her never to postpone urination and to empty her bladder completely.
- Tell the male patient that prompt treatment of predisposing conditions, such as chronic prostatitis, helps prevent recurrent UTIs.

EACHING AID

Self-care tips for urinary tract infections

Dear Patient:

Here's some advice to help you treat your urinary tract infection (UTI) and keep it from coming back.

Treatment guidelines
● Take any prescribed medicine exactly as your doctor directs. Unless your doctor tells you otherwise, take the entire amount prescribed, even if you feel better after a few days. This will ensure that all of the infection-causing germs are killed. If you stop taking your medicine too soon, you run the risk of the infection coming back.
● Place a warm heating pad on your abdomen and sides or try a warm sitz bath to soothe pain and burning sensations. Or, ask your doctor to prescribe a pain reliever.

Diet tips
● Drink 10 to 14 glasses of fluid daily to increase urine flow and flush out germs.
● Eat foods and drink fluids with high acid content to acidify your urine and inhibit urinary tract germs. Some high-acid foods are meats, nuts, plums, prunes, and whole-grain breads and cereals. Some high-acid drinks are cranberry and other fruit juices.
    A note of caution: If you're taking a sulfonamide drug (such as Gantrisin or Gantanol) to treat your infection, avoid cranberry juice because its high acid content can interfere with the action of the drug.
● Limit your intake of milk, cheese, and other products with a high calcium content.
● Avoid caffeine, carbonated beverages, and alcohol; these substances irritate the bladder.

Prevention tips
● Practice sensible hygiene. For example, wipe from front to back each time you go to the bathroom. This reduces the chance that germs from your bowel will enter your urinary tract.
● Change your underpants daily.
● Wear cotton undergarments because cotton "breathes." This enhances ventilation, which deters germ growth.
● Avoid tight slacks or nylon pantyhose, which prevent air circulation and encourage germs to multiply and grow.
● Take showers instead of baths because germs in the bath water can enter your urinary tract.
● Avoid bubble baths, bath oils, perfumed vaginal sprays, and strong bleaches and cleansing powders in the laundry. These products can irritate the skin of your crotch, which may trigger germ growth and infection.
● Urinate frequently (every 3 hours) to completely empty your bladder.
● Use the bathroom as soon as you sense the need. Delayed urination is a major cause of UTIs.
● Urinate after sex. This will help rid your urinary tract of germs.

When to call the doctor
● Call your doctor right away if you suspect you have a new or recurring UTI.
● Call the doctor if you notice symptoms such as an increased urge to urinate, increased urination (especially at night), pain when you urinate, or bloody or cloudy urine.

12

Managing cancer

*P*rimarily a disease of older adults, cancer is second only to cardiovascular disease as the leading cause of death in the United States (over 400,000 deaths annually). More than 67% of patients who die of cancer are over age 65. During the last 65 years, the age-adjusted cancer death rate has continually increased, mostly because of deaths from lung cancer. If lung cancer deaths were calculated separately, the cancer death rate for males would be unchanged during the same time period, while the rate for women would show a slight decrease. The most common cancers in geriatric patients are breast, lung, prostate, and colorectal cancer; these diseases progress more slowly in this population.

Cancer occurs as a malignant transformation (carcinogenesis) of normal cells, causing the cells to enlarge and divide more rapidly than normal and lose their ability to function normally. The characteristic feature of cancer is the cell's ability to proliferate — rapidly, uncontrollably, and independently — from a primary site to other tissues where it establishes secondary foci (metastases).

Although the exact cause of cancer is unknown, current evidence indicates that carcinogenesis results from a complex interaction of carcinogens and accumulated mutations in several genes. Smoking is believed to be a major contributing factor. Researchers believe that genes within the cell are transformed by irritants, such as cigarette smoke, or transform on their own from an inherited defect.

This chapter discusses the types of cancer that commonly affect older adults.

SKIN CANCER

The most common type of cancer in human beings, skin cancer strikes an estimated 500,000 people annually in the United States. Chronic exposure to ultraviolet radiation from the sun is thought to be the most common cause. People with light skin, hair, and eyes; those who tend to freckle or burn easily; and those with a history of working outdoors or living in equatorial regions have an increased risk of developing skin cancer. The disease is more common on exposed areas of skin, such as the head, neck, and dorsal surface of the hands. Because exposure to ultraviolet rays is thought to be cumulative, the incidence of skin cancer increases with age.

The two most common types of skin cancer, basal cell carcinoma and squamous cell carcinoma, have a high cure rate and usually remain localized. Malignant melanoma, the most lethal type, is relatively rare, accounting for only 1% to 2% of all malignant tumors.

Basal cell carcinoma is a slow-growing, destructive skin tumor that usually occurs in people over age 40. The two major types of basal cell epithelioma are noduloulcerative and superficial. *Squamous cell carcinoma*, which arises from keratinizing epidermal cells, is an invasive tumor with the potential for metastasis. Lesions on sun-damaged skin tend to be less invasive and less likely to metastasize than lesions on unexposed skin. Notable exceptions are squamous cell lesions on the lower lip and the ears;

almost invariably, these are markedly invasive metastatic lesions with a poor prognosis. *Melanoma,* which arises from a melanin-producing cell or melanocyte, is slightly more common in women than in men. Peak incidence occurs between ages 50 and 70, although the incidence in younger age-groups is increasing.

Common sites for melanoma are the head and neck in men, the legs in women, and the backs of people exposed to excessive sunlight. Up to 70% of malignant melanomas arise from a preexisting nevus. Melanomas seldom appear in the conjunctiva, choroid, pharynx, mouth, vagina, or anus.

There are four types of melanomas. Superficial spreading melanoma, the most common type (accounting for 50% to 70% of cases), usually develops between ages 40 and 50. Nodular melanoma, accounting for 12% to 30% of cases, usually develops between ages 40 and 50. It grows vertically, invades the dermis, and metastasizes early. Acrallentiginous melanoma is the most common melanoma among Hispanics, Asians, and Blacks, accounting for 35% to 60% of melanomas in these populations. In whites, it represents 2% to 8% of the cases. It occurs on the palms and soles and in sublingual locations. Lentigo maligna melanoma is relatively rare, accounting for 10% to 15% of cases. This is the most benign, the slowest growing, and the least aggressive of the four types. It usually occurs in areas heavily exposed to the sun in people ages 60 to 70.

Causes

Prolonged sun exposure is the most common cause of skin cancer; 90% of tumors occur on sun-exposed areas of the body. Arsenic ingestion, radiation exposure, burns, immunosuppression and, rarely, vaccinations are other possible causes. Melanoma occurs slightly more often within families, and people who have had one melanoma are at greater risk of developing a second.

Some experts hypothesize that basal cell epithelioma originates when undifferentiated basal cells become carcinomatous instead of differentiating into sweat glands, sebum, and hair. Squamous cell carcinoma may begin with induration and inflammation of a preexisting premalignant lesion. When

squamous cell carcinoma arises from normal skin, the nodule grows slowly on a firm, indurated base. Untreated, this nodule eventually ulcerates and invades underlying tissues.

Melanoma spreads through the lymphatic and vascular systems and metastasizes to the regional lymph nodes, skin, liver, lungs, and central nervous system (CNS). Its course is unpredictable, however, and recurrence and metastasis may not occur for more than 5 years after resection of the primary lesion. The prognosis varies with the tumor thickness. In most patients, superficial lesions are curable, whereas deeper lesions tend to metastasize.

Assessment findings

The patient may report an odd-looking skin lesion or a sore that did not heal, prompting him to seek medical care. He may also report changes in a preexisting skin marking, such as a mole, birthmark, scar, freckle, or wart. The history may also disclose prolonged exposure to the sun at some time in the patient's life or other risk factors for this disease.

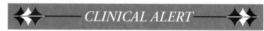

CLINICAL ALERT

Suspect melanoma when any preexisting skin lesion or nevus enlarges, changes color, becomes inflamed or sore, itches, ulcerates, bleeds, changes texture, or shows signs of surrounding pigment regression.

Basal cell lesions on the face, particularly the forehead, eyelid margins, and nasolabial folds, will appear as small, smooth, pinkish, and translucent papules in the early (noduloulcerative) stage. Telangiectatic vessels cross the surface, and the lesions may be pigmented. As the lesions enlarge, their centers become depressed and their borders become firm and elevated. These ulcerated tumors are called rodent ulcers.

Inspection of the chest and back may disclose multiple oval or irregularly shaped, lightly pigmented plaques, which may have sharply defined, slightly elevated, threadlike borders (superficial basal cell epitheliomas). Inspection of the head and neck may show waxy, sclerotic, yellow to white plaques without distinct borders. These plaques may resemble small patches of scleroderma and may suggest scle-

---

Documenting skin lesions

To aid diagnosis, describe lesions accurately, keeping in mind that two or more types can coexist. Primary skin lesions appear on previously healthy skin in response to disease or external irritation. In some cases, lesions change during the natural course of a disease. Scratching, rubbing, or applying medication also can alter the original lesion. Modified lesions are described as secondary lesions.

Begin by observing the patient's overall appearance from a distance of 3' to 6' (1 to 2 m) noting complexion, general color, color variations, and general appearance. Because abnormal skin variations are identified by their description, note changes in pigmentation (areas that are lighter or darker than the rest of the skin), freckles, moles (nevi), and tanning (usually considered normal variations). Although usually benign, nevi that occur in large numbers (over 40) or that change in size and appearance may indicate cancer.

Morphology
Document the lesion's size (measure and record its dimensions), shape or configuration, color, elevation or depression, pedunculation (connection to the skin by a stem or stalk), and texture. Document the color, consistency, and odor of any exudate.

Distribution
Note the pattern and location on first inspection. Document the extent and pattern of involvement.

Configuration
Accurately describing the arrangement of lesions in relation to each other may help determine their cause. Document the pattern as discrete, confluent, grouped, diffuse, linear, annular, or arciform.

---

rosing basal cell epitheliomas (morphea-like epitheliomas).

Squamous cell lesions on the face, ears, dorsa of the hands and forearms, and other sun-damaged skin areas may appear scaly and keratotic with raised, irregular borders. In late disease, the lesions grow outward (exophytic), are friable, and tend toward chronic crusting. As the disease progresses and metastasizes to the regional lymph nodes, the patient may complain of pain and malaise. He may also complain of anorexia and resulting fatigue and weakness.

In superficial spreading melanoma, inspection may reveal lesions on the ankles or the inside surfaces of the knees. These lesions may appear red, white, or blue over a brown or black background. They may have an irregular, notched margin. Palpation may reveal small, elevated nodules that may ulcerate and bleed. These lesions may grow horizontally for years, but when vertical growth occurs, the prognosis worsens.

In nodular melanoma, inspection of the knees and ankles may reveal a uniformly discolored nodule that may appear grayish and resemble a blackberry.

Occasionally, this melanoma is flesh-colored, with flecks of pigment around its base, which may be inflamed. Palpation may disclose polypoidal nodules that resemble the surface of a blackberry.

In acral lentiginous melanoma, inspection may show pigmented lesions on the palms and soles and under the nails. The color may resemble a mosaic of rich browns, tans, and black. Inspection of the nail beds may reveal an irregular tan or brown stain that diffuses from the nail bed.

In lentigo maligna melanoma, the patient history may reveal a long-standing lesion that has now ulcerated. Inspection may disclose a large lesion (3 to 6 cm) that appears as a freckle of tan, brown, black, whitish, or slate color on the face, back of the hand, or under the fingernails. The lesion may have irregular scattered black nodules on its surface. Palpation may reveal a flat nodule with smaller nodules scattered over the surface.

Document the color, morphology, distribution, and configuration of the lesion. For guidelines on what to include in your documentation, see *Documenting skin lesions.*

Diagnostic tests

Incisional or excisional biopsy and histologic studies provide a definitive diagnosis and staging of skin cancer (although basal cell carcinoma may be diagnosed from its appearance). Baseline laboratory studies may include complete blood count with differential, erythrocyte sedimentation rate, platelet count, liver function studies, and urinalysis.

Depending on the depth of melanoma invasion and any metastatic spread, baseline diagnostic studies may also include chest X-rays, computed tomography (CT) scans of the chest and abdomen, and a gallium scan. Signs of bone metastasis may require a bone scan; CNS metastasis may require a CT scan of the brain. Magnetic resonance imaging (MRI) also may be used to assess metastasis.

Treatment

Depending on the size, location, and depth of the lesion, treatment for basal cell and squamous cell carcinoma may include curettage and electrodesiccation, chemotherapy, surgical excision, radiation therapy, chemosurgery, or cryotherapy.

Curettage and electrodesiccation offers good cosmetic results for small lesions. Topical fluorouracil is often used for superficial lesions. This drug produces marked local irritation or inflammation in the involved tissue but no systemic effects. Microscopically controlled surgical excision carefully removes recurrent lesions until a tumor-free plane is achieved. Radiation therapy is used if the tumor location requires it and for older or debilitated patients who might not tolerate surgery.

Chemosurgery, which consists of periodic application of a fixative paste (such as zinc chloride) and subsequent removal of fixed pathologic tissue, may be necessary for persistent or recurrent lesions. Cryotherapy freezes the cells with liquid nitrogen and kills them.

Malignant melanoma always requires surgical resection to remove the tumor (with a 3- to 5-cm margin and possibly regional lymphadenectomy). The extent of resection depends on the size and location of the primary lesion. Closure of a wide resection may necessitate a skin graft. If so, plastic surgery techniques provide excellent cosmetic repair.

Deep primary melanoma lesions may warrant adjuvant chemotherapy, typically with dacarbazine or carmustine. After surgical removal of a mass, intra-arterial isolation perfusion is performed to prevent recurrence and metastasis. During this therapy, chemotherapeutic agents are infused in arteries that feed the tumor area. Although still experimental, immunotherapy, consisting of treatment with bacille Calmette-Guérin (BCG) vaccine, offers hope to patients with advanced melanoma. In theory, immunotherapy combats cancer by boosting the body's disease-fighting systems.

Chemotherapy as a primary treatment is useful only in melanoma that has metastasized. Dacarbazine and the nitrosoureas have generated some response. Radiation therapy also is reserved for metastatic disease. It doesn't prolong survival but may reduce tumor size and relieve pain. Regardless of treatment, melanomas require close, long-term follow-up care to detect metastasis and recurrence. Statistics show that about 13% of recurrences develop more than 5 years after primary surgery.

Complications

Disease progression can lead to disfiguring lesions of the eyes, nose, and cheeks. Squamous cell carcinoma can progress to lymph node involvement and visceral metastasis, resulting in respiratory problems. Melanoma has a strong tendency to metastasize, and complications result from disease progression to the lungs, liver, or brain.

Nursing interventions

● Although disfiguring lesions are distressing, try to accept the patient as he is in order to increase his self-esteem and to strengthen your relationship with him. Listen to his fears and concerns, and offer reassurance when appropriate. Remain with him during periods of severe stress and anxiety. Provide positive reinforcement as he makes an effort to adapt.
● Arrange for the patient to interact with others who have a similar problem. Help him and his family members set realistic goals and expectations. When the patient is ready, involve him and his family

members whenever possible in making decisions about his care.

● After surgery, take precautions to prevent infection. Keep the wound dry and clean, and check dressings often for excessive drainage, foul odor, redness, and swelling. Coordinate a consistent care plan for changing the patient's dressings. A standard routine helps the patient and his family members learn how to care for the wound.

◆◆——— CLINICAL ALERT ———◆◆

If odor is a problem, try controlling it with balsam of Peru, yogurt flakes, oil of cloves, or other odor-masking substances, even though they may be ineffective for long-term use. Topical or systemic antibiotics also control odor temporarily and eventually alter the lesion's bacterial flora.

● If surgery included lymphadenectomy, apply a compression stocking and instruct the patient to keep the extremity elevated to minimize lymphedema.

● Watch for complications of treatment, including infection and local skin irritation from chemotherapeutic agents applied topically. Watch for radiation's adverse effects, such as nausea, vomiting, hair loss, malaise, and diarrhea. Provide reassurance and comfort measures when appropriate.

● If the patient is receiving systemic chemotherapy, watch for associated complications, such as mouth sores, hair loss, weakness, fatigue, and anorexia. Offer orange or grapefruit juice or ginger ale to help relieve nausea and vomiting.

● Provide periods of rest between procedures if the patient tires easily. Provide small, frequent meals consisting of high-protein, high-calorie foods if the patient is anorexic. Consult with the dietitian to incorporate foods that the patient enjoys into his diet.

● In advanced metastatic disease, control and prevent pain with regularly scheduled administration of analgesics. If the patient is dying, identify the needs of the patient, his family members, and friends, and provide appropriate support and care.

Patient teaching

● Explain all procedures and treatments to the patient and his family members. Encourage them to ask questions, and then answer them honestly. Tell the patient what to expect before and after surgery, what his wound will look like, and what type of dressing he'll have.

◆◆——— CLINICAL ALERT ———◆◆

If the patient is to have a skin graft, warn him that the donor site for the graft may be as painful as the tumor excision site, if not more so.

● Instruct the patient to eat frequent, small, high-protein meals. Advise him to consume eggnog, pureed foods, and liquid protein supplements if the lesion has invaded the oral cavity and is causing difficulty eating.

● To prevent disease recurrence, tell the patient to avoid excessive sun exposure and to use a strong sunscreen or a sunshade to protect his skin from damage by ultraviolet rays. Direct him to wear protective clothing (hats, long sleeves) whenever he's outdoors.

● Emphasize the need for close follow-up care to detect recurrences early. Explain that recurrences and metastases often occur years later, so follow-up must continue for years. Teach the patient how to recognize the signs of recurrence by periodically examining his skin for precancerous lesions; if he finds any, urge him to contact his doctor at once.

● Advise the patient to relieve local inflammation from topical fluorouracil with cool compresses or with a corticosteroid ointment. Instruct the patient with noduloulcerative basal cell epithelioma to wash his face gently when ulcerations and crusting occur; scrubbing too vigorously may cause bleeding from the wounds.

● Teach the patient and his family members relaxation techniques to help relieve anxiety. Encourage the patient to continue these after he is discharged. As appropriate, direct the patient and his family members to hospital and community support services — for example, social workers, psychologists, cancer support groups, or a hospice.

Breast cancer

Although breast cancer may develop any time after puberty, about 70% of cases occur in women over age 50 and about 20% in women under age 30. This disease rarely occurs in men. Five-year survival rates have shown steady improvement — from 53% in the 1940s to 70% in the 1980s and 76% in the 1990s — because of earlier diagnosis and better treatment. Mortality, however, hasn't changed in the past 50 years.

The most reliable breast cancer detection method is regular breast self-examination, followed by immediate professional evaluation of any abnormality. As a person ages, the breasts decrease in size and breast tissue is replaced with fat, which makes identification of palpable tumors easier. Another detection method, mammography, is probably responsible for the increase in reported cases. The American Cancer Society estimates diagnosis of over 214,000 new cases in the United States during 1996.

Unfortunately, many older women do not receive regular mammograms, even when recommended by health care professionals, either because they're afraid — of radiation, of discovering cancer, or of discomfort during the procedure — or because they're embarrassed about exposing their breasts.

Mammograms also can be expensive. Medicare covers 80% of the cost, leaving the patient responsible for the remainder, unless she has supplemental coverage. The nurse has an important responsibility to help dispel the patient's fears of the test and explain the benefits of early detection.

Causes

The causes of breast cancer remain elusive. Significant risk factors include a family history of breast cancer (mother, sister, grandmother, aunt) and being a woman over age 45 and premenopausal. Other risk factors may include a long menstrual cycle, early onset of menses, or late onset of menopause; first pregnancy after age 35; a high-fat diet; a history of endometrial or ovarian cancer; radiation exposure; estrogen therapy; antihypertensive therapy; alcohol and tobacco use; and preexisting fibrocystic breast disease. The recent discovery of the breast cancer gene BRCA 1 confirms the theory that the disease can be inherited from either the mother or the father.

About half of all breast cancers develop in the upper outer quadrant. Growth rates vary: Theoretically, a slow-growing breast cancer may take up to 8 years to become palpable at $\frac{3}{8}$" (1cm). Breast cancer spreads by way of the lymphatic system and the bloodstream through the right side of the heart to the lungs and to the other breast, chest wall, liver, bone, or brain. Survival time depends on tumor size and the number of involved lymph nodes.

Breast cancer is classified by histologic appearance and the lesion's location. Adenocarcinoma, also called ductal carcinoma, arises from the epithelium. Intraductal carcinoma develops within the ducts and includes Paget's disease. Infiltrating breast carcinoma occurs in the breast's parenchymal tissue. Inflammatory breast cancer is a rare type that grows rapidly and causes overlying skin to become edematous, inflamed, and indurated. Lobular carcinoma in situ involves the lobes of glandular tissue. Medullary or circumscribed breast cancer is an enlarging tumor with a rapid growth rate.

In addition to these classifications, staging helps to define the cancer's extent. The most common system for staging, both before and after surgery, is the TNM (tumor, node, metastasis) system, which looks at the size of the tumor, the number of lymph nodes involved, and the extent of any metastasis.

Assessment findings

The patient typically reports that she detected a painless lump or mass in her breast or that she noticed a thickening of breast tissue. In other cases, a mammogram detects the lesion before it becomes palpable. The patient's history may indicate several risk factors for breast cancer.

Inspection may reveal a nipple discharge (clear, milky, or bloody), nipple retraction, scaly skin around the nipple, and skin changes, such as dimpling, peau d'orange, or inflammation. Arm edema, also identified on inspection, may indicate advanced nodal involvement.

Palpation of the breast may reveal a hard lump, mass, or thickening of breast tissue. Palpation of the cervical supraclavicular and axillary nodes may also reveal lumps or enlargement.

Diagnostic tests

Most breast lumps are detected by women doing breast self-examinations. All women should perform a monthly breast self-examination, and The American Cancer Society recommends additionally a yearly clinical exam and a yearly mammogram for women over age 50. Mammography is considered the essential test for breast cancer and can detect a tumor too small to palpate.

Fine-needle aspiration and excisional biopsy provide cells for histologic examination to confirm the diagnosis. Ultrasonography can distinguish between a fluid-filled cyst and a solid mass.

To rule out chest metastasis, a chest X-ray will be ordered. Scans of the bone, brain, liver, and other organs are performed to detect distant metastases. Laboratory tests, such as alkaline phosphatase levels and liver function studies, can also uncover distant metastases.

A hormonal receptor assay of tumor tissue can determine whether the tumor is estrogen- or progesterone-dependent. This test helps the doctor decide whether the patient should receive hormone-blocking therapy.

Treatment

The type of treatment chosen usually depends on the disease's stage and type, the woman's age and menopausal status, and the disfiguring effects of the surgery. Therapy may include any combination of surgery, radiation, chemotherapy, and hormonal therapy.

Surgical options include lumpectomy, partial mastectomy, total mastectomy, and modified radical mastectomy. For a lumpectomy, the surgeon makes a small incision near the nipple to remove the tumor, surrounding tissue and, possibly, nearby lymph nodes. Lumpectomy is used for patients with small, well-defined lesions. Fewer than 20% of cancer patients undergo this operation.

In some cases, the surgeon will perform a lumpectomy by freezing the tumor with a cryoprobe (which chills the tumor to -292° F (-180° C), thawing the tumor, and then repeating the procedure four more times. Finally, he refreezes the tumor and then performs the surgery. This cell-destroying technique, called cryolumpectomy, is recommended only for small, early primary tumors.

In a partial mastectomy, the surgeon removes the tumor along with a wedge of normal tissue, skin, fascia and, possibly, axillary lymph nodes. With a total or simple mastectomy, the entire breast is removed. The surgeon uses this procedure if the cancer appears confined to breast tissue and no lymph node involvement is detected. After mastectomy, reconstructive surgery can create a breast mound if the patient desires it and if she doesn't have advanced disease.

In a modified radical mastectomy, the surgeon removes the entire breast, axillary lymph nodes, and the lining that covers the chest muscles. This procedure differs from radical mastectomy in that it preserves the patient's pectoral muscles. Modified radical mastectomy has replaced radical mastectomy as the most widely used surgical procedure for treating breast cancer.

Before or after tumor removal, primary radiation therapy may be effective for a patient who has a small, early-stage tumor without distant metastases. Radiation therapy is also used to prevent or treat local recurrence. Furthermore, preoperative breast irradiation helps to "sterilize" the field, making the tumor more manageable surgically, especially in inflammatory breast cancer.

Chemotherapy may be administered either as adjuvant therapy or as primary therapy. It usually consists of a combination of drugs, such as cyclophosphamide, fluorouracil, methotrexate, doxorubicin, vincristine, and prednisone. A typical regimen used for both premenopausal and postmenopausal women is cyclophosphamide, methotrexate, and fluorouracil. The patient may base her decision to undergo chemotherapy on several factors, including the cancer's stage and hormonal receptor assay results.

Hormonal therapy lowers levels of estrogen and

other hormones suspected of nourishing breast cancer cells. For example, antiestrogen therapy (specifically tamoxifen, which is most effective against tumors identified as estrogen-receptor–positive) is used in postmenopausal women. Alternatively, the patient may receive antiandrogen therapy (aminoglutethimide) or androgen (fluoxymesterone), estrogen (diethylstilbestrol), or progestin (megestrol) therapy.

Complications
Disease progression and metastasis lead to site-specific complications, including infection, decreased mobility if the disease metastasizes to the bone, central nervous system effects if the tumor metastasizes to the brain, and respiratory problems if it spreads to the lungs.

Nursing interventions
• Evaluate the patient's feelings about her illness, and determine her level of knowledge. Listen to her concerns, and stay with her during periods of severe anxiety.
• Administer ordered analgesics as required. Monitor and record their effectiveness.
• Perform comfort measures, such as repositioning, to promote relaxation and relieve anxiety.
• If immobility develops late in the disease, prevent complications by frequently repositioning the patient, using a convoluted foam mattress, and providing skin care (particularly over bony prominences).
• Watch for treatment complications, such as nausea, vomiting, anorexia, leukopenia, thrombocytopenia, GI ulceration, alopecia, and bleeding. Provide comfort measures and prescribed treatments to relieve these complications.
• Following surgery, inspect the dressing anteriorly and posteriorly. Record the amount and color of drainage, and report excessive bleeding promptly. Drainage usually appears bloody during the first 4 hours, then becomes serous.
• Monitor the patient's vital signs.
• If a general anesthetic was given during surgery, monitor intake and output for at least 48 hours.

◆◆ ——— *CLINICAL ALERT* ——— ◆◆

Prevent lymphedema of the arm, which may be an early complication of lymph node dissection, by helping the patient with arm-strengthening exercises. Such prevention is crucial because lymphedema can't be treated effectively.
• Use strict aseptic technique when changing dressings or I.V. tubing or performing any invasive procedure. Monitor temperature and white blood cell count closely. Inspect the incision.
• Encourage the patient and her partner to look at her incision as soon as feasible — if possible, when the first dressing is removed.

Patient teaching
• Clearly explain all procedures and treatments. Besides the usual preoperative teaching, show the mastectomy patient how to ease postsurgical pain by lying on the affected side or by placing a hand or pillow on the incision. Point out where the incision will be. Inform the patient that after the operation, she'll receive analgesics because pain relief encourages coughing and turning and promotes well-being. Explain that a small pillow placed under the arm anteriorly may provide comfort.
• Tell her that she may move about as soon as possible, usually after the effects of the anesthetic subside or the first evening after surgery. Explain that she may have an incisional drain or some type of suction to remove accumulated fluid, to relieve tension on the suture line, and to promote healing.
• Urge the patient to avoid activities that may injure her arm and hand on the side of her surgery. Caution her not to let blood be drawn from or allow injections into that arm. She should also refuse to have blood pressure taken or I.V. therapy administered on the affected arm. To help prevent lymphedema, instruct the patient to exercise her hand and arm on the affected side regularly and to avoid activities that might allow infection of this hand or arm. Tell her that infection increases the risk of lymphedema. Reinforce your teaching by providing her with a copy of the teaching handout *Strengthening your arm and shoulder.*

TEACHING AID

Strengthening your arm and shoulder

Dear Patient:

After a mastectomy, you need to strengthen your arm and shoulder muscles. When your doctor gives you the go-ahead, do the exercises below daily. They'll help increase your mobility by preventing your arm and shoulder muscles from stiffening and becoming shorter. Daily exercises also help maintain muscle tone and improve your circulation.

Follow these instructions, doing each exercise as many times as your nurse or doctor directs.

Wall climb

Stand facing a wall, with your toes as close to the wall as possible and your feet apart. Bend your elbows slightly. Then place your palms against the wall at shoulder level.

Flexing your fingers, work your hands up the wall until you fully extend your arms. Then work your hands back down to the starting point.

Pendulum swings

Place your unaffected arm on the back of a chair. Bend forward from the waist, and let your affected arm hang loosely.

First, swing your arm from left to right in front of you. Make sure the movement comes from your shoulder joint and not from your elbow.

Second, maintaining the same position, trace small circles with your arm. Again, make sure the motion comes from your shoulder joint. (As your arm relaxes, the size of the circle will probably increase.) Then circle in the opposite direction.

Third, swing your arm forward and backward from your shoulder within your range of comfort.

Pulley

Drape a rope over your shower curtain rod (or through an overhead pulley, hook, or loop). Hold the opposite ends of the rope in each hand.

With your arm outstretched, use a seesaw motion to slide the rope back and forth over the rod.

Rope turns

Tie a rope to a doorknob; then stand facing the door. Hold the rope's free end in the hand of your affected side. Place your other hand on your hip. Extend your affected arm slightly to the side away from your body. Now turn the rope, making as wide a swing as possible. Start slowly, and increase your speed as your arm grows stronger.

• Inform the patient that she may experience "phantom breast syndrome," a tingling sensation in the area where the breast was removed.

• If a mastectomy was performed, give the patient the names of local agencies or stores that supply breast prostheses and bras. Refer her to a local chapter of Reach for Recovery. Explain that with slight changes in her wardrobe, she will still be able to dress fashionably.

• Women who have had breast cancer in one breast have a higher risk of developing cancer in the other breast or of developing recurrent cancer in the chest wall. For this reason, urge the patient to continue self-examination of the other breast and to comply with recommended follow-up treatment.

• Teach the patient relaxation techniques to help relieve anxiety, and encourage her to continue these after she is discharged.

• As appropriate, direct the patient and her family member to hospital and community support services — for example, social workers, psychologists, cancer support groups, or a hospice.

PROSTATIC CANCER

The most common cancer in men over age 50, prostatic cancer is a leading cause of male cancer death. Adenocarcinoma is the most common form; only seldom does prostatic cancer occur as a sarcoma. About 85% of prostatic cancers originate in the posterior prostate gland; the rest grow near the urethra. Prostatic cancer seldom results from the benign hyperplastic enlargement that commonly develops around the prostatic urethra in older men.

Slow-growing prostatic cancer seldom produces signs and symptoms until it's well advanced. Typically, when primary prostatic lesions spread beyond the prostate gland, they invade the prostatic capsule and then spread along the ejaculatory ducts in the space between the seminal vesicles or perivesicular fascia. When prostatic cancer is treated in its localized form, the 5-year survival rate is 70%; after metastasis, it's less than 35%. When prostatic cancer is

fatal, death usually results from widespread bone metastases.

Prostatic cancer accounts for about 22% of all cancers. Incidence is highest among blacks and lowest among Asians; it appears unrelated to socioeconomic status or fertility.

Causes
Risk factors for prostatic cancer include age (the cancer seldom develops in men under age 40) and infection. In addition, researchers suspect that androgens may speed tumor growth.

Assessment findings
The patient may report urinary problems, such as dysuria, frequency, retention, back or hip pain, and hematuria. These complaints may indicate advanced disease, with back or hip pain signaling bone metastasis. The patient usually has no signs or symptoms in the early stages.

Inspection may reveal edema of the scrotum or leg in advanced disease. Palpation of the prostate during digital rectal examination (DRE) may detect a nonraised, firm, nodular mass with a sharp edge (in early disease) or a hard lump (in advanced disease).

Diagnostic tests
DRE is the standard screening test. Blood tests may show elevated levels of prostate-specific antigen (PSA). Although most men with metastasized prostatic cancer will have an elevated PSA level, the finding also occurs with other prostatic diseases. So the PSA level should be assessed in light of DRE findings. The American Cancer Society recommends a yearly DRE with palpation of the prostate and a yearly PSA test.

Transrectal prostatic ultrasonography may be used for patients with abnormal DRE and PSA test findings. A bone scan and excretory urography may be ordered to determine the disease's extent. The TNM method is used to stage prostate cancer.

Treatment
Therapy varies by cancer stage and may include prostatectomy, radiation, orchiectomy (removal of

the testes) to reduce androgen production, and hormonal therapy with synthetic estrogen (diethylstilbestrol). Radical prostatectomy is usually effective for localized lesions without metastasis. A transurethral resection of the prostate may be performed to relieve an obstruction.

Radiation therapy may cure locally invasive lesions in early disease and may relieve bone pain from metastatic skeletal involvement. It also may be used prophylactically for patients with tumors in regional lymph nodes. Alternatively, internal beam radiation may be recommended because it permits increased radiation to reach the prostate but minimizes the surrounding tissues' exposure to radiation.

If surgery, radiation, and hormonal therapy aren't feasible or successful, chemotherapy may be tried. Chemotherapy for prostatic cancer (combinations of cyclophosphamide, doxorubicin, fluorouracil, cisplatin, and vincristine) offers limited benefits. Research continues to seek the most effective chemotherapeutic regimen.

Complications

Progressive disease can lead to spinal cord compression, deep vein thrombosis, pulmonary emboli, and myelophthisis.

Nursing interventions

● At all times, encourage the patient to express his fears and concerns, including those about changes in his sexual functioning due to surgery. Offer reassurance when possible.
● Allow the patient's family members to assist in his care, and encourage them to provide psychological support.
● Administer ordered analgesics as necessary, and provide comfort measures to reduce pain. Encourage the patient to identify care measures that promote his comfort and relaxation.
● After prostatectomy, regularly check the dressing, incision site, and drainage systems for excessive blood. Also watch for signs of bleeding (pallor, restlessness, falling blood pressure, and rising pulse rate). Be alert for signs of infection (fever, chills, inflamed incision area). Maintain adequate fluid intake (at least 2,000 ml daily). Give antispasmod-

ics, as ordered, to control postoperative bladder spasms. Also provide analgesics as needed. Because urinary incontinence commonly follows prostatectomy, keep the patient's skin clean and dry.
● After suprapubic prostatectomy, keep the skin around the suprapubic drain dry and free from drainage and urine leakage. Encourage the patient to begin perineal exercises between 24 and 48 hours after surgery.
● Provide meticulous catheter care. After prostatectomy, a patient usually has a three-way catheter with a continuous irrigation system. Check the tubing for kinks, mucus plugs, and clots, especially if the patient complains of pain. Warn him not to pull on the tubes or the catheter.
● After transurethral resection, watch for signs of urethral stricture (dysuria, decreased force and caliber of urine stream, and straining to urinate). Also observe for abdominal distention (a result of urethral stricture or catheter blockage by a blood clot). Irrigate the catheter as ordered.
● After perineal prostatectomy, avoid taking the patient's temperature rectally or inserting an enema or other rectal tubes. Provide pads to absorb draining urine. Assist the patient with frequent sitz baths to relieve pain and inflammation.

✦✦— CLINICAL ALERT —✦✦

After perineal or retropubic prostatectomy, reassure the patient that urine leakage after catheter removal is normal and will subside in time.

● After radiation therapy, watch for common adverse effects, including proctitis, diarrhea, bladder spasms, and urinary frequency.

✦✦— CLINICAL ALERT —✦✦

Internal radiation of the prostate almost always results in cystitis during the first 2 to 3 weeks of therapy.

● Encourage the patient to drink at least eight 8-oz glasses (2,000 ml) of fluid daily. Administer analgesics and antispasmodics to decrease his discomfort.
● If the patient receives diethylstilbestrol, watch for adverse effects (gynecomastia, fluid retention, nausea, vomiting). Also be alert for signs of thrombo-

phlebitis (pain, tenderness, swelling, warmth, redness in calf).

Patient teaching

• Before surgery, discuss the expected results. Explain that radical surgery always produces impotence. Up to 7% of patients experience urinary incontinence.

• To help minimize incontinence, teach the patient how to do perineal exercises while he sits or stands. To develop his perineal muscles, tell him to squeeze his buttocks together and hold this position for a few seconds, then relax. He should repeat this exercise 10 times as frequently as the doctor orders.

• Prepare the patient for postoperative procedures, such as dressing changes and intubation.

• If appropriate, discuss the adverse effects of radiation therapy. All patients who receive pelvic radiation will develop such symptoms as diarrhea, urinary frequency, nocturia, bladder spasms, rectal irritation, and tenesmus. Teach the patient how to follow a bland, low-fat, low-residue, low-gluten diet. Explain the action and adverse effects of any antiemetic or antidiarrheal medications ordered by the doctor. Provide the patient with a copy of the teaching handout *Caring for yourself during pelvic radiation*.

• Encourage the patient to maintain as nearly normal a lifestyle as possible during recovery. When appropriate, refer him to the social services department, local home health care agencies, hospices, and other support organizations.

COLORECTAL CANCER

The second most common visceral cancer in the United States and Europe, colorectal cancer occurs equally in men and women but is more common in those over age 40. Malignant tumors of the colon or rectum are almost always adenocarcinomas. About half of these are sessile lesions of the rectosigmoid area; the rest are polypoid lesions.

Colorectal cancer progresses slowly, remaining localized for a long time. Unless the tumor has metastasized, the 5-year survival rate is relatively high: about 80% for rectal cancer and more than 85% for colon cancer. If left untreated, the disease is invariably fatal.

Causes

Although the exact cause of colorectal cancer is unknown, studies show a greater incidence in higher socioeconomic groups, suggesting a relation to diet (excessive intake of animal fat, particularly beef, and low intake of fiber). Other factors that increase the risk of developing colorectal cancer include a history of digestive tract diseases, ulcerative colitis (cancer usually starts in 11 to 17 years), and familial polyposis (cancer almost always develops by age 50).

Assessment findings

The most common sign of colorectal cancer is a change in bowel habits.

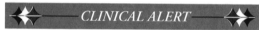
CLINICAL ALERT

The older adult may ignore bowel symptoms, believing them to be from constipation, poor diet, or hemorrhoids. Evaluate the patient's responses to your questions carefully.

Signs and symptoms depend on the tumor's location. If the tumor develops on the colon's right side, the patient probably won't have signs and symptoms in the early stages because the stool is still in liquid form in that part of the colon. He may have a history of black, tarry stools, however, and report anemia, abdominal aching, pressure, and dull cramps. As the disease progresses, he may complain of weakness, diarrhea, obstipation, anorexia, weight loss, and vomiting.

A tumor on the left side of the colon causes symptoms of obstruction even in the early disease stages because stools are more completely formed when they reach this part of the colon. The patient may report rectal bleeding (often ascribed to hemorrhoids), intermittent abdominal fullness or cramping, and rectal pressure.

As the disease progresses, obstipation, diarrhea, or ribbon- or pencil-shaped stools may develop. The patient may note that the passage of flatus or stool

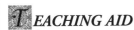EACHING AID

Caring for yourself during pelvic radiation

Dear Patient:

Your doctor has ordered radiation therapy to treat your cancer. This therapy often causes unpleasant side effects. Fortunately, you can sometimes prevent them. Other times, you can do things to make yourself more comfortable. Follow the advice below.

Eat smart

Radiation to the pelvic area can sometimes cause diarrhea and crampy abdominal pain. Avoid foods and beverages that irritate your stomach, such as those listed below, to reduce these side effects.
● Avoid spicy and fried foods.
● Avoid foods with high amounts of gluten, such as wheat grain products and other foods that produce gas, such as onions, peas, and beans.
● Avoid high-fiber foods, such as fresh fruits, vegetables, and whole grain cereals.
● Stay away from extremely hot or cold foods, which can produce gas.
● Avoid carbonated, caffeinated, and alcoholic beverages, which increase intestinal activity.

So what should I eat?

● Bland foods, such as white bread, chicken, and Jell-O, are usually best tolerated.
● Jelly on bread makes a nice snack.
● Most types of fish are good sources of low-fat protein.
● Diet supplements, such as Isocal, Sustacal, or Ensure, may be ordered by your doctor to prevent you from losing weight.

Minimize tiredness

● Limit activities, especially strenuous ones.
● Get more sleep.
● If possible, schedule radiation treatments at your convenience.
● Ask for help from family and friends, such as pitching in with daily chores or driving you to the hospital. Most people are glad to help out; they just need to be asked.
● Intercourse may be painful during pelvic radiation, but usually improves after treatment ends.

Take care of your skin

Because the radiation passes through your skin to get to your tumor, your skin may feel dry and itchy, but it should return to normal after the radiation ends. Take the following steps to combat dryness:
● Check your skin daily for any red or dry areas. If you find any, inform your doctor and the nurse at the radiation department.
● Keep the area clean and dry. Wash it with mild soap and water. Pat the skin dry; don't rub it. Rubbing will damage the skin more.
● If your skin is itchy, dust a little cornstarch on it. Use only a small amount; don't let the cornstarch form small caked areas.

relieves his pain. He may also report obvious bleeding during defecation and dark or bright red blood in the feces or in the mucus in or on the feces.

A patient with a rectal tumor may report a change in bowel habits, often beginning with an urgent need to defecate on arising ("morning diarrhea") or obstipation alternating with diarrhea. He also may notice blood or mucus in the stools and complain of a sense of incomplete evacuation. Late in the disease, he may complain of pain that begins as a feeling of rectal fullness and progresses to a dull, sometimes constant ache confined to the rectum or sacral region.

Inspection of the abdomen may reveal distention or visible masses. Abdominal veins may appear enlarged and visible from portal obstruction. The inguinal and supraclavicular nodes may also appear enlarged. You may note abnormal bowel sounds on abdominal auscultation. Palpation may reveal abdominal masses. Right-side tumors usually feel bulky; tumors of the transverse portion are more easily detected.

Diagnostic tests

Several tests support a diagnosis of colorectal cancer. A digital rectal examination detects suspicious rectal and perianal lesions, identifying almost 15% of colorectal cancers. A fecal occult blood test detects blood in stools, a warning sign of rectal cancer. The American Cancer Society recommends that these tests be performed yearly on men and women over age 50.

Proctoscopy or sigmoidoscopy, both of which permit visualization of the lower GI tract, can detect up to 66% of colorectal cancers. The American Cancer Society recommends that this test be performed every 3 to 5 years in people over 50. Colonoscopy permits visual inspection and photography of the colon up to the ileocecal valve and provides access for polypectomies and biopsies of suspected lesions.

Excretory urography verifies bilateral renal function and allows inspection for displacement of the kidneys, ureters, or bladder by a tumor pressing against these structures. Barium enema studies, using a dual contrast of barium and air, allow the location of lesions that aren't detectable manually or visually.

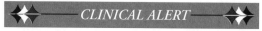

CLINICAL ALERT

Barium studies shouldn't precede colonoscopy or excretory urography because barium sulfate interferes with these tests.

A CT scan allows better visualization if a barium enema yields inconclusive results or if metastasis to the pelvic lymph nodes is suspected. Carcinoembryonic antigen, although not specific or sensitive enough for early diagnosis of colorectal cancer, permits patient monitoring before and after treatment to detect metastasis or recurrence.

Treatment

The most effective treatment for colorectal cancer is surgery to remove the malignant tumor and adjacent tissues as well as any lymph nodes that may contain cancer cells. Adjuvant therapy includes chemotherapy, radiation therapy, or both.

The type of surgery depends on the tumor's location. Tumors in the cecum and ascending colon require a right hemicolectomy (for advanced disease), which may include resection of the terminal segment of the ileum, cecum, ascending colon, and right half of the transverse colon with corresponding mesentery. Surgery for proximal and middle transverse colon tumors is a right colectomy that includes the transverse colon and mesentery corresponding to midcolic vessels, or segmental resection of the transverse colon and associated midcolic vessels. Surgery for sigmoid colon tumors usually is limited to the sigmoid colon and mesentery.

For tumors in the upper rectum, surgery usually involves anterior or low anterior resection. A newer method, using a stapler, allows for much lower resections than previously possible. Abdominoperineal resection and permanent sigmoid colostomy are required for tumors in the lower rectum.

Chemotherapy is used if the patient has metastasis, residual disease, or a recurrent inoperable tumor. A commonly used regimen consists of fluorouracil combined with levamisole or leucovorin. Researchers are also evaluating the effectiveness of fluorouracil with recombinant interferon alfa-2a. Radiation therapy, used before or after surgery, induces tumor regression.

Complications

As the tumor grows and encroaches on the abdominal organs, abdominal distention and intestinal obstruction occur. Anemia may develop if rectal bleeding isn't treated.

Nursing interventions

● Before colorectal surgery, monitor the patient's diet modifications, and administer laxatives, enemas, and antibiotics, as ordered. These measures help clean the bowel and decrease the risk of abdominal and peritoneal cavity contamination during surgery.

● After surgery, monitor vital signs, intake and output, and fluid and electrolyte balance. Also monitor for complications, including anastomotic leaks, hemorrhage, irregular bowel function, phantom rectum, ruptured pelvic peritoneum, stricture, urinary dysfunction, and wound infection.

● Care for the patient's incision and, if appropriate, his stoma. To decrease discomfort, administer ordered analgesics as necessary, and perform comfort measures such as positioning.

● Encourage the patient to look at the stoma and to participate in its care as soon as possible. Consult with an enterostomal therapist, if available, for instructions on setting up a postoperative regimen for the patient.

● Teach proper hygiene and skin care. Allow the patient to shower or bathe as soon as the incision heals.

● Watch for adverse effects of radiation therapy (nausea, vomiting, hair loss, malaise), and provide comfort measures and reassurance.

● During chemotherapy, watch for complications (such as infection) and expected adverse effects. Prepare the geriatric patient for these problems. Take steps to reduce these effects — for example, by having the patient rinse his mouth with normal saline mouthwash to prevent ulcers.

● To help prevent infection, use strict aseptic technique when caring for I.V. catheters and providing wound care. Change I.V. tubing and sites according to facility policy. Have the patient wash his hands before and after meals and after going to the bathroom.

● For the older patient — who's already coping with many age-related bodily changes — a colostomy may threaten his self-concept and pose major adjustment problems. He may feel isolated from what he views as normal society. He may be afraid to socialize, fearful of the reactions of others or of embarrassing episodes. Arthritic fingers, poor eyesight, and reduced energy reserves can hamper his ability to care for the colostomy. He may perceive the resultant need for assistance as a significant loss of independence.

● Listen to the patient's fears and concerns, and stay with him during periods of severe stress and anxiety. Encourage him to identify actions and care measures that will promote his comfort and relaxation. Whenever possible, include family members in care decisions.

Patient teaching

● Throughout therapy, answer the patient's questions, and tell him what to expect from surgery and other treatments. If appropriate, explain that the stoma will be red, moist, and swollen; reassure the patient that postoperative swelling eventually will subside.

● Show the patient a diagram of the intestine as it appears before and after surgery, stressing how much of the bowel will remain intact. Supplement your teaching with instruction booklets (available for a fee from the United Ostomy Association and free from various companies that manufacture ostomy supplies). Arrange a postsurgical visit from a recovered ostomy patient. Prepare the patient for the I.V. lines, nasogastric tube, and indwelling urinary catheter he'll have postoperatively.

● Preoperatively, teach the patient the coughing and deep-breathing exercises that he should perform postoperatively. Explain to his family members that their positive reactions will foster the patient's adjustment.

● If appropriate, instruct the patient with a sigmoid colostomy to perform his own irrigation as soon as he's able after surgery. Advise him to schedule irrigation for the time of the day when he normally evacuates. Many patients find that irrigating every 1 to 3 days is necessary for regulation.

• Direct the patient to follow a high-fiber diet. If flatus, diarrhea, or constipation occur, tell him to eliminate suspected causative foods from his diet. Explain that he may reintroduce them later. Teach him which foods may alleviate constipation, and encourage him to increase his fluid and fiber intake. If diarrhea is a problem, advise the patient to try eating applesauce, bananas, or rice. Caution him to take laxatives or antidiarrheal medications only as prescribed by his doctor.

• When appropriate, explain that after several months, many patients with an ostomy establish control with irrigation and no longer need to wear a pouch. A stoma cap or gauze sponge placed over the stoma protects it and absorbs mucoid secretions. Explain that before achieving such control, the patient can resume physical activities provided that he's not at risk for injuring the stoma or surrounding abdominal muscles. If the patient wants to swim, he can place a pouch or stoma cap (if regulated) over the stoma. He should avoid heavy lifting, which can cause herniation or prolapse through weakened muscles in the abdominal wall. Suggest that he consider a structured, gradually progressive exercise program to strengthen abdominal muscles. Such a program can be instituted under a doctor's supervision.

• Emphasize the importance of keeping follow-up appointments. Anyone who has had colorectal cancer has an increased risk of developing another primary cancer. The patient should have a yearly screening (sigmoidoscopy, digital rectal examination, occult blood test) and follow-up testing.

• If the patient will undergo radiation therapy or chemotherapy, explain the treatment to him. Make sure he understands the adverse effects that usually occur and the measures he can take to prevent them or decrease their severity.

• If appropriate, suggest counseling to deal with the patient's sexual and self-esteem concerns. Some men are impotent for a time after colostomy.

ESOPHAGEAL CANCER

Most common in men over age 60, esophageal cancer is nearly always fatal. The disease occurs worldwide, most commonly in Japan, Russia, China, the Middle East, and in parts of South Africa, where it has reached almost epidemic proportions. In the United States, more than 8,000 cases of esophageal cancer are reported annually. Men are affected more often than women, and the disease is also more common in blacks and alcoholics.

Esophageal tumors are usually fungating and infiltrating. In most cases, the tumor partially constricts the lumen of the esophagus; it metastasizes early by way of the submucosal lymphatic system, often fatally invading adjacent vital intrathoracic organs. The liver and lungs are the usual sites of distant metastases; less common sites include the bone, kidneys, and adrenal glands.

Most cases (98%) arise in the squamous cell epithelium; few are adenocarcinomas and fewer still, melanomas and sarcomas. About half the squamous cell cancers occur in the lower portion of the esophagus, 40% in the midportion, and the remaining 10% in the upper or cervical esophagus. Regardless of cell type, the prognosis for esophageal cancer is poor: 5-year survival rates are less than 5%, and most patients die within 6 months of diagnosis.

Causes

Although the cause of esophageal cancer is unknown, several predisposing factors have been identified. These include chronic irritation from heavy smoking or excessive use of alcohol; stasis-induced inflammation, as occurs in achalasia or stricture; previous head and neck tumors; and nutritional deficiency, as occurs in untreated sprue and Plummer-Vinson syndrome.

Assessment findings

Early in the disease, the patient may report a feeling of fullness, pressure, indigestion, or substernal burning. He may also tell you he uses antacids to relieve GI upset. Later, he may complain of dysphagia and weight loss. The degree of dysphagia varies, depending on the extent of disease. At first, the dysphagia is mild, occurring only after the patient eats solid foods, especially meat. Later, the patient has difficulty swallowing coarse foods and, in some cases, liquids.

The patient may complain of hoarseness (from laryngeal nerve involvement), a chronic cough (possibly from aspiration), anorexia, vomiting, and regurgitation of food (resulting from the tumor size exceeding the limits of the esophagus). He may also complain of pain on swallowing or pain that radiates to his back. In the late stages of the disease, the patient appears very thin, cachexic, and dehydrated.

Diagnostic tests

X-rays of the esophagus with barium swallow and motility studies delineate structural and filling defects and reduced peristalsis. Chest X-rays or esophagography may reveal pneumonitis.

Esophagoscopy, punch and brush biopsies, and exfoliative cytologic tests confirm the presence of esophageal tumors. Bronchoscopy (usually performed after esophagoscopy) may reveal tumor growth in the tracheobronchial tree.

Endoscopic ultrasonography of the esophagus combines endoscopy and ultrasound technology to measure the tumor's depth of penetration. A CT scan may help diagnose and monitor esophageal lesions. MRI permits evaluation of the esophagus and adjacent structures.

Liver function studies and other laboratory tests may reveal abnormalities. If so, a liver scan and a mediastinal tomography scan can help reveal the extent of the disease.

Treatment

Esophageal cancer usually is advanced when diagnosed, so surgery and other treatments can only relieve disease effects.

Palliative therapy consists of treatment to keep the esophagus open, including dilatation of the esophagus, laser therapy, radiation therapy, and insertion of prosthetic tubes (such as the Celestin tube) to bridge the tumor. Radical surgery can excise the tumor and resect either the esophagus alone or

the stomach and esophagus. Chemotherapy and radiation therapy can slow the tumor's growth.

Gastrostomy or jejunostomy can help provide adequate nutrition. A prosthesis can be used to seal any fistula that develops. Endoscopic laser treatment and bipolar electrocoagulation can help restore swallowing by vaporizing cancerous tissue. If the tumor is in the upper esophagus, however, the laser can't be positioned properly. Analgesics are used for pain control.

Complications

Direct invasion of adjoining structures may lead to severe complications, such as mediastinitis, tracheoesophageal or bronchoesophageal fistula (causing an overwhelming cough when swallowing liquids), and aortic perforation with sudden exsanguination. Other complications include an inability to control secretions, obstruction of the esophagus, and loss of lower esophageal sphincter control, which can result in aspiration pneumonia.

Nursing interventions

● Monitor the patient's nutritional and fluid status, and provide him with high-calorie, high-protein foods. If he's having trouble swallowing solids, puree or liquefy his food, and offer a commercially available nutritional supplement. As ordered, provide tube feedings and prepare him for supplementary parenteral nutrition.

● To prevent food aspiration, place the patient in Fowler's position for meals and allow him plenty of time to eat. If he regurgitates food, provide mouth care.

● If the patient has a gastrostomy tube, feed him slowly, by gravity, in prescribed amounts (usually 200 to 500 ml).

✦✦ ─── CLINICAL ALERT ─── ✦✦

Offer the patient something to chew before each feeding. This promotes gastric secretions and provides some semblance of normal eating.

● Administer ordered analgesics for pain relief as necessary. Provide comfort measures, such as repositioning, and distractions to help decrease discomfort.

• After surgery, monitor the patient's vital signs, fluid and electrolyte balance, and intake and output. Immediately report any unexpected changes in his condition. Monitor him for such complications as infection, fistula formation, pneumonia, empyema, and malnutrition.

• After radiation therapy, monitor the patient for such complications as esophageal perforation, pneumonitis and fibrosis of the lungs, and myelitis of the spinal cord.

• After chemotherapy, take steps to decrease adverse effects, such as providing normal saline mouthwash to help prevent mouth ulcers. Allow the patient plenty of rest, and administer prescribed medications to reduce adverse effects. Protect him from infection.

• If an anastomosis to the esophagus was performed, position the patient flat on his back to prevent tension on the suture line. Watch for signs of an anastomotic leak.

• If the patient had a prosthetic tube inserted, make sure it doesn't become blocked or dislodged. This could cause a perforation of the mediastinum or precipitate tumor erosion.

• Throughout therapy, answer the patient's questions, and tell him what to expect from surgery and other therapies. Listen to his fears and concerns, and stay with him during periods of severe anxiety.

• Encourage the patient to identify actions and care measures that will promote his comfort and relaxation. Whenever possible, include the patient and family members in care decisions.

• Because the prognosis with this disease is poor, the patient may refuse any treatment. If so, respect his wishes.

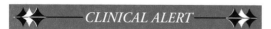

CLINICAL ALERT

If a question arises about the patient's competence to refuse treatment, remember that an adult who can consent to treatment is also qualified to refuse it.

Patient teaching

• Explain the procedures that the patient will undergo after surgery: closed chest drainage, nasogastric suctioning, and insertion of gastrostomy tubes. If appropriate, instruct the family members in gastrostomy tube care: checking tube patency before each feeding, providing skin care around the tube, and keeping the patient upright during and after feedings. Reinforce your teaching by giving them a copy of the teaching handout *How to care for your gastrostomy tube.*

• Stress the need to maintain adequate nutrition, and ask a dietitian to instruct the patient and his family members. If the patient has difficulty swallowing solids, instruct him to puree or liquefy his food and to follow a high-calorie, high-protein diet to minimize weight loss. Also, recommend that he add a commercially available high-calorie supplement to his diet.

• Encourage the patient to follow as normal a routine as possible after recovery from surgery and during radiation therapy and chemotherapy. Tell him that this will help him maintain a sense of control and reduce the complications associated with immobility. Advise him to rest between activities and to stop any activity that tires him or causes pain.

• Refer the patient and his family members to appropriate organizations, such as the American Cancer Society, community support groups, home health care agencies, and hospices.

LEUKEMIA

Beginning as a malignant proliferation of white blood cell (WBC) precursors, or blasts, in bone marrow or lymph tissue, leukemia results in an accumulation of these cells in peripheral blood, bone marrow, and body tissues.

The most common forms of leukemia in the older adult population are acute myeloblastic (myelogenous) leukemia (AML), which causes rapid accumulation of myeloid precursors (myeloblasts), and chronic lymphocytic leukemia (CLL). This accumulation is marked by the uncontrollable spread of abnormal, small lymphocytes in lymphoid tissue, blood, and bone marrow.

Acute leukemia ranks twentieth among causes of

How to care for your gastrostomy tube

Dear Patient:

Use these guidelines to review what the nurse taught you about caring for your gastrostomy tube.

Checking tube position

Make sure the tube is in place. Look for a mark in indelible ink on the tube where it should exit from your body.

If you can't see the mark, the tube is slipping too far into your body. If you see more tube below the mark than usual, the tube is pulling out of your body. Either way, contact the doctor immediately before trying to administer feedings or medicine through the tube.

Once you're sure the tube is positioned correctly, remove the gauze from the tube opening and unclamp the tube.

Clearing the tube

● Pour 2 tablespoons (3 milliliters) of water into the funnel or syringe used for feeding or giving medicine. Let the water flow into the stomach by gravity.

● Reclamp the tube, and remove the funnel or syringe. (If you lose the clamp, fold the tube and fasten it with a rubber band.)

● Cover the end of the tube with a gauze pad. Then wrap a rubber band around the pad to hold it in place.

● Wash the funnel or syringe thoroughly.

Changing the dressing

Change your dressing daily, or whenever it's wet or soiled. Don't use scissors to remove the old dressing; you might cut the tube accidentally.

● First, carefully clean the skin around the tube with mild soap and warm water. Then rinse and dry the skin thoroughly.

● Position two 4" x 4" gauze pads, cut halfway through the middle, around the tube so the slit sides overlap; this will protect the skin from gastric leakage.

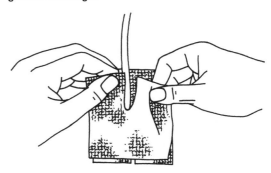

● Then cover the slit pads with uncut gauze pads, and secure them with hypoallergenic tape.

Caring for your skin

● Keep the skin around your stomach opening clean and dry to avoid skin irritation and infection. Check it several times a day.

● If you see any leakage of food or medicine around the tube, immediately apply a warm, moistened towel to soften any encrusted fluid, and wash, rinse, and dry the skin. Then call the doctor.

● If the skin becomes irritated, dust it with karaya gum powder.

● Call the doctor if the skin around the tube feels sore, looks red, or seems puffy, or if you feel any discomfort in your stomach.

cancer-related death in people of all ages. In the United States, an estimated 11,000 people develop acute leukemia annually. Untreated, the disease is invariably fatal, usually because of complications resulting from leukemic cell infiltration of bone marrow or vital organs. With treatment, the prognosis varies.

CLL occurs most commonly in older adults, almost always in men over age 50. According to the American Cancer Society, CLL accounts for almost one-third of new leukemia cases annually. It's the most benign and the most slowly progressive form of leukemia. However, the prognosis is poor if anemia, thrombocytopenia, neutropenia, bulky lymphadenopathy, or severe lymphocytosis develops. Gross bone marrow replacement by abnormal lymphocytes is the most common cause of death, usually within 4 to 5 years of diagnosis.

Causes

The exact cause of acute leukemia is unknown; however, viruses, genetic abnormalities, exposure to radiation (especially if prolonged) or to certain chemicals and drugs, and chronic exposure to benzene are likely contributing factors. Although the pathogenesis isn't clearly understood, immature, nonfunctioning WBCs appear to accumulate first in the tissue where they originate (lymphocytes in lymph tissue, granulocytes in bone marrow). These immature WBCs then spill into the bloodstream and, from there, infiltrate other tissues.

The cause of CLL is also unknown, but researchers suspect heredity may play a part because a higher incidence has been recorded within families. Undefined chromosomal abnormalities and certain immunologic defects, such as ataxia-telangiectasia or acquired agammaglobulinemia, are also suspected. CLL doesn't seem to result from radiation exposure.

Assessment findings

Acute leukemia follows an aggressive course in the older patient. His history usually shows a sudden onset of high fever and abnormal bleeding, such as bruising after minor trauma, nosebleeds, gingival bleeding, purpura, ecchymoses, and petechiae. He may also report fatigue and night sweats. More in-

sidious symptoms include weakness, lassitude, recurrent infections, chills, and possibly abdominal or bone pain. When assessing the patient, you may note tachycardia and, during auscultation, decreased ventilation, palpitations, and a systolic ejection murmur.

Inspection of a patient with acute leukemia may reveal pallor. On palpation, you may note lymph node enlargement as well as liver or spleen enlargement.

In the early stages of CLL, the patient usually complains of fatigue, malaise, fever, weight loss, and frequent infections. Inspection may reveal macular or nodular eruptions, evidence of skin infiltration. Palpation may detect enlarged lymph nodes, liver, and spleen, along with bone tenderness and edema from lymph node obstruction. As the disease progresses, you may note anemia, pallor, weakness, dyspnea, tachycardia, palpitations, bleeding, and infection from bone marrow involvement. You may also see signs of opportunistic fungal, viral, or bacterial infections, usually in late stages.

Diagnostic tests

Bone marrow aspiration showing a proliferation of immature WBCs confirms acute leukemia. If the aspirate is dry or free of leukemic cells but the patient has other typical signs of leukemia, a bone marrow biopsy — usually of the posterior superior iliac spine — should be performed. Blood counts show thrombocytopenia and neutropenia, and a WBC differential determines the cell type. Lumbar puncture detects meningeal involvement, and cerebrospinal fluid analysis detects abnormal WBC invasion of the central nervous system.

Typically, CLL is an incidental finding during a routine blood test that reveals numerous abnormal lymphocytes. In the early stages, the patient has a mildly but persistently elevated WBC count. Granulocytopenia is the rule, although the WBC count climbs as the disease progresses. Blood studies also reveal a hemoglobin count under 11 g/dl, hypogammaglobulinemia, and depressed serum globulin levels. Other common developments include neutropenia (less than 1,500/mm^3), lymphocytosis (more than 10,000/mm^3), and thrombocytopenia (less than 150,000/mm³).

For both types of leukemia, bone marrow aspiration and biopsy show lymphocytic invasion and a CT scan identifies affected organs.

Treatment

Systemic chemotherapy aims to eradicate leukemic cells and induce remission. It's used when fewer than 5% of blast cells in the marrow and peripheral blood are normal. The specific chemotherapeutic regimen varies with the diagnosis.

For meningeal infiltration in AML, the patient receives an intrathecal instillation of methotrexate or cytarabine with cranial radiation. Systemic treatment for AML consists of a combination of I.V. daunorubicin and cytarabine. If these fail to induce remission, treatment includes some or all of the following: a combination of cyclophosphamide, vincristine, prednisone, and methotrexate; high-dose cytarabine alone or with other drugs; amsacrine; etoposide; and azacytidine and mitoxantrone.

Systemic chemotherapy for CLL includes alkylating agents, usually chlorambucil or cyclophosphamide, and sometimes corticosteroid (prednisone) when autoimmune hemolytic anemia or thrombocytopenia occurs.

Treatment for either type may also include antibiotic, antifungal, and antiviral drugs and granulocyte injections to control infection, as well as transfusions of platelets to prevent bleeding and of red blood cells (RBCs) to prevent anemia. Bone marrow transplantation is performed in some patients.

Radiation therapy can help relieve symptoms in CLL. It's generally used to treat enlarged lymph nodes, painful bony lesions, or massive splenomegaly. When CLL causes obstruction or organ impairment or enlargement, local radiation therapy can reduce organ size, and splenectomy can help relieve the symptoms. Allopurinol can prevent hyperuricemia, a relatively uncommon finding.

Complications

The most common complication is infection, which can be fatal. In the end stage of the disease, possible complications include anemia, progressive splenomegaly, leukemic cell replacement of the bone marrow, and profound hypogammaglobulinemia, which usually results in fatal septicemia.

Nursing interventions

● Develop a plan of care for the leukemic patient that maximizes comfort, minimizes the adverse effects of chemotherapy, promotes preservation of veins, manages complications, and provides teaching and psychological support. Before treatment begins, help establish an appropriate rehabilitation program for the older adult during remission.

● Watch for signs of meningeal infiltration (confusion, lethargy, headache). If it develops, the patient will need intrathecal chemotherapy. After intrathecal drug instillation, place the patient in Trendelenburg's position for 30 minutes. Make sure he receives enough fluids, and keep him supine for 4 to 6 hours. Check the lumbar puncture site often for bleeding.

● Take steps to prevent hyperuricemia, a possible result of rapid leukemic cell lysis due to chemotherapy. Make sure the patient receives about 2 liters of fluid daily, and give him acetazolamide, sodium bicarbonate tablets, and allopurinol, as ordered. Check the patient's urine pH level often; it should be above 7.5. Watch for a rash and other hypersensitivity reactions to allopurinol.

● If the patient receives daunorubicin or doxorubicin, watch for early indications of cardiotoxicity, such as arrhythmias and signs of heart failure.

● Monitor the patient's temperature every 4 hours. If it rises over 101° F (38.3° C) and the WBC count decreases, he'll need prompt antibiotic therapy.

● After bone marrow transplantation, keep the patient in a sterile room, administer antibiotics, and transfuse packed RBCs as necessary.

● Administer prescribed analgesics as needed, and monitor their effectiveness. Provide comfort measures, such as position changes and distractions, to alleviate the patient's discomfort.

● Be alert for adverse effects of treatment, and take measures to prevent or alleviate them. For instance, you can control mouth ulceration by checking often for obvious ulcers and gum swelling and by providing frequent mouth care and saline rinses. Check the rectal area daily for induration, swelling, erythema, skin discoloration, and drainage.

• To control infection, place the patient in a private room and impose reverse isolation if necessary (although the benefits of reverse isolation are controversial). Coordinate care so that the patient doesn't come into contact with staff members who also care for patients with infections or infectious diseases. Screen staff members and visitors for contagious diseases. Don't use an indwelling urinary catheter or give I.M. injections; they provide an avenue for infection. If the patient does develop signs of infection — a temperature over 100° F (37.8° C), chills, or redness or swelling of any body part — report them at once.

• Clean the patient's skin daily with mild soap and water, and provide frequent soaks if ordered. Keep the perianal area clean, apply a mild lotion or cream to keep the skin from drying and cracking, and thoroughly clean the skin before all invasive skin procedures. Change I.V. tubing according to your facility's policy. Use strict aseptic technique and a metal scalp vein needle (metal butterfly needle) when starting an I.V. line. If the patient is receiving total parenteral nutrition, provide scrupulous subclavian catheter care.

• Watch for bleeding. If it occurs, apply ice compresses and pressure, and elevate the extremity. Don't give the patient aspirin or aspirin-containing drugs. Also, don't administer rectal suppositories, take a rectal temperature, or perform a digital rectal examination.

• Watch for signs of thrombocytopenia (easy bruising and nosebleeds, bleeding gums, black, tarry stools) and anemia (pale skin, weakness, fatigue, dizziness, palpitations).

• Establish a trusting relationship to promote communication. Allow the patient and his family members to express their anger, anxiety, and depression. Let the family members participate in the patient's care as much as possible.

• The elderly patient with leukemia may feel frightened, so take time to listen to his fears. Try to keep his spirits up by improving his personal appearance, providing a pleasant environment, and asking questions about his family. If possible, provide opportunities for his favorite activities. Minimize stress by

maintaining a calm, quiet atmosphere that's conducive to rest and relaxation.

• If the patient doesn't respond to treatment and has reached the terminal phase of the disease, he'll need supportive nursing care. Take steps to manage pain, fever, and bleeding; make sure the patient is comfortable; and provide emotional support for him and his family members. If he wishes, provide for religious counseling. Discuss the option of home or hospice care.

Patient teaching

• Describe the disease course, diagnostic tests, and treatments as well as their adverse effects.

• Teach the patient and his family members how to recognize signs and symptoms of infection (fever, chills, cough, sore throat). Warn the patient about to be discharged to avoid coming in contact with obviously ill people, especially children with common contagious childhood diseases. Reinforce your instructions by providing him with a copy of the teaching handout *How to avoid infection.*

• Inform the patient that drug therapy is tailored to his type of leukemia and usually consists of a combination of drugs. Teach him about the ones he'll receive, including possible adverse effects and the measures he can take to prevent or alleviate them.

• Tell the patient that if the chemotherapy causes weight loss and anorexia, he'll need to eat and drink high-calorie, high-protein foods and beverages. If he loses his appetite, advise him to eat small, frequent meals. If the chemotherapy and adjunctive prednisone instead cause weight gain, he'll need dietary counseling.

• If the patient receives cranial radiation, explain what the treatment is and how it will help him. Be sure to discuss potential adverse effects and the steps he can take to minimize them.

• If the patient needs a bone marrow transplant, reinforce the doctor's explanation of the procedure, including possible benefits and adverse effects. Teach him about total-body irradiation and the chemotherapy that he'll undergo before transplantation. Also tell him what to expect after the transplantation.

• Instruct the patient to use a soft toothbrush and to

EACHING AID

How to avoid infection

Dear Patient:

As your doctor and nurse have explained, you have an increased risk of getting an infection. Here are some simple steps you can take to protect yourself.

Follow your doctor's directions

- Be sure to take all your medications exactly as prescribed. Don't stop taking your medication unless your doctor tells you to do so.
- Keep all medical appointments so that your doctor can monitor your progress and the drug's effects.
- If you need to go to another doctor or to a dentist, explain that you're receiving an immunosuppressant drug.
- Wear a medical identification tag or bracelet that says you are taking an immunosuppressant drug.

Avoid sources of infection

- To minimize your exposure to infections, avoid crowds and people who have colds, the flu, chickenpox, shingles, or other contagious illnesses.
- Check with your doctor before you get any immunizations, especially live-virus vaccines. These contain weakened but living viruses that can cause illness in anyone who's taking an immunosuppressant drug. And avoid contact with anyone who has recently been vaccinated.
- Examine your mouth and skin daily for lesions, cuts, or rashes.
- Wash your hands thoroughly before preparing food. To avoid ingesting harmful organisms, thoroughly wash and cook all food before you eat it.

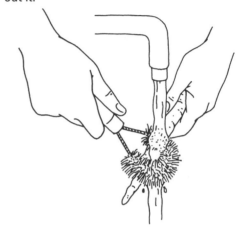

Recognize hazards

- Learn to recognize the early signs and symptoms of infection: sore throat, fever, chills, and a tired or sluggish feeling. Call your doctor immediately if you think you're coming down with an infection.
- Treat minor skin injuries with a triple antibiotic ointment such as Neosporin. If the injury is a deep one, or if it becomes swollen, red, or tender, call your doctor at once.

Perform routine hygiene

- Practice good oral and personal hygiene, especially hand washing. Report any mouth sores or ulcerations to your doctor.
- Don't use commercial mouthwashes if they have high alcohol and sugar content, because they may irritate your mouth and promote bacterial growth.

avoid hot, spicy foods and commercial mouthwashes to prevent irritating the mouth ulcers that typically result from chemotherapy.

• Warn the patient to take care to prevent bleeding because his blood may not have enough platelets to clot properly. Tell him to avoid aspirin and aspirin-containing drugs, and teach him how to recognize drugs that contain aspirin. Teach him the signs of abnormal bleeding (bruising, nosebleeds, petechiae) and how to apply pressure and ice to stop such bleeding. Urge him to report excessive bleeding or bruising to his doctor.

• Advise the patient to limit his activities and to plan rest periods during the day. Stress the importance of follow-up care, frequent blood tests, and taking all medications exactly as prescribed. Teach the patient the signs of recurrence (swollen lymph nodes in the neck, axilla, and groin; increased abdominal size or discomfort), and tell him to notify his doctor immediately if these signs occur.

• As appropriate, refer the patient and his family members to the social services department, home health care agencies, hospices, support groups, and the American Cancer Society.

LUNG CANCER

The most common forms of lung cancer are squamous cell (epidermoid) carcinoma, small-cell (oat-cell) carcinoma, adenocarcinoma, and large-cell (anaplastic) carcinoma. The most common site is the wall or epithelium of the bronchial tree.

The prognosis depends on the cancer's extent when diagnosed and the cells' growth rate, but it's usually poor. Only about 13% of patients with lung cancer survive 5 years after diagnosis. Although the disease is largely preventable, it's the most common cause of cancer-related death in men. In women, lung cancer ranks just ahead of breast cancer as a leading cause of cancer-related death.

Causes
Lung cancer's exact cause remains unclear. Risk factors include a history of smoking, exposure to carcinogenic and industrial air pollutants (asbestos, arsenic, chromium, coal dust, iron oxides, nickel, radioactive dust, uranium), and genetic predisposition.

Assessment findings
Because early lung cancer may cause no symptoms, the disease is commonly advanced when diagnosed. While taking the patient's history, be sure to assess his exposure to carcinogens. If he's a smoker, determine pack years (the number of packs smoked daily multiplied by the number of years smoked).

The patient's chief complaints may include coughing (induced by tumor stimulation of nerve endings), hemoptysis, dyspnea (from the tumor occluding airflow), and sometimes hoarseness (from the tumor or tumor-bearing lymph nodes pressing on the laryngeal nerve). On inspection, you may notice the patient becoming short of breath when he walks or exerts himself. You may also observe finger clubbing; edema of the face, neck, and upper torso; dilated chest and abdominal veins (superior vena cava syndrome); weight loss; and fatigue.

Palpation may reveal enlarged lymph nodes and an enlarged liver. Percussion findings may include dullness over the lung fields in a patient with pleural effusion. Auscultation may disclose decreased breath sounds, wheezing, and pleural friction rub (with pleural effusion).

Diagnostic tests
Chest X-rays usually show an advanced lesion and can detect a lesion up to 2 years before signs and symptoms appear. They also can indicate tumor size and location. Cytologic sputum analysis, which is 75% reliable, requires a sputum specimen expectorated from the lungs and tracheobronchial tree, not from postnasal secretions or saliva.

Bronchoscopy can identify the tumor site, and bronchoscopic washings provide material for cytologic and histologic studies. The flexible fiber-optic bronchoscope increases test effectiveness. Needle biopsy of the lungs relies on biplanar, fluoroscopic visual control to locate peripheral tumors before withdrawing a tissue specimen for analysis. This procedure allows a firm diagnosis in 80% of patients.

Tissue biopsy of metastatic sites (including supraclavicular and mediastinal nodes and pleura) helps to assess the disease's extent. Based on histologic findings, staging determines the disease's extent and prognosis and helps direct treatment. Thoracentesis allows chemical and cytologic examination of pleural fluid.

Additional studies include chest tomography, bronchography, esophagography, and angiocardiography (contrast studies of the bronchial tree, esophagus, and cardiovascular tissues). Tests to detect metastases include a bone scan (abnormal findings may lead to a bone marrow biopsy, which is typically recommended for patients with small-cell carcinoma), a CT scan of the brain, liver function studies, and gallium scans of the liver and spleen.

Treatment

Various combinations of surgery, radiation therapy, and chemotherapy improve the prognosis and prolong patient survival. Because lung cancer is usually advanced at diagnosis, most treatment is palliative.

Surgery is the primary treatment for stage I, stage II, or selected stage III squamous cell carcinomas, adenocarcinomas, and large-cell carcinomas unless the tumor is inoperable or other conditions (such as cardiac disease) rule out surgery. Surgery may consist of partial lung removal (wedge resection, segmental resection, lobectomy, or radical lobectomy) or total removal (pneumonectomy or radical pneumonectomy).

Preoperative radiation therapy may reduce tumor bulk to allow for surgical resection and may also improve response rates. Radiation therapy is ordinarily recommended for stage I and stage II lesions if surgery is contraindicated and for stage III disease that's confined to the involved hemothorax and the ipsilateral supraclavicular lymph nodes. Radiation therapy usually begins about 1 month after surgery (to allow the wound to heal). It's directed at the chest area most likely to develop metastasis.

Chemotherapeutic drug combinations of fluorouracil, vincristine, mitomycin, and cisplatin have a response rate of 30% to 50% but have a minimal

effect on long-term survival. Promising drug regimens for treating small-cell carcinomas include cyclophosphamide, doxorubicin, and vincristine; cyclophosphamide, doxorubicin, vincristine, and etoposide; and etoposide, cisplatin, cyclophosphamide, and doxorubicin.

Immunotherapy is investigational. Nonspecific regimens using bacille Calmette-Guérin (BCG) vaccine or, possibly, *Corynebacterium parvum* offer the most promise. In laser therapy, also largely investigational, a laser beam is directed through a bronchoscope to destroy local tumors.

Complications

When the primary tumor spreads within the chest, complications may include tracheal obstruction, esophageal compression with dysphagia, phrenic nerve paralysis with hemidiaphragm elevation and dyspnea, sympathetic nerve paralysis with Horner's syndrome, eighth cervical and first thoracic nerve compression with ulnar and Pancoast's syndrome (shoulder pain radiating to the ulnar nerve pathways), lymphatic obstruction with pleural effusion, and hypoxemia. Other complications are anorexia and weight loss, sometimes leading to cachexia, finger clubbing, and hypertrophic osteoarthropathy. Endocrine syndromes may involve production of hormones and hormone precursors.

Nursing interventions

- Provide comprehensive supportive care and patient teaching to minimize complications and speed the older patient's recovery from surgery, radiation therapy, or chemotherapy. Urge the patient to voice his concerns, and schedule time to answer his questions. Be sure to explain procedures before performing them, to reduce his anxiety.
- Before and after surgery, give ordered analgesics as necessary.
- After thoracic surgery, maintain a patent airway, and monitor chest tubes to reestablish normal intrathoracic pressure and prevent postoperative and pulmonary complications. Check vital signs and watch for and report abnormal respiration and other changes.
- Suction the older patient often, and encourage

him to begin deep-breathing and coughing exercises as soon as possible. Check secretions often.

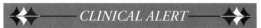
CLINICAL ALERT

Sputum will appear thick and dark with blood initially, but it should become thinner and grayish yellow within 1 day.

● Monitor and document the color of closed chest drainage. Keep chest tubes patent and draining effectively. Watch for fluctuations in the water-seal chamber on inspiration and expiration, indicating that the chest tube remains patent. Watch for air leaks and report them immediately.

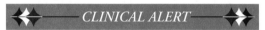
CLINICAL ALERT

Position the older adult on the surgical side to promote drainage and lung reexpansion.

● Watch for and report any foul-smelling discharge or excessive drainage on surgical dressings. Usually, you'll remove the dressing after 24 hours, unless the wound appears infected.

● Monitor intake and output and maintain adequate hydration. Watch for and be prepared to treat infection, shock, hemorrhage, atelectasis, dyspnea, mediastinal shift, and pulmonary embolism.

● To help prevent pulmonary embolism, apply antiembolism stockings and encourage the patient to perform range-of-motion (ROM) exercises.

● For the older adult receiving chemotherapy, ask the dietary department to provide soft, nonirritating, protein-rich foods. Encourage the patient to eat high-calorie, between-meal snacks. Give antiemetics and antidiarrheals as needed. Schedule care to help the patient conserve his energy. Impose reverse isolation if bone marrow suppression develops during treatment.

● Provide meticulous skin care for the patient receiving radiation therapy to help minimize skin breakdown.

Patient teaching

● Before surgery, supplement and reinforce the doctor's explanations of the disease and the operation itself. Teach the older adult about postoperative procedures and equipment, including urinary catheterization, insertion of chest tubes and endotracheal tubes, dressing changes, and I.V. therapy. Teach him how to cough and breathe deeply from the diaphragm and how to perform ROM exercises. Reassure him that analgesics and proper positioning will help to control postoperative pain.

● Warn an outpatient to avoid wearing tight clothing, getting a sunburn, or applying harsh ointments on his chest. Teach him exercises to prevent shoulder stiffness and how to use an incentive spirometer to keep his lungs aerated.

● If the patient is receiving chemotherapy or radiation therapy, explain the possible adverse effects and tell him which he should report to the doctor. Teach him ways to avoid complications such as infection.

● Teach high-risk geriatric patients how to reduce their chances of developing lung cancer or recurrent cancer. Refer smokers to local branches of the American Cancer Society or Smokenders. Provide information about group therapy, individual counseling, and hypnosis. Urge all heavy smokers over age 40 to have a chest X-ray annually and cytologic sputum analysis every 6 months. Also encourage older people who have recurring or chronic respiratory tract infections, chronic lung disease, or a nagging or changing cough to seek prompt medical evaluation.

13

Managing diabetes

A chronic disease of insulin deficiency or resistance, diabetes mellitus is characterized by disturbances in carbohydrate, protein, and fat metabolism. Insulin's role in the body is to transport glucose into the cells for fuel or for storage as glycogen; it also stimulates protein synthesis and free fatty acid storage in the adipose tissues. Insulin deficiency compromises the body tissues' ability to access essential nutrients for fuel and storage. Because the incidence of diabetes increases with age, health care professionals who care for older people must have a thorough understanding of this common disease.

Diabetes takes two primary forms: type I, insulin-dependent diabetes mellitus, and the more prevalent type II, non-insulin-dependent diabetes mellitus. Several secondary forms are linked to such conditions as pancreatic disease, hormonal or genetic syndromes, and ingestion of certain drugs or chemicals. Among older adults, type II diabetes is the more common.

TYPE II DIABETES MELLITUS

As the body ages, the cells become more resistant to insulin, reducing the older adult's ability to metabolize glucose. In addition, the release of insulin from the pancreatic beta cells is reduced and delayed. The result of these combined processes is hyperglycemia.

In the older patient, sudden concentrations of glucose cause increased and more prolonged hyperglycemia.

Diabetes affects almost one in five people ages 65 and over. Because symptoms are vague, researchers believe many more older people probably have undiagnosed type II diabetes. Additionally, over 40% of people this age have some form of glucose intolerance.

Causes
Type II diabetes in older persons is caused by abnormal insulin secretion, resistance to insulin action in target tissues, and faulty hepatic gluconeogenesis. The primary cause of hyperglycemia in older adults is increased insulin resistance in the peripheral tissues. Although the actual number of insulin receptors decreases slightly with age, resistance is believed to occur after insulin binds with the receptor. Additionally, the beta cells in the islets of Langerhans are less sensitive to high glucose levels, delaying the production of insulin. Some older adults are also unable to inhibit glucose production in the liver.

Obesity, reduced physical activity, coexisting illnesses, and poor eating habits also increase the risk of type II diabetes in older adults.

Assessment findings
The symptoms of type II diabetes are usually vague and develop gradually. Affected geriatric patients often have a family history of diabetes mellitus or another endocrine disease; have had a recent, severe

viral infection, stress, or trauma; or are taking drugs that increase blood glucose levels.

In older adults, the classic symptoms of diabetes, polydipsia and polyuria, may be absent; nonspecific complaints may be the only clues to the disease. Often, home care or community nurses are the first to suspect a problem. The patient may report loss of appetite, incontinence, and decreased vision. He or a caregiver may report his confusion or even delirium. Constipation or abdominal bloating may result from gastric hypotonicity.

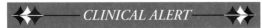

Because their thirst mechanism functions less effectively, older people may not report polydipsia, a hallmark of diabetes in younger adults.

Ophthalmologic examination may show retinopathy or cataract formation. Inspection may reveal skin changes, especially on the legs and feet, due to impaired peripheral circulation. The patient may also have a chronic skin condition, such as cellulitis or a nonhealing wound. Palpation may reveal poor skin turgor and dry mucous membranes, related to dehydration. Decreased peripheral pulses, cool skin, and decreased reflexes may also be palpable, and the patient may complain of peripheral pain or numbness. Auscultation may reveal orthostatic hypotension.

Diagnostic tests

Fasting serum glucose levels and glucose tolerance tests provide the definitive diagnosis for diabetes. Older people may have a near-normal fasting glucose level but prolonged hyperglycemia after eating. Therefore, the 2-hour postprandial serum glucose test and the oral glucose tolerance test are more helpful in diagnosing their diabetes.

For several days before a glucose tolerance test, the older adult should consume at least 5 oz (150 g) of carbohydrates daily (10.5 oz [300 g] if he's malnourished). Age-related gradients are used to interpret the results. For each decade after age 55, 10 mg/dl is added to the standard values at the first, second, and third hours. So a glucose level that would be significantly elevated for a 35-year-old

person would be normal for an 85-year-old.

Diagnosis is usually made when one of the following three criteria are met:
● random plasma glucose concentrations ≥ 200 mg/dl
● fasting blood glucose concentrations ≥ 140 mg/dl
● plasma glucose concentrations after oral glucose intake ≥ 200 mg/dl.

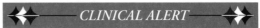

Urine testing for glucose is of little value in assessing the older person. Because the renal threshold for glucose increases with age, older adults can be hyperglycemic without having glucose spill into their urine.

Blood testing for glycosylated hemoglobin (hemoglobin A or HbA$_{1C}$), which reflects the average level of serum glucose within the previous 3 months, is usually performed to monitor the effectiveness of diabetic therapy.

Treatment

Effective treatment of diabetes is aimed at achieving optimal blood glucose levels and decreasing complications. Depending on the nature of the disease, treatment may be basic or aggressive. Type I diabetics need insulin and close monitoring of serum glucose levels. Type II diabetics may require oral antidiabetic drugs or may be controlled by diet and lifestyle changes alone.

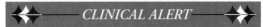

Diabetes is not a static disease: type II may progress to type I, and the type I person's need for insulin may be only temporary (as in steroid-induced diabetes).

Oral antidiabetic drugs stimulate endogenous insulin production and may increase insulin sensitivity at the cellular level. The patient's other medications must also be considered when developing a drug regimen.

A dietitian can develop an individualized diet to meet the patient's needs. The diet should meet nutritional guidelines, control blood glucose levels, and maintain appropriate body weight. The dietitian estimates the patient's total daily energy requirements, based on his ideal body weight, then develops a diet that provides the proper carbohydrate, protein, and fat content. For the obese older person, weight loss is also a dietary goal. To improve the patient's compliance, discuss and plan the diet with him and incorporate as many of his preferences as possible.

Exercise is an important tool in managing type II diabetes. Physical activity increases insulin sensitivity, improves glucose tolerance, and promotes weight control. Research also suggests that moderate exercise can delay or prevent the onset of type II diabetes in high-risk groups. When you plan an exercise program for an older person, make sure the level of exertion matches his level of fitness.

Treatment of older adults is also based on symptoms. Optimal blood glucose control is essential to help prevent the acute and chronic complications of diabetes.

Complications

Hypoglycemia is a potential complication for diabetics who are treated with insulin or oral antidiabetic drugs. It may be caused by excessive insulin administration, inadequate caloric intake, alcohol consumption, or excessive exercise. Older adults are more sensitive to low blood glucose levels than younger adults. Their hypoglycemic symptoms may range from mild to severe and may go unrecognized until the condition is life-threatening.

You may encounter two other metabolic complications of diabetes: Diabetic ketoacidosis (DKA), characterized by severe hyperglycemia, is a life-threatening condition. It usually occurs in people with type I diabetes, but may occasionally affect people with type II diabetes who are under extreme physical or emotional stress. Hyperosmolar hyperglycemic nonketotic syndrome (HHNS), also known as hyperosmolar coma, is the most common acute metabolic complication seen in older diabetics.

People with diabetes mellitus also have a greater risk of developing various chronic illnesses affecting virtually all body systems. In the older population, macrovascular and microvascular complications are accelerated because of preexisting cardiovascular effects of aging. The most common chronic complications include peripheral and autonomic neuropathy, peripheral vascular disease, cardiovascular disease, retinopathy, nephropathy, and diabetic dermopathy.

Peripheral neuropathy usually affects the hands and feet and may cause numbness or pain and possibly skin lesions. Autonomic neuropathy manifests itself in several ways, including gastroparesis (delayed gastric emptying which leads to a feeling of nausea and fullness after meals), nocturnal diarrhea, impotence, and orthostatic hypotension.

Older diabetics have 10 times the incidence of hypertension found in nondiabetic older adults. This results in a greatly increased risk of transient ischemic attacks and cerebrovascular accident, coronary artery disease and myocardial infarction, cerebral atherosclerosis, progression of retinopathy and neuropathy, cognitive impairment, and central nervous system depression.

Hyperglycemia impairs an older adult's resistance to infection, because the glucose content of the epidermis and urine encourages bacterial growth. This makes the older person susceptible to skin and urinary tract infections and vaginitis.

Nursing interventions

Although diabetes is managed similarly in all age-groups, management of older patients requires special consideration and adjustment. Keep in mind that older people are likely to resist drastic lifestyle changes. You may need to adapt your interventions to the individual and compromise to achieve treatment goals.
● Initially, you'll need precise records of vital signs, weight, fluid intake, urine output, and caloric intake. When a therapeutic regimen has been established, monitor serum glucose or glycosylated hemoglobin levels every 6 to 8 weeks.
● Monitor for acute complications of diabetic therapy, especially hypoglycemia (slow cerebration, dizziness, weakness, pallor, tachycardia, diaphoresis, seizures, and coma), which requires that you give the patient carbohydrates immediately in the form of fruit juice, hard candy, honey or, if he's unconscious, glucagon or I.V. dextrose. Also be alert for signs of HHNS (urinary incontinence, abdominal

discomfort, neurologic abnormalities, and stupor).
● Your patient may have cardiovascular complications, such as cerebrovascular, coronary artery, and peripheral vascular impairment, and peripheral and autonomic nervous system effects. Look for signs of diabetic neuropathy (numbness or pain in the hands and feet, footdrop, and neurogenic bladder). Also watch for signs of urinary tract and vaginal infections.
● Provide meticulous skin care, especially to the feet and legs. Treat all injuries, cuts, and blisters promptly. Avoid constricting hose, slippers, or bed linens. Refer the older adult to a podiatrist for regular foot and nail care, if needed.
● Encourage your patient to verbalize his feelings about diabetes and its effects on his lifestyle and life expectancy.
● Offer emotional support and a realistic assessment of his condition. Explain that with proper treatment, he can have a near-normal lifestyle and life expectancy.
● Help the older adult develop new coping strategies. Refer him and his family members to a counselor, or encourage them to join a support group if appropriate.

Patient teaching
The current trend of shorter hospital stays for serious medical conditions means patients leave acute care facilities earlier and sicker than ever before. So, patient teaching, which used to be completed in the hospital, must now be accomplished in other settings. Health care professionals in home care, doctor's offices, and community care settings must recognize their responsibility for continued patient teaching. Armed with a thorough understanding of diabetes, the older patient can better control his condition and take measures to prevent acute complications and hospitalization.

The older adult's ability to learn about his disease and comply with the treatment regimen may be affected by his cognitive ability, memory, and level of interest; the presence of depression, anxiety, pain, visual impairment (inability to see the insulin syringe, medicine bottle, or glucometer), or hearing impairment; his level of dexterity (may be affected

by arthritis, neuropathy, or paralysis); the cost of diabetes management; and the availability of support systems.

Your teaching may be directed at the patient, his family members, or any other caregiver. Here are some of the most important patient-teaching points:
● Teach the patient about the disease process, and stress the importance of carefully following the prescribed treatment plan. Tailor your teaching to the patient's needs, abilities, and developmental stage. Discuss diet, medications (including administration techniques), exercise, monitoring techniques, hygiene, and how to prevent, recognize, and treat hypoglycemia and hyperglycemia.
● Encourage your patient to keep all doctor's and laboratory test appointments and to maintain a log of blood glucose results. Explain that he can still do the things he enjoys, including traveling and eating out. Give him the teaching handouts *Travel tips for diabetic patients* and *Diet-conscious tips for dining out,* pages 251 and 252.
● To encourage compliance with necessary lifestyle changes, explain how blood glucose control affects long-term health. Encourage the patient to use a glucometer at home (see *Testing your blood glucose levels,* page 253). Tell him about assistive devices that may make compliance easier, such as magnifying attachments for the syringe and nonslip pads and holders for patients with weak arms.
● Teach your patient self-care measures to avoid complications, and give him the teaching handout *Preventing diabetic complications,* page 254.
● Instruct the patient in foot care. Tell him to wash his feet daily, carefully dry between his toes, and inspect for corns, calluses, redness, swelling, bruises, and breaks in the skin. Urge him to report any skin changes to the doctor. Advise him to wear comfortable, nonconstricting shoes and never to walk barefoot. Reinforce your teaching by giving him a copy of the handout *Taking care of your feet,* page 255.
● Teach your patient how to manage his diabetes when he has a minor illness, such as a cold, the flu, or an upset stomach. Give him a copy of the teaching handout *Managing diabetes during illness,* pages 256 and 257.

(Text continues on page 258.)

EACHING AID

Travel tips for diabetic patients

Dear Patient:

If you enjoy travel, diabetes needn't cramp your style — as long as you plan ahead and make the following adjustments.

Before you go

Visit your doctor for a general checkup, travel guidelines, and prescriptions (for example, antidiarrheal medication). Ask for a note describing your condition, the type of medications you're taking, and any allergies you have.

Unless you travel by car, pack your diabetic supplies in a carry-on bag in case your luggage is lost or delayed. Be sure to pack enough medication to last for the entire trip.

If you travel by boat or plane, ask your doctor if you can use an antiemetic (a medication that prevents vomiting), such as Dramamine. Take the medication 4 hours before departure and as often as needed thereafter.

If your medication dosage must be adjusted across time zones, ask your doctor exactly how much medication to take. Remember to ask for return-trip guidelines too.

In a country where English isn't spoken, learn to say the following sentences, or write them on a card:

- I am a diabetic.
- Please get me a doctor.
- Sugar or orange juice, please.

During your trip

Follow your diabetic diet while en route. If you travel by boat or plane, call ahead and request special diabetic meals. After boarding, identify yourself to the steward, and explain what time you must eat so your meals and snacks can be ready.

Regardless of how you travel, always carry some simple carbohydrate snacks, such as sugar cubes, hard candy, an apple, or an orange, in case a meal or snack is delayed or you have an unexpected low blood sugar reaction. On a car trip where you can't stop every few hours for a snack or a meal, carry food with you.

Some precautions

Wear sturdy, comfortable shoes to avoid foot injury — avoid new shoes or open-toed sandals.

Plan your activities carefully; excessive exercise can cause your blood glucose level to fall dangerously low. If you take a home glucose monitor with you, be sure to monitor your blood glucose levels daily.

Wear a medical information bracelet or carry a card that identifies you as a diabetic and lists your medications. And make sure your traveling companions know you're a diabetic and know how to treat you for low blood glucose levels in case you should become unconscious.

Bon voyage!

Diet-conscious tips for dining out

Dear Patient:

When you try to lose weight or maintain your ideal weight, dining out may pose a dilemma. But it doesn't have to. Just keep these tips in mind.

Plan ahead

If you can, check the restaurant's menu a day or two before you eat there, so you'll know your choices. If the menu doesn't list anything you want, choose another restaurant.

Before you leave home, eat some raw vegetables or an apple to take the edge off your appetite. That way you'll be less inclined to overeat.

Choose healthful foods

Select an entree of broiled, poached, or steamed (rather than sautéed or fried) chicken or fish. Or choose pasta with sauce on the side. If you want beef, order a lean cut. Because most restaurant portions are at least 6 ounces, (170 grams) eat only half of what you're served. Your portion should be no larger than a deck of cards. You can ask to take the other half home.

Complement the entree with a baked or boiled potato and a salad. Opt for fresh fruit for dessert, or choose sherbet or angel food cake. If you're very hungry, have a clear soup or raw vegetables as an appetizer.

Choose a calorie-free dinner beverage, such as seltzer, water, black coffee, or tea, and limit yourself to one cocktail. Better yet, avoid alcohol entirely. Its effects may undermine your willpower.

Skip fatty foods

Trim visible fat from meats. Add little or no margarine to your baked potato. Stay away from gravies and cream sauces. Ask that your salad dressing be served on the side so you can control the amount you use, or create your own with vinegar or lemon juice and oil. At salad bars, watch out for calorie-packed toppings, such as bacon, nuts, croutons, and cheese.

Be firm

Tell the waiter you're on a special diet. Ask him to recommend dishes that are prepared without butter, oil, or sauces. Remember, many people are health-conscious these days, and your waiter is probably accustomed to such requests.

Don't hesitate to return food that's not prepared the way you requested. After all, you're paying for the meal.

Special tips

● Think twice before you order such "diet platters" as a hamburger and a scoop of cottage cheese. Both of these foods are loaded with fat and calories.
● If you wish to cut down on portion sizes, choose an appetizer as the main course, order a la carte, or share food with a companion.
● Don't rush through your meal. Your brain doesn't know that you're full until 20 minutes after you've eaten enough. Eating slowly gives you time to feel full without overeating.
● If you decide to splurge on a big meal, don't blame yourself. Just go back to your diet and avoid the temptation to continue overeating.

EACHING AID

Testing your blood glucose levels

Dear Patient:

Testing your blood glucose (sugar) levels daily will tell you whether your diabetes is under control. Follow these steps to learn how to obtain blood and then perform the test.

Getting ready

1. First, assemble the necessary equipment: your glucose meter, a lancet, and a vial with reagent strips.
2. Remove a reagent strip from the vial. Then replace the cap, making sure it's tight.
3. Turn on the glucose meter and insert the reagent strip according to the manufacturer's instructions. Then wait for the display window to show that the meter is ready for the blood sample.

Obtaining blood

1. Choose a site on the end or side of any fingertip. Wash your hands thoroughly and dry them. To enhance blood flow, hold your finger under warm water for a minute or two.
2. Hold your hand below your heart, and milk the blood toward the fingertip that you plan to pierce. Squeeze that fingertip with the thumb of the same hand. Place your fingertip (with your thumb still pressed against it) on a firm surface, such as a table.
3. Twist off the lancet's protective cap. Then grasp the lancet and quickly pierce your fingertip, just to the side of the finger pad (as shown at the top of the next column), where you have more blood vessels and fewer nerve endings.

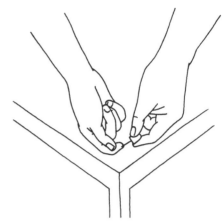

4. Remove your thumb from your fingertip to permit blood flow. Then milk your finger gently until you get a large hanging drop of blood.

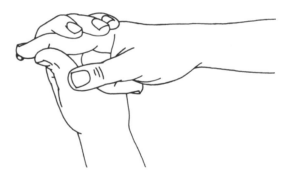

Testing blood

1. When the display window indicates that the meter is ready, touch the drop of blood to the reagent strip at the indicated spot. The drop of blood will automatically start the meter's timer.
2. After the meter has finished the test, you can read the results from the display window. The meter will automatically store the date, time, and results of the test.

EACHING AID

Preventing diabetic complications

Dear Patient:

There's no way around it. Controlling your diabetes means checking your blood glucose (sugar) levels daily and making the following good health habits a way of life.

Care for your heart
Because diabetes raises your risk of heart disease, take care of your heart by following these American Heart Association guidelines:
● Maintain your normal weight.
● Exercise regularly, following your doctor's recommendations.
● Help control your blood pressure and cholesterol levels by eating a low-fat, high-fiber diet as your doctor prescribes.

Care for your eyes
Have your eyes examined by an ophthalmologist at least once a year. He may detect any damage that could cause blindness, before symptoms appear. Early treatment may prevent further damage.

Care for your teeth
Schedule regular dental checkups and follow good home care to minimize dental problems related to diabetes, such as gum disease and abscesses. If you experience any bleeding, pain, or soreness in your gums or teeth, report this to the dentist immediately. Brush your teeth after every meal and floss daily. If you wear dentures, clean them thoroughly every day and make sure they fit properly.

Care for your skin
Breaks in your skin can increase your risk of infection. Check your skin daily for cuts and irritated areas and see your doctor if necessary. Bathe daily with warm water and mild soap and pat your skin dry thoroughly, taking extra care between your toes and in any other areas where skin surfaces touch. Then, apply a lanolin-based lotion to prevent dryness. Always wear cotton underwear to allow moisture to evaporate and help prevent skin breakdown.

Care for your feet
Diabetes can reduce blood flow to your feet and dull their ability to feel heat, cold, or pain. Follow your health care professional's instructions on daily foot care, and take precautions to prevent foot problems.

Check your urine
Because symptoms of kidney disease usually don't appear until the problem is advanced, your doctor will check your urine routinely for protein, which can signal kidney disease. Don't delay telling your doctor if you have symptoms of a urinary tract infection (burning, painful, or difficult urination or blood or pus in the urine).

Get regular checkups
See your doctor regularly so that he can detect early signs of complications and start treatment promptly.

EACHING AID

Taking care of your feet

Dear Patient:

Because you have diabetes, your feet require meticulous daily care. Why? Diabetes can reduce the blood supply to your feet, so normally minor injuries, such as an ingrown toenail or a blister, can lead to a dangerous infection. Diabetes also reduces sensation in your feet, allowing you to burn or chill them without feeling it. To prevent foot problems, follow these instructions.

Routine care

● Wash your feet in warm, soapy water every day. To prevent burns, use a thermometer to check the water temperature first.

● Dry your feet thoroughly by blotting them with a towel. Be sure to dry between the toes.

● Apply oil or lotion to your feet immediately after drying to prevent evaporating water from drying your skin and to keep your skin soft. But don't put lotion between your toes.

● If your feet perspire heavily, use a mild foot powder, sprinkled lightly between your toes and in your socks and shoes.

● File your nails even with the end of your toes; don't cut them. And don't cut the corners of your nails or file them shorter than the ends of your toes. If your nails are too thick, tough, or misshapen to file, consult a podiatrist. Also, don't dig under toenails or around cuticles.

● Exercise your feet daily to improve circulation. Sitting on the edge of the bed, point your toes upward, then downward, 10 times. Then make a circle with each foot, 10 times.

Special precautions

● Make sure your shoes fit properly. Buy only leather shoes (because leather allows air in and out), and break in new shoes gradually, increasing wearing time by a half hour each day. Check worn shoes frequently for rough spots in the lining.

● Wear clean cotton socks daily. Don't wear socks with holes or darns that have rough, irritating seams.

● Consult a podiatrist for treatment of corns and calluses. Self-treatment or application of caustic agents may be harmful.

● If your feet are cold, wear warm socks or slippers and use extra blankets in bed. Avoid using heating pads and hot water bottles; these devices may cause burns.

● Check your feet daily for cuts, cracks, blisters, or red, swollen areas.

● If you cut your foot, no matter how slightly, contact your doctor. Meanwhile, wash the cut thoroughly and apply a mild antiseptic. Avoid harsh antiseptics, such as iodine, which can cause tissue damage.

● Don't wear tight-fitting garments or engage in activities that can decrease circulation. Specifically, avoid wearing elastic garters, sitting with your knees crossed, picking at sores or rough spots on your feet, walking barefoot, or applying adhesive tape to your feet.

TEACHING AID

Managing diabetes during illness

Dear Patient:

Minor illness — a cold, the flu, an infection, or an upset stomach — can drastically alter your ability to control your blood glucose (sugar) levels. As your body attempts to compensate for the stress of an illness, your blood glucose levels may rise. To prevent this, maintain your usual medication schedule and pattern of meals and snacks, if possible, and follow these guidelines:

● If you have a home glucose monitor, check your glucose level every 8 hours.

● Call the doctor if you can't eat or keep down any food or liquids, if you can't eat normally for more than 24 hours, or if you have a fever.

● If you live alone, arrange for someone to check on you several times daily.

In addition, use this list of foods and liquids to guide you through the stages of recovery. Just follow the instructions, starting at your stage of the illness. Note that you might not start at stage 1. You can start with stage 3, for instance, depending on your symptoms. Also, if your symptoms get worse and you can't tolerate the recommended foods, you may drop back one stage until you feel better.

Stage 1

Your symptoms: severe nausea and vomiting, severe diarrhea, fever

Allowable foods and beverages: orange, grapefruit, or tomato juice; soup; broth; tea; coffee; cola

Special instructions: Sip a teaspoon of liquid

every 10 to 15 minutes. If you can't tolerate this, call your doctor. Advance to stage 2 when nausea and diarrhea stop (or almost stop) and you're no longer vomiting.

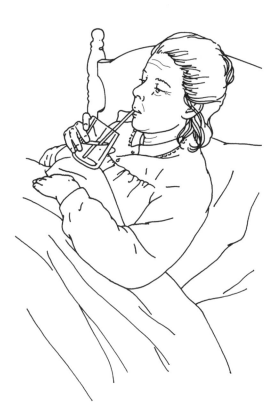

Stage 2

Your symptoms: little or no appetite, occasional diarrhea, fatigue, fever

Allowable foods and beverages: creamed soup, mashed potatoes, cooked cereal, plain

T *EACHING AID*

Managing diabetes during illness (continued)

yogurt, bananas, fruit-flavored gelatins, juice, broth, regular soft drinks

Special instructions: Take ½ to 1 cup of food or beverage every 1 to 2 hours. Because fever causes you to perspire and lose body fluids, you should also continue to sip an unsweetened beverage (tea or coffee without sugar, water, or diet soft drinks, for example) every 10 to 15 minutes.

You're ready to advance to stage 3 when you've consumed the suggested amount of food and liquids several times and your symptoms are improving.

Stage 3

Your symptoms: limited appetite, small meals tolerated, sluggishness, slight fever, able to sit up or walk

Allowable foods and beverages: Use your diabetic meal plan to guide you through this stage of your recovery. (If you don't have one, talk to a diet counselor.) You can skip the protein and fat groups listed on your meal plan.

● Milk list — Eat one of these foods instead of drinking 1 cup of milk: ½ cup of eggnog or sweetened custard or 1 cup of creamed soup or plain yogurt.

● Bread and cereal list — You can eat one of the following foods instead of one bread or starch serving: ¼ cup of sherbet; ½ cup of cooked cereal, mashed potatoes, ice cream or fruit-flavored gelatin; ¾ cup of a regular soft

drink; 1 cup of noodle soup; or five salted crackers.

● Vegetable list — Eat a half serving from the bread and cereal serving list in your meal plan.

● Fruit list — You can eat any of these foods instead of one fruit serving: ¼ cup of grape or prune juice; ⅓ cup of apple juice; ½ cup of unsweetened applesauce, a regular soft drink, or orange or grapefruit juice; ½ of a banana or an ice pop; or 2 tsp of honey

Special instructions: Eat as many meals and snacks as your meal plan calls for.

Advance to stage 4 when your appetite increases and you can follow your diabetic meal plan without any problems. If you still have a fever, drink several extra glasses of water, unsweetened tea or coffee, or diet soft drink daily.

Stage 4

Your symptoms: general sick feeling, stomach upset by heavy or spicy foods

Allowable foods and beverages: Use food lists on your regular meal plan. Choose foods that don't give you problems. For protein, try cottage cheese, broiled fish, or baked chicken. Eat fruit, vegetables, starch, and protein in moderation.

Special instructions: Eat at regular meal and snack times. Use your regular diabetic meal plan if you have no problems for a day with the easier-to-digest foods.

- Describe the signs and symptoms of diabetic neuropathy to your patient, and emphasize the need for precautions, because decreased sensation can mask injuries.
- Urge the older adult to visit his doctor for annual eye examinations to detect diabetic retinopathy early.
- For careful dietary control of sugar intake, teach the patient and his family members how to monitor the diet and use food exchange lists. Show them how to read labels in the supermarket to identify fat, carbohydrate, protein, and sugar content.
- Teach the patient and family members to use a home glucose monitor, if prescribed. Then have them give a return demonstration of the procedure to confirm that they understand it. Arrange for a visiting nurse to check on the patient's technique after discharge.
- Encourage the patient and family members to contact the American Association of Diabetes Educators and the American Diabetes Association for additional information.

HYPEROSMOLAR HYPERGLYCEMIC NONKETOTIC SYNDROME

Also known as hyperosmolar coma or hyperosmolar nonketotic coma, this acute metabolic complication of diabetes is a medical emergency. It's also the most common complication affecting older diabetes patients. Hyperosmolar hyperglycemic nonketotic syndrome (HHNS) is characterized by severe hyperglycemia (blood glucose levels exceeding 800 mg/dl), hyperosmolarity (serum osmolarity exceeding 280 mOsm/L), and severe dehydration from osmotic diuresis. The syndrome frequently causes impaired consciousness — typically coma or near coma.

When it's not diagnosed early enough for effective treatment, HHNS carries a high mortality rate.

Pathophysiology

HHNS begins with insulin deficiency, which hinders glucose uptake by fat and muscle cells, and causes glucose to accumulate in the blood. At the same time, the liver responds to the demands of the energy-starved cells by converting glycogen to glucose and releasing glucose into the blood, further increasing the blood glucose level. When this level exceeds the renal threshold, excess glucose is excreted in the urine.

The insulin-deprived cells respond by rapidly metabolizing protein, which depletes intracellular potassium and phosphorous and liberates too many amino acids. The liver converts these amino acids into urea and glucose.

The result of these grossly elevated blood glucose levels is increased serum osmolarity and glucosuria, which lead to osmotic diuresis. The massive fluid loss from diuresis causes electrolyte imbalances and dehydration, which further increase osmolarity and diuresis. The glomerular filtration rate decreases and the amount of glucose excreted diminishes, further raising the serum glucose level.

Unabated, the cycle continues, causing additional hyperosmolarity and dehydration.

Causes

Various acute and chronic illnesses and other conditions — such as acute pancreatitis, severe burns, uremia, hypothermia, and thyrotoxicosis — can precipitate HHNS by causing stress, which increases the older person's insulin needs. Previously undiagnosed or untreated diabetes (possibly because the older patient doesn't buy medications or take them regularly) is a common cause of HHNS. In addition, the use of alcohol or certain drugs (including phenytoin, thiazide diuretics, steroids, mannitol, propranolol, immunosuppressants, diazoxide, glucagon, furosemide, ethacrynic acid, and cimetidine) may precipitate HHNS. Certain medical procedures, such as peritoneal dialysis, total parenteral nutrition, prolonged mannitol-induced diuresis, and nasogastric tube feedings with high-protein mixtures, also increase the risk of HHNS.

Assessment findings

The symptoms of HHNS are usually insidious, and the older adult may attribute them to other causes. He may report urinary incontinence, abdominal discomfort, and nausea or vomiting. The caregiver may report a change in level of consciousness. In some cases, the first signs of HHNS are stupor and lethargy.

Inspection reveals a rapid respiratory rate, poor skin turgor, and possibly tacky mucous membranes. Auscultation may reveal hypotension and decreased bowel sounds.

Diagnostic tests

Random blood glucose testing reveals extreme hyperglycemia. Arterial blood gas analysis reveals mild metabolic acidosis.

Treatment

Treatment of HHNS involves fluid and electrolyte replacement and insulin therapy; fluid replacement is even more important than insulin therapy. Expect to give abundant I.V. fluids — hypotonic saline solution or, if the patient has hypovolemic shock, isotonic saline solution. Insulin therapy immediately follows.

A low insulin dosage, usually given by continuous infusion, gradually decreases hyperglycemia and hyperosmolarity. Electrolyte replacement aims to replace ions lost through osmotic diuresis. Normal saline solution replaces sodium and chloride. Once fluid replacement begins to shift potassium back to the cells and lower the serum potassium level, parenteral potassium replacement is ordered.

Complications

HHNS can cause a coma, hypovolemic shock, stroke, and myocardial infarction. Without treatment, it's almost always fatal.

Nursing interventions

- Check for a patent airway and adequate circulation.
- Administer I.V. fluids as ordered.

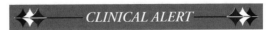

CLINICAL ALERT

Because the older adult is at higher risk for fluid overload, be sure to assess his fluid tolerance while you administer fluids. Also assess his lungs for crackles. Notify the doctor immediately if you find them, and be prepared to slow the infusion rate.

- Begin the insulin infusion as ordered.

CLINICAL ALERT

Patients with HHNS are more sensitive to insulin than patients with diabetic keto-acidosis, so expect to give them less insulin. Monitor blood glucose levels closely to help avoid hypoglycemia, and document the infusion rate and blood glucose levels regularly (see *Documenting continuous insulin infusion,* page 260). When the blood glucose level approaches 250 mg/dl, you'll probably give I.V. glucose and discontinue the insulin infusion. Give further insulin subcutaneously, as ordered.

- Monitor your patient's electrolyte levels every 4 hours, and administer replacement therapy as ordered. Be alert for signs of hypokalemia (cardiovascular irregularities, arrhythmias, decreased peristalsis, and weakness).
- Record your patient's vital signs every 15 minutes until he's stable. Report any drop in blood pressure or increase in heart rate or respiratory rate to the doctor. Monitor level of consciousness and intake and output.

Patient teaching

- Review with the patient the importance of taking prescribed medications on time. If the doctor has ordered home glucose monitoring, make sure the patient is comfortable using the device and have him do a return demonstration. Arrange for a visiting nurse to check on his technique and disease knowledge.
- For a newly diagnosed diabetic patient, your

𝒞HARTING GUIDE

Documenting continuous insulin infusion

A continuous medication infusion requires careful documentation. The rate of the infusion as well as any change and the reason for the change should be documented hourly. With a continuous insulin infusion, blood glucose levels should be documented in the same place. An I.V. flow sheet, like the one below, can easily be adapted to serve both purposes.

Date _11/25/96_

Patient name: _Harold Grunkle_

Solutions: A _NSS – 1,000 ml_

B _50 units insulin in 100 ml D_5W_

C _____

D _____

Time	Sol. A START TIME: 8:00am	Sol. B. START TIME: 8:00am	Blood glucose
10:00 a.m.	100	8	580
11:00 a.m.	100	8	380
11:15 a.m.	100	↓6	

Document the I.V. infusion rate every hour. Designate one column of the flow sheet for blood glucose results. Document the blood glucose level in that column, next to the time when it was taken. In many cases, you will perform the test, and it will take a few minutes to communicate the result to the doctor and receive new orders. In the example above, the patient's blood glucose taken at 11:00 a.m. was 380. At 11:15 the nurse changed the infusion rate to 6 ml/hr to comply with the doctor's order in response to the test. She started a new line with that time entry and continued to take hourly blood glucose measurements.

teaching should include information about diet, medications, exercise, monitoring techniques, hygiene, and how to prevent and recognize hypoglycemia and hyperglycemia. Use the teaching handouts in this section to reinforce your teaching.

● Stress the importance of keeping follow-up appointments with the doctor. To encourage compliance with lifestyle changes, emphasize the importance of blood glucose control in maintaining long-term health.

≈ *14* ≈

Responding to drug and alcohol abuse

Substance abuse, including both drug abuse and misuse and alcohol abuse, is a widespread but often hidden problem in the geriatric population. Its magnitude is unknown because older people typically deny it and many caregivers don't recognize it. Yet it's likely to keep growing as the number of older adults in the U.S. increases.

More than 32 million Americans are now over age 65, and this age group will increase to about 50 million over the next 30 years. Four out of five older people have at least one chronic medical condition, and 35% have three or more. To treat these conditions, the average older person takes 3 to 12 prescription drugs per year, according to a 1995 study, and 1 to 4 nonprescription drugs. This widespread drug use sets the stage for both misuse and abuse.

In addition, many older people abuse alcohol, either to ease the pain of advancing age or because they've always had an alcohol problem. And mixing drugs with alcohol causes special problems, including potentially lethal interactions, that are exacerbated by the age-related physiologic changes that affect the older adult's tolerance of drugs and alcohol. (For more about these changes, see Chapter 16.)

DRUG ABUSE AND MISUSE

A 1979 federal government study defined *drug abuse* as the "nontherapeutic use of any psychoactive substance — including alcohol — in such a manner as to adversely affect some aspect of the user's life. The use pattern may be habitual or occasional. The user may obtain the substance from legitimate prescriptions, friends, nonprescription preparations, or illegal channels."

Drug misuse, defined as the "inappropriate use of drugs for therapeutic purposes," may include inappropriately prescribing drugs for oneself, taking medications prescribed for other people, or failing or forgetting to take drugs according to the doctor's instructions (noncompliance).

Incidence

The incidence of drug dependence in older adults is not as well documented as that of alcohol abuse. However, we do know that only about 60% of older people take their prescribed medications properly and that approximately 30% of all medications they take are nonprescription preparations.

Very few older adults are reported to use illegal substances (such as marijuana, heroin, cocaine, or LSD). This may be because older adults simply "outgrow" the desire to take such drugs or because addicts tend to die before reaching old age. Or the problem may simply be under-reported because elderly drug abusers have escaped treatment or contact with law enforcement.

Studies also indicate that older men tend to misuse psychoactive substances more than women, except for psychotropic drugs, such as Haldol.

Risk factors for substance abuse in older adults

Older people may become dependent on drugs or alcohol for many reasons. Look for the following risk factors when assessing your patient for substance abuse.

Predisposing factors
- Family history (alcohol)
- Previous substance abuse
- Previous pattern of substance consumption (alone or with others)
- Personality traits (sedative-hypnotics and anxiolytics)

Factors that may increase substance exposure and consumption
- Gender (men: alcohol and illicit drugs; women: sedative-hypnotics and anxiolytics)

- Chronic illness with pain (opioid analgesics); insomnia (hypnotic drugs); anxiety (anxiolytics)
- Excessive administration of "as-needed" drugs by caregivers, for example, for sleep or pain (institutionalized older people)
- Life stressors, losses, and social isolation (alcohol used to numb self and deal with emotional pain)
- Family collusion and drinking partners (alcohol)
- Discretionary time and money (alcohol)

Factors that may increase the effects and abuse potential of substances
- Age-associated drug sensitivity (pharmacokinetic and pharmacodynamic factors)
- Chronic medical illnesses
- Other medications (alcohol-drug or drug-drug interactions).

Adapted with permission from Atkinson, R.M., and Ganzini, L. "Substance Abuse," in *The American Psychiatric Press Textbook of Geriatric Neuropsychiatry.* Edited by Coffey, C.E., et al. Washington, D.C.: The American Psychiatric Press, Inc., 1994.

Causes

Information excess, self-medication, polypharmacy, and misreading symptoms are factors that contribute to drug abuse or misuse in older adults. (See *Risk factors for substance abuse in older adults.*)

Information excess

Older adults typically suffer from several chronic disorders at once, some of which require lifelong drug therapy. This translates to frequent doctor's visits and much information to learn about prescribed medications. Older people take longer to process new information because of age-related sensory deficits and changes in short-term memory. They also may be poorly educated and hard to teach. What's more, people who live alone make more medication errors, which can lead to more drug interactions. This is especially true in the rapidly growing home care population.

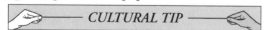 ─── *CULTURAL TIP* ───

Many older people have cultural attitudes and beliefs that may make compliance even harder.

For example, patients from Eastern cultures may prefer alternative therapies such as meditation over conventional drug therapy to treat various conditions.

An older adult may stop taking a drug when his symptoms subside even though the drug has been prescribed for long-term use. In addition, he may suspect that anything that happens after he takes the medication was caused by it.

Self-medication

An older person may be able to comprehend and follow instructions, but this is ineffective unless he can afford the treatment and has access to a doctor. If money and accessibility of medical care are significant obstacles, the patient may be drawn by necessity or convenience to self-medication with nonprescription preparations. Symptoms for which an older person might seek nonprescription drugs are chronic pain, insomnia, indigestion, and constipation.

Eventually the older person's medicine cabinet or

bedside table may contain dozens of containers filled with prescription and nonprescription drugs, some of which may have been prescribed originally for a spouse or another family member. In many cases, the person buys new medications without discarding old ones and rarely — if at all — checks expiration dates, setting up a very dangerous situation, especially for the patient who is cognitively impaired.

Polypharmacy

Older patients who are being treated for multiple disorders or who buy nonprescription drugs for other reasons may fall into a pattern of inappropriate and excessive drug use, called *polypharmacy.* This puts him at high risk for drug interactions and adverse reactions. (See *Risk factors for polypharmacy.*)

Interactions. The drugs most commonly used by older patients are antihypertensives, cardiac drugs, and diuretics. A person who takes two or more drugs concurrently may experience any of the following reactions: *indifference* (no interactive effect); *synergism* (a combined effect greater than the sum total of each individual drug's effects), which is rare; *potentiation* (increased action as a result of the drug combinations); and *antagonism* (negation or reduction of effect of either drug). Any of these effects can occur against the background of altered drug metabolism characteristic of aging.

Adverse reactions. The risk of adverse drug reactions increases with each drug the patient takes. Common adverse reactions include confusion, dizziness, anorexia, incontinence, weakness, immobility, and rashes. The safest approach is to follow the "rule of five": No more than five drugs at the lowest dose should be prescribed.

Many prescription and nonprescription drugs can cause a one-time reaction or symptoms of substance abuse related to repeated overmedication or taking a large quantity one time only. Such drugs include anesthetics, analgesics, anticholinergics, anticonvulsants, antihistamines, antihypertensives, cardiovascular drugs, antimicrobials, antiparkinsonian agents, chemotherapeutic drugs, corticosteroids, GI prepa-

> ### *Risk factors for polypharmacy*
>
> Many factors can contribute to polypharmacy in older adults. The more risk factors that exist, the greater the person's risk of polypharmacy. The most common risk factors include:
> - increased age
> - multiple symptoms
> - multiple medical conditions
> - many prescriptions
> - multiple doctors
> - lack of a primary provider to coordinate therapy
> - use of several pharmacies
> - changes in drug regimen
> - hoarding of medications
> - self-treatment.

rations, muscle relaxants, nonsteroidal anti-inflammatory drugs, antidepressants, and disulfiram.

Nonprescription preparations that contain bromide (such as Bromo-Seltzer and Sominex) can mimic a wide variety of psychiatric problems, including organic brain syndrome, because the bromide accumulates in the body. Antihistamines and other drug classes can cause confusion. (See *Drugs that cause confusion in older adults,* page 264.)

Psychotropic and cardiovascular drugs — taken by 75% of nursing home residents — are responsible for the most serious adverse drug reactions in older adults. For example, a patient who is taking an antihypertensive may suffer a hypertensive crisis from taking a nonprescription cold product such as Robitussin, Nyquil, or Comtrex.

Generic substitution adds a final element of unpredictability. The Food and Drug Administration's "20/20 rule" states that a generic drug must be shown to be equivalent to the proprietary drug in an amount plus or minus 20%. This means that a generic substitute may deliver 20% more or less than the therapeutic dose of the brand name product.

Misinterpretation

Misinterpretation of an older adult's numerous vague symptoms can misdirect drug therapy. For

---

Drugs that cause confusion in older adults

The following drug classes can cause confusion in older adults:
- antiarrhythmics
- anticholinergics
- antiemetics
- antihistamines
- antihypertensives
- antiparkinsonian agents
- antipsychotics
- diuretics
- histamine blockers
- narcotic analgesics
- sedative-hypnotics
- tranquilizers.

---

example, exposure to heavy metals, rat poisons, or volatile substances such as household gas and paint may cause impaired cognition, hallucinations, delusions, and even seizures. A doctor who fails to detect the underlying cause of these symptoms might prescribe drug therapy when simply removing the toxic substances would resolve the problem.

For more information about drug therapy in older adults, see Chapter 16.

Assessment findings

When assessing your older patient for drug abuse, you'll need to be aware of how age-related physiologic changes affect drug pharmacokinetics — specifically, absorption, distribution, metabolism, and elimination.

The signs and symptoms of drug abuse — depression, confusion, anorexia, weakness, ataxia, tremor, constipation, diarrhea, and urine retention — can also be manifestations of other problems. So you'll need to carefully evaluate your patient to rule out any other imitative medical problems.

Patient history

Obtaining an accurate and thorough history is crucial in assessing an older person for drug abuse or misuse. But you'll need to deal with certain barriers that older people present, such as sensory losses (especially hearing), cognitive impairment, and physical debility. In addition, the older patient may fail to disclose signs and symptoms of drug abuse because he thinks they're a manifestation of the normal aging process. To overcome these barriers, you'll need to be patient; face the older patient when you interview him; ask simple, direct questions; and show respect for the person's intelligence and experience.

A thorough drug history should include all prescription and nonprescription drugs currently taken, the current drug schedule, the patient's knowledge of diseases and medications, any adverse reactions or other problems the patient experienced while taking the medications, the number of prescribing doctors, the number of pharmacies used, the patient's ability to pay for prescriptions, the patient's use of other drugs (including alcohol, caffeine, and nicotine), his level of impairment (including physical, mental, and sensory), his level of compliance, his beliefs about medications, his educational level, and his previous compliance with treatment regimens. Whenever possible, include family members or appropriate caregivers in your history taking.

Be alert for clues suggesting special needs or problems that may contribute to noncompliance, such as the following:
- medication that requires equipment the patient does not own
- medication regimen that doesn't fit the patient's lifestyle (for example, a schedule requiring medication to be taken with meals three times daily when the patient only eats two meals per day)
- unclear instructions
- instructions that are not in the patient's native language
- patient's reporting that instructions were given in a noisy, hurried, or busy atmosphere.

Also be alert for possible limitations that might interfere with compliance, such as inability to open childproof containers because of joint disease; inability to get to the pharmacy to have a prescription filled; lack of proper storage facilities (such as a refrigerator for storing suspensions); and inability to swallow tablets or capsules.

Treatment

The key to treatment of drug abuse and misuse is prevention, which is achieved largely through education — of both health care providers and elderly patients themselves. Health care professionals need to become informed about the serious problem of polypharmacy among the elderly. Factors that commonly hinder diagnosis and proper treatment of drug misuse include focusing only on the older patient's admitting condition, reluctance to intervene, and attributing presenting symptoms as secondary to multiple health problems and perceptual impairment rather than to drug use.

All health care professionals — doctors, pharmacists, and nurses — must collaborate in an effort to simplify the medication regimens of elderly patients whenever possible. The concept of "counterdetailing," a face-to-face educational session between the doctor and a clinical pharmacist, has been proposed to reduce the prescription of targeted drugs.

And older patients themselves must be educated about their medications, including the importance of taking all drugs exactly as prescribed. They must also learn not to expect a prescription for treatment of every symptom.

Complications

Negative consequences of drug abuse and misuse in older adults include deteriorating health; development of drug dependence; drug sensitivity, leading to reactions that mimic other illnesses, especially mental illness; and suicide. Note that barbiturates are the most prevalent means of suicide among older people.

Nursing diagnoses

For your patient diagnosed with drug abuse, you'll need to identify nursing diagnoses and establish goals. The three most appropriate nursing diagnoses for the patient with drug abuse are knowledge deficit, noncompliance, and risk for injury.

Nursing interventions

Patient education is one of the most important aspects of nursing interventions for drug abuse. Teaching is most effective when provided in small incre-

ments of specific information. For older adults, "unlearning" previously stored information is the most difficult type of learning.

Additional interventions include simplifying the patient's drug regimen and modifying his self-medication routines.

◆◆ ── CLINICAL ALERT ── ◆◆

The Omnibus Budget Reconciliation Act (OBRA) established specific guidelines for use of antipsychotics and benzodiazepines in long-term care settings. These guidelines call for careful and well-documented use of all psychotropic medications. The long-acting benzodiazepines include Valium, Dalmane, Tranxene, Doral, Centrax, Paxipam, and Klonopin. OBRA guidelines state that benzodiazepines cannot be given for more than 10 consecutive days for sleep or for more than 4 consecutive months for anxiety or dementia unless gradual dose reduction is attempted and function improvement with long-acting benzodiazepines is noted.

Patient teaching

Older patients and their families need to learn about medications and about normal and abnormal changes associated with aging. In these times of scarce medical resources, consumers are becoming more responsible for their own education. Senior centers, Over 50 Clubs, and publications by insurance providers are useful vehicles for disseminating drug information. Nurses in doctor's offices have a unique opportunity to educate patients at routine visits before problems occur.

When teaching an older patient and his family, use a variety of methods, including written and verbal instructions; multiple sessions, which allow information to be broken down into small parts to improve comprehension; and demonstrations by patient and family to ensure that they understand what you've taught.

Make sure your teaching about drugs includes:
● name of medication
● class of drug
● purpose

- proper administration
- potential adverse effects
- precautions
- proper storage.

Pharmaceutical company package inserts are a helpful source of information but often use language geared to the professional. Instead, provide medication sheets written in layman's terms using a simple format to facilitate comprehension. Many pharmacies also supply a helpful fact sheet with every prescription that includes warnings about possible adverse effects and drug interactions.

Simplifying the drug regimen
The goal of simplifying the drug regimen is to improve the patient's compliance. Work with the doctor to try to reduce the number of times per day the patient must take his medications. Arrange the dosage schedule to match the patient's lifestyle, taking into consideration his usual activities of daily living (ADLs), nutritional status, functional limitations, and the availability of resources and support people.

Encourage the patient and family to use one pharmacy for all prescriptions. Many pharmacies now keep computerized records that can alert the pharmacist and, in turn, the patient, to possible interactions, contraindications, and other problems.

Use compliance aids, such as calendars, dispenser packs, blister packs, telephone calls from family members or friends, and beepers or timers, to help the patient who has difficulty remembering. Make sure the plan is individualized. The patient may have an effective reminder system in place and may just need some reinforcement.

Modifying self-medication practices
When helping a patient improve self-medication practices, be sure to do the following:
- Help the patient identify his self-medication practices, including types of nonprescription drugs used, frequency, and rationale for use.
- Encourage proper selection of drugs by reading labels and checking with the pharmacist or doctor before taking any nonprescription drugs.
- Suggest using nonpharmacologic therapies, such as heat or cold applications and exercise for arthritis

and dietary changes for insomnia; be sure to instruct the patient in all aspects of these therapies to minimize the risk of injury.
- Educate the patient about the potential hazards of self-medication, especially if he's already taking prescription medications or if he drinks.
- Provide written instructions, and ask the patient to repeat them to you to ensure his comprehension.
- Encourage the patient to check all old medications for name and date and to discard outdated ones.
- Instruct the patient to avoid caffeine and alcohol, to decrease daytime sleep, and to establish a daily routine that includes exercise early in the day. This will encourage a normal wake-sleep pattern and reduce the need for sleeping medications.
- Periodically review the patient's entire drug regimen as part of a routine evaluation. Ask the patient or a family member to bring in all medications — both prescription and nonprescription — to which the patient has access. Evaluate the regimen for drugs with no obvious indication, duplicate medications, use of medications with adverse interactions, contraindicated drugs, inappropriate drug dosages, and drugs used to counteract adverse effects of other prescribed drugs. Determine whether drugs prescribed for short-term relief of symptoms can be discontinued. To ensure a thorough and accurate evaluation, make sure you know the patient's diagnosis and the lowest effective drug dosage to treat the diagnosis, know the optimal administration routes, report adverse reactions immediately, and use "as needed" medications sparingly and only for the prescribed purpose.
- Educate the patient about the hazards of altering dosages, discontinuing medications without the doctor's approval, and supplementing prescribed drug therapy with nonprescription preparations without the health care team's knowledge.

ALCOHOL ABUSE

Research suggests that alcoholism affects 2% to 10% of adults over age 60. More than half of all geriatric hospital admissions are due to alcohol-related problems; according to the National Institute on Alcohol Abuse and Alcoholism, the figure may be as high as 70%.

Causes

A significant number of people begin drinking heavily after age 60. Because these older adults have no history of substance abuse and have shown no signs of alcohol abuse before age 60, researchers theorize that the excessive drinking is a direct response to the stressors associated with aging. The late-onset type of alcoholism is known as reactive, or Type II, alcoholism. (See *Stressors that lead to alcoholism in older adults.*)

In reactive alcoholism, the proportion of patients with a family history of alcoholism is less than 40%. A recent study of older alcoholics showed that 97% of the subjects had depression as a primary diagnosis and alcoholism as a secondary diagnosis. The researchers believed this was due to depression masking alcoholism.

Assessment findings

Symptoms of alcohol abuse are easy to miss in older adults because of multiple preexisting conditions that may cause similar symptoms. So you'll need to be especially alert for clues that may arise in the patient history or physical exam.

Patient history

The patient history may yield such clues as problems in caring for himself, injuries, infections, malnutrition, sensory alterations, anxiety, and sleep disturbances. Suspect alcohol abuse if the history includes loss of a spouse, financial duress, isolation due to immobility, recent retirement, and lack of close relatives.

Physical examination

When performing the assessment, be alert for the following clues:
● Treatment of a normally treatable medical disease is ineffective.
● The patient complains of insomnia or chronic fatigue associated with poor sleep.

Stressors that lead to alcoholism in older adults

Researchers believe that many older people start drinking heavily as a response to the stresses of aging. These include:
● physical changes that can cause immobility, isolation, loss of health, and sometimes chronic pain
● emotional losses, such as loss of spouse, friends, family, and coworkers; loss of purpose, identity, fulfillment, and self-esteem associated with working
● feelings of helplessness
● loss of routine
● boredom
● financial worries.

● The patient complains of diarrhea or urinary incontinence and exhibits weight loss or malnutrition on inspection.
● The patient exhibits signs of trauma, such as frequent falls, accidents, bruising, or fractures.
● The patient exhibits noticeable deterioration in cognitive function, including confusion and short-term memory loss.
● The patient frequently complains of anxiety and requests or uses antianxiety agents, hypnotics, or sedatives.
● The postoperative patient exhibits unexplained agitation, anxiety, and confusion or a new onset of seizure activity, especially without a history of cerebrovascular disease.

Assessment findings include repeated falls or fractures, burns, pressure ulcers, recurrent lung infections, weight loss or other signs of malnourishment, self-neglect, multiple spider nevi, bruising, scarring, gastric distress, poor appetite, motor disturbances (apraxia, ataxia), memory loss, insomnia or other inconsistent sleeping patterns, and depression.

During the assessment, keep in mind the normal, age-related physiologic changes. These include decreased gastric pH, slower regeneration of organ cells, decrease in circulating blood, decreased metabolism, decreased rate of excretion, increase in the percentage of fat cells, decreased body water, and lean body mass. Because of these changes, the reactive alcoholic will show signs of toxicity sooner than the younger, healthy adult.

Because of decreased peristalsis and slow regeneration of GI organ cells, the reactive alcoholic may have gastritis, peptic ulcers, malnutrition, or GI hemorrhage. Gait disturbances may be due to a thiamine deficiency.

In assessing the cardiovascular system, you may detect peripheral edema, arrhythmias, or cardiomegaly. Because of the liver's vascularity and its intricate relationship to the cardiovascular system, signs of liver damage, such as jaundice and ascites, may also be present. Peripheral neuropathy and tremors may be due to alcohol consumption.

Other findings may include palmar erythema and hepatomegaly in late-stage alcohol dependence.

Laboratory findings

In older patients, laboratory findings may not indicate problems until alcoholism has become advanced. Specific laboratory tests used to detect alcohol abuse include gamma-GT (GGT), aspartate aminotransferase, and mean corpuscular volume (MCV). GGT is particularly sensitive to the effects of alcohol; elevated GGT levels may persist for more than 60 hours following moderate alcohol intake. Levels above 24 U/L in females and above 37 U/L in males may indicate alcohol abuse. Aspartate aminotransferase levels above 20 U/L may indicate acute hepatic disease. MCV, the ratio of hematocrit to the RBC count, indicates the size of red blood cells and helps to diagnose anemia, a consequence of alcoholism. Normal MCV is 84 to 99 fl.

In addition, approximately half of all alcohol abusers experience malabsorption of folate, vitamin B (thiamine), vitamin B_{12}, and fat. Malabsorption may result from mucosal damage in the intestine, increased GI motility, and reduced biliary and pancreatic secretions. Accelerated osteoporotic changes may also occur.

Assessment tools

Various assessment tools have been developed for evaluating alcohol abuse, including the Michigan Alcohol Screening Test, the CHARM questionnaire, and the CAGE questionnaire. One of these assessment tools should be incorporated into the health history completed on admission to the facility.

The Michigan Alcohol Screening Test (MAST) consists of a 25-item questionnaire. It's easy to use because it takes less than 10 minutes to complete, requires no special training to administer, is suitable for administration in a variety of settings and has a high level of validity.

The most recent variation of the MAST test is the MAST-G, which was developed to evaluate late-onset alcoholism in older adults. However, this test is still new and validation studies are still in progress. (See *MAST-G: Alcoholism screening test for older adults.*)

The CHARM and CAGE questionnaires are brief, unscored surveys that provide some standardization for health histories. The CHARM questionnaire uses the acronym CHARM to elicit information about alcohol and prescription drug use in older patients. (See *The CHARM questionnaire,* page 270.) The CAGE questionnaire, which asks only four questions, is very effective in identifying alcoholics in clinical settings.

The *Diagnostic and Statistical Manual of Mental Disorders,* 4th edition *(DSM-IV),* cites seven criteria for establishing a diagnosis of substance dependence. Three or more of the seven criteria must be manifested at any one time in the same year to establish a diagnosis of dependence. Researchers of geriatric alcoholism, however, think that applying the *DSM-IV* criteria to older people is difficult because the emphasis is on consequences that they don't experience.

Although these assessment tools are excellent and proven, they merely provide a standard framework for health histories. Remember that denial may distort the patient's responses to the questions, thus invalidating the findings.

If you're a home health nurse, you can search for more clues in the patient's home environment. Cigarette burns in the upholstery and poor housekeeping combined with failure to respond to traditional treatments for presenting symptoms (such as Maalox for GI upset or Elavil for depression) may point to substance abuse.

CHARTING GUIDE

MAST-G: Alcoholism screening test for older adults

Use this tool, known as MAST-G, to help assess your older patient for possible alcohol abuse. Score each "yes" answer with one point; give each "no" answer a zero. Five or more "yes" responses indicates that the patient has an alcohol problem.

	YES (1)	NO (0)
1. After drinking, have you ever noticed an increase in your heart rate or beating in your chest?	____	____
2. When talking with others, do your ever underestimate how much you actually drink?	____	____
3. Does alcohol make you sleepy so that you often fall asleep in your chair?	____	____
4. After a few drinks, have you sometimes not eaten or been able to skip a meal because you didn't feel hungry?	____	____
5. Does having a few drinks help decrease your shakiness or tremors?	____	____
6. Does alcohol sometimes make it hard for you to remember parts of the day or night?	____	____
7. Do you have rules for yourself that you won't drink before a certain time of the day?	____	____
8. Have you lost interest in hobbies or activities you used to enjoy?	____	____
9. When you wake up in the morning, do you ever have trouble remembering part of the night before?	____	____
10. Does having a drink help you sleep?	____	____
11. Do you hide your alcohol bottles from family members?	____	____
12. After a social gathering, have you ever felt embarrassed because you drank too much?	____	____
13. Have you ever been concerned that drinking might be harmful to your health?	____	____
14. Do you like to end your evening with a nightcap?	____	____
15. Did you find that your drinking increased after someone close to you died?	____	____
16. In general, would you prefer to have a few drinks at home rather than go out to social events?	____	____
17. Are you drinking more now than in the past?	____	____
18. Do you usually take a drink to relax or calm your nerves?	____	____
19. Do you drink to take your mind off your problems?	____	____
20. Have you ever increased your drinking after experiencing a loss in your life?	____	____
21. Do you sometimes drive when you've had too much to drink?	____	____
22. Has a doctor or a nurse ever said they were worried or concerned about your drinking?	____	____
23. Have you ever made rules to manage your drinking?	____	____
24. Does having a drink help when you feel lonely?	____	____

Adapted with permission from Beresford, T.P. "Alcoholism in the Elderly," *International Review of Psychiatry* 5:477-83, 1993.

HARTING GUIDE

The CHARM questionnaire

This questionnaire asks five questions, using the acronym CHARM, to assess older adults for substance abuse.

C = Cut down?
H = How do you use?
A = Anyone concerned?
R = Relief use?
M = More than intended?

C "Have you ever **cut** down or quit drinking?"
"When, in your life, would you say your drinking was the heaviest?"
"Have you thought recently that you should cut down?"

H "**How** do you use your alcohol?"
"What are your rules about alcohol use?"
"Has your drinking changed in the last 3 months? Year?"

A "Has **anyone** ever seemed concerned about your drinking?"
People have different feelings about drinking alcohol.
How do your friends and family view your drinking?"
"Have you ever had health problems that caused your doctor to ask you to alter your drinking habits?"

R "Have you ever used alcohol to **relieve** problems?" (Look for social or emotional discomfort, such as loneliness or depression.)
"When you drink alcohol, what's usually the reason?"
"Do you ever have a drink when you feel lonely or upset?"
"How is your sleep?"
"What do you use to help you fall asleep?"

M "Do you ever drink **more** than you intended? What were the circumstances?"
"Most people have times when they drink more than they intended to.
What situations might cause you to drink more than you expected to?"

Adapted with permission from Sumnicht, G. *Sailing White Horses: Adventures with Older Substance Abusers*. Madison, Wis.: PICADA, 1991.

Treatment

The prognosis for late-onset alcoholics is better than for other alcoholics if they receive treatment. Unfortunately, by the time the older person is treated for dependence, permanent damage has already occurred in many cases.

Once the person has decided to stop drinking, the health care team must carefully manage the withdrawal process to achieve detoxification. (De-toxification in a treatment center is necessary only if the patient has a medical illness that requires monitoring.) Another important step is identifying sources of stress and helping patients find ways to regain control over their lives.

Confronting the patient

The Johnson method detailed in the book *I'll Quit Tomorrow* has been a favored approach in home care. In this approach, family members and others with influence over the patient confront him with the facts about his addiction and the behavior it causes. The goal is to encourage the patient to confront the consequences of his behavior and thus motivate him to seek help. The Johnson method differs from the Alcoholics Anonymous (AA) approach in that the support team does not wait for the patient to hit "rock bottom" before beginning interventions.

Dealing with physical withdrawal

The standard therapy for alcoholism is detoxification, administration of vitamin C and B-complex vitamins (especially thiamine), and fluid replacement. Treatment of coexisting psychiatric disorders (such as anxiety and affective disorder) and cognitive impairment may be necessary during acute withdrawal.

Signs and symptoms of alcohol withdrawal include tachycardia, hypertension, shortness of breath, headache, nausea, irritability, psychomotor agitation, and sleep disturbances. In severe withdrawal, alcohol withdrawal syndrome (delirium tremens) occurs from increased activity of the autonomic nervous system. Depression, anxiety, distorted perception, and hallucinations may be manifestations of neuron excitation.

Withdrawal may be more severe if the patient is also experiencing concomitant malnutrition, physical illness, emotional stress, depression, social isolation, and fatigue.

The benzodiazepines lorazepam (Ativan) and oxazepam (Serax) are the drugs of choice for short-term administration to patients undergoing drug withdrawal. (Dosage for older adults is one-half to one-third the normal adult dosage.) However, these drugs may raise problems of their own regarding dependence and compliance, and their use must be closely monitored.

Some researchers advocate using chlordiazepoxide hydrochloride (Librium) to treat symptoms of alcohol withdrawal in older adults because it produces a smoother withdrawal without cumulative sedation and it promotes less dependence than long-acting benzodiazepines such as diazepam. But others do

not advocate treatment with benzodiazepines unless the patient has significant withdrawal symptoms, such as marked diaphoresis, tremors, agitation, or cardiac irregularities such as tachycardia. Clonidine (Catapres) patches may be substituted for benzodiazepines in moderate withdrawal cases. Clonidine controls autonomic nervous system excitation, insomnia, and anxiety but will not inhibit the tremors of alcohol withdrawal syndrome.

Detoxification should be achieved, if possible, without the use of disulfiram because of the risk of liver damage.

If the patient is debilitated, thiamine treatment should begin. The thiamine should be administered before any I.V. dextrose to avoid Wernicke's encephalopathy caused by depletion of marginal stores of thiamine. Thiamine should then be given orally along with multivitamins.

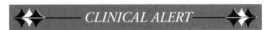
CLINICAL ALERT

Because the older patient may be more sensitive to these drugs, withdrawal may take longer (weeks or months) and be more severe than in younger adults.

Changing the patient's outlook

By working cooperatively with the doctor, family members, home health care agencies, social agencies, and senior citizen centers, you may be able to help the patient develop a positive attitude toward life and reduce his need to drink. In the institutional setting, you'll need to surrender some of your control over the patient and make him responsible for his addiction. For long-term success, the recovering patient must learn to fill the place alcohol once occupied in his life with something constructive.

Other strategies for coping with the psychological aspects of alcoholism include AA, adverse conditioning, behavioral psychotherapy, and psychosocial approaches. The AA program encourages the patient to learn about his disease, confront his denial, change his attitudes and lifestyle, and make a commitment to recovery. Some older adults find this program unappealing because of the stigma surrounding stereotypical alcoholics. One way to deal with this reluctance is to help older people form their own AA chapter.

Adverse conditioning associates alcohol with negative sights, smells, tastes, and thoughts to evoke negative reinforcement. Behavioral psychotherapy establishes behavioral goals and a time frame in which to complete the goals, which may range from total abstinence to holistic networking (group treatment through the support of others).

The psychosocial approach is the most widely used in treatment programs because it addresses through talk therapy the social and psychological stressors associated with aging. This approach can center on the individual, group, or family and often can take place within the patient's facility. Geriatric group programs restore members' capacity to enter into relationships, improve self-image and communication, and provide catharsis.

Other options
Day treatment programs developed specifically for reactive older alcoholics have been particularly successful because of the program structure. These programs focus on three areas: primary health needs and risk reduction; education about the physical, emotional, and psychosocial needs of the older patient; and skill-building in individual coping and socialization.

Inpatient programs, some of which embrace the AA philosophy, also are available. These programs designed for older alcoholics typically last 90 to 120 days and deal with the older person's special problems, including physical disabilities, cognitive impairment, aphasia, and sensory deficits. They also provide physical therapy, occupational therapy, special diets, and adaptive equipment. These programs provide sufficient time to integrate new information and make the behavioral changes necessary to achieve sobriety.

Complications
The older alcoholic may suffer permanent damage in a relatively short period because of the normal physiologic changes connected with aging and because it takes less alcohol to cause toxicity. Hepatotoxicity, nephrotoxicity, GI toxicity, and cerebral toxicity put the patient at risk for permanent cognitive impairment, decreased liver and kidney function, and GI damage leading to ulcers and hemorrhage. (See *Complications of alcohol use*.)

Alcohol can increase the metabolism of other drugs, such as anticonvulsants (Dilantin), anticoagulants (Coumadin), and antidiabetic drugs (Orinase). The combination of alcohol and diuretics can lower blood pressure, which is already compromised in an older person and may be labile. Motor, sensory, verbal, and global deficits are marked in alcoholics and very marked in the older alcoholic.

Other physical complications may include the following:
- *Subacute organic mental syndrome* is related to active alcohol abuse. Symptoms include confusion, memory loss, decreased verbal fluency, and loss of visual-spatial and problem-solving skills. Symptoms subside after 3 to 4 weeks of abstinence.
- *Wernicke's syndrome,* which occurs secondary to thiamine deficiency, is marked by true delirium with clouding of alertness, focal neurologic deficits, ataxia, and ophthalmoplegia.
- *Korsakoff's syndrome* is characterized by profound anterograde and retrograde amnesia, although sensorium and verbal fluency are intact.
- *Alcoholic polyneuropathy* causes decreased sensation in the extremities, fine motor dysfunction, and weakness, especially in the lower extremities and hands. When slight to moderate, it usually resolves almost completely within 6 months of alcohol abstinence and rehabilitation.
- *Alcoholic dementia* may be diagnosed if organic mental syndrome does not clear up after alcohol abstinence lasting 3 weeks. In this case, the patient will demonstrate symptoms of memory loss, aphasia, and apraxia.
- *Marchiafava-Bignami disease* is a rare disorder that causes demyelination of the corpus callosum in chronic alcoholics (predominantly males). Nutritional factors may be involved. Symptoms include agitation and confusion with progressive dementia and frontal release signs (altered impulses control judgment). The patient may recover after several months, but the disease may also progress to seizures, coma, and death. Although it first appeared

Complications of alcohol use

Alcohol can damage body tissues by its direct irritating effects, changes that take place in the body during its metabolism, aggravation of existing deisease, accidents occurring during intoxication, and interactions between the substance and drugs. Such tissue damage can cause the following complications:

Cardiopulmonary complications
- Cardiac arrhythmias
- Cardiomyopathy
- Chronic obstructive pulmonary disease
- Essential hypertension
- Increased risk of tuberculosis
- Pneumonia

Hepatic complications
- Alcoholic hepatitis
- Cirrhosis
- Fatty liver

GI complications
- Chronic diarrhea
- Esophageal cancer
- Esophageal varices
- Esophagitis
- Gastric ulcers
- Gastritis
- GI bleeding
- Malabsorption
- Pancreatitis

Neurologic complications
- Alcoholic dementia
- Alcoholic hallucinosis
- Alcohol withdrawal delirium
- Korsakoff's syndrome
- Peripheral neuropathy
- Seizure disorders
- Subdural hematoma
- Wernicke's encephalopathy

Psychiatric complications
- Amotivational syndrome
- Depression
- Fetal alcohol syndrome
- Impaired social and occupational functioning
- Multiple substance abuse
- Suicide

Other complications
- Beriberi
- Hypoglycemia
- Leg and foot ulcers
- Prostatitis

among red wine drinkers in Italy, Marchiafava-Bignami disease has been reported in many other countries and with many other alcoholic beverages.

Nursing diagnoses

For the alcoholic patient, nursing diagnoses may include but not be limited to the following:
- Altered cerebral, renal, cardiopulmonary, and GI tissue perfusion
- Altered nutrition: Less than body requirements
- Altered role performance
- Anxiety
- Fluid volume deficit
- Impaired adjustment
- Impaired social interaction
- Ineffective individual coping
- Ineffective family coping
- Knowledge deficit of substance abuse
- Noncompliance
- Powerlessness
- Risk for infection
- Risk for injury
- Self-care deficit
- Sensory or perceptual alterations
- Situational low self-esteem
- Social isolation
- Spiritual distress

Nursing interventions

Nursing care of the older alcoholic must focus on both his physical and psychological needs. You'll need to ensure the patient's safety and take care of any physical problems while helping him confront the stressors that cause him to drink and develop positive coping skills. Whenever possible, encourage the patient and his family to participate in planning and implementing the patient's care.

Acute intoxication or withdrawal

● Carefully monitor the patient's mental status, heart rate, breath sounds, blood pressure, and temperature every 30 minutes to 6 hours, depending on the severity of his signs and symptoms.

● Assess the patient for signs of inadequate nutrition and dehydration. Institute seizure precautions and administer prescribed drugs to treat withdrawal.

Chronic alcohol abuse

● Orient the patient to reality because he may have hallucinations and may try to harm himself or others. Minimize noise and shadows to delusions and hallucinations. Use restraints only to protect the patient or others.

● Approach the patient in a nonthreatening way. Limit sustained eye contact, which he may perceive as threatening. Listen attentively, respond with empathy, and explain all procedures even if the patient is verbally abusive.

● Monitor the patient for signs of depression or impending suicide.

● Help him accept his drinking problem and the need for abstinence.

● Refer the patient to AA, and offer to arrange a visit from an AA member. Refer spouses of alcoholics to Al-Anon and adult children of alcoholics to the National Association for Children of Alcoholics.

Johnson method of confrontaion

● Before confronting the patient, evaluate his level of denial, significant relationships, history of alcohol abuse, and previous social and recreational activities. Also assess the support team's knowledge and beliefs about alcoholism because their attitudes can significantly affect the outcome.

● Encourage positive health behaviors and offer emotional support in a calm, nonjudgmental man-

ner. Present various treatment options. Avoid being vague. Be prepared for rationalization as a defense, and prepare in advance solutions to the excuses the patient may offer to avoid seeking help. You'll need to break down his defenses to motivate him to seek help before he suffers permanent damage.

● Once the motivation process has begun, long-term goals should focus on increasing the patient's socialization and support network, improving his diet, and implementing an exercise program. A multidisciplinary approach is essential. Support groups, such as AA, Seniors for Sobriety, and Helping Hands, can offer large-print materials and peer support, and can fill the gaps that exist in treatment after acute detoxification.

Patient teaching

● Educate the patient and his family about the need to abstain permanently from alcohol.

● Explain to the patient and family that relapses may occur. Help them develop a plan of action.

PREVENTING SUBSTANCE ABUSE

There is an urgent need to educate health care providers about assessment and early intervention for drug and alcohol abuse in the geriatric setting. Recent studies have found that nursing curricula provide almost no education about the addictive process. Nurse clinicians confirm that they are ill-prepared to diagnose and care for addicted people.

Older patients frequently seek medical help for anxiety, depression, or confusion. Without proper screening, they're often misdiagnosed and given drugs as treatment, which may make their problems worse. Doctors need accurate reports from nursing staff to prescribe appropriate treatment. Home health employees, especially aides who spend the most time with the patient, should be adequately trained to report changes in the patient's nutritional status, mental status, sleep patterns, and ADLs.

Detecting elder abuse and neglect

Elder abuse and neglect is a serious and prevalent problem for older people in home, community, and institutional settings. Reported instances of abuse and neglect involve people of both sexes; both well and frail; and all racial, ethnic, and socioeconomic groups. Frail older people who live alone are particularly vulnerable to self-neglect, and those who become dependent on others for care are at higher risk for abuse by either a family member or a caregiver who is under intense strain.

Although abuse and neglect of older people is not a new phenomenon, it recently has received more attention. Yet, despite growing awareness of this problem by health care professionals, the abuse remains extremely difficult to detect.

Older people are given inadequate care for reasons beyond abuse and neglect, such as ignorance, disability, poverty, lack of access to care, and poor caregiver training. It's up to professionals who care for aging adults to determine when inadequate care is actually due to abuse or neglect.

Incidence
In a 1988 survey of 2,020 older adults living in Boston, 3.2% of the people reported having been abused, either physically (about two-thirds of the cases) or verbally. A 1989 study of abuse in nursing homes found that 36% of the nurses and assistants had seen at least one incident of physical abuse, and 81% had observed at least one incident of psychological abuse in the previous year. Excessive restraint was the most common type of physical abuse reported; yelling was the most common psychological abuse.

Determining the actual incidence of elder abuse and neglect is difficult. Health care professionals may fail to identify and report the problem for any of several reasons: denial of the extent of the problem in society; ignorance of signs and symptoms; difficulty in identifying abuse without obvious signs of battering; ignorance of reporting laws and procedures; and ageism (incidents in which the older person's reports of abuse are ignored because he's labeled "demented"). In other cases, the abused older adult may be unwilling or unable to report the problem for fear of retaliation, not having his basic needs met, and being institutionalized or abandoned. When the abusive person is an offspring, the parent may be reluctant to report the abuse because of shame and embarrassment and feeling that he has failed as a parent. Finally, in some cases the older person is physically unable to report the abuse because of illness or such impairments as dementia or aphasia.

Definitions and types
Definitions and categories of elder abuse vary from state to state and among agencies. The U.S. Department of Health and Human Services defines abuse as "the willful infliction of injury, unreasonable confinement, intimidation, or punishment with resulting physical harm or pain or mental anguish, or deprivation by an individual, including a caretaker,

of goods or services that are necessary to attain or maintain physical, mental, and psychosocial well-being." The Federal government defines neglect, on the other hand, as any "failure to provide goods and services necessary to avoid physical harm, mental anguish, or mental illness." It's neglect, too, when an older person doesn't receive adequate care — for example, if he's left in soiled clothing for extended periods of time.

At the state level, Ohio, for example, defines abuse as "knowingly causing physical harm or recklessly causing serious physical harm to a resident by physical contact with the resident or by the use of physical or chemical restraint, medication, or isolation as punishment, for staff convenience, excessively, as a substitute for treatment, or in amounts that preclude habilitation and treatment." Ohio defines neglect as "recklessly failing to provide a resident with any treatment, care, goods, or service necessary to maintain the health or safety of the resident when the failure results in serious physical harm to the resident."

Common elements of all these definitions of abuse are:
- an action
- committed knowingly
- against another individual
- and causing harm to that individual.

Neglect, on the other hand, contains the following common elements:
- failure to provide treatment, care, goods, or a service
- for another person
- which omission leads to harm for that individual.

The absence of a standard definition of abuse makes it even more urgent that you be vigilant for signs of abuse as you assess and treat older adults.

Abuse and neglect include physical abuse, psychological abuse, financial exploitation, physical neglect, psychological neglect, self-neglect, and violation of rights.

Causes

What specific characteristics put an older person at risk for mistreatment? Studies have shown that cognitive impairment (for example, dementia) and

shared living arrangements are the risk factors most likely to predispose older people to mistreatment. The extreme psychological and physical demands placed on a caregiver by a cognitively impaired person, who may exhibit aggressive, disruptive, and hostile behaviors, predispose the older adult to mistreatment by a fatigued and demoralized caregiver. And, shared living arrangements increase the opportunities to develop stress and tension that escalate to episodes of abuse, particularly if an older person is heavily dependent on a caregiver.

What specific characteristics of caregivers put them at risk for mistreating an older person? Abusers often have a history of family violence, alcoholism or drug addiction, or mental illness. Additionally, abusers may be unduly dependent on the older person for either housing or financial support. Isolation is another factor that may contribute to elder abuse. In many cases, the caregiver has no support system of family or friends with whom to share concerns, and the elder also has no family, friends, or neighbors who visit (see *Risk factors for elder abuse*).

IDENTIFYING ABUSE AND NEGLECT

A team approach, with its collaborative style, is generally believed to be the best method of detecting elder abuse and neglect. Researchers have suggested that a geriatric interdisciplinary team, consisting of a doctor, a nurse, and a social worker, can detect signs of elder abuse more effectively than a single health care professional.

Using a systematic approach — as provided by a written protocol, for example — can also help the assessment process (see *Protocol for identifying and assessing elder abuse and neglect,* pages 278 to 280).

The identification process begins when a health care professional first comes in contact with an older person. The most common settings are the emergency room, the doctor's office, or the home. Each setting requires different skills for detecting and assessing abuse and neglect. For example, an older

Risk factors for elder abuse

The following risk factors are most likely to contribute to abuse of elderly people.

RISK FACTOR	MECHANISM
Poor health and functional impairment in the older person	Disability reduces the older person's ability to seek help and defend himself.
Cognitive impairment in the older person	Aggressive or disruptive behavior resulting from dementia may precipitate abuse. Higher rates of abuse have been found among patients with dementia.
Substance abuse or mental illness on the part of the abuser	Abusers are likely to abuse alcohol or drugs and to have serious mental illness, which in turn leads to abusive behavior.
Dependence of the abuser on the victim	Many abusers depend on the victim financially — for housing and other forms of financial support. Abuse results from attempts by a relative (especially an adult child) to obtain resources from the older person.
Shared living arrangement	Older adults who live alone are much less likely to be abused. A shared living situation provides greater opportunities for tension and conflict, which generally precede incidents of abuse.
External factors causing stress	Stressful life events and continuing financial strain decrease the family's resistance and increase the likelihood of abuse.
Social isolation	Older people with few social contacts are more likely to be victims of abuse. Isolation reduces the likelihood that abuse will be detected and stopped. In addition, social support can buffer the effects of stress.
History of violence	Particularly among spouses, a history of violence in the relationship may predict abuse in later life.

Adapted with permission from Lachs, M.S., and Pillemer, K. "Abuse and neglect of elderly persons," *The New England Journal of Medicine* 332(7):437-43, February 16, 1995.

person who arrives in the emergency room because of an urgent problem may have overt signs of physical abuse, such as bruises, making detection easier. But a visit to the doctor's office can be scheduled when overt signs of physical abuse are less noticeable or have healed, making abuse harder to detect. The home health care nurse, on the other hand, has the advantage of observing the older person in his own surroundings but must complete the initial evaluation without another team member's assessment and opinion.

In any setting, psychological abuse and exploitation are more difficult to identify than physical abuse. Self-neglect is similarly challenging to identify and usually involves a number of ethical considerations as well.

Elder interview

The initial interview is conducted in a private setting by either a doctor, a nurse, or person from the home care environment, such as a social worker or another team member. Both the older person and the caregiver are present.

Certain clues should alert you to suspect elder abuse and neglect. For example, older people who seek medical care long after an injury has occurred may be abuse victims. Lacerations and fractures that have healed without appropriate medical treatment

(Text continues on page 280.)

Protocol for identifying and assessing elder abuse and neglect

Use the following guidelines to help you evaluate the possibility of abuse or neglect in your patient.

Tools
Sketch sheet or trauma graph
- tape measure
- camera, film, flash
- paper and pen
- consent and release-of-information forms.

Taking the history
Follow these guidelines when interviewing patient and caregiver.
- Examine patient alone.
- Explain to caregiver that you'll interview her separately after interviewing the older person.
- Work questions into conversation in relaxed manner. Provide support to geriatric patient and caregiver.
- Don't be judgmental or allow personal feelings to interfere with providing optimal care. Don't *prematurely* diagnose the older person as a victim of elder abuse or neglect.
- Pay special attention to trauma, burns, nutrition, recent change in condition, and financial status.
- Interview collateral contacts (visiting nurse, neighbors, friends) as soon as possible to obtain additional information.

Presentation
The following factors may suggest abuse or neglect.
- Patient brought into emergency department by someone other than caregiver
- Prolonged interval between trauma or illness and presentation for medical care (for example, gross decubiti)
- Suspicious history: The older adult is new to system with history of "doctor hopping." Description of how injury occurred does not match physical findings; patient has injuries not mentioned in history or has history of previous similar episodes; too many "explained" injuries or inconsistent explanations over time.
- Medication bottles or patient's pharmacy profile indicates that medications are not being taken or given as prescribed.

Functional evaluation
- Administer Mini-Mental State Examination or Dementia Scale to determine current mental status.
- Collect pertinent data (length of time at residence, medical insurance source, income sources).
- Assess older person's ability to perform activities of daily living.
- Ask older person to describe a typical day to determine degree of independence, most frequent and significant contacts, who and how often seen.
- Ask older person about role expectations of self and caregiver.
- Have older person report any recent crisis in family life.
- Ask if there is alcohol use, drug use, mental illness, or dysfunctional behavior among household or family members.
- Ask directly if the older person has experienced any of the following:
— being shoved, shaken, or hit (record verbatim; when, where on body, examine body)
— being left alone, tied to chair or bed, or locked in room (record verbatim; when and duration)
— having money or property taken or signed over to someone else. Determine current assets, financial status (specify).
— withholding of food, medication, or medical care; being oversedated with medication or alcohol.
— being threatened or feeling afraid of caregiver.
- Assess how the older person responds in above situations.
- Ask patient how he copes with stress and upsetting incidents.
- Assess degree of patient's dependence on caregiver alone for financial, physical, or emotional support.

Physical examination
- If injury is due to an accident, document circumstances.
- Examine closely for effects of undermedication or overmedication; assess nutrition, hygiene, and personal care for evidence of abuse or neglect (such

Protocol for identifying and assessing elder abuse and neglect (continued)

as dehydration or malnourishment without illness-related cause).
● Assess for the following:
— burns (unusual location or type)
— physical or thermal injury on head, scalp, or face
— bruises and hematomas (unusual location, bruise in shape of fingerprints, presence of other injuries in different stages of resolution)
— mental status and neurologic examination changes from previous level
— fractures, falls, or evidence of physical restraint (such as contractures)
— ambulation status (poor ambulation may suggest sexual assault).
● Observe and document:
— size, color, shape, and location of injury (use sketch sheet or take photographs)
— no new lesions during patient's hospitalization
— family or caregiver(s) do not visit or show concern
— abnormal or suspicious behavior of older person (extremely fearful or agitated, overly quiet and passive, or expressing fear of caregiver)
— clinician's intuition that all is not well between patient and caregiver
— patient-caregiver interaction (for example, is yelling at each other a long-term pattern with which both are comfortable or a "new" behavior that may indicate escalation toward more abusive acts?)

Diagnostic tests
In a medical setting, diagnostic procedures may include the following:
● radiologic screening for fractures or evidence of physical restraint
● metabolic screening for nutritional, electrolyte, or endocrine abnormality
● toxicology screening or drug levels for over- or undermedication
● hematology screening for coagulation defect when abnormal bleeding or bruising is documented
● Computed tomography scan for head trauma or

major change in neurologic status
● pelvic exam to rule out venereal disease from sexual assault.

Caregiver interview
Begin by thanking the caregiver for waiting while you interviewed the older person. Explain that you need the caregiver's help; that you're performing an assessment of the older person's current situation to determine what services are appropriate at this time. Ask for the caregiver's perception of how things are going. Then proceed with the following questions.
● Tell me what you want me to know about the patient.
● What is her medical condition? What medicine does she take?
● What kind of care does she require?
● How involved are you with her everyday activities and care?
● What do you expect her to do for herself?
— Do you do these things now?
— Are you able to do them?
— Have you had any difficulties? If so, what kind? Please describe how you spend a typical day.
● How do you cope with having to care for your mother all the time?
● Do you have supports or respite care? What and when? Are there other siblings who help?
● What responsibilities do you have outside the home? Do you work? What are your hours? What do you do?
● Would you mind telling me what your income is? (If this question seems touchy to the caregiver, say, "I just wondered if your family can afford the pills she needs to take." At the same time, assess the caregiver's degree of dependence on the older person's income, pensions, assets.)
● Is the older person's Social Security check directly deposited in the bank?
● Who owns this house? Do you pay rent? Whose name is on the deed?
● If you help your mother pay her bills, how do you do it? Is your name on her account? Do you have power of attorney? Does it have a durable clause? When did you get it?
Save more delicate questions for last.
● You know those bruises on your mother's arms (head,

(continued)

Protocol for identifying and assessing elder abuse and neglect *(continued)*

nose, etc.); how do you suppose she got them? (Document response verbatim. If possible, ask caregiver to demonstrate how injury may have happened.)

- Your mother seems rather undernourished and thin; how do you think she got this way?
- Is there any reason why you waited this long to seek medical care for your mother?
- Caring for someone as impaired as your mother is a difficult task. Have you ever felt so frustrated with her that you pushed her a little harder than you expected? How about hitting or slapping her? What were the circumstances? (Record verbatim.)
- Have you ever had to tie your mother to a bed or chair, or lock her in a room when you go out at night?
- Have you ever yelled at her or threatened her verbally?

Be alert for the following signs of a high-risk situation.

- Alcohol use, drug abuse, or mental illness in caregiver's residence.
- Caregiver is alienated or socially isolated, or has poor self-image.
- Caregiver is young or immature, and behavior indicates own dependency needs have not been met.
- Caregiver is forced by circumstances to care for patient who is unwanted.
- Caregiver is unemployed, without sufficient funds, and dependent on patient for housing and money. Caregiver's or patient's poor health or chronic illness may exacerbate poor relationship.
- Caregiver exhibits abnormal behavior (for example, is frustrated, secretive, or overly hostile; shows little concern; demonstrates poor self-control; "blames" older person; exhibits exaggerated defensiveness and denial; avoids facial or eye contact with older person).

Collateral contacts
Interview about a dozen collateral contacts promptly, before caregiver attempts to collude with patient.

Forming a diagnosis
Integrate patient history, physical examination, caregiver history, and collateral contact information to diagnose patient. Based on your assessment findings, the diagnosis may be expressed as follows:

- No evidence for elder abuse or neglect
- Suspicion of neglect
- Suspicion of abuse
- Strong evidence of abuse or neglect
- Gross neglect.

Adapted with permission from Quinn, M.J., and Tomita, S. *Elderly Abuse and Neglect.* New York: Springer Publishing, 1986.

---

may indicate abuse. Additionally, abuse and neglect may be suspected in situations where a caregiver insists on providing the older person's medical history rather than allowing the older adult to speak for himself. A caregiver may also provide implausible explanations for illnesses or injuries or insist that the older person is "accident prone."

Also suspect elder neglect if frail or cognitively impaired older people are not accompanied to appointments by their caregivers. Repeated admissions, numerous emergency visits, and readmissions for medical noncompliance may also be indicators of elder abuse or neglect.

Following the initial interview, the aging adult and caregiver are questioned separately, because the older person may be afraid to speak openly in the caregiver's presence. The health care provider interviews the older person while a social worker interviews the caregiver. If only one health care professional is available, this individual should explain the procedure of separate interviews at the start of the process.

Questions to ask
Interviewing a possible abuse victim is challenging. You'll need to create a relaxed environment for the

older person, ask frank questions in a sensitive manner (incorporating the questions throughout the conversation), and allow the older adult sufficient time to respond. The following are some suggested questions:

- Has anyone at home ever hurt you?
- Has anyone ever touched you without your consent?
- Has anyone ever made you do things you didn't want to do?
- Has anyone taken anything that was yours without asking?
- Has anyone ever scolded or threatened you?
- Have you ever signed any documents that you didn't understand?
- Are you afraid of anyone at home?
- Are you alone a lot?
- Has anyone ever failed to help you take care of yourself when you needed help?
- Does anyone help you with your finances?

If an older person answers "yes" to any of the above questions, ask him for additional details about the incident. It also may be helpful to ask if the older person believes that future mistreatment is preventable.

Caregiver interview

A health care professional who interviews a caregiver suspected of abuse should be familiar with the causes of abuse, know the key questions to ask, and use one of the screening tools available for assessing caregiver stress. The interview should be conducted in a relaxed and private setting. Start the interview by putting the caregiver at ease. Once again, be direct yet sensitive in asking for information. Start with general questions; then proceed to more specific ones. And always allow sufficient time for the caregiver to respond.

Try to identify any physical, mental, emotional, social, or economic factors that may be causing the caregiver's abusive behavior. Ask the caregiver to describe, in her own words, her responsibilities in the caregiving role. Ask if she has support systems, such as family, friends, or community assistance. Can she take any time off for recreational activities

or just to unwind? If so, how does she plan for and accomplish these breaks? Determine if the caregiver can accurately identify the older person's medical and social needs. Does the older person have a family doctor? A doctor is important for ongoing care. If the older person shows signs of dementia, ask the caregiver to describe his behavior on a typical day. Does the older person demonstrate abusive, hostile, or threatening behavior toward the caregiver?

Document the caregiver's nonverbal behavior during the interview. Do you maintain good eye contact? What is the caregiver's tone of voice? Consider her personal history. Can she meet her own needs? Does she have another job outside the home? Assess the caregiver's use of drugs or alcohol, and determine whether she or others in the household have any mental health problems.

Document any signs of financial or material abuse or neglect. Financial responsibilities usually are linked to legal matters. Coercing the older person to change a will or sign contracts may be a sign of financial abuse. Other marks of financial abuse or neglect are a lack of amenities, a pattern of spending changes, numerous unpaid bills when someone is designated to pay them, forging of checks, and increased use of automatic teller machines when the older person is homebound.

Use a tool, such as the Caregiver Strain Index (CSI) or the Zarit Scale, to determine the caregiver's level of stress. The CSI, developed in 1983, helps quantify stress levels of a primary caregiver who is responsible for a medically ill person. It evaluates three areas: the patient's characteristics, the caregiver's subjective perceptions of the relationship, and the caregiver's physical and emotional health. More than six "yes" answers indicates an increased level of stress (see *Caregiver strain index,* page 282).

The Zarit Scale was developed in 1985 to help evaluate the burden of caregivers of older adults with dementia. This tool helps measure the caregiver's health, psychological well-being, financial situation, and social support network as well as the relationship between a caregiver and the older person (see *Zarit scale: Caregiver burden interview,* pages 283 and 284).

CHARTING GUIDE

Caregiver strain index

This questionnaire helps to evaluate the stress level of a primary caregiver who is caring for a medically ill person.

I am going to read a list of things that other people have found to be difficult when helping out after someone comes home from the hospital. *Would you tell me whether any of these apply to you?* (Give examples.)

	Yes = 1	No = 0
Sleep is disturbed (for example, because _____ is in and out of bed or wanders around at night).	_____	_____
It is inconvenient (for example, because helping takes so much time or it's a long drive over to help).	_____	_____
It is a physical strain (for example, because of lifting in and out of a chair).	_____	_____
It is confining (for example, helping restricts free time).	_____	_____
There have been family adjustments (for example, because helping has disrupted routine and reduced privacy).	_____	_____
There have been changes in personal plans (for example, had to turn down a job or could not go on vacation).	_____	_____
There have been other demands on my time (for example, from other family members).	_____	_____
There have been emotional adjustments (for example, because of severe arguments).	_____	_____
Some behavior is upsetting (such as incontinence, trouble remembering things, or accusing people of taking things).	_____	_____
It is upsetting to find that _____ has changed so much from his former self. (He is a different person than he used to be.) There have been work adjustments (for example, because of having to take time off).	_____	_____
Caring for _____ is a financial strain. I feel completely overwhelmed (for example, because of worrying about _____ and concerns about how I will manage).	_____	_____

Total score (count "yes" responses): _____

Reprinted with permission from Robinson, B.C. "Validation of a Caregiver Strain Index." *Journal of Gerontology* 38(3):344-48, May 1983.

COMPREHENSIVE ASSESSMENT

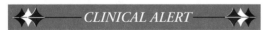

CLINICAL ALERT

Abuse or neglect is rarely the victim's chief complaint.

After the interviews of both the older person and the caregiver, a comprehensive assessment is the next step. This includes preassessment strategies and an evaluation of functional, cognitive, and psychosocial domains. An evaluation for dementia is also part of the cognitive assessment.

Assessment strategies

Knowledge and preparation are essential for an accurate, comprehensive assessment. Prior to meeting the older person, you must be aware of the targeted symptoms that need assessment and organize the

CHARTING GUIDE

Zarit scale: Caregiver burden interview

This questionnaire was designed to help evaluate the stress level of caregivers of people with dementia. Ask the caregiver to circle the answer to each question that best reflects how she feels. Then add up the score to determine her stress level.

Key: **0 = Never**   **1 = Rarely**   **2 = Sometimes**   **3 = Quite frequently**   **4 = Nearly always**

1. Do you feel that your relative asks for more help than he/she needs?

     0   1   2   3   4

2. Do you feel that because of the time you spend with your relative you don't have enough time for yourself?

     0   1   2   3   4

3. Do you feel stressed between caring for your relative and trying to meet other responsibilities for your family or work?

     0   1   2   3   4

4. Do you feel embarrassed over your relative's behavior?

     0   1   2   3   4

5. Do you feel angry when you're around your relative?

     0   1   2   3   4

6. Do you feel that your relative currently affects your relationship with other family members or friends in a negative way?

     0   1   2   3   4

7. Are you afraid of what the future holds for your relative?

     0   1   2   3   4

8. Do you feel that your relative is dependent upon you?

     0   1   2   3   4

9. Do you feel strained when you're around your relative?

     0   1   2   3   4

10. Do you feel your health has suffered because of your involvement with your relative?

     0   1   2   3   4

11. Do you feel that you don't have as much privacy as you would like because of your relative?

     0   1   2   3   4

12. Do you feel that your social life has suffered because you are caring for your relative?

     0   1   2   3   4

13. Do you feel uncomfortable about having friends over because of your relative?

     0   1   2   3   4

14. Do you feel that your relative seems to expect you to take care of him/her as if you were the only one he/she could depend on?

     0   1   2   3   4

15. Do you feel that you don't have enough money to care for your relative in addition to the rest of your expenses?

     0   1   2   3   4

(continued)

Zarit scale: Caregiver burden interview (continued)

Key:	0 = Never	1 = Rarely	2 = Sometimes	3 = Quite frequently	4 = Nearly always

16. Do you feel that you will be unable to take care of your relative much longer?

     0   1   2   3   4

17. Do you feel that you have lost control of your life since your relative's illness?

     0   1   2   3   4

18. Do you wish you could just leave the care of your relative to someone else?

     0   1   2   3   4

19. Do you feel uncertain about what to do about your relative?

     0   1   2   3   4

20. Do you feel you should be doing more for your relative?

     0   1   2   3   4

21. Do you feel you could do a better job in caring for your relative?

     0   1   2   3   4

22. Overall, how burdened do you feel in caring for your relative?

     0   1   2   3   4

Scoring key:

  0-20 Little or no burden

21-40 Mild to moderate burden

41-60 Moderate to severe burden

61-88 Severe burden

---

equipment necessary to document suspected abuse or neglect, including a camera, film, a tape measure, and forms for consent and release of information.

In cases of suspected abuse and neglect, the older person may not be able to provide a thorough history. To identify mistreatment, you'll need astute observation skills, use of pertinent assessment tools, and accurate documentation. Some states have specific documentation guidelines, but the medical record should be clear and explicit and should include the following:

• chief complaint and description of the abusive event or neglectful situation, using the patient's own words whenever possible rather than the interviewer's assessment

• complete medical history

• relevant social history

• a detailed description of any injuries, including type, number, size, location, stages of healing, color, resolution, possible causes, and any explanations given (including, where applicable, a body chart or drawing showing the location and nature of the injuries and evidence of any old injuries that may have resulted from abuse)

• an opinion on whether the injuries were adequately explained

• results of all pertinent laboratory and other diagnostic procedures

• color photographs and imaging studies, if applicable

• if the police were called, the name of the investigating officer and any actions taken
• quotations or verbatim comments made by the patient.

Functional assessment

Begin the functional assessment by evaluating activities of daily living (ADLs). A recommended tool is the ADL Checklist developed in 1963 by Katz et al. ADLs include bathing, dressing, grooming, eating, toileting, walking, transferring, and maintaining bowel and bladder continence. Instrumental activities of daily living (IADLs), more sophisticated levels of function, also should be assessed. These include the older person's capacity to shop, prepare meals, perform housework, handle finances, use the telephone, take medications, and arrange transportation. For more information about these tools, see Chapter 2. An older adult who is dependent on a caregiver for any ADLs or IADLs may be at increased risk for abuse because of the added strain placed on the caregiver.

Assessing hearing and vision

If the screenings indicate impaired hearing or vision, determine if the older person has the appropriate aids. If he doesn't have hearing aids or eyeglasses, determine whether he chooses to purchase them and can afford them. Suspect financial or material neglect if the older adult requires eyeglasses or hearing aids, wishes to have them, and can afford them, yet has neither. Suspect material neglect if he has the proper aids but they're not functioning properly.

Assessing mobility

Balance and gait disorders are common problems for older people. Determine whether the older adult has an increased risk of falling and whether he uses an assistive device, such as a cane, walker, or wheelchair. Is the device with him? Does he own the proper assistive device? If not, does he wish to purchase one and learn to use it? Can he afford it? If the older person wants the device and can afford it but does not have one, financial neglect may be the reason.

If the dependent older person requires 24-hour supervision for impaired mobility, assess whether he is receiving the appropriate assistance. If he's not, determine whether he is competent to refuse care or whether the care is being withheld because the caregiver refuses to pay for it, even though funds are available. Again, financial neglect may be the reason.

Assessing nutritional status

Determine the older person's nutritional status by evaluating his height and weight and dietary intake (get a diet history if possible). Also ask his usual weight and compare it to the current weight. If there's a discrepancy between the two weights, evaluate for possible medical causes before you consider that the weight discrepancy may be due to neglect.

Assessing continence

If the older person is incontinent, determine if the problem is new or chronic. If it's chronic, find out how he manages the problem. Incontinence is a major source of caregiver stress. Consider physical neglect if the caregiver is capable of care but does not provide it, as evidenced by skin breakdown. Suspect financial neglect if the older person can afford proper supplies, such as protective undergarments, but the caregiver is not purchasing them.

Cognitive assessment

Identifying impaired cognition in an older person has important implications when abuse or neglect is suspected. Depending on the level of impairment, the older person may not be able to explain the cause of a problem, for example, what caused the bruises discovered during the physical assessment. In addition, older people do not present with problems in the same way as younger adults. For example, an older patient who is dehydrated may display signs of confusion rather than complain of thirst.

Begin with the simplest screening test, such as the clock drawing test. Instruct the older adult to draw the face of a clock with all 12 hours and to place the hour and minute hands on a specified time, such as 2:35. If he performs poorly on this test, he'll need further testing, such as the Mini-Mental State Examination (see Chapter 2).

Assessing for dementia

Dementia is a clinical syndrome involving a loss of intellectual function and memory impairment that's severe enough to cause dysfunction in daily living and possible self-neglect, especially when an older adult lives alone. Any mention of possible abuse or neglect by the older person must be taken seriously and evaluated further. Because of the behavior and personality changes associated with this illness — such as violent outbursts — the caregiver of a demented older adult should be evaluated for stress.

Psychosocial assessment

This part of the comprehensive assessment evaluates coping style, depression, living arrangements, and formal and informal support systems. In assessing the older person's coping style, ask him to relate how he has handled difficult situations or personal losses in the past.

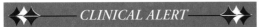

CLINICAL ALERT

Depression is a treatable problem that is often overlooked in older adults. But it's important to evaluate older people for depression, especially in cases of possible abuse or neglect. A depressed older person may not have the energy to do anything about the problem (see Chapter 4 for more information on assessing for depression).

Evaluating your patient's living arrangements may uncover possible financial abuse, particularly if a caregiver is financially dependent on the older adult. Directly ask the older person if the current living arrangements are satisfactory. Ask who else lives in the home. If the older adult owns the home, determine if the caregiver is living there out of choice or necessity. Find out if the older person or caregiver requires cohabitation or if it's a mutually agreed upon arrangement.

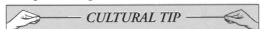

CULTURAL TIP

Be aware of possible cultural influences on living arrangements. Sharing a home with an adult child is more common among certain ethnic groups. For example, many black older people live with family members, and approximately three-fourths of Hispanic older adults live with a family member.

Finally, assess the older person's support services. An informal network of family and friends can provide valuable services for an older person, as can neighbors, church members, and community services. Ask the older person how often friends and neighbors visit. Inquire about any religion-affiliated sources of support. Suspect psychological abuse or neglect when a caregiver leaves an older person alone for long periods of time, ignores his needs for companionship, prevents his friends from visiting, or fails to inform the older person of changes in routines or plans.

Determine if formal services, such as visiting nurse services, are needed and if they are in place. If there's a discrepancy between need and services provided, suspect financial or material abuse or neglect. For example, note when an older person needs, wants, and can afford services, but the caregiver is not providing them. Also suspect financial abuse or neglect if unnecessary services are being provided or exorbitant prices are being charged.

Physical examination

When you perform the physical examination, use a standard examination form and begin by describing the person's general appearance. A physically abused or neglected older person may exhibit unshaven or uncombed hair; poor skin hygiene; an unkempt or unclean body; patches of hair missing; a foul odor; unexplained bruises or bruises in various stages of healing; burns from cigarettes, ropes, or chains; and injuries reflecting the outline of an object, such as a belt or handprint. In addition, he may offer explanations that don't match the injury.

Use a head-to-toe approach, moving downward on the body so you don't miss any important indicators. Bruises on the face or handprints on the neck may indicate physical abuse.

Assess the skin carefully and note any signs, such as bruises or skin breakdown. Document how old the bruises seem to be and whether there are injuries in different stages of resolution. Proceed down the body, paying attention to unusual areas of injuries.

Check the upper inner arms and thighs for bruises. Check bony prominences for skin breakdown, the coccyx for decubitus ulcers, and the heels of both feet for signs of ulcers; positive findings may reflect the effects of physical immobility or they may signal neglect.

Assess for dehydration and malnutrition. Signs of physical neglect may include weight loss, poor skin turgor, decubitus ulcers, poor personal hygiene, or failure to comply with medical treatment.

Diagnostic tests

Inform the older adult and caregiver about any ordered laboratory tests or X-ray procedures. Diagnostic tests that may rule out suspected abuse or neglect include:
- X-ray for fractures
- computed tomography scan of the head to detect neurologic changes or head trauma
- blood tests, including complete blood count, serum electrolyte levels, coagulation studies, iron studies, vitamin B_{12} levels, thyroid hormone levels, drug toxicology screening, and screening for tertiary syphilis, hepatitis, and anemia
- urinalysis. Obtain a urine specimen for culture and sensitivity if a urinary tract infection is suspected. For males, obtain a voided specimen; for females, consider a straight catheterization sample.

FORMULATING INTERVENTIONS

After the physical examination and before meeting with the older person and caregiver, hold a brief interdisciplinary meeting. The meeting is to ensure that all team members who participated in the evaluation agree with the findings and to formulate recommendations for halting the abuse or neglect. The team members should individualize the recommendations, based on the needs and strengths of the older person and his caregiver, rather than trying to fit the older adult into an established plan of care.

True geriatric patient care means respecting the older person, helping him define realistic goals, and then providing the support he needs to achieve those goals. In choosing interventions for abuse, you should be guided primarily by the following criteria: the safety needs of the older patient; his rights to self-determination, autonomy, and freedom of choice; and the legal requirements for reporting abuse and neglect.

A variety of social and legal interventions can be used to either stop current mistreatment or reduce the risk of potential abuse or neglect. Each intervention has advantages and limitations. Aside from weighing the practical pros and cons, the health care team will also need to consider the ethical implications of various interventions and ensure that the older person maintains his autonomy in the decision-making process.

Ethical concerns

Ethical dilemmas — situations requiring a choice between what seem to be two equally desirable or undesirable alternatives — may develop at any point during the comprehensive assessment. An example of a desirable choice would be an older adult obliged to chose to live with one of two children he likes. Both children want him, but they live in different states. An example of an undesirable choice would be deciding whether to move to a nursing home or remain in an abusive situation. In such situations, your role is to help the older person understand all his options and to support him in his decision.

Autonomy and informed consent

Autonomy is defined as "the duty to respect persons and their right to self-determination regarding the course of their lives and issues concerning the integrity of their bodies and minds." Preserving an older person's autonomy means you allow him to select treatment options, even when the choice is not in his best interests, and respect his values, even when they differ from yours.

The concept of informed consent is a part of autonomy; it means that the older person receives enough information about the results of the assessment to make decisions. The information you present must be in terms that the older person can understand. Consider these five fundamental issues

of informed consent:
- Is the older adult capable of understanding the situation?
- Is he able to express a preference?
- Has he received accurate information about the benefits and risks?
- Are there clear options? Does the older person understand them?
- What happens when his preferences are contrary to the doctor's or family members'?

Steps for planning interventions

You need to answer four critical questions in order to create the most appropriate treatment plan for an abused or neglected older adult. They are:
- Is abuse or neglect suspected?
- Is your geriatric patient in immediate danger?
- Is he willing to accept services voluntarily?
- Does your patient have the capacity to make decisions?

(See *Steps to follow in suspected elder abuse.*)

Is abuse suspected?

If the answer is *no* (after interviews and comprehensive assessment), but the health care team has found inadequate care or the potential for abuse and neglect, the team develops a treatment and follow-up plan based on the identified needs and strengths of the older person and any caregiver involved. The plan typically includes referrals to a home health care agency, legal services, hotlines, and other community resources. However, if the inadequate care is related to a caregiver, the caregiver should be referred to appropriate training and self-help programs. You should then review the proposed service plan with the older person (and caregiver if one is involved) and formulate a contract for care and follow-up.

If abuse *is* suspected, you are legally obligated to report it to the designated state agency; usually Adult Protective Services (APS). If the abused older person lives in a long-term facility, the reporting mechanism may vary. The Older Americans Act of 1978 established a Long-Term Care Ombudsman program that investigates all complaints made by residents against a nursing facility.

Is the older adult in immediate danger?

Ensuring a mistreated older person's safety should be your first concern. If you believe imminent danger *does not* exist, devise a service plan and negotiate its acceptance with the older person and caregiver.

If imminent danger *does* exist, you must arrange to have the older person removed from the dangerous setting immediately. If he has significant injuries due to physical abuse, hospitalization achieves this goal. If hospitalization is not an option, devise a plan of immediate separation. APS staff members will work with you to place an abused older person in a safe environment, such as foster home, adult group home, or nursing facility, if he cannot remain in his home or is living in the home of the abuser. In certain cases, however, the older person can remain at home, if support services are provided. For example, an older person who is malnourished from self-neglect secondary to a new diagnosis of early dementia may be able to remain at home with support from a helpful neighbor, a meals-on-wheels program, a daily telephone-call program, and adult daycare services.

Will the older person accept the service plan?

The ultimate goal of the service plan is to achieve a level of care that is satisfactory to the older person. Exercising his right of self-determination, he may choose to remain in an abusive situation. However, if you have good negotiating skills, present enough easily understood information, and demonstrate respect and compassion, you can usually persuade him to take at least one step toward improving his situation. An older adult may be more willing to accept services when he's informed enough to help in decision making.

Does the older person have the capacity to make decisions?

Whenever an abused older person refuses services, his competence to make decisions must be evaluated to ensure his safety. This is especially important when dealing with cognitively impaired people who can't speak for themselves.

When an older patient *does* have decision-making capacity, is not in imminent danger, and refuses

Steps to follow in suspected elder abuse

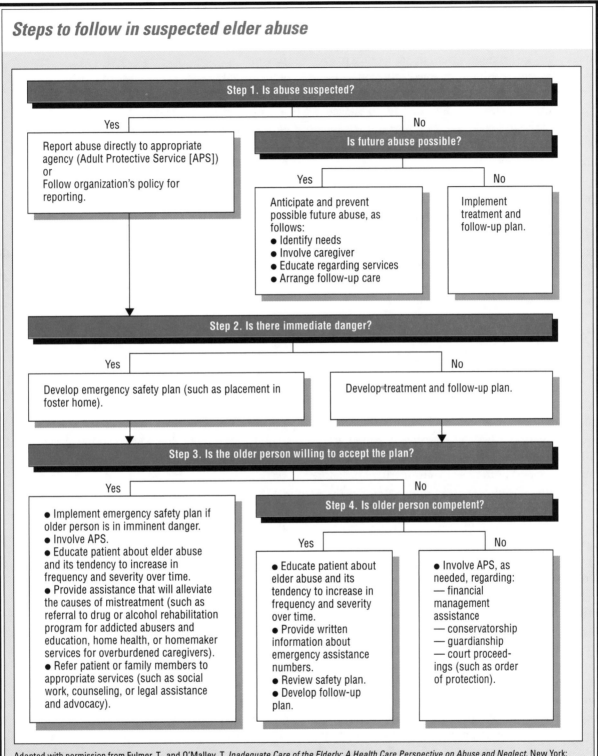

Step 1. Is abuse suspected?

Yes → Report abuse directly to appropriate agency (Adult Protective Service [APS]) or Follow organization's policy for reporting.

No → **Is future abuse possible?**

Yes → Anticipate and prevent possible future abuse, as follows:
- Identify needs
- Involve caregiver
- Educate regarding services
- Arrange follow-up care

No → Implement treatment and follow-up plan.

Step 2. Is there immediate danger?

Yes → Develop emergency safety plan (such as placement in foster home).

No → Develop treatment and follow-up plan.

Step 3. Is the older person willing to accept the plan?

Yes →
- Implement emergency safety plan if older person is in imminent danger.
- Involve APS.
- Educate patient about elder abuse and its tendency to increase in frequency and severity over time.
- Provide assistance that will alleviate the causes of mistreatment (such as referral to drug or alcohol rehabilitation program for addicted abusers and education, home health, or homemaker services for overburdened caregivers).
- Refer patient or family members to appropriate services (such as social work, counseling, or legal assistance and advocacy).

No → **Step 4. Is older person competent?**

Yes →
- Educate patient about elder abuse and its tendency to increase in frequency and severity over time.
- Provide written information about emergency assistance numbers.
- Review safety plan.
- Develop follow-up plan.

No →
- Involve APS, as needed, regarding:
— financial management assistance
— conservatorship
— guardianship
— court proceedings (such as order of protection).

Adapted with permission from Fulmer, T., and O'Malley, T. *Inadequate Care of the Elderly: A Health Care Perspective on Abuse and Neglect.* New York: Springer Publishing Co., 1987, and Ohio State Medical Association and Ohio Department of Human Services. *Ohio Physician's Elder Abuse Prevention Project-Trust Talk: Break the Silence, Begin the Cure.* Columbus, Ohio: Ohio State Medical Association, 1994.

services, you must honor this choice. Then document the service plan, the patient's refusal, the evaluation of his capacity to make decisions, any educational instructions given, the follow-up plan, and the referral to APS in the medical record. Give him emergency numbers to call and a list of suitable community agencies, in case he decides to take advantage of them. Finally, send a report of the situation and the team's follow-up recommendations to the doctor.

When the older person *does not* have decision-making capacity, is not in imminent danger, and refuses services, you must intervene on his behalf by reporting the situation to APS. In some states, APS will begin an investigation within 24 hours for emergency situations and, otherwise, within 3 working days. Various legal interventions may be implemented, depending on the individual case.

Education

Regardless of whether the older adult consents to or refuses interventions, he needs education about the incidence of mistreatment and the tendency for it to increase over time. In teaching older adults, it's useful to provide both written and oral information. If the older person is hearing-or vision-impaired, use a voice amplifier or large-print instructions. Always ask the older adult to repeat your instructions before the teaching session is over. In some cases, you'll need to provide instructions to the caregiver rather than the older person. In that case, the same principles apply.

Social interventions

When the suspected cause of abuse or neglect is primarily social in nature, the social worker becomes the lead person on the interdisciplinary team and works most directly with the older person and caregiver. The other team members stay involved in order to monitor health issues and provide support for the social plan as needed. The older adult's social needs and use of appropriate services is evaluated regularly, either by telephone or periodic follow-up visits with the patient or the involved community professionals.

Each service plan is developed to match the identified needs and strengths of both the abused and the abuser. All social plans should include the following:
- identified needs
- goals to meet the needs
- actions of all involved
- timeline for achievement of goals
- follow-up review date.

The older person's financial resources and the availability of community-based resources, particularly for home-bound patients, are pertinent when you select social interventions. If the geriatric patient is eligible for Medicaid, the social worker can help him obtain and complete Medicaid forms. If he is not eligible for Medicaid, the social worker can tell him about other available financial resources. If community-based support services are not available, the older person may have to begin planning for long-term care in a nursing facility.

Support services can be organized into four categories: health supports, social resources, assistive services, and housing support. (For a more comprehensive list of support services, see *Services for older people*.)

A 1989 study of 204 abused and neglected older people found that the most frequently used service was case management — defined as coordination of services and monthly monitoring by a health care professional — followed by homemaking assistance and legal services. Meal assistance, guardianships, and institutional placements were also used frequently.

Legal interventions

You can use a variety of legal interventions when working with abused older people. These include services and protections provided under the Adult Protective Services Law and the Domestic Violence Law as well as powers of attorney, representative payeeship, guardianship, conservatorship, and civil commitment (involuntary hospitalization). However, taking legal action requires serious and careful thought to avoid infringing on an older adult's rights and freedoms.

Services for older people

Health services
- Home health care services (nursing; social work; physical, occupational, speech, and respiratory therapists; medical equipment suppliers)
- Local senior outreach programs (parish nurse programs; health assessments such as blood pressure and cholesterol tests at community events)
- Adult day care (services offered by nursing homes, integrated delivery networks, and retirement communities)
- Adult day hospitals (mental health, rehabilitation)
- Telephone help lines (cancer help lines, "Ask a nurse" lines; lines sponsored by local chapters of the Alzheimer's Association).

Social services
- Meals on wheels
- Adult day care
- Respite care
- Homemaker services (light housekeeping and meal preparation)

- Mental health counseling
- Volunteer home visitors
- Telephone help lines and reassurance programs
- Support groups
- Community talks
- Senior citizen groups
- Transportation services.

Additional assistive services
- Adult Protective Services (in each state, listed under Department of Health and Human Services)
- Legal services (attorneys specializing in elder law).

Living options
- Group homes, congregate living
- Senior apartment complexes
- Continuing care retirement communities
- Assisted living facilities
- Nursing facilities.

Experts recommend that you consider three questions when suggesting a specific legal option:
- Is the older adult unable to make or carry out decisions about major issues (such as health care, housing, living arrangements, and sale or management of property and money) on his own behalf?
- Is there a risk to his health and safety? Is there a risk of theft or loss of property or money because he is unable to act effectively on his own behalf?
- Do the actions that someone else would have to take on the older adult's behalf require legal authority?

You always should try to implement the least restrictive legal interventions; those that least limit an older person's right to make decisions and that least restrict his personal freedoms. For example, if guardianship is necessary, consider using a limited guardianship — for only specific areas of asset management and personal decision-making, as needed — rather than a full guardianship. For a more in-depth discussion of legal issues, see Chapter 20.

Intervening in acute-care facilities

Acute-care facilities should have abuse and neglect policies that include reporting obligations and the steps to follow when abuse or neglect is suspected. The policy should clarify at least the following elements: definitions of types of abuse and neglect; the legal obligation of health care professionals to report abuse, even if only suspected; and the names of those who should receive the report, both internally and in the community.

Because abuse and neglect are hard to detect, the policy should include a written protocol for the systematic identification of mistreatment. A specific form for documenting findings is important to guide you through the abuse protocol and includes the older person's demographic data; the type of abuse or neglect; the name and address of the alleged abuser, if known; a brief description of the situation; the names of the individuals contacted at APS and law enforcement agencies; and any other actions taken. The completed form is sent to the appropriate person for follow-up, usually a social worker or the geriatric assessment team.

Some acute-care facilities have an Adult Protection Team consisting of APS workers, ethicists, nurses, doctors, social workers, local police, and possibly an elder care attorney. The team's purpose is to monitor the management of geriatric mistreatment cases, to educate and guide reporting procedures, and to consult with all health care professionals.

Intervening in long-term care facilities

The Omnibus Budget Reconciliation Act of 1987 has had the greatest impact on the nursing home industry since Medicare and Medicaid in 1965. Its primary aim was to prevent substandard care, abuse, and neglect. The law established a set of residents' rights, one of which is the right to be free from abuse and neglect. It also mandated tighter rules for enforcing nursing home compliance with regulations; nurse aide training requirements; and a registry of nurse aides with a record of abuse or neglect. The law heightened the awareness of health care professionals and consumers, not only to the serious problem of elder abuse and neglect in institutions, but also to the means to detect or prevent abuse in long-term care settings.

Nursing homes are obligated to have a policy on reporting abuse and to thoroughly investigate all reports of abuse in a timely manner. The policy must include the same elements contained in the policies of acute-care facilities.

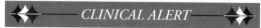

CLINICAL ALERT

All reports of abuse, even if unsubstantiated, must be reported to the state agency or agencies responsible for nursing facilities.

To improve the detection of abuse or to prevent it, nursing homes need to be extremely careful in selecting personnel; to provide adequate training in abuse detection, reporting, and prevention strategies; to teach all staff members the necessary job skills for working with a vulnerable, aged population that is highly dependent on the staff and that may exhibit behavioral problems secondary to dementia; to teach staff members how to deal with anger and stress effectively; to provide adequate supervision by professional staff; to avoid excessive use of overtime and double shifts; and to recruit a pool of volunteers to support staff members during peak activities, such as meal times.

Educational sessions for the residents, family members, and the community on various issues of elder care may be helpful.

16

Administering and monitoring medications

our out of five people over age 65 have at least one chronic disorder. This helps explain why the aged consume more drugs than any other age-group. Although older people represent only about 12% of the population, they take 30% to 40% of the prescription drugs issued. That's about 400 million prescriptions a year.

The drugs most commonly prescribed for older patients include cardiovascular drugs (such as antiarrhythmics, alpha and beta blockers, and digitalis preparations), antihypertensives, analgesics, antiarthritics, sedatives, tranquilizers, laxatives, and antacids.

In older people with chronic disorders, drug therapy can help extend and enhance the quality of life. For instance, drugs are often used successfully to manage arthritis, diabetes, heart disease, glaucoma, osteoporosis, and hypertension. However, the danger for older adults lies in concurrent use of multiple drugs to manage multiple disorders. Consider the example of an 85-year-old female with adult-onset diabetes mellitus, osteoporosis, glaucoma, and hypertension. She takes tolbutamide for diabetes, conjugated estrogens and calcium supplements for osteoporosis, timolol for glaucoma, and triamterene with hydrochlorothiazide for hypertension. If she developed congestive heart failure, arthritis, or a peptic ulcer, she might add three or more drugs to her treatment regimen.

Managing multiple treatments obviously requires careful planning and special monitoring to avoid serious adverse reactions and drug interactions. Fur-

ther complicating the picture, the older adult's reaction to drugs is typically very different from the younger adult's.

AGE-RELATED CHANGES AND DRUG THERAPY

Drug therapy for older people presents special problems caused by age-related physical changes. These changes affect drug absorption, distribution, metabolism, and excretion. The changes also facilitate adverse reactions, which may interfere with compliance. Careful dosage adjustments and close monitoring are crucial to ensure an older person's safety and the efficacy of drug therapy.

Pharmacokinetic changes
The aging process alters body composition and triggers changes in the digestive system, liver, and kidneys. These, in turn, affect drug dosages and administration techniques (see *How age affects drug action*, page 294).

Age-related changes influence a drug's pharmacokinetics (how a drug is absorbed into the blood stream, distributed throughout the body, metabolized, and eliminated). These normal physiologic changes in the older person are exacerbated by acute or chronic diseases. Together, these factors can increase the risk of drug toxicity and adverse reactions.

How age affects drug action

As the body ages, body structures and systems change. This affects how the body responds to medications. Here are some changes that commonly and significantly affect medication administration.

Body composition

As a person grows older, total body mass and lean body mass tend to decrease while body fat tends to increase. Total body water decreases and the amount of plasma albumin available for binding with drugs diminishes. These factors affect the relationship between a drug's concentration and solubility in the body.

Digestive system

Decreases in gastric acid secretion and GI motility reduces the body's ability to absorb many drugs well.

This can cause problems with certain drugs, such as digoxin, whose narrow therapeutic range is tied closely to absorption.

Hepatic system

Advancing age reduces the blood supply to the liver, and certain liver enzymes become less active. As a result, the liver loses some of its ability to metabolize drugs. With reduced liver function, higher levels of a drug remain in circulation, causing more intense drug effects. This increases the risk of drug toxicity.

Renal system

Kidney function also diminishes with age. This alone may impair drug elimination by 50% or more. In many cases, decreased kidney function leads to increased blood levels of certain drugs.

Absorption

In older adults, several factors often alter absorption of drugs administered by oral, I.M., or subcutaneous (S.C.) routes. Absorption of oral drugs may be slowed by mucosal atrophy, decreased gastric emptying, decreased gastric acid secretion and higher pH, reduced splanchnic blood flow, duodenal diverticula, and decreased GI motility. However, because transit time is slowed, oral drugs remain in the system longer, so complete absorption is still possible.

Absorption of drugs given I.M. and S.C. may be delayed by reduced blood flow and altered capillary wall permeability. However, because muscle mass generally decreases with aging, an I.M. injection also may be absorbed faster by an older adult.

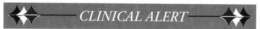

CLINICAL ALERT

Don't give I.M. injections in muscle masses that aren't used, such as the thigh of a wheelchair-bound patient.

Distribution

Age-related changes in body composition include relatively increased body fat and decreased body water, which alter the distribution patterns for most drugs. In an older patient, a highly fat-soluble drug such as diazepam has an increased volume of distribution and a prolonged distribution phase, which prolongs half-life and duration of action. In contrast, a highly water-soluble drug, such as gentamicin, has a decreased volume of distribution; more of the drug remains in the bloodstream, which increases the risk of drug toxicity.

Aging also reduces plasma levels of albumin, a blood protein that binds with and transports many drugs. As a result, more unbound drug may circulate in the bloodstream. This increases the pharmacologic action of drugs that are protein-bound, heightening the risk of adverse effects and drug toxicity. Multiple drug regimens may compete for protein binding sites, and some drugs may be displaced, resulting in increased free serum concentration of those drugs.

Additional factors that can alter drug distribution include declining cardiac output, poor nutrition, extremes of body weight, dehydration, electrolyte and mineral imbalances, inactivity, and prolonged bed rest.

Detecting age-related adverse reactions to drugs

The physiologic changes of aging make older adults more susceptible to drug-induced illnesses and adverse reactions than younger adults. Other conditions common to many older patients also increase the risk of adverse reactions.

To help prevent these problems or detect them early, check the patient's history for the following risk factors:
- altered mental status
- financial problems
- frail health

- history of previous adverse reactions
- history of allergies
- multiple chronic illnesses
- patient is a woman
- patient lives alone
- polypharmacy or complex medication regimens
- poor nutritional status
- renal failure
- small build
- treatment by several doctors.

Perhaps the most significant factor is physical size; older patients typically are smaller than younger patients. So if an older patient receives the same drug dose as a younger patient, the older person's typically lower fluid volume can result in higher blood drug levels.

Metabolism

Alterations in drug metabolism increase the risk of drug accumulation, prolonged half-life and toxicity. Aging reduces the liver's ability to metabolize drugs, and liver disease can further compromise liver function. So can other diseases that reduce hepatic blood flow, such as congestive heart failure.

Drug metabolism by the liver depends primarily on two processes: blood flow and metabolic enzyme action. Because aging reduces hepatic blood flow, less drug is delivered to be metabolized into inactive compounds.

Hepatic enzymes metabolize drugs in two major pathways or phases, which operate less efficiently with the diminished liver mass and altered nutritional status that accompany aging. Phase I reactions (oxidation, reduction, or hydrolysis of drug molecules) are affected more than phase II reactions (coupling of the drug or its metabolite with an acid to produce an inactive compound). Thus, aging leads to different clinical effects, depending on whether a drug is metabolized in phase I, phase II, or both.

Excretion

Most drugs are excreted through the kidneys. With aging, glomerular filtration and tubular secretion decline progressively. Renal function is also impaired by dehydration and cardiovascular and renal diseases. Keep in mind that an older patient has a smaller renal reserve than a younger patient, even if blood urea nitrogen and serum creatinine levels appear normal. In an older patient who's receiving drugs that aren't metabolized, expect to see signs and symptoms of toxicity due to delayed drug clearance and excretion.

Adverse drug reactions

Even if an older adult receives the optimum drug dosage for his age and condition, he's still at risk for an adverse drug reaction. Ongoing physiologic changes, poor compliance with the drug regimen, and greater drug consumption help explain why about 40% of the people who experience adverse drug reactions are over age 60. (See *Detecting age-related adverse reactions to drugs*.)

Although many drugs can cause adverse reactions, most of the serious reactions experienced by older people result from relatively few drugs: diuretics, antihypertensives, digitalis glycosides, corticosteroids, sleeping aids, and nonprescription drugs.

Probably the most troublesome problem with drug therapy in older patients is the potential for misdiagnosing or failing to detect an adverse reac-

How drug action is altered in older adults

Differences in the way older persons absorb, distribute, metabolize, and eliminate drugs can alter the effects of medications. The age related differences are listed below.

Absorption

- Change in quality and quantity of digestive enzymes
- Increased gastric pH
- Decrease in number of absorbing cells
- Decreased GI motility
- Decreased intestinal blood flow
- Decreased GI emptying time

Distribution

- Decreased cardiac output and reserve
- Decreased blood flow to target tissues, liver, and kidneys
- Decreased distribution space and area
- Decreased lean body mass
- Increased adipose stores
- Decreased plasma protein (decreases protein binding drugs)
- Decreased total body water

Metabolism

- Decreased microsomal metabolism of drug
- Decreased hepatic biotransformation

Elimination

- Decreased renal excretion of drug
- Decreased respiratory and vital capacity with increased carbon dioxide retention
- Decreased number of receptors
- Variability in receptor sensitivity

tion. Signs and symptoms of adverse drug reactions (such as confusion, depression, drowsiness, urine retention, weakness, and lethargy) are typically blamed on disease or the aging process. If an adverse drug reaction is undetected or misidentified, the patient usually keeps taking the drug. Careful nursing assessment can help identify drug-related adverse effects so that the dosage can be reduced or the drug replaced with a safer alternative. (See *How drug action is altered in older adults.*)

Drug interactions

Many potent drugs commonly used by older adults can interact to cause hazardous effects. For example, cimetidine interacts with many drugs, including aminophylline, phenytoin, antidepressants, and propranolol; anticholinergics, such as antidepressants and certain tranquilizers, can have additive effects when used concurrently; and digoxin can become more toxic when taken with diuretics or other drugs that decrease the body's potassium levels.

To prevent harmful drug interactions, be aware of all the medications your patient is taking and keep in mind that they may be taking several drugs prescribed independently by several doctors.

◆◆ ——— *CLINICAL ALERT* ——— ◆◆

The fewest drugs possible should be given at the lowest dosages possible to minimize risk to the patient.

Pharmacodynamic changes

A drug's action in the body and its interaction with body tissues (its pharmacodynamics) change significantly in older people. Age-related changes in tissue sensitivity to drugs can enhance some drug effects. This is especially true for barbiturates such as pentobarbital, benzodiazepines such as diazepam, and alcohol.

Age-related changes in the number or function of tissue and organ receptors can alter a drug's effect. The number and function of beta receptors decreases with age, thereby affecting drugs that stimulate or block beta receptors. Such drugs include the bronchodilator metaproterenol and propranolol, a drug that decreases cardiac output and myocardial oxygen consumption.

Similarly, age-related changes in cholinergic and dopaminergic receptors in the nervous system may influence the effect of drugs such as phenothiazines, chlorpromazine, and other psychoactive agents. Receptor changes may contribute to adverse neurologic effects including extrapyramidal adverse effects, such as dystonia and akathisia, and tardive dyskinesia. To compensate for pharmacodynamic changes, older patients commonly require lower dosages of many drugs than younger patients.

Problems of polypharmacy

An older person with multiple physical dysfunctions or symptoms may take prescribed drugs from several doctors at once for acute or chronic ailments. He might also self-medicate with nonprescription drugs to relieve common complaints, such as indigestion, dizziness, constipation, and insomnia. This multiple-drug use, known as polypharmacy, is a serious problem in geriatric care. If the older patient and his doctors fail to communicate and make adjustments regarding concurrent drug use, the patient might fall into a pattern of inappropriate and excessive drug use that puts his health and safety at risk and confounds therapeutic goals (see *Dealing with polypharmacy*).

ENHANCING PATIENT COMPLIANCE

Getting an older patient to follow your medication instructions can be a challenge. Older patients may have many reasons for noncompliance, such as poor vision or hearing, physical disability, or failure to understand the importance of taking the medication. The danger is that noncompliance may lead to unsuccessful treatment and an apparent lack of therapeutic response. Furthermore, the doctor might misinterpret the inadequate response and increase the drug dosage or prescribe a second drug, compounding the patient's problems.

Dealing with polypharmacy

Older patients who have multiple disorders sometimes obtain prescriptions from three or four doctors and three or four pharmacies. They might neglect to inform each doctor of the various drugs they are already taking; conversely, a doctor might fail to discontinue any previous drugs the patient is taking. Older patients might also take one or more nonprescription drugs to relieve common complaints such as stomach ache, dizziness, or constipation. Besides the unnecessary expense, this behavior (called polypharmacy) increases the risk of adverse drug reactions and interactions.

Identifying polypharmacy
Because of your close contact with patients, you are the health care team member who is best able to recognize polypharmacy. Suspect excessive use of drugs if your patient uses:
- several (usually 10 or more) drugs for no logical reason; for example, laxatives that are not needed
- duplicate drugs, such as sleep sedatives and tranquilizers
- an inappropriate dosage
- contraindicated drugs
- drugs to treat adverse reactions.

To avoid such problems, make sure your older patient understands why he must take all of his medications and how to take them correctly. To ensure compliance, enlist the help of family members, the pharmacist, and other caregivers to tailor supervision and teaching to fit each patient's needs.

Monitoring medication administration

Giving medications to an older patient requires the same basic steps as for any other patient but with certain, additional precautions. Use the following guidelines to modify your approach.

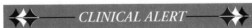
CLINICAL ALERT

Before giving any medication to an older adult, be sure to confirm the patient's identity by checking his identification band and comparing it to the name on the medication record. An older person may be disoriented or confused, especially in a new setting. Also, a hearing deficit can cause the patient to mistakenly answer to a name that isn't his.

If the doctor specifies that a medication be taken before meals, be sure to give it when the patient's stomach is empty. Because older people produce less gastric acid, optimum drug absorption may depend on having the stomach free of food. Also, try to schedule medication administration to interfere as little as possible with the older patient's normal activities. For example, give a diuretic early in the day to prevent the patient from getting up at night to urinate.

Advise the patient to contact you or his doctor before taking any nonprescription drugs to avoid adverse drug interactions. If necessary, regularly monitor serum levels of drugs, such as digoxin or potassium, to avoid toxicity.

To avoid improper storage and possible drug deterioration, advise the patient to keep all prescribed drugs in their original containers. Keep in mind that some drugs deteriorate when exposed to light; others decompose if they come in contact with other drugs — in a pillbox, for example. Before the patient stores drugs together, advise him to consult his pharmacist or doctor.

Suggest a storage area that's well-lighted but protected from direct sunlight. It should not be the bathroom medicine cabinet or a spot near the kitchen sink because these may be too warm or humid. And it should not be the patient's bedside table; if drugs are kept at the bedside, the patient could give himself an accidental overdose by taking them before he's fully awake and alert.

If your older patient is discharged from the facility with a new drug regimen, schedule follow-up care by a visiting nurse to assess his ability to follow the regimen and to monitor his response to therapy.

Impaired physical mobility can decrease a patient's ability to self-administer medication. For example, pill bottles routinely come with childproof safety caps, which many older people have difficulty opening. When an older adult requests them, most pharmacies provide containers that are easier to open.

When the doctor advises discontinuing a drug, instruct the patient to discard it — in the toilet, if possible. This prevents others from using the drug and ensures that the patient won't continue taking it by mistake.

Recognizing adverse reactions

Older adults are especially susceptible to adverse drug effects, such as urticaria and rashes, impotence, incontinence, and GI upset. When other, more serious, adverse effects occur, you must be able to recognize them and intervene appropriately (see *Recognizing common adverse reactions in older adults*).

Tailoring your teaching

The abilities and needs of older adults differ from those of younger people. Therefore, tailor your style of teaching to take into account older patients' learning, motivational, and social differences. To teach successfully, keep in mind how the aging process may affect a person's mental capacity, sensory perception, and psychomotor function.

Changes in mental capacity

A person's intellectual ability changes with age. Some factors of intelligence, such as those associated with experience and learning over time, increase with age. And, as degenerative processes occur, some mental processes decline, causing such changes as slowed processing time and slowed response time. You can maximize your older patient's learning ability by asking him what he knows about the drugs he's taking before you begin your teaching and by using concrete examples the person will understand and relate to — for example, saying "two tablespoons" in describing a measure rather than "30 cc." To prevent confusion, be sure to label each medication bottle. And plan to provide written material to reinforce your oral instructions.

Older people generally need more time to process and react to information, especially when learning something new and complex, such as a new drug schedule or the difference between a drug's actions and its adverse effect. Adapt your teaching by avoiding long lists of directions. Instead, divide your instructions into short, discrete steps, and wait for

Recognizing common adverse reactions in older adults

Common signs and symptoms of adverse reactions to medications include hives, impotence, incontinence, stomach upset, and rashes. Older persons are especially susceptible and may experience serious adverse reactions such as orthostatic hypotension, dehydration, altered mental status, anorexia, blood disorders, and tardive dyskinesia.

Additional adverse reactions, such as anxiety, confusion, and forgetfulness, could be mistakenly dismissed as typical behavior rather than recognized as drug effects.

Orthostatic hypotension

Marked by light-headedness or faintness and unsteady footing, orthostatic hypotension is a common adverse effect of antidepressants, antihypertensives, antipsychotics, and sedatives.

To prevent accidents, such as falls, warn the patient not to sit up or get out of bed too rapidly. Instruct him to call for assistance in walking if he feels dizzy or faint.

Dehydration

If your patient is taking diuretics, such as hydrochlorothiazide, be alert for dehydration and electrolyte imbalance. Monitor blood levels and provide potassium supplements, as ordered.

Oral dryness can result from many medications. If anticholinergic medications cause dryness, suggest sucking on sugarless candy for relief.

Altered mental status

Agitation or confusion can follow ingestion of alcohol or anticholinergic, antidiuretic, antihypertensive, antipsychotic, antianxiety, or antidepressant medications. Paradoxically, depression is a common adverse effect of antidepressants.

Anorexia

This is a warning sign of toxicity, especially from digitalis glycosides, bronchodilators, and antihistamines.

Blood disorders

If the patient takes an anticoagulant, such as warfarin, watch for signs of easy bruising or bleeding (such as excessive bleeding after toothbrushing). Easy bruising or bleeding could be a sign of other problems such as blood dyscrasias or thrombocytopenia. Drugs that can cause these reactions include several antineoplastic agents such as methotrexate, antibiotics like nitrofurantoin, and anticonvulsants such as valproic acid and phenytoin. Tell a patient who bruises easily to report this sign to his doctor immediately.

Tardive dyskinesia

Characterized by abnormal tongue movements, lip pursing, grimacing, blinking, and gyrating motions of the face and extremities, this disorder can be triggered by psychotropic drugs such as haloperidol or chlorpromazine.

---

your patient to respond to or repeat each one.

Remember that an older patient may confuse a word or symbol you've just taught with a similar word or symbol you're introducing. For example, in a discussion about blood sugar levels, he might confuse the terms *hyperglycemia* and *hypoglycemia*. Wait for a response before introducing a new concept or definition, and whenever possible, use appropriate, common lay terms, such as "high blood sugar" and "low blood sugar."

Because a person's short-term memory decreases with age, give older patients more time to comprehend what you've said, and repeat your demonstra-

tions. Also, devise clues to help them remember information, such as colors or shapes of tablets linked to times. Older people are especially anxious about making mistakes on "tests," asking too many questions, or hurting your feelings if they can't grasp the information, so they may need extra time to answer your questions. And don't hesitate to repeat information if the older adult seems hesitant.

Sensory losses

An older patient who routinely fails to respond to you or who responds inappropriately may have hearing loss. The ability to discriminate high-frequency sounds diminishes around age 50 and declines greatly after age 65. Severe impairment can make the patient feel isolated, suspicious, or even paranoid. The older person may nod his head and agree with everything you say when you look like you're expecting a response.

If the patient speaks loudly or tilts his head when listening, assess him for deafness. Also check the ears for excessive cerumen, a common, reversible cause of hearing loss.

During teaching sessions, make sure an older person with a chronic hearing problem uses a hearing aid, if available. Face the patient when you talk. Speak slowly, clearly, and in a normal tone; don't raise your voice.

Vision loss, in the form of cataracts and presbyopia, prevents many older people from reading the small print on drug containers or glossy labels. Diabetic retinopathy and macular degeneration also cause vision problems. Yellowing of the ocular lens produces color distortion, affecting your patient's ability to visually differentiate pills. And the drugs themselves may affect your patient's vision. For example, phenylbutazone, an anti-inflammatory drug, may cause blurred vision.

Impaired vision may prevent your patient from learning from videos, closed-circuit TV, or filmstrips. He may not be able to read written instructions or measure specific doses using a syringe.

When you're teaching, make sure the older adult has access to eyeglasses, contact lenses, or other vision-enhancers, such as a magnifying glass. Use large teaching aids with oversized print. If your patient doesn't suffer from color distortion, use colors in the teaching aids; however, remember to select easily distinguished colors with sufficient contrast to help the older person differentiate between printed text and background. Make sure that reading lights are properly placed and supply bright but diffused light.

Loss of flexibility and fine motor skills

Aging gradually diminishes a person's muscle strength and endurance. This can limit flexibility and prevent him from completing tasks that require fine motor skills. In fact, many older people can't turn a dial or knob effectively. Check for such limi-

tations before giving your patient a videocassette, tape recorder, or audiocassette for self-paced learning and before demonstrating how to perform a procedure.

Loss of flexibility and fine motor skills can also impede a person's ability to open drug containers or handle and pick up pills. If you doubt your older patient's ability to use the containers, have him open and close one in your presence. Make this demonstration part of every self-medication program before an older patient's discharge from a facility or upon his admission to the home care agency. If he can't manage and there are no children in the household, tell him to ask his pharmacist for nonchild-proof drug containers.

Fostering motivation

Conduct teaching sessions when the older adult is alert and ready to learn. Make an appointment, and keep sessions brief. Break down compliance skills into appropriate components, and teach just a few at each session.

Make sure the patient hasn't recently taken medication that impairs his concentration or just finished a strenuous activity that saps his energy. Find out if he has other immediate concerns, and try to address them. Also find out what activities and lifestyle the patient wants to maintain after returning home. This will help you present information in a way that makes it important to him.

Be supportive. Positive reinforcement increases your patient's confidence about taking medication.

List the nursing diagnoses that your teaching can correct. Identify these problems, and ask the patient if he wants to overcome them. Explain the relationship between the prescribed medication and the patient's desire to overcome health problems.

List health habits that will help keep him well. Explain how the things you're teaching will help achieve this goal. If your patient doesn't see himself as having a role in his own health care (believing instead that the doctor holds control), tell him that the doctor feels that the medication will help him.

Some older people adapt to their conditions so well that they don't consider them problems and don't want to learn about them. Convincing such a person that you're teaching him something useful is only half the battle. You may also have to convince him that the methods you're teaching are in his best interest. To gain his confidence, start by asking about his sleeping, eating, and other health habits. Ask him what he knows about a technique or health care tip before you explain it. List any of his health beliefs that will reinforce or hinder your teaching, and discuss these beliefs with him before you teach something new.

With the older adult's permission, include family members or other caregivers in teaching sessions, and enlist their support. However, explain how important it is for the patient to participate in his own care. This might prevent family members from needlessly taking over the responsibility of administering the patient's drugs.

Other obstacles, such as a lack of resources, can sabotage your patient's motivation. If you can detect these problems, you might be able to reduce or overcome them. For example, if the older person can't afford the prescribed medication, help him find out if relatives or a social service agency can help. If he doesn't have transportation to the pharmacy or the doctor's office, find out if a friend, family member, or transportation service can help.

Promoting compliance

To foster compliance in the older adult, first determine his ability to comply; then intervene to prevent noncompliance.

Assessing compliance ability

After learning your patient's health and drug history, determine his previous success in adhering to treatment plans. Ask him about all drugs — prescription and nonprescription — he takes currently and those he has taken in the past. If possible, ask to see samples. Have the patient name each drug and tell you why, when, and how often he takes it. Find out if he has drugs that are prescribed by more than one doctor. Also ask if he's taking any drugs originally prescribed for another person or family member (this is not uncommon).

Evaluate the older person's cognitive skills. Can he remember to take prescribed drugs on time and

regularly? Can he remember where he stored his drugs? Also evaluate his physical ability to comply. Can he read drug labels and directions? Does he identify drugs by sight or by touch? Can he open drug containers easily?

Assess the older adult's beliefs concerning drug use. For example, he may believe that chronic medication use implies that he's sick or weak and therefore may take medications erratically.

Ask questions to help you identify possibly harmful food or drug interactions that may interfere with compliance (such as those caused by alcohol or caffeine). Assess the older person's lifestyle. Does he live with family or friends? Does he live alone or with a debilitated spouse?

Preventing noncompliance

If your facility has a specially designed computer program, use it to help prevent possible drug interactions. Enter all the data you've collected on drug dosage, frequency, and administration route into a master file of drugs commonly used by older patients. From this information, the computer compiles a list of the older person's medications, potential interactions, possible adverse effects, and suggested ways he can handle any adverse effects. (If you lack a computer, you can compile a similar list using a reputable drug reference.)

Then review the findings with the patient and give him the list. If he knows what to expect, he's more likely to comply with treatment. Advise him about specific food-drug interactions, and provide a list of foods and beverages to avoid. As your patient receives drugs, new or familiar, name them, explain their intended effect, and describe possible adverse reactions to watch for and report.

Encourage the patient to purchase drugs from only one pharmacy, preferably one that maintains a drug profile for each customer. Advise him to consult the pharmacist, who can warn him about potentially harmful drug or food interactions before they occur.

If the older adult's forgetfulness interferes with compliance, devise a system for helping him remember to take his drugs properly. Suggest that he purchase or make a scheduling aid, such as a calendar, checklist, alarm wristwatch, or compartmented drug container (see *Using compliance aids*). If he simply can't remember to take his drugs on time and in the right amounts, or can't remember where he stored them, explore his family's ability to help. If he lives alone or with a debilitated spouse, he may need continuing support from a visiting nurse or another caregiver. Refer him to appropriate community resources for supervision to avoid drug misuse.

To circumvent noncompliance caused by visual impairment, provide dosage instructions in large print, if necessary.

To correct problems related to dosage form and administration, help the patient find easier ways to take the drug. For example, if he can't swallow tablets or capsules, see about switching to a liquid or powdered form of the drug. Or suggest that he slide the tablet down with soft foods such as applesauce. Keep in mind that some drug forms — for example, enteric-coated tablets, timed-release capsules, or sublingual or buccal tablets — should not be crushed. Doing so may affect absorption and effectiveness. Also, some crushed drugs taste bitter or can stain teeth or irritate oral mucosa.

To alter eating habits that lead to noncompliance, emphasize which drugs the patient must take with food and which he must take on an empty stomach. Explain that taking some drugs on an empty stomach may cause nausea, whereas taking some drugs on a full stomach may interfere with absorption. Also find out whether the older person eats regularly or skips meals. If he skips meals, he may be skipping doses, too. As needed, help him coordinate his drug administration schedule with his eating habits.

If mobility or transportation deters compliance, help the older adult locate a pharmacy that delivers. Consider using a mail-order pharmacy.

Help your patient evaluate misguided beliefs about sickness and the use of medications. Emphasize the medication's ability to enhance his health.

If financial considerations prevent compliance, help the older adult explore new ways to manage. Perhaps he's trying to save money by not having prescriptions filled or refilled or by taking fewer doses than ordered to make the drug last longer. Suggest using less expensive generic equivalents of name-brand drugs whenever possible. Also explore ways that family members can help, or refer the older person to the social service department and appropriate community agencies. For example, many states have programs to help low-income, older people buy needed drugs.

Documenting drug therapy and teaching

Follow the standard procedure for documenting medication administration. Document all assessment findings and laboratory test results in the older person's chart. Record all medications, instructions, and teaching materials given to the patient, family members, or other caregivers. Keep a record of all drugs, dosages, and adverse reactions and interventions. Describe the older person's understanding of his drug regimen. Finally, note all health and social service agency referrals.

ADMINISTERING MEDICATIONS

Whether you're delivering your patient's medications or preparing him to self-administer, keep in mind the age-related factors that may require modification of the procedures. Before administering any drug, be sure to verify the order on the older person's medication record by checking it against the doctor's order.

Check the label three times before administering the drug to make sure you're giving the prescribed medication. Check when you take the container from the shelf or drawer, again before you place the medication in the medication cup, and again before returning the container to the shelf or drawer. If you're administering a unit-dose medication, check the label a fourth time at the patient's bedside immediately after readying the medication and before discarding the wrapper.

Confirm the patient's identity by asking his name, but don't rely on an older adult's response. Also check the name, room number, and bed number on his wristband.

Assess the older person's condition, including

Using compliance aids

To help your patient safely comply with oral or inject-able drug therapy, you or a family member could pre-measure doses for him, using compliance aids like those shown below or ones you create yourself. Most pharmacies or community service agencies can sup-ply similar aids.

One-day pill pack
A plastic box with four lidded medication compart-ments marked "breakfast," "lunch," "dinner," and "bedtime" helps the older person see whether he's taken all the medications prescribed for one day. The lids may also be embossed with braille characters if needed.

The patient, caregiver, or visiting nurse must remember to fill the device each day. Being small, the device doesn't hold many tablets or capsules.

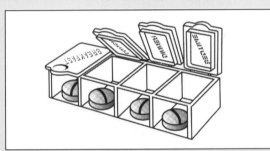

Seven-day pill reminder
The boxes shown here can help the patient remember if he has taken all the tablets and capsules prescribed for each day of the week. Each box has seven medica-tion compartments marked with the initials for each day of the week (in both braille characters and printed letters).

Like the one-day pill container, this device is inap-propriate for large numbers of tablets or capsules, or for tablets and capsules that must be taken at different times each day.

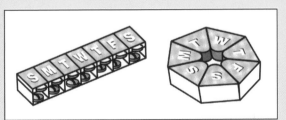

Homemade dosing aids
Show the patient and his caregivers how to make their own compliance aids by labeling clean, empty jars; extra prescription bottles (obtainable from the pharmacist); or envelopes with the drug name, the time of day, and the day of the week to take the medication. Recommend using a separate container for each time, and fill this container every morning with the correct dose of each medication.

Syringe-filling device
This device precisely measures insulin doses for a visually impaired diabetic person. Designed for use with a disposable U-100 syringe and an insulin bottle, the device is set by the caregiver to accommodate the syringe's width. She then positions the plunger at the point determined by the dose and tightens the stop. When the device is set, the patient can draw up the precise dose ordered for each injection.

There are several drawbacks to this device: it can't be used if insulin needs to be mixed or if doses vary; the settings must be checked and adjusted whenever the syringe size or type is changed; and the screws must be checked regularly because they loosen with repeated use.

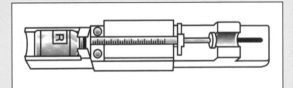

Syringe scale magnifier
This device helps a visually impaired diabetic patient read syringe markings, thereby enabling him to fill his own syringe. The plastic magnifier snaps onto the syringe barrel. This device may be impractical for a patient with arthritis who can't easily attach the magnifier to the syringe.

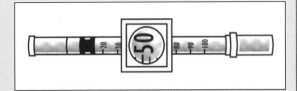

level of consciousness and vital signs, as needed. Changes in his condition may warrant withholding medication or changing the form or dosage.

Be sure to wash your hands with warm water and soap and to provide privacy for your patient. Explain the purpose of the medication, the reason for the procedure, and the steps involved in the procedure.

Giving oral medications

Because giving drugs orally is usually the safest, most convenient, and least expensive method, most drugs are administered by this route.

Oral drugs are sometimes prescribed in higher dosages than their parenteral equivalents because after absorption through the GI system they are immediately broken down by the liver, before they reach the systemic circulation. However, oral dosages normally prescribed for adults may be dangerous for the older adult.

Oral administration is contraindicated for unconscious patients; in some cases it is contraindicated in patients with nausea and vomiting and in those unable to swallow.

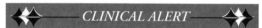

CLINICAL ALERT

Remember that dosages for an older adult may need to be reduced because of age-related changes affecting the drug's pharmacokinetics.

Equipment

Patient's medication record and chart ∎ prescribed medication ∎ medication cup.

Optional supplies include an appropriate vehicle (such as jelly, pudding, or applesauce) for crushed pills; juice, a drinking straw, and water or milk for liquid medications; and mortar and pestle for crushing pills.

Implementation

● Give the patient his medication and, as needed, an appropriate food or liquid to aid swallowing, minimize adverse effects, or promote absorption. Suggest that he take a few sips of fluid first, if not contraindicated, to moisten the mucous membranes and aid in swallowing. Keep in mind that older adults have

decreased saliva production, which might cause a dry mouth.

● Help the older person place the medication in his mouth. If he has difficulty swallowing (common in older people because of a diminished gag reflex and decreased saliva production), have him place the medication on the back of his tongue and drink some fluid. If necessary, gently massage the upper neck area just below the chin or have him use the chin tuck method to aid swallowing.

● If appropriate, crush the medication to facilitate swallowing. (See *Altering tablets and capsules.*)

● If the older person has dentures, encourage him to wear them as much as possible to maintain the gum line and the fit of the dentures. You needn't remove them for medications unless they fit poorly and collect debris in loose-fitting areas.

● Always give the most important medication first, and allow time for the patient to take it. Should he tire or refuse to take any more medications, he'll already have taken the most important ones.

● Stay with the older adult until he has swallowed the drug. If he seems confused or disoriented, check his mouth to make sure he has swallowed it.

● Return and reassess the patient's response within 1 hour after giving the medication. Monitor the patient frequently for adverse effects or signs of toxicity.

Special considerations

Make sure you have a written order for every medication given. Verbal orders should be signed by the doctor within the specified time period. (Hospitals usually require a signature within 24 hours; long-term care facilities, within 48 hours.)

Keep in mind that administration of any narcotic drug must be cosigned by another nurse, as mandated by law.

If the patient questions you about his medication or the dosage, check his medication record again. If the medication is correct, reassure him. Make sure you tell him about any changes in his medication or dosage. Instruct him, as appropriate, about possible adverse reactions. Ask him to report anything that he feels may be an adverse effect.

To avoid damaging or staining the older person's

Altering tablets and capsules

When caring for an older person, you may crush tablets or capsules so he can swallow them more easily. But first find out whether a liquid preparation of the same drug is available. If not, determine whether crushing will affect the drug's action, and follow these guidelines.

Which forms shouldn't be altered

Avoid crushing sustained-release (extended-release or controlled-release) drugs. However, some of these drugs can be scored and broken. Also avoid crushing capsules that contain tiny beads of medication. You could empty the beads into a beverage, pudding, or applesauce, however.

Don't crush or score enteric-coated tablets, which usually are shiny or candy-coated, because they are designed to prevent GI upset. Finally, avoid altering buccal and sublingual tablets.

Crushing tablets

If you need to crush a tablet, try to use a chewable form, which is easier to crush. Then use a mortar and pestle or a pill crusher, or press the tablet between two spoons, or place it in a small plastic bag and crush it with a rolling pin. Once the tablet is crushed, give the patient a drink to wet the esophagus. Unless contraindicated, mix the medication with 1 tsp or 1 tbs of pureed fruit or pudding.

Breaking tablets

If you need to break a tablet, use one that's scored. Use an instrument that can't cause injury, such as a spatula.

If a tablet isn't scored, it should be crushed, weighed, and dispensed by the pharmacist. Also follow this procedure when breaking a tablet into smaller pieces than the score allows or when giving the patient part of a capsule.

---

teeth, give acid or iron preparations through a straw. An unpleasant-tasting liquid is usually more palatable if taken through a straw because the liquid contacts fewer taste buds. If the older person has dentures, make sure that he's wearing them to ensure proper sealing of the mouth around the straw. Be sure to clean the dentures well after he has taken liquid medications such as iron, which may stain the dentures.

Giving buccal, sublingual, and translingual medications

Certain drugs are given buccally, sublingually, or translingually to prevent their destruction or transformation in the stomach or small intestine. These drugs act quickly because the oral mucosa's thin epithelium and abundant vasculature allow direct absorption into the bloodstream.

Equipment

Patient's medication record and chart ■ prescribed medication ■ medication cup.

Implementation

● Inspect the patient's oral cavity for problems, such as irritation, inflammation, or receding gingival tissue that might interfere with absorption. Older people experience changes in the oral mucosa with thinning of the epithelium and decreased vascularity.

● *For buccal administration*, place the tablet in the buccal pouch, between the cheek and gum. For sublingual administration, place the tablet under the tongue. Make sure that the patient keeps his dentures in place. (See *Placing drugs in the oral mucosa*, page 306.)

● Instruct the patient to keep the medication in place until it dissolves completely to ensure absorption.

● Caution him against chewing the tablet or touching it with his tongue to prevent accidental swallowing. Make sure that the geriatric patient completely understands not to chew or swallow the medication.

● Tell him not to smoke before the drug has dissolved because nicotine's vasoconstrictive effects slow absorption.

Placing drugs in the oral mucosa

Buccal and sublingual administration routes allow some drugs, such as nitroglycerin or methyltestosterone, to enter the bloodstream rapidly without being degraded in the GI tract. To give a drug sublingually, place it under the patient's tongue, as shown below, and ask him to leave it there until it's dissolved.

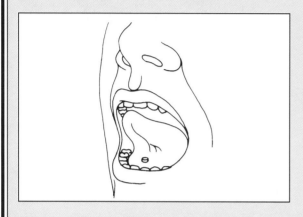

To give a drug buccally, insert it between the patient's cheek and teeth, as shown below. Ask him to close his mouth and hold the tablet against his cheek until the tablet is absorbed.

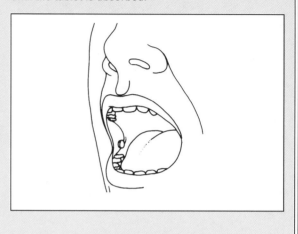

● *For translingual administration,* tell the older person to hold the medication canister vertically, with the valve head at the top and the spray orifice as close to his mouth as possible. Instruct him to spray the dose onto his tongue by pressing the button firmly.

Special considerations

Don't give liquids after administering these drugs because some buccal tablets may take up to 1 hour to be absorbed. In that case, the patient should rinse his mouth with water between doses. Tell the angina patient to wet the nitroglycerin tablet with saliva and keep it under the tongue until fully absorbed. Some buccal medications can irritate the mucosa. Provide thorough mouth care after each dose to prevent this and promote circulation to the gums and oral cavity.

Alternate sides of the mouth for repeat doses to prevent excessive irritation of the same site. Sublingual medications — for example, erythrityl tetranitrate (Cardilate) — may cause a tingling sensation under the tongue. If the patient finds this annoying, try placing the drug in the buccal pouch instead.

Giving topical medications

Applied directly to the skin surface, topical medications include lotions, pastes, ointments, creams, powders, shampoos, and aerosol sprays. The medication is absorbed through the epidermal layer into the dermis. The extent of absorption depends on the vascularity of the region.

Except for nitroglycerin and certain supplemental hormone replacements, topical medications are commonly used for local, rather than systemic, effects. Ointments have a fatty base, which is an ideal vehicle for such drugs as antimicrobials and antiseptics. Topical medications are usually applied two or three times a day to achieve a therapeutic effect.

Equipment

Patient's medication record and chart ■ prescribed medication ■ sterile tongue blades ■ gloves ■ 4" x 4" sterile gauze pads ■ transparent semipermeable dressing ■ adhesive tape ■ solvent.

Implementation

- Make sure that the patient thoroughly understands your explanation of the procedure; after discharge, he must apply the medication by himself.
- Put a glove on your dominant hand.
- Help the patient assume a comfortable position that provides access to the area to be treated.
- Expose the area to be treated. Make sure the skin or mucous membrane is intact (unless you're treating a skin lesion, such as an ulcer). Applying medication to broken or abraded skin can cause unwanted systemic absorption and further irritation.
- If necessary, clean the skin of debris, including crusts, epidermal scales, and old medication. Use a gentle cleaning motion to prevent further breakdown. An older person's skin loses elasticity and can be dry and fragile, prone to becoming irritated and broken down more easily. Change your glove if it becomes soiled.
- *To apply a paste, cream, or ointment,* first open the container. Then place the lid or cap upside down to prevent contamination of the inside surface.
- Remove a tongue blade from its sterile wrapper and cover one end with medication from the tube or jar. Then, transfer the medication from the tongue blade to your gloved hand.
- Apply the medication to the affected area with long, smooth strokes that follow the direction of hair growth. This technique avoids forcing medication into hair follicles, which can cause irritation and lead to folliculitis. Avoid excessive pressure when applying the medication because it could abrade the skin.
- To prevent contamination of the medication, use a new tongue blade each time you remove medication from the container.
- To protect applied medications and prevent them from soiling the patient's clothes, tape a sterile gauze pad or transparent semipermeable dressing over the treated area.

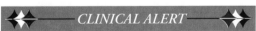
CLINICAL ALERT

Use paper tape rather than adhesive tape to secure dressings. Paper tape is less irritating to the skin and easier on the skin when it's removed.

- After applying topical medication to a patient's hands, cover them with white cotton gloves; after treating the feet, apply terry cloth scuffs.
- Assess the older person's skin for signs of irritation, allergic reaction, or breakdown.
- *To remove ointment,* wash your hands; then rub solvent on them and apply it liberally to the treated area in the direction of hair growth. Or saturate a sterile gauze pad with the solvent, and use this pad to gently remove the ointment. Remove excess oil by gently wiping the area with the sterile gauze pad. An older person's skin is fragile, so don't rub briskly to remove the medication because you could irritate the skin.

Special considerations

Manual dexterity and movement may be diminished in an older person. If the patient is expected to apply the medication at home, assess his ability to handle the needed equipment. Make sure he can open the tube or jar and is able to reach the affected area.

Giving rectal medications

Rectal medications may be supplied as suppositories or as ointment. A rectal suppository may be inserted to stimulate peristalsis and defecation or to relieve pain, vomiting, and local irritation. Because peristalsis is diminished in older people, rectal suppositories are commonly used to facilitate bowel elimination.

Because insertion of a rectal suppository may stimulate the vagus nerve, be especially alert with the older person who has cardiac disease. Suppositories are contraindicated in patients with potential cardiac arrhythmias, and may be contraindicated in patients with recent rectal or prostate surgery because of the risk of local trauma or discomfort during insertion.

An ointment used to produce local effects may be applied externally to the anus or internally to the rectum to reduce inflammation or relieve pain and itching.

Equipment and preparation

Patient's medication record and chart ■ rectal suppository or tube of ointment and ointment applicator ∎ 4" x 4" gauze pads ∎ gloves ∎ water-soluble lubricant. A bedpan is optional.

Store rectal suppositories in the refrigerator until needed to prevent softening and possible decreased effectiveness of the medication. A softened suppository is also difficult to handle and insert. To harden it again, hold the suppository (in its wrapper) under cold running water.

Implementation

● Provide privacy. While any patient may be uncomfortable with intrusive procedures, the older person may be particularly self-conscious and embarrassed. Take special care to expose only the area necessary and to keep the patient warm.

● *To insert a rectal suppository,* first place the patient on his left side in Sims' position. Then drape him with the bedcovers to expose only the buttocks.

● Put on gloves.

● Remove the suppository from its wrapper, and generously lubricate it with water-soluble lubricant. The older person requires additional lubrication because of the possibility of hemorrhoids, which can make the insertion uncomfortable.

● Lift the patient's upper buttock with your non-dominant hand to expose the anus.

● Instruct the patient to take several deep breaths through his mouth to help relax the anal sphincters and reduce anxiety or discomfort during insertion.

● Using the index finger of your dominant hand, insert the suppository — tapered end first — about 3" (8 cm), until you feel it pass the internal anal sphincter. Direct the tapered end toward the side of the rectum so it contacts the membranes.

● After inserting the suppository past the sphincter, hold it in place for a minute or two to ensure that it does not slide out because relaxation of the rectal sphincter occurs with aging.

● Tell the patient to squeeze the buttocks to-gether, if possible, to help keep the suppository in place.

● Ensure the patient's comfort. Encourage him to lie quietly and, if applicable, to retain the suppository for the appropriate length of time. A suppository administered to relieve constipation should be retained as long as possible (at least 20 minutes) to be effective. Press on the anus with a gauze pad if nec-essary until the urge to defecate passes.

● Discard the used equipment.

● *To apply a rectal ointment,* for external application, wear gloves or use a gauze pad to spread medication over the anal area.

● For internal application, attach the applicator to the tube of ointment and liberally coat the applicator with water-soluble lubricant.

● Use approximately 1" (2.5 cm) of ointment. To gauge how much pressure to use during application, squeeze a small amount from the tube before you attach the applicator.

● Lift the patient's upper buttock with your non-dominant hand to expose the anus.

● Instruct the patient to take several deep breaths through his mouth to relax the anal sphincters and reduce anxiety or discomfort during insertion.

● Gently insert the applicator, directing it toward the umbilicus.

● Slowly squeeze the tube to eject the medication.

● Remove the applicator and place a folded 4" x 4" gauze pad between the patient's buttocks to absorb excess ointment.

● Disassemble the tube and applicator. Recap the tube, and clean the applicator thoroughly with soap and warm water.

Special considerations

Instruct the patient to avoid expelling the suppository. However, if he has difficulty retaining it, place him on a bedpan, or help him to the commode or bathroom.

Make sure the patient's call button is handy and watch for his signal because he may be unable to suppress the urge to defecate. For example, a patient with proctitis has a highly sensitive rectum and may not be able to retain a suppository for long.

Be sure to inform the patient that the suppository may discolor his next bowel movement. Anusol suppositories, for example, can give feces a silver-gray pasty appearance.

If the patient is to use rectal medications at home, teach him all about the procedure.

Be sure to assess the patient's manual dexterity to determine his ability to complete the task. Diminished fine motor coordination might interfere with the patient's ability to manipulate the tube and applicator, remove the suppository from its wrapper, or reach the site of insertion. If appropriate, enlist the help of a family member or other caregiver.

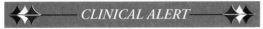

CLINICAL ALERT

Keep in mind that older people may become embarrassed at the prospect of having someone help them with this very personal procedure. This may be even more true if the family member is a son or daughter. Reinforce the need to protect the older person's privacy and self-esteem.

Giving vaginal medications

With reduced estrogen secretion, older women experience changes in the vagina, such as increased vaginal alkalinity and a thinning of the vaginal epithelium. This increases their risk for atrophic vaginitis (treatable with estrogen) and infection requiring vaginal medications.

Vaginal medications usually come with a disposable applicator that enables placement of medication in the anterior and posterior fornices. Vaginal administration is most effective when the patient can remain lying down afterward to retain the medication.

Equipment

Patient's medication record and chart ■ prescribed medication ■ applicator (if necessary) ■ gloves ■ water-soluble lubricant ■ small sanitary pad.

Implementation

● If possible, plan to give vaginal medications at bedtime, when the patient is recumbent.
● Provide privacy. The older woman may be extremely self-conscious and embarrassed.
● Ask the patient to void.
● Ask if she would rather insert the medication herself. If so, provide appropriate instructions. If not, proceed with the following steps.
● Help her into the lithotomy position.
● Expose only the perineum.
● *To insert a vaginal suppository*, remove the suppository from the wrapper and lubricate it with water-

soluble lubricant. (Because the older woman's tissues are more fragile and easily irritated, use a liberal amount of lubricant to minimize tissue trauma and increase ease of insertion.) Put on gloves and expose the vagina. (The labia of the older woman may appear flatter and less elastic.) With an applicator or the forefinger of your free hand, insert the suppository about 2" (5 cm) into the vagina, then remove the applicator. To prevent the medication from soiling the patient's clothing and bedding, provide a sanitary pad. Help her return to a comfortable position, and advise her to remain in bed as much as possible for the next several hours to promote drug absorption.
● *To insert ointments, creams, or gels*, first insert the plunger into the applicator. Then fit the applicator to the tube of medication. Gently squeeze the tube to fill the applicator with the prescribed amount of medication. Lubricate the applicator. Put on gloves and expose the vagina. Insert the applicator as you would a small suppository, and administer the medication by depressing the plunger on the applicator. Then remove the applicator. To prevent the medication from soiling the patient's clothing and bedding, provide a sanitary pad. Help the patient return to a comfortable position, and advise her to remain in bed as much as possible for the next several hours to promote drug absorption.
● After vaginal insertion, remove and discard your gloves, and wash your hands thoroughly. Wash the applicator with soap and warm water and store it, unless it's disposable. If the applicator can be used again, label it so it will be used only for the same patient.

Special considerations

If possible, teach the older woman how to insert a vaginal medication. She may have to administer it herself after discharge.

Be sure to assess the older woman's manual dexterity. Decreased fine motor coordination can interfere with her ability to manipulate the tube and applicator, remove the suppository from the wrapper, or reach the insertion site.

If the patient has mobility problems, suggest that she insert the medication while sitting on the toilet or edge of the bed and then lie down after insertion. Enlist the aid of a family member or another caregiver, if necessary. Remember that the older woman may be embarrassed by having someone help her with this very personal task, especially if the helper is a son or daughter. Stress the need to protect the patient's privacy and self-esteem.

Watch for increased irritation. Vaginal medications may cause local irritation.

Giving transdermal medications

Transdermal drugs are conveyed directly into the bloodstream from an adhesive disk or patch or a measured dose of ointment on the skin. This system delivers medication in a constant, controlled manner to provide a prolonged systemic effect. However, age-related changes in older persons, such as vascular changes resulting in a decreased blood supply, can affect drug absorption through the skin.

Medications available in transdermal form include nitroglycerin, used to control angina; estradiol for postmenopausal hormone replacement; clonidine, used to treat hypertension; nicotine, for smoking cessation; and fentanyl, a narcotic analgesic used to control chronic pain.

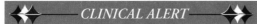
CLINICAL ALERT

Be especially alert when using fentanyl patches with older adults. Some have died of overdoses after using a fentanyl patch, so the manufacturer advises restricting the use of this patch to people with severe chronic pain that can't be managed with less powerful drugs.

Equipment
Patient's medication record and chart ■ prescribed medication (disk or ointment) ■ application strip or measuring paper (for nitroglycerin ointment) ■ adhesive tape ■ plastic wrap (optional for nitroglycerin ointment) or semipermeable dressing. Gloves are optional.

Implementation
● Put on gloves, if necessary. Remove any previously applied medication.
● *To apply a transdermal ointment,* place the pre-scribed amount of ointment on the application strip or measuring paper, taking care not to get any on your skin. Apply the strip to any dry, hairless area of the body. Avoid skin that is loose or hanging, which can interfere with adherence and absorption. Don't rub the ointment into the skin. Tape the application strip and ointment to the skin. If desired, cover the strip with plastic wrap, and tape the wrap in place.
● *To apply a transdermal disk,* open the package and remove the disk. Without touching the adhesive surface, remove the clear plastic backing. Apply the disk to a dry, hairless area.
● After applying transdermal medications, store the medication as ordered.
● Instruct the patient to keep the area around the disk or ointment as dry as possible.
● If you didn't wear gloves, wash your hands immediately after applying the disk or ointment to avoid absorbing the drug yourself.
● Monitor the patient closely for possible adverse reactions. An older person is at risk because of age-related changes affecting pharmacokinetics.
● If the patient is using transdermal nitroglycerin, assess his vital signs frequently after application, noting any changes in blood pressure.

CLINICAL ALERT

Institute safety precautions to minimize the older person's risk of falling as a result of orthostatic hypotension. Warn the patient to change positions slowly and to dangle his legs before getting out of bed.

● Assess the patient for dry mouth and dizziness. Offer ice chips or hard candy to alleviate dry mouth. Help him get out of bed and ambulate to prevent injury.

Special considerations
Contraindications for transdermal applications are the same for older adults as for any adult. It is extremely important to alternate the application sites to avoid skin irritation.

Instruct the patient using scopolamine disks not to drive or operate machinery until his response to the drug has been determined.

Warn a patient using clonidine disks to check

with his doctor before using any nonprescription cough preparations because these may counteract the effects of the drug.

Giving eye medications

Eye medications — drops, ointments, and disks — serve diagnostic as well as therapeutic purposes. Understanding the ocular effects of medications is important because certain drugs can cause eye disorders or have serious ocular effects. For example, anticholinergics, which are often used during eye examinations, can precipitate acute glaucoma in persons who are predisposed to the disorder.

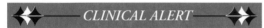
CLINICAL ALERT

Many older people require more than one type of eye medication in the same eye. Some eye medications are compatible and may be given together; others are not. Accurate timing of administration is crucial.

Equipment and preparation

Patient's medication record and chart ■ prescribed eye medication ■ gloves ■ warm water or normal saline solution ■ sterile gauze pads ■ facial tissues. Ocular dressings are optional.

Verify the order on the patient's medication record by checking it against the doctor's order on his chart. Make sure the medication is labeled for ophthalmic use. Then check the expiration date. Remember to date the container the first time you use the medication. After it's opened, an eye medication may be used for a maximum of 2 weeks to avoid contamination.

Inspect ocular solutions for cloudiness, discoloration, and precipitation (some eye medications are suspensions and normally appear cloudy). Don't use any solution that appears abnormal. If the tip of an eye ointment tube has crusted, turn the tip on a sterile gauze pad to remove the crust.

Implementation

● Make sure you know which eye to treat; different medications or doses may be ordered for each eye.
● Put on gloves.
● If the patient is wearing an eye dressing, remove it

by gently pulling it down and away from his forehead. Take care not to contaminate your hands.
● Remove any discharge by cleaning around the eye with sterile gauze pads moistened with warm water or normal saline solution. With the patient's eye closed, clean from the inner to the outer canthus, using a fresh sterile gauze pad for each stroke.
● To remove crusted secretions around the eye, moisten a gauze pad with warm water or normal saline solution. Ask the patient to close the eye, and then place the gauze pad over it for a minute or two. Remove the pad, and then reapply moist sterile gauze pads, as necessary, until the secretions are soft enough to remove without traumatizing the mucosa.
● Have the patient sit or lie in the supine position. Instruct him to tilt his head back and toward the side of the affected eye so excess medication can flow away from the tear duct, minimizing systemic absorption through the nasal mucosa.
● Remove the dropper cap from the medication container, if necessary, and draw the medication into it. Be careful to avoid contaminating the dropper tip or bottle top.
● Before instilling the eyedrops, tell the patient to look up and away. This moves the cornea away from the lower lid and minimizes the risk of touching the cornea with the dropper if the patient blinks.
● *To instill eyedrops,* first steady the hand holding the dropper by resting it against the patient's forehead. Then, with your other hand, gently pull down the lower lid of the affected eye and instill the drops in the conjunctival sac. Avoid placing the drops directly on the eyeball.
● Because an older person's eyes have less subcutaneous fat in the orbit, they're more sunken, which limits their upward gaze. Arthritic changes in the neck add to the difficulty of positioning the eyes to receive eyedrops. If possible, administer eyedrops while the patient is lying supine. Administer the drops quickly after positioning because the impulse to blink increases as time goes on.
● After administering the drops, apply gentle pressure over the inner canthus to prevent eyedrops from flowing into the tear duct. If more than one medication is being instilled, wait a few moments

between drugs because the fluids could overflow if given concurrently.

• *To apply eye ointment,* first squeeze a small ribbon of medication on the edge of the conjunctival sac from the inner to the outer canthus. Cut off the ribbon by turning the tube. Steady the hand holding the medication tube by bracing it against the patient's forehead or cheek.

• After instilling eyedrops or eye ointment, instruct the patient to close his eyes gently, without squeezing the lids shut. If you instilled drops, tell the patient to blink. If you applied ointment, tell him to roll his eyes behind closed lids to help distribute the medication over the surface of the eyeball.

• Use a clean tissue to remove any excess solution or ointment leaking from the eye. Use a fresh tissue for each eye to prevent cross-contamination.

• Apply a new eye dressing if necessary.

• Return the medication to the storage area. Make sure you store it according to the label's instructions.

• Wash your hands.

Special considerations

When administering an eye medication that might be absorbed systemically (such as atropine), gently press your thumb on the inner canthus for 1 to 2 minutes after instilling drops while the patient closes his eyes. This helps prevent medication from flowing into the tear duct.

Teach the patient how to instill eye medications so that he can continue treatment at home, if necessary. Review the procedure and then ask him to demonstrate it. (Provide the teaching aid *Administering eyedrops.*)

Make sure that the older person can identify the eye medication container. Often, eyedrops and ointments are supplied in small bottles or tubes that are difficult to handle and are labeled with very small print. If the older person has difficulty with this, devise an identification system to help him.

Note that instilling some eye medications can cause transient burning, itching, and redness. Rarely, systemic effects occur. Warn the patient not to rub the eye and to take safety precautions to minimize the risk of injury.

Giving ear medications

Eardrops may be instilled to treat infection and inflammation, to soften cerumen for later removal, to produce local anesthesia, or to facilitate removal of an insect trapped in the ear. Eardrops are usually contraindicated if a patient has a perforated eardrum; however, they may be permitted with certain medications if sterile technique is used. Other conditions also prohibit instillation of certain medications into the ear. For instance, drops containing hydrocortisone are contraindicated if the patient has herpes, another viral infection, or a fungal infection.

Equipment and preparation

Patient's medication record and chart ■ prescribed eardrops ■ light source ■ facial tissue or cotton-tipped applicator. Optional supplies include cotton balls and a bowl of warm water.

Warm the medication to body temperature in the bowl of warm water, or carry it in your pocket for 30 minutes before administering it to avoid adverse effects (such as vertigo, nausea, and pain) from instilling cold eardrops. The older person's ability to detect temperature changes is diminished, so test the temperature of the medication by placing a drop on your wrist. (If the medication is too hot, it can burn the patient's eardrum.) Before using a glass dropper, make sure it's not chipped, to avoid injuring the ear canal.

Verify the order on the patient's medication record by checking it against the doctor's order.

Implementation

• Have the patient lie on the side opposite the affected ear.

• Straighten the patient's ear canal. Pull the auricle of the ear up and back.

• Using a light source, examine the ear canal for drainage or cerumen. Accumulated cerumen is common in the older patient and can reduce the medication's effectiveness. Clean the canal with the tissue or cotton-tipped applicator as needed.

• Compare the label on the eardrops to the order on the patient's medication record. Check the label again while drawing the medication into the dropper. Finally, check the label before returning the

*T*EACHING AID

Administering eyedrops

Dear Patient:

Your doctor has prescribed eyedrops for you. Here's how to instill the drops in your eye.

1. Wash your hands thoroughly.

2. Hold the medication bottle up to the light and examine it. If the medication is discolored or contains sediment, don't use it. Instead, take it back to the pharmacy and have it examined.

If the medication looks okay, warm it to room temperature by holding the bottle between your hands for 2 minutes.

3. Moisten a rayon cosmetic puff or a tissue with water, and clean any secretions from around your eyes. Wipe outward in one motion, starting from the side near your nose. Use a fresh rayon puff or tissue for each eye.

4. Squeeze the bulb of the eyedropper and slowly release it to fill the dropper with medication. Then stand or sit before a mirror or lie on your back, whichever is most comfortable.

5. Tilt your head slightly backward and toward the eye you're treating. Pull down your lower eyelid.

6. Position the dropper over the space that you've exposed between your lower lid and the white of your eye. Steady your hand by resting two fingers against your cheek or nose.

7. Look up at the ceiling. Then squeeze the prescribed number of drops into the space.

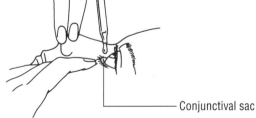

Conjunctival sac

Take care not to touch the dropper to your eye, eyelashes, or finger.

Close your eye briefly, but don't squeeze it shut. Wipe away excess medication with a clean tissue.

8. Release the lower lid. Try to keep your eye open and not blink for at least 30 seconds. Apply gentle pressure to the corner of your eye at the bridge of your nose for 1 minute, as shown below. This will prevent the medication from being absorbed through your tear duct.

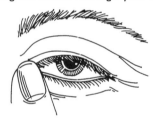

9. Repeat the procedure in the other eye, if the doctor orders.

10. Recap the bottle and store it away from light and heat.

If you're using more than one kind of drop, wait 5 minutes before you use the next one.

Important: Call your doctor immediately if you notice any of these effects: _____

_____

_____

And remember, never put medication in your eyes unless the label reads "For Ophthalmic Use" or "For Use in Eyes."

Additional instructions:

_____

_____

eardrops to the shelf or drawer.

• To avoid damaging the ear canal with the dropper, gently support the hand holding the dropper against the patient's head. Straighten the patient's ear canal again and instill the ordered number of drops. To prevent discomfort, aim the dropper so that the drops fall against the sides of the ear canal, not on the eardrum. Hold the ear canal in position until you see the medication disappear down the canal. Then release the ear.

• Instruct the patient to remain on his side for 5 to 10 minutes to allow the medication to run down into the ear canal.

• If ordered, tuck the cotton ball loosely into the opening of the ear canal to prevent the medication from leaking out. Be careful not to insert it too deeply into the canal, which could prevent drainage of secretions and increase pressure on the eardrum.

• Clean and dry the outer ear.

• Wash your hands.

• If ordered, repeat the procedure in the other ear after 5 to 10 minutes.

• Assist the patient into a comfortable position.

Special considerations

Some conditions make the normally tender ear canal even more sensitive, so be especially gentle when performing this procedure. For instance, to avoid injuring the eardrum, never insert a cotton-tipped applicator into the ear canal past the point where you can see the tip. If cleaning is necessary, apply eardrops to soften cerumen; then irrigate the ear as ordered to facilitate its removal.

If the patient has vertigo, keep the side rails of his bed up and assist him during the procedure, as necessary. Also, move slowly and unhurriedly to avoid exacerbating his vertigo.

Teach the older person how to instill the eardrops correctly so that he can continue treatment at home, if necessary. Review the procedure and let him try it himself while you observe.

Giving subcutaneous injections

A drug moves into the bloodstream more rapidly when it's injected into the adipose (fatty) tissues beneath the skin, than when it's given by mouth.

S.C. injection allows slower, more sustained drug infusion than I.M. injection; it also causes minimal tissue trauma and minimizes the risk of striking large blood vessels and nerves.

Drugs and solutions for S.C. injection are injected through a relatively short needle, using meticulous sterile technique. The most common S.C. injection sites are the outer aspect of the upper arm, anterior thigh, loose tissue of the lower abdomen, buttocks, and upper back. S.C. injection is contraindicated in sites that are inflamed, edematous, scarred, or covered by a mole, birthmark, or other lesion. It may also be contraindicated in patients with impaired coagulation mechanisms.

Equipment and preparation

Patient's medication record and chart ■ prescribed medication ■ needle of appropriate gauge and length ■ gloves ■ 1- to 3-ml syringe ■ alcohol sponges. Optional equipment includes an antiseptic cleaning agent, filter needle, insulin syringe, and insulin pump.

Select a needle of the proper gauge and length. Usually, a 25 to 27 G, ½" needle works well. However, if the patient is obese or heavy, a ⅝" needle may be needed. Use a 27 G needle for a very thin older patient.

Remember to check the label on the medication container against the medication record. Read the label again as you draw up the medication for injection. Follow the same procedure for verifying the order and drawing up the medication as you would for any adult.

Implementation

• Select an appropriate injection site. Closely inspect the patient for the best site available. With a decrease in body mass and loss of subcutaneous tissue, the deltoid area may not be an appropriate site for some older people. Rotate sites according to a schedule for patients who require repeated injections. Use different areas of the body unless contraindicated by the specific drug. (Heparin, for example, should be injected only in certain sites.)

• Put on gloves.

• Position and drape the patient if necessary.

• Clean the injection site with an alcohol sponge, beginning at the center of the site and moving outward in a circular motion. Allow the skin to dry before injecting the drug to avoid a stinging sensation from introducing alcohol into subcutaneous tissues.

• Loosen the protective needle sheath.

• With your nondominant hand, grasp the skin around the injection site firmly to elevate the subcutaneous tissue, forming a 1" (2.5-cm) fat fold. Because the older patient has a decrease in subcutaneous tissue, you might need to grasp a larger area to obtain adequate subcutaneous tissue.

• Holding the syringe in your dominant hand, insert the loosened needle sheath between the fourth and fifth fingers of your other hand while still pinching the skin around the injection site. Pull back the syringe with your dominant hand to uncover the needle by grasping the syringe like a pencil. Don't touch the needle.

• Position the needle with its bevel up.

• Tell the patient he'll feel a prick as the needle is inserted.

• Insert the needle quickly in one motion at a 45- to 90-degree angle, depending on the subcutaneous tissue at that site. (See *Giving subcutaneous injections*.)

• Release the patient's skin to avoid injecting the drug into compressed tissue and irritating nerve fibers.

• Pull back the plunger slightly to check for blood return. If no blood appears, begin injecting the drug slowly. If blood appears upon aspiration, withdraw the needle, prepare another syringe, and repeat the procedure.

• Don't aspirate for blood return when giving insulin or heparin. It's not necessary with insulin and may cause a hematoma with heparin.

• After injection, remove the needle gently but quickly at the same angle used for insertion.

• Cover the site with an alcohol sponge, and massage the site gently (unless you have injected a drug that contraindicates massage, such as heparin or insulin) to distribute the drug and facilitate absorption.

• Remove the alcohol sponge and check the injec-

Giving subcutaneous injections

Before giving the injection, elevate the subcutaneous tissue at the site by grasping it firmly.

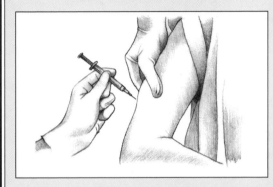

Insert the needle at a 45- or 90-degree angle to the skin surface, depending on needle length and the amount of subcutaneous tissue at the site. Some medications, such as heparin, should always be injected at a 90-degree angle.

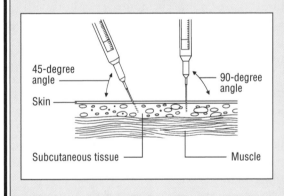

---

tion site for bleeding or bruising. Because of vascular changes, older people are more subject to bruising and hematomas.

• Dispose of the injection equipment according to facility policy. To avoid needle-stick injuries, don't resheath the needle.

Special considerations

If the medication is available in prefilled syringes, adjust the angle and depth of insertion according to needle length. If this is not possible, you might have to transfer the medication to another syringe with an appropriately sized needle attached.

To establish more consistent blood insulin levels when giving *insulin injections*, rotate injection sites within anatomic regions. Follow the same procedure and precautions as you would for any adult when administering insulin to an older person.

The preferred site for *heparin injections* is the lower abdominal fat pad, 2" (5 cm) beneath the umbilicus, between the right and the left iliac crests. Injecting heparin into this area, which isn't involved in muscular activity, reduces the risk of local capillary bleeding. Always rotate the sites from one side to the other.

Don't administer any injection within 2" of a scar, a bruise, or the umbilicus.

Don't aspirate to check for blood return when giving heparin injections because this may cause bleeding into the tissues at the site. Older patients are especially prone to this because of vascular changes. For the same reason, don't rub or massage the site after the heparin injection. Rubbing can cause localized minute hemorrhages or bruises. If the patient bruises easily, apply ice to the site for the first 5 minutes after the heparin injection to minimize local hemorrhage, then apply pressure.

If the older person is to receive S.C. heparin injections at home, make sure that he and a family member or other caregiver are able to demonstrate the procedure for preparing and administering the injection. If the patient's vision is impaired, suggest using assistive devices such as a scale magnifier or syringe filling device.

Encourage the patient to record the site used for the heparin injection. Marking a body diagram and noting the date of the injection on the diagram helps him remember where the last injection was given.

If the patient is allowed to use the deltoid muscle site for heparin injections and has difficulty doing this, suggest using the wall to help elevate the subcutaneous tissue. Show him how to rotate the shoulder of the selected arm towards the body. Then have him lean against the wall so that the deltoid area is exposed, clean the site, and inject the drug.

Giving intramuscular injections

I.M. injections deposit medication deep into muscle tissue, which is well vascularized and can absorb it quickly. This route of administration provides rapid systemic action and absorption of relatively large doses (up to 5 ml in appropriate sites). I.M. injections are recommended for patients who are uncooperative because the method eases administration and ensures absorption. They're also suitable for patients who can't take medication orally and for drugs that are altered by digestive juices. Because muscle tissue has few sensory nerves, I.M. injection allows less painful administration of irritating drugs.

I.M. injections require sterile technique to maintain the integrity of muscle tissue. Choose the site for an I.M. injection carefully, taking into account the older adult's general physical status and the purpose of the injection. Don't administer I.M. injections at inflamed, edematous, or irritated sites or at those containing moles, birthmarks, scar tissue, or other lesions.

I.M. injections may also be contraindicated in patients with impaired coagulation mechanisms and in those with occlusive peripheral vascular disease, edema, or shock because these conditions impair peripheral absorption. Oral or I.V. routes are preferred for drugs that are poorly absorbed by muscle tissue, such as phenytoin, digoxin, chlordiazepoxide, diazepam, and haloperidol.

Equipment and preparation

Patient's medication record and chart ■ prescribed medication ■ diluent or filter needle (if needed) ■ 3- to 5-ml syringe ■ 20G to 25G, 1" to 3" needle ■ gloves ■ alcohol sponges.

Follow the same procedure for verifying the order and drawing up the medication for the older person as for any adult.

Implementation

● Select an appropriate injection site (see *Modifying intramuscular injections*). Remember to always rotate injection sites for people who require repeated injections.
● Position and drape the patient appropriately, making sure the site is well exposed and lighting is adequate. Ensure the patient's privacy. Older patients often are self-conscious about any exposure.

Modifying intramuscular injections

Before you give an I.M. injection to an older person, consider the physical changes that accompany aging and choose your equipment, site, and technique accordingly.

Choosing a needle

An older person usually has less subcutaneous tissue and less muscle mass than a younger adult — especially in the buttocks and deltoids. So you might need to use a shorter needle than you would for a younger adult.

Selecting a site

An older patient typically has more fat around the hips, abdomen, and thigh areas. This makes the vastus lateralis muscle and ventrogluteal area (gluteus medius and minimus, but not gluteus maximus muscles) primary injection sites. The ventrogluteal site is preferred because it is easily accessed without repositioning the patient excessively, and is free from major nerves and blood vessels. The muscle remains large enough for injection even in very slender patients and is located well away from areas of contamination if the patient is incontinent. The deltoid site is usually a poor site for all but infrequent administration of very small amounts.

You should be able to palpate the muscle in these areas easily. However, if the patient is extremely thin, gently pinch the muscle to elevate it and to avoid putting the needle completely through it (which will alter the absorption and distribution of the drug).

Caution: Never give an I.M. injection in an immobile limb because of poor drug absorption and the risk that a sterile abscess will form at the injection site.

Checking technique

To avoid inserting the needle in a blood vessel, pull back on the plunger and look for blood before injecting the drug. Because of age-related vascular changes, older patients are also at greater risk for hematomas. To check bleeding after an I.M. injection, you may need to apply direct pressure over the puncture site for a longer time than usual. Gently massage the injection site to aid drug absorption and distribution. However, avoid site massage with certain drugs given by the Z-track injection technique, such as iron dextran or hydroxyzine hydrochloride.

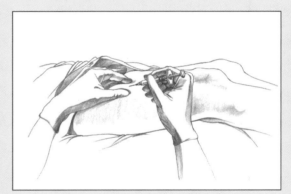

This illustration shows an injection given in the vastus lateralis.

● Loosen the protective needle sheath, but don't remove it.
● After selecting the injection site, gently tap it to stimulate nerve endings and minimize pain when the needle is inserted. Then clean the skin at the site with an alcohol sponge. Move the sponge outward in a circular motion to a circumference of about 2" (5 cm) from the injection site. Then allow the skin to dry to avoid introducing alcohol into the needle puncture, which causes pain. Keep the alcohol sponge for later use.
● Put on gloves. With the thumb and index finger of

your nondominant hand, gently stretch the skin of the injection site taut.
● Holding the syringe in your dominant hand, remove the needle sheath by slipping it between the free fingers of your other hand and then drawing back the syringe.
● Position the syringe at a 90-degree angle to the skin surface, with the needle a couple of inches from the skin. Because the older person frequently has a decrease in muscle mass, the site of the injection and the length of the needle should be appropriate for his size. Even for older adults, the ventrogluteal site

provides a well developed muscle free of nerves and blood vessels. If the needle length cannot be chosen, such as in the case of commercially pre-filled unit dose syringes, alter the angle of injection when entering the muscle mass. Patients who are wheelchair-bound have atrophied lower extremity muscles, so that the deltoid may be a better choice for them if the volume of the injection is 1 ml or less.

● Tell the patient that he will feel a prick as you insert the needle. Then quickly and firmly thrust the needle through the skin and subcutaneous tissue, deep into the muscle.

● Support the syringe with your nondominant hand, if desired. Pull back slightly on the plunger with your dominant hand to aspirate for blood. If no blood appears, place your thumb on the plunger rod and slowly inject the medication into the muscle. A slow, steady injection rate allows the muscle to distend gradually and accept the medication under minimal pressure. You should feel little or no resistance against the force of the injection. The air bubble in the syringe should follow the medication into the injection site.

◆◆ CLINICAL ALERT ◆◆

If blood appears in the syringe on aspiration, the needle is in a blood vessel. If this occurs, stop the injection, withdraw the needle, prepare another injection with new equipment, and inject another site. Don't inject the bloody solution.

● After the injection, gently but quickly remove the needle at the same angle that it was inserted.

● Using a gloved hand, cover the injection site immediately with the used alcohol sponge, apply firm but gentle pressure, and unless contraindicated, massage the relaxed muscle to help distribute the drug and promote absorption. Some authorities recommend using a dry sterile sponge and applying gentle pressure at the site without massaging it because this could cause tissue irritation. Check your facility's policy.

● Remove the alcohol sponge and inspect the injection site for signs of active bleeding or bruising. If bleeding continues, apply pressure to the site; if bruising occurs, you may apply ice.

● Watch for adverse reactions at the site for 30 minutes after the injection.

● Discard all equipment according to standard precautions and your facility's policy. Don't attempt to recap needles; dispose of them in an appropriate sharps container to avoid needle-stick injuries.

Special considerations

Never inject a drug into sensitive muscles, especially those that twitch or tremble when you assess site landmarks and tissue depth with your fingertips. Injections in these trigger areas may cause sharp or referred pain, such as the pain caused by nerve trauma.

Keep a rotation record that lists all available injection sites, divided into various body areas, for patients who require repeated injections. Rotate from a site in the first area to a site in each of the other areas. Then return to a site in the first area that is at least 1" (2.5 cm) away from the previous injection site in that area.

If the patient has experienced pain or emotional trauma from repeated injections, try numbing the area before cleaning it by holding ice on it for several seconds. If you must inject more than 5 ml of solution, divide the solution and inject it at two separate sites. Always encourage the patient to relax the muscle you'll be injecting because injections into tense muscles are more painful and might bleed more readily.

I.M. injections can damage local muscle cells, causing elevated levels of serum creatine kinase (CK), which can be confused with the elevated enzymes resulting from damage to cardiac muscle, as in myocardial infarction. To distinguish between skeletal and cardiac muscle damage, diagnostic tests for suspected myocardial infarction must identify the isoenzyme of CK specific to cardiac muscle (CK-MB) and include tests for lactate dehydrogenase and aspartate aminotransferase. If it's important to measure these enzyme levels, suggest that the doctor switch to I.V. administration and adjust dosages accordingly.

Note that because older patients have decreased muscle mass, I.M. medications can be absorbed more quickly than expected, and you may see more immediate effects than anticipated. Monitor the patient closely.

Giving medications through enteral tubes

Drugs may be given through nasogastric (NG) tubes, gastrostomy tubes or, in certain cases, gastrostomy feeding buttons. The following section focuses on the NG tube and provides additional information on giving drugs through a gastrostomy tube and gastrostomy feeding button.

Besides providing an alternate means of nourishment, the NG tube allows direct instillation of medication into the GI system of a patient who can't ingest it orally. Before instillation, the patency and positioning of the tube must be carefully checked because this procedure is contraindicated if the tube is obstructed or improperly positioned or if the patient is vomiting or his bowel sounds are absent.

Oily medications and enteric-coated or sustained-release tablets are contraindicated for instillation through an NG tube. Oily medications cling to the sides of the tube and resist mixing with the irrigating solution. And crushing enteric-coated or sustained-release tablets to facilitate transport through the tube destroys their intended effect. (See *Giving medications through an NG tube.*)

Equipment and preparation

Patient's medication record and chart ▪ prescribed medication ▪ towel or linen-saver pad ▪ 50- or 60-ml piston type catheter-tip syringe ▪ feeding tubing ▪ two 4" x 4" gauze pads ▪ stethoscope ▪ gloves ▪ diluent ▪ cup for mixing medication and fluid ▪ spoon ▪ 50 ml of water ▪ rubber band ▪ gastrostomy tube and funnel (if needed). Optional equipment includes pill-crushing equipment (mortar and pestle, for example) and a clamp (if not already attached to tube).

For maximum control of suction, use a piston syringe instead of a bulb syringe. The liquid for diluting the medication can be juice, water, or a nutritional supplement.

Gather the necessary equipment for use at the patient's bedside. Liquids should be at room temperature. Administering cold liquid through the NG

Giving medications through an NG tube

Holding the nasogastric (NG) tube at a level above the patient's nose, pour up to 30 ml of diluted medication into the syringe barrel. To prevent air from entering the patient's stomach, hold the tube at a slight angle and add more medication before the syringe empties. If necessary, raise the tube slightly higher to increase the flow rate. But be careful not to raise it too high. Older patients are at risk for cramping.

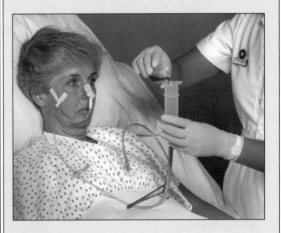

After you've delivered the whole dose, position the patient on her right side, with her head slightly elevated, to minimize esophageal reflux.

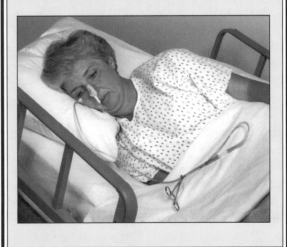

tube can cause abdominal cramping. Although this is not a sterile procedure, make sure the cup, syringe, spoon, and gauze are clean.

If the prescribed medication is in tablet form, crush the tablets to ready them for mixing in a cup with the diluting liquid.

Implementation

- Put on gloves.
- Detach the tube from the patient's gown. To avoid soiling the sheets during the procedure, fold back the bed linens to the patient's waist and drape his chest with a towel or linen-saver pad.
- Elevate the head of the bed so the patient is in Fowler's position, as tolerated.
- Observe the tube at the nares. When the tube is first inserted and placement checked by X-ray, document the length of the external segment. Compare the length of the external segment now with that of the initial insertion. Note whether the tape securing the tube to the patient's face is in position. If the length of the external segment of the tube has increased, the tube may be out of place. If this occurs, notify the doctor.
- If the length of the external segment is accurate, and after unclamping the tube, take the 50- or 60-ml syringe and create a 10-cc air space in its chamber. Then attach the syringe to the end of the tube.
- Auscultate the patient's abdomen about 3" (8cm) below the sternum with the stethoscope. Then gently insert the 10 cc of air into the tube. You should hear the air bubble entering the stomach. If you hear this sound, gently draw back on the piston of the syringe. The appearance of gastric contents implies that the tube is patent and in the stomach. (However, only an X-ray positively confirms the tube's position.) If no gastric contents appear when you draw back on the piston, the tube may have risen into the patient's esophagus, in which case you'll have to advance it before proceeding.
- If you meet resistance when aspirating for stomach contents, stop the procedure. Resistance may indicate a nonpatent tube or improper tube placement. (Keep in mind that some smaller NG tubes can collapse when aspiration is attempted.) If the tube seems to be in the stomach, resistance probably

means the tube is lying against the stomach wall. To relieve resistance, withdraw the tube slightly or turn the patient.

- After you establish that the tube is patent and in the correct position, clamp the tube, detach the syringe, and place the end of the tube on the 4" x 4" gauze pad.
- Mix the crushed tablets with the diluent. If the medication is in capsule form, open the capsules and empty their contents into the liquid. Pour liquid medications directly into the diluting liquid. Stir well with the spoon. (If the medication was in tablet form, make sure the particles are small enough to pass through the eyes at the distal end of the tube.) Keep in mind that you need enough diluent to dissolve the medication, but not too much, which could result in fluid overload in the older patient.
- Reattach the syringe, without the piston, to the end of the tube and open the clamp.
- Deliver the medication slowly and steadily. Don't allow it to flow in too quickly; because of age-related changes in the GI tract, older patients are at risk for cramping.
- If the medication flows smoothly, slowly add more until the entire dose has been given. If the medication doesn't flow properly, don't force it. It may be too thick to flow through the tube. If so, dilute it with water, being careful not to overload the patient with fluid. If you suspect tube placement is inhibiting flow, stop the procedure and reevaluate the placement.
- Watch the patient's reaction throughout the procedure. If he shows any sign of discomfort, stop the procedure immediately.
- As the last of the medication flows out of the syringe, start to irrigate the tube by adding 30 to 50 ml of water. Irrigation clears medication from the sides of the tube and from the distal end, reducing the risk of clogging.
- When the water stops flowing, quickly clamp the tube. Detach the syringe and dispose of it properly.
- Fasten the NG tube to the patient's gown.
- Remove the towel or linen-saver pad and replace the bed linens.
- Leave the patient in Fowler's position, or have him lie on his right side with the head of the bed par-

Giving medications through a gastrostomy tube

Surgically inserted into the stomach, a gastrostomy tube reduces the risk of fluid aspiration into the lungs, a constant danger with a nasogastric (NG) tube.

To administer medication by this route, prepare the patient and medication as you would for an NG tube. Then gently lift the dressing around the tube to assess the skin for irritation caused by gastric secretions. Report any redness or irritation to the doctor. If there is no irritation, follow these steps:

- Remove the dressing that covers the tube. Then remove the dressing or plug at the tip of the tube and attach the syringe or funnel to the tip.
- Release the clamp and instill about 10 ml of water into the tube through the syringe to check for patency. If the water flows in easily, the tube is patent. If it flows in slowly, raise the funnel to increase pressure. If the water still doesn't flow properly, stop the procedure and notify the doctor.
- Pour up to 30 ml of medication into the syringe or funnel. Tilt the tube to allow air to escape as the fluid flows downward. Just before the syringe empties, add medication as needed.

- After giving the medication, pour in about 30 ml of water to irrigate the tube.
- Tighten the clamp, place a 4" x 4" gauze pad on the end of the tube, and secure it with a rubber band.
- Cover the tube with two more 4" x 4" gauze pads, and secure them firmly with tape.
- Keep the head of the bed elevated for at least 30 minutes after the procedure to aid digestion.

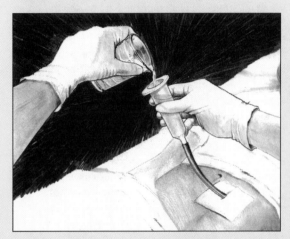

tially elevated. Have him maintain this position for at least 30 minutes after the procedure to facilitate the downward flow of medication into his stomach and to prevent esophageal reflux.

- You may be asked to deliver medications through a gastrostomy tube or gastrostomy feeding button. (See *Giving medications through a gastrostomy tube* and *Giving medications through a gastrostomy feeding button,* page 322.)

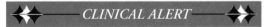
◆◆——— CLINICAL ALERT ———◆◆

If the feeding button pops out during the procedure, reinsert it, estimate the amount of medication already delivered, and resume. Be aware of your facility's policy regarding reinsertion. Some facilities only allow specially trained personnel to reinsert them (see *Reinserting a gastrostomy feeding button,* page 323).

- Once daily, clean the peristomal skin with mild

soap and water or povidone-iodine, and let the skin air-dry for 20 minutes, to avoid skin irritation. Also clean the site whenever spillage occurs.

Special considerations

To prevent instillation of too much fluid (more than 400 ml of liquid at one time for an adult), plan the drug instillation so that it doesn't coincide with the patient's regular NG tube feeding, if possible. Be sure to calculate the patient's fluid needs based on his condition. Take into consideration the amount of fluid used for irrigation.

When you must schedule a tube feeding and medication instillation simultaneously, administer the medication first to ensure that the patient receives the prescribed drug therapy, even if he can't tolerate an entire feeding. Remember to avoid giving him foods that may interact adversely with the medication.

Giving medications through a gastrostomy feeding button

The gastrostomy feeding button is an alternative feeding device for an ambulatory patient receiving long-term enteral feedings. Approved by the Food and Drug Administration for 6-month implantation, the feeding button can be used to replace a gastrostomy tube if necessary.

The button has a mushroom dome at one end and two wing tabs and a flexible safety plug at the other. When inserted into an established stoma, the button lies almost flush with the skin, with only the top of the safety plug visible.

The button usually can be inserted into a stoma in less than 15 minutes. Besides its cosmetic appeal, the device is easily maintained, reduces skin irritation and breakdown, and is less likely to dislodge and move than an ordinary feeding tube. A one-way, antireflux valve mounted just inside the mushroom dome prevents accidental leakage of gastric contents. The device usually requires replacement after 3 to 4 months, most often because the antireflux valve wears out. To administer medication by this route:

- Gather the necessary equipment: water-soluble lubricant, gloves, medication accessories (including adapter, feeding catheter, medication, diluent, syringe), catheter clamp, cleaning equipment (including water, a syringe, cotton-tipped applicator, pipe cleaner, and mild soap or povidone-iodine solution). Optional: pump to provide continuous infusion over several hours.

- Ask the doctor to order the liquid form of the drug, if possible. If not, you may administer a tablet or capsule through the button if the drug is dissolved in 30 to 50 ml of warm water.
- Attach the adapter and feeding catheter to the syringe. Clamp the catheter. Then draw up the dissolved medication into a syringe and inject it into the feeding tube.
- Open the safety plug and attach the adapter and feeding catheter to the button. Allow the medication to flow into the patient slowly, to prevent cramping and possible fluid overload.
- Next, withdraw the medication syringe and flush the tube with 50 ml of warm water.
- After administration, clean the inside of the feeding catheter with a cotton-tipped applicator and water to preserve patency and to dislodge any particles. Remove the adapter and feeding catheter. The antireflux valve should prevent gastric reflux. Then snap the safety plug in place to keep the lumen clean and prevent leakage if the antireflux valve fails.
- If the patient feels nauseated or vomits after feeding, vent the button with the adapter and feeding catheter to control emesis.
- Wash the catheter and syringe in warm soapy water and rinse thoroughly. Clean the catheter and adapter with a pipe cleaner. Rinse well before using for the next dose. Soak the equipment once a week according to the manufacturer's recommendations.

If the patient receives continuous tube feedings, stop the feeding and check the quantity of residual stomach contents. Although older people have decreased gastric emptying, the amount of residual that would alert you to withhold medications and feedings is usually 100 ml. However, check your facility's policy for the exact standard. An excessive amount of residual contents might indicate intestinal obstruction or paralytic ileus.

If the NG tube is attached to suction, be sure to turn off the suction for 20 to 30 minutes after administering the medication.

If possible, teach the patient who requires long-term treatment to instill the medication himself.

Have him observe you as you perform the procedure several times before you allow him to try it himself.

Be sure to remain with the patient when he performs the procedure for the first few times so you can provide assistance and answer any questions. As the patient performs the procedure, give him positive reinforcement and correct any errors in his technique, as necessary.

Giving medications through a peripheral I.V. site

I.V. medications are given through a peripheral I.V. site using one of three methods: direct or bolus, intermittent or piggyback, and continuous. The

Reinserting a gastrostomy feeding button

If your patient's gastrostomy button pops out — for example, from coughing — you or the patient will need to reinsert it. Here are the steps to follow.

Collect the equipment
● Gather gloves, the gastrostomy button (shown at right), mild soap and water, an obturator, water-soluble lubricant, and if necessary, the ordered medication, a catheter adapter, and a catheter.

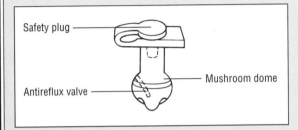

● Before reinsertion, wash your hands and put on gloves; then wash the button with soap and water and rinse it thoroughly.

Insert the button
● Check the depth of the stoma to make sure you have a button of the correct size. Then clean around the stoma with soap and water and let it air dry.
● Lubricate the obturator with water-soluble lubricant and distend the button several times to ensure patency of the antireflux valve.
● Lubricate the mushroom dome and stoma. Gently push the button through the stoma and into the stomach, as shown below.

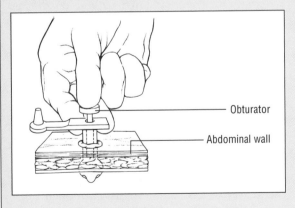

● Remove the obturator by rotating it gently as you withdraw it to keep the antireflux valve from adhering. If the valve sticks nonetheless, gently push the obturator back into the button until the valve closes.
● After removing the obturator, check the valve to make sure it's closed. Then close the flexible safety plug, which should be relatively flush with the skin surface, as shown below.

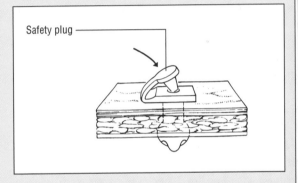

● If you need to administer the drug right away, open the safety plug and attach the adapter and catheter, as shown here. Deliver the drug as ordered.

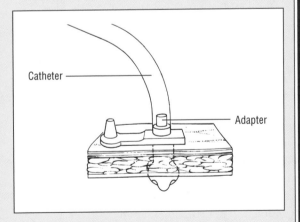

bolus method delivers a one-time dose of a drug whereas the intermittent and continuous methods deliver the necessary dose over a given period.

Follow the same procedure for reconstituting, mixing, and adding medications to an I.V. solution for an older person as you would for any adult.

Giving a bolus injection

A bolus injection is given directly through a primary I.V. tubing or through an intermittent infusion device such as a heparin lock. Because it allows the patient more freedom to move around, a heparin lock is used more often than a keep-vein-open line.

Equipment. Patient's medication record and chart ■ alcohol sponges ■ needle (20 G or smaller) with a syringe containing normal saline solution ■ syringe containing the prescribed drug ■ saline- or heparin-filled syringe for flushing ■ tape.

If the drug you're giving isn't compatible with the primary solution, you'll need another syringe filled with saline flush solution. Needleless systems are available to prevent accidental needle sticks. The procedure for using them is the same as for using syringes with needles. Check with your facility for availability and recommendations.

Implementation. *To give a bolus through a primary I.V. line,* first put on gloves. Then close the flow clamp on the I.V. tubing and clean the port closes to the insertion site with alcohol sponge.

● Puncture the center of the port with the needle attached to the medication syringe. Aspirate slightly to check for a blood return. Be especially careful not to manipulate the venipuncture site since the older patient's veins are very fragile.

● Inject the medication slowly over the recommended time interval. Observe the site as you are injecting for any puffiness or swelling which might indicate possible infiltration. If this occurs, stop the injection and evaluate the I.V. site; if necessary, remove the I.V. and restart in another area.

● Remove the syringe and the needle and clean the post with an alcohol sponge.

● *To give a bolus through a heparin lock,* first put on gloves. Then wipe the injection port of the heparin

lock with an alcohol sponge and insert the needle attached to the saline-filled syringe.

● Check for a blood return. If none appears, apply a tourniquet tightly above the injection site, keeping it in place for about 1 minute, then aspirate again. If blood still doesn't appear, remove the tourniquet and inject the saline solution. Monitor the patient's skin under the tourniquet to minimize the risk of bruising and possible injury.

● If you feel resistance or see swelling, stop the injection immediately. Resistance indicates occlusion; swelling indicates infiltration. If these occur, insert a new heparin lock.

● If you feel no resistance, watch for signs of infiltration, such as stiffness or pain at the site, as you slowly inject the saline solution. If these occur, insert a new heparin lock.

● If you aspirate blood, slowly inject the saline solution and continue observing for signs of infiltration. The saline solution flushes out any heparin solution that's incompatible with the medication.

● Withdraw the needle and the syringe.

● Insert the needle attached to the medication syringe.

● Inject the medication at the required rate. Then remove the needle from the injection port. Watch the patient closely for his response to the medication and for any adverse reactions.

● Insert the needle of the remaining saline-filled syringe into the injection port and slowly inject the saline solution. This flushes all the medication through the device.

● Remove the needle and insert and inject the heparin or saline flush solution to prevent clotting in the device.

● Discard all uncapped needles immediately to prevent needle sticks.

Giving an intermittent infusion

The most common way to administer I.V. drugs, intermittent infusion allows you to maintain therapeutic blood levels using small volumes (25 to 250 ml) over several minutes to a few hours. You can deliver an intermittent infusion through a piggyback line or intermittent infusion device called a heparin lock, or through a primary line.

For all its convenience, intermittent administration carries certain risks. When you're giving a dose through the primary I.V. line, both drugs or solutions must be compatible. Repeated needle sticks into the ports increase the risk of contaminating the tubing or heparin lock cap.

Equipment. Patient's medication record and chart ■ prescribed medication in a piggyback minibag ■ piggyback tubing ■ 20 G needle (or smaller) or a recessed needle device ■ syringe filled with 1 ml of heparin or saline flush ■ two needles with syringes filled with 2 ml of normal saline solution ■ alcohol sponges ■ I.V. pole.

Be sure to use the appropriate amount of fluid for the piggyback medication. Follow the manufacturer's guidelines, but also keep in mind the older patient's size, body mass, and fluid status. If a drug can be given in 100- to 250-ml volume, using 100 ml might be more appropriate for the older patient to prevent fluid overload.

◆◆ ── *CLINICAL ALERT* ── ◆◆

Consult a doctor before rapidly administering a volume of 250 ml I.V. That volume can be too much fluid for the patient to handle, placing him at risk for fluid overload.

Implementation. Follow these steps.
● *To give a piggyback infusion through a heparin lock,* first remove the I.V. administration tubing from the box.
● Straighten the tubing and close the roller clamp. Remove the protective cap from the end, and attach the 20 G needle. You may also use a needleless system or a click-lock I.V. system.
● Remove the protective cap from the diaphragm of the minibag and remove the cap from the I.V. tubing spike. Insert the spike into the diaphragm of the minibag. Hang the bag on the I.V. pole.
● Squeeze the drip chamber of the I.V. tubing and allow the chamber to fill halfway.
● Remove the cap from the needle or needleless/recessed needle system and open the roller clamp when the solution reaches the tip of the needle. Cover the needle with its protective cap.

● Clean the port on the heparin lock with an alcohol sponge. Remove the needle cap and insert it into the heparin lock. Securely tape this connection to reduce the risk of dislodging the needle. Check the I.V. site for infiltration.
● Adjust the roller clamp to infuse the medication over the recommended time interval. Keep in mind the patient's fluid status when determining the length of time for the infusion.
● When the infusion is complete, remove the needle from the heparin lock. Clean the heparin lock port with an alcohol sponge and inject the saline solution. Follow with a heparin flush, if used.
● Discard any uncapped needles immediately to avoid needle sticks.
● *To give a piggyback infusion through a primary line,* follow the first four steps for administering a piggyback infusion through a heparin lock.
● Clean the Y-port above the roller clamp of the primary I.V. tubing with an alcohol sponge. Insert the needle of the piggyback tubing into the port and tape the connection securely.
● Hang the primary I.V. bag or bottle lower than the minibag, using the extension hook included in the piggyback tubing box.
● Open the roller clamp on the piggyback tubing. Adjust the roller clamp of the primary bag to set the infusion rate of the minibag. To avoid fluid overload and adverse reactions, don't allow the infusion to run too fast.

◆◆ ── *CLINICAL ALERT* ── ◆◆

While the minibag is infusing, the primary I.V. solution will not run.

● When the minibag is finished, the primary I.V. solution resumes; be sure to readjust the rate of the primary solution.

Giving a continuous infusion
A continuous, or primary, I.V. infusion helps maintain a constant therapeutic drug level. This method may be the least irritating to the patient. It is probably more convenient for you because you'll spend less time mixing solutions and hanging bags than with the intermittent infusion method. And less handling means a lower infection risk. However,

fluid overload can occur if the rate and volume aren't carefully monitored. Also, vein selection and maintenance of the I.V. site might be difficult because of the condition of the older person's veins.

Equipment. Patient's medication record and chart ■ prescribed medication in a container of I.V. solution ■ administration set ■ gloves ■ infusion pump or controller, if appropriate.

Implementation. Attach the administration set to the solution container and prime the tubing.
• Attach the tubing to the pump or controller, if appropriate.
• Put on gloves and remove the protective cap at the end of the administration set. Then attach the set to the venipuncture device.
• Begin the infusion and regulate the flow for the ordered rate.
• Frequently monitor the flow rate and the patient.

Special considerations
Maintain an accurate intake and output record, and be alert for excessive fluid retention. When a patient receives small amounts hourly, an excessive total daily volume might not be obvious.

Giving a large volume of fluid can change a patient's electrolyte levels. Be sure to check these frequently.

When you're giving a bolus injection of a drug that's incompatible with dextrose 5% in water, flush the device with normal saline solution.

If the patient feels a burning sensation during the heparin injection, stop and check the needle placement. If the needle is in the vein, inject heparin at a slower rate to minimize irritation. If the needle isn't in the vein, remove and discard the needle. Then select a new site and restart the procedure.

Keep in mind that drugs given by bolus injection produce an immediate effect. Be alert for signs of adverse reactions. Check the condition of the patient's veins. Often they're fragile and easily injured, making routine site rotation difficult.

Whenever you insert or remove a needle from a heparin lock, be sure to stabilize the device to prevent trauma to the vein and dislodgment. Be pre-

pared to use an armboard to stabilize the I.V. site, or cover the area with stockinette to prevent the patient from manipulating the area.

If the older person is confused and tries to handle or pull out the I.V. line, don't immediately assume that restraints are needed. First, find out why he is interfering with the I.V. line. There may be a complication at the site or another problem that you can correct. If you can't identify a correctable problem, try to distract the patient from focusing on the I.V. line. Cover the area with stockinette to keep it out of sight, and give the patient other objects to manipulate if he seems to need something to do with his hands. An armboard is often not helpful because the patient may try to remove it as well. If the patient persists in endangering the I.V. line, put a mitt on his non-I.V. hand to prevent him from grasping at the tubing and the dressing. As a last resort, apply a soft wrist restraint on the patient's non-I.V. arm, but only after you obtain a doctor's order.

Consider using restraints only when other alternatives have failed. Be aware that most confused patients become more confused and combative when restrained, and may be at risk for aspiration, falls, and injury to the restrained limb. Release the restraint and reposition the patient at least every 2 hours.

Giving medications through a central venous catheter
A central venous (CV) line may be inserted in a patient who needs multiple transfusions of fluid, blood or blood products, antibiotics, chemotherapy or total parenteral nutrition. These infusions can be given for short or prolonged periods, using a single-lumen or multilumen catheter. A single-lumen catheter allows infusions of just one solution at a time. A multilumen catheter allows simultaneous infusion of several solutions regardless of their compatibility.

The doctor inserts the CV line directly into the patient's subclavian or internal jugular vein. Depending on the type, the line terminates in the superior vena cava. Drugs may be administered by continuous or intermittent infusion through the CV line. A bolus dose can be given through an injection cap on the catheter.

For a patient who needs CV therapy for 5 days to several months, or who requires repeated venous access, a peripherally inserted central catheter (PICC) line may be used. A PICC line helps to prevent complications that can occur with a CV line. It's easier to insert than other CV devices and provides safe, reliable access for drugs and blood sampling. A patient receiving PICC therapy must have a peripheral vein large enough to accept a 14 G or 16 G introducer needle and a 3.8 G to 4.8 G catheter. The doctor or specially trained nurse inserts a PICC via the basilic, median antecubital basilic, cubital, or cephalic vein. The PICC is then threaded to the superior vena cava or subclavian vein or to a noncentral site, such as the axillary vein.

Giving a continuous infusion

When giving an I.V. solution by continuous infusion (usually longer than 30 minutes), first prepare the solution and tubing. To ensure accurate delivery of the solution, use a volumetric control device.

Equipment. Patient's medication record and chart ▪ prescribed solution or medication ▪ administration set ▪ filter, if appropriate ▪ gloves ▪ flushing solution (saline and heparin) ▪ alcohol sponges ▪ smooth-edged clamp (if lacking on the catheter).

Implementation. Put on gloves and clamp the catheter.
● Remove the cap from the catheter tip and insert the tubing into the catheter. Tape over any non-luer-lock connections to prevent disconnection.

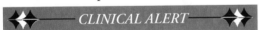
CLINICAL ALERT

If a clamp isn't available, have the patient perform Valsalva's maneuver to prevent an air embolism. As he bears down and takes a deep breath, remove the cap and plug in the I.V. tubing. Valsalva's maneuver is contraindicated if the patient is at risk for arrhythmias.
● After administering the drug or fluid, flush the CV catheter.
● Wipe the injection cap with alcohol.
● Insert a syringe with sterile normal saline solution into the cap and gently flush the catheter.

● Clean the injection cap again, insert a syringe filled with heparin solution, and flush a second time. As you withdraw the syringe containing the flush solution, continue to put pressure on the plunger to prevent blood from entering the catheter. Be sure to check your facility's policy for flushing a CV catheter.

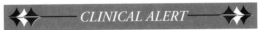
CLINICAL ALERT

If your patient has a Groshong catheter, you don't need heparin flush solution. Because of the Groshong catheter's pressure-sensitive valve, flush with 5 ml of sterile normal saline solution every 7 days. If the patient is receiving highly viscous fluids or if blood samples were drawn through the catheter, flush with 20 ml of the sodium chloride solution to prevent crystallization of the catheter tip.

Giving an intermittent infusion

Antibiotics and other drugs may be given intermittently through a CV line, typically for 40 to 60 minutes. You either inject a drug into an existing I.V. line that feeds into the CV line or administer it through an injection cap.

Equipment. Patient's medication record and chart ▪ prescribed medication ▪ I.V. tubing ▪ short needle (1" or less) ▪ two 3- to 5-ml syringes filled with sterile normal saline solution ▪ heparin solution ▪ alcohol sponges.

Implementation. Attach a needle or appropriate needleless system to the end of the I.V. tubing.
● Put on clean gloves and clean the injection cap with an alcohol sponge.
● If you're uncertain about compatibility, flush the catheter with 3 to 5 ml of sterile sodium chloride solution.
● Plug the needle into the injection cap and start the infusion at the desired rate. Tape over any non-luer-lock connections.
● When the infusion is complete, close the roller clamp on the I.V. tubing. Unplug the needle and discard it.
● Clean the injection cap with alcohol and flush

with 3 to 5 ml of the sterile sodium chloride solution, according to facility policy.

Giving a bolus injection

A bolus injection allows rapid I.V. drug administration. It may be used in an emergency to provide immediate drug effect. Alternatively, it may be used to achieve peak drug levels in the bloodstream or to deliver drugs that can't be diluted , such as diazepam and phenytoin. It may also be used to administer drugs that can't be given I.M. because they're toxic to muscle tissue or because the patient's ability to absorb them is impaired.

Equipment. Patient's medication record and chart ■ syringe with prescribed drug ■ alcohol sponges ■ two 3 to 5 ml syringes with sterile normal saline solution ■ heparin solution ■ gloves.

Implementation. Put on clean gloves.
● Clean the injection cap with an alcohol sponge and flush it with the sterile saline solution.
● Insert the needle of the syringe containing the drug, then slowly inject the drug according to the manufacturer's directions or your facility's policy.
● Withdraw the needle and discard it.
● Clean the injection cap again with an alcohol sponge.
● Inject the cap with 3 to 5 ml of sterile sodium chloride solution. Clean the cap a third time and inject it with heparin solution according to your facility's policy.

Giving medication through a PICC line

As with any CV line, be sure to check for blood return and flush with normal saline solution before administering a drug through a PICC line.

Equipment. Patient's medication record and chart ■ syringe with prescribed medication ■ two 3-ml syringes filled with sterile normal saline solution ■ gloves.

Implementation. Clamp the 7" (17.5 cm) extension tubing, and connect the empty syringe to the tubing. Release the clamp and aspirate slowly to verify blood return. Flush with 3 ml of normal saline solution; then administer the drug.
● After giving the drug, flush the PICC again with 3ml of normal saline solution. (And remember to flush with the same solution between infusions of incompatible drugs or fluids.)

Special considerations

During continuous infusion, monitor your patient's fluid status closely for signs of overload.

When your patient is receiving antibiotics every 4hours, monitor him for bleeding because he may be receiving more heparin than is therapeutic.

For a hospitalized patient receiving intermittent PICC therapy, flush the catheter with 6 ml of normal saline solution and 6 ml of heparin (10 units/ml) after each use. For catheters that aren't being used, a weekly flush of 2 ml (1,000 units/ml) of heparin maintains patency.

Remember to add an extension set to all PICC lines so you can start and stop an infusion away from the insertion site. An extension set also makes using a PICC line easier for the patient who is to administer infusions himself.

Assess the catheter insertion site through the transparent semipermeable dressing every 24 hours. Look at the catheter and check for any bleeding, redness, drainage, or swelling. Ask your patient if he's having any pain associated with therapy. Although bleeding is common for the first 24 hours after insertion, excessive bleeding after that must be evaluated.

Giving medications through a vascular access port

A vascular access device is surgically implanted under local anesthesia by a doctor. The device consists of a silicone catheter attached to a reservoir, which is covered with a self-sealing silicone rubber septum. Such a device is used most commonly when an external CV catheter is not desirable for long term I.V. therapy. The most common type of vascular access device is a vascular access port (VAP). One- and two-piece units with single or double lumens are available. (See *Understanding vascular access ports.*)

VAPs come in two basic types: top entry (such as

Understanding vascular access ports

Typically, a vascular access port (VAP) is used to deliver intermittent infusion of medication, chemotherapy, or blood products. Because the device is completely covered by the patient's skin, it reduces the risk of extrinsic contamination. Patients sometimes prefer this type of central line because it doesn't alter the body image and requires less routine catheter care.

The VAP consists of a catheter connected to a small reservoir. A septum designed to withstand multiple punctures seals the reservoir.

VAPs come in two basic designs: top entry and side entry. In a top-entry port, the needle is inserted perpendicular to the reservoir. In a side-entry port, the needle is inserted into the septum nearly parallel to the reservoir. (A needle stop prevents the needle from coming out the other side.)

TOP-ENTRY VAP

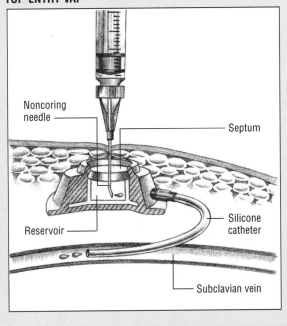

Noncoring needle
Septum
Reservoir
Silicone catheter
Subclavian vein

SIDE-ENTRY VAP

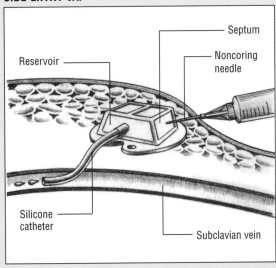

Septum
Noncoring needle
Reservoir
Silicone catheter
Subclavian vein

Med-i-Port, Port-A-Cath, and Infuse-A-Port) and side entry (such as S.E.A. Port). The VAP reservoir can be made of titanium (such as Port-A-Cath), stainless steel (such as Q-Port), or molded plastic (such as Infuse-A-Port). The type of port and catheter size to be used depends on the patient's therapeutic needs.

Implanted in a pocket under the skin, a VAP functions much like a long-term CV catheter, except that it has no external parts. The attached indwelling catheter tunnels through the subcutaneous tissue so the catheter tip lies in a central vein (the subclavian vein, for example). A VAP can also be used for arterial access or can be implanted into the epidural space, peritoneum, or pericardial or pleural cavity.

Typically, VAPs deliver intermittent infusions. Most often used for chemotherapy, a VAP can also deliver I.V. fluids, medications, or blood products. You can also use a VAP to obtain blood samples.

VAPs offer several advantages, including minimal activity restrictions, few self-care measures for the patient to learn and perform, and few dressing changes (except when used to maintain continuous infusions or intermittent infusion devices). Implanted devices are easier to maintain than external devices. For instance, they require heparinization only once after each use (or periodically if not in use). They also pose less risk of infection because they have no exit site to serve as an entry for micro-organisms.

Because VAPs create only a slight protrusion under the skin, many patients find them easier to accept than external infusion devices. But because the device is implanted, the older person might find it more difficult to manage, particularly if he must administer medication or fluids daily or frequently, or if his fine motor skills and manual dexterity are impaired. Some persons who fear or dislike needle punctures could be uncomfortable using a VAP and might require a local anesthetic. In addition, im-plantation and removal of the device requires sur-gery and hospitalization. The comparatively high cost of VAPs makes them worthwhile only for pa-tients who require infusion therapy for at least 6 months.

Implanted VAPs are contraindicated in patients who have been unable to tolerate other implanted devices and in those who may develop allergic reac-tions.

Equipment and preparation

Patient's medication record and chart.
For a bolus injection: Extension set ■ 10-ml syringe filled with normal saline solution ■ clamp ■ syringe containing prescribed medication. A sterile needle filled with heparin flush solution is optional.

For a continuous infusion: Prescribed I.V. solution or medication ■ I.V. administration set ■ filter, if ordered ■ extension set ■ clamp ■ 10-ml syringe filled with normal saline solution ■ antimicrobial ointment ■ adhesive tape ■ sterile 2" x 2" gauze pad ■ sterile tape ■ transparent semipermeable dressing.

Some facilities use an implantable port access kit.

Confirm the size and type of the device and the insertion site with the doctor. Attach the tubing to the solution container, prime the tubing with fluid, fill the syringes with saline or heparin flush solution, and prime the noncoring needle and extension set. All priming must be done using strict aseptic tech-nique, and all tubing must be free of air. After

you've primed the tubing, recheck all connections for tightness. Make sure that all open ends are cov-ered with sealed caps.

Implementation

The VAP can be used immediately after placement, although some edema and tenderness might persist for about 72 hours. This makes the device initially difficult to palpate and slightly uncomfortable for the patient.

● Using aseptic technique, inspect the area around the port for signs of infection or skin breakdown.
● Place an ice pack over the area for several minutes to alleviate possible discomfort from the needle puncture. Or administer a local anesthetic after cleaning the area.
● Wash your hands thoroughly and put on sterile gloves. Keep the gloves on throughout the proce-dure.
● Clean the area with an alcohol sponge, starting at the center of the port and working outward with a firm, circular motion over a 4" to 5" (10- to 13-cm) diameter. Repeat this procedure twice.
● If your facility's policy calls for a local anesthetic, check the patient's record for possible allergies. As indicated, anesthetize the insertion site by injecting 0.1 ml of lidocaine (without epinephrine).

Accessing a top-entry port. Palpate the area over the port to locate the port septum.
● Anchor the port with your nondominant hand. Then, using your dominant hand, aim the needle at the center of the device.
● Insert the needle perpendicular to the port sep-tum. Push the needle through the skin and septum until you reach the bottom of the reservoir.
● Check needle placement by aspirating for blood return.
● If you're unable to obtain blood, remove the needle and repeat the procedure. Inability to obtain blood may indicate that the catheter is lodged against the vessel's wall. Ask the patient to raise his arms, perform Valsalva's maneuver (if not contrain-dicated), or change position to free the catheter. If you still don't get a blood return, notify the doctor; a coating of fibrin (fibrin sleeve) on the distal end of

the catheter may be occluding the opening.
• Flush the device with normal saline solution. If you detect swelling or if the patient reports pain at the site, remove the needle and notify the doctor.

Accessing a side-entry port. To gain access to a side-entry port, follow the same procedure as with a top-entry port; however, insert the needle parallel to the reservoir instead of perpendicular to it.

Giving a bolus injection. Attach the 10-ml syringe filled with saline solution to the end of the extension set and remove all the air. Now attach the extension set to the noncoring needle. Check for blood return. Then flush the port with normal saline solution, according to your facility's policy. (Some require flushing the port with a sterile needle of heparin solution first.)
• Clamp the extension set and remove the saline syringe.
• Connect the medication syringe to the extension set. Open the clamp and inject the drug, as ordered.
• Examine the skin surrounding the needle for signs of infiltration, such as swelling or tenderness. If you note these signs, stop the injection and intervene appropriately.
• When the injection is complete, clamp the extension set and remove the medication syringe.
• Open the clamp and flush with 5 ml of normal saline solution after each drug injection to minimize drug incompatibility reactions.
• Flush with heparin solution, as your institution's policy directs.

Giving a continuous infusion. Remove all air from the extension set by priming it with an attached syringe of normal saline solution. Now attach the extension set to the noncoring needle.
• Flush the port system with normal saline solution. Clamp the extension set and remove the syringe.
• Connect the administration set, and secure the connections with sterile tape if necessary.
• Unclamp the extension set and begin the infusion.
• Apply a small amount of antimicrobial ointment to the insertion site.
• Affix the needle to the skin. Then apply a trans-parent semipermeable dressing.
• Examine the site carefully for infiltration. If the patient complains of stinging, burning, or pain at the site, discontinue the infusion and intervene appropriately.
• When the solution container is empty, obtain a new I.V. solution container, as ordered.
• Flush with heparin solution as facility policy directs.

Special considerations

After the device is implanted, monitor the site for signs of hematoma and bleeding. Edema and tenderness may persist for about 72 hours. The incision site requires routine postoperative care for 7 to 10 days. You'll also need to assess the implant site for signs of infection, device rotation, or skin erosion. You don't need to apply a dressing to the wound site except during infusions or to maintain an intermittent infusion device.

While the patient is hospitalized, a luer-lock injection cap may be attached to the end of the extension set to provide ready access for intermittent infusions. Besides saving nursing time, a luer-lock cap reduces the discomfort of accessing the port, and prolongs the life of the port septum by decreasing the number of needle punctures.

If your patient is receiving a continuous or prolonged infusion, change the dressing and needle every 5 to 7 days. Also change the tubing and solution as you would for a long-term CV infusion. If your patient is receiving an intermittent infusion, flush the port periodically with heparin solution. When the VAP isn't being used, flush it every 4 weeks. During the course of therapy, you might have to clear a clotted VAP, as ordered.

Besides performing routine care measures, be prepared to handle several common problems that could arise during infusion with a VAP. These include an inability to flush the VAP, withdraw blood from it, or palpate it.

Home care

A home care patient needs thorough teaching about procedures and follow-up visits from a home care nurse, to ensure safety and successful treatment.

If the patient will be accessing the port himself, explain that the most uncomfortable part of the procedure is inserting the needle into the skin. Once the needle has penetrated the skin, the patient will feel mostly pressure. Eventually, the skin over the port will become desensitized from frequent needle punctures. Until then, the patient may want to use a topical anesthetic.

Stress the importance of pushing the needle into the port until the patient feels the needle bevel touch the back of the port. Many patients tend to stop short of the back of the port, leaving the needle bevel in the rubber septum.

Teach the patient not to pull on or manipulate the device, which can lead to "twiddler's syndrome" (this occurs when the patient plays with the port area, causing the VAP to rotate or the catheter to migrate). Loop and tape the catheter securely using a transparent semipermeable membrane dressing.

Stress the importance of flushing the port as scheduled. If possible, instruct a family member in all aspects of care, especially if the patient has decreased fine motor skills and manual dexterity.

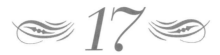

Guiding bladder and bowel retraining

Habitual and automatic patterns of elimination are established as a person grows and develops. These patterns are influenced by various factors such as diet, fluid intake, activity level, lifestyle, and advancing age.

In older people, two of the most common elimination problems are bladder and bowel incontinence. These problems may result from age- or disease-related changes in GU or GI system function, or, less often, from changes in other body systems, such as the musculoskeletal and nervous systems. If elimination problems are severe enough, they can have serious psychosocial effects and threaten the person's ability to function and survive.

INCONTINENCE

In older adults, incontinence commonly follows any loss or impairment of urinary or anal sphincter control. The incontinence may be transient or established.

Urinary incontinence

Approximately 10.3 million adults experience some form of urinary incontinence; this number includes about 50% of the 1.6 million people in extended-care facilities and 15% to 30% of older people living in the community.

Causes

Urinary incontinence can have many causes, including confusion, depression, dehydration, fecal impaction, restricted mobility, various disorders, urethral sphincter damage, and certain drugs. (See also Chapter 11.)

Assessment findings

• Ask the patient when he first noticed urine leakage and whether it began suddenly or gradually. Have him describe his typical urinary pattern: Does incontinence usually occur during the day or at night? Ask him to rate his urinary control: Does he have moderate control, or is he completely incontinent? If he sometimes urinates with control, ask him to identify when and how much he usually urinates. Use an incontinence monitoring record.

• Evaluate related problems, such as urinary hesitancy, frequency, urgency, nocturia, and decreased force or interrupted urine stream. Ask the patient to describe any previous treatment he had for incontinence or measures he performed by himself.

• Ask about medications, including nonprescription drugs. Review his medication and diet history for drugs and foods that affect digestion and elimination.

• Assess the patient's environment. Is a toilet or commode readily available, and how long does the patient take to reach it? Once the patient is in the bathroom, assess manual dexterity: How easily does he manipulate his clothes; what assistive devices could he use?

- Evaluate the patient's mental status and cognitive function.
- Quantify his normal daily fluid intake.
- Review the patient's medical history, noting especially the number and route of births and any incidence of urinary tract infections (UTI), prostate disorders, spinal injury or tumor, cerebrovascular accident, or bladder, prostate, or pelvic surgery. Check for a history of disorders such as delirium, dehydration, urine retention, restricted mobility, fecal impaction, infection, inflammation, or polyuria.
- For the examination, protect the patient's bed with an incontinence pad.
- Inspect the urinary meatus for obvious inflammation or anatomic defects. Have the patient bear down while you note any urine leakage. Gently palpate the abdomen for bladder distention, which signals urine retention. If possible, have the patient examined by a urologist.
- Obtain specimens for laboratory tests, as ordered.

Treatment

If the patient's incontinence is acute, treating the underlying disorder generally resolves it. Chronic incontinence could require behavioral, pharmacologic, or surgical treatments. As a general rule, the least invasive treatment is selected. Many forms of urinary incontinence respond to behavioral methods, such as bladder retraining and Kegel exercises.

Fecal incontinence

Although not usually a sign of serious illness, fecal incontinence can seriously impair an older patient's physical and psychological well-being. It affects up to 10% of nursing home residents and 3% to 4% of older people in the community.

Causes

Fecal incontinence may occur gradually (as in dementia) or suddenly (as in spinal cord injury). Most commonly, it results from fecal stasis and impaction accompanying reduced activity, inappropriate diet, untreated painful anal conditions, or chronic constipation. Fecal incontinence can also result from chronic laxative use; reduced fluid intake; neuro-

logic deficits; and pelvic, prostatic, or rectal surgery as well as medications, such as antihistamines, psychotropics, and iron preparations.

A person with fecal incontinence might not be aware of the need to defecate. If he can't get to the bathroom or use a commode or bedpan on his own, he may lose rectal sensitivity from having to suppress the urge while waiting for help. Musculoskeletal changes also can affect a person's ability to assume a comfortable position, interfering with the frequency and effectiveness of bowel elimination.

Assessment findings

- Ask the patient with fecal incontinence to identify its onset, duration, and severity. Also have him identify any discernible incontinence patterns. For instance, determine whether it occurs at night. Keep a bowel record for 1 week.
- Focus the history on GI, neurologic, and psychological disorders. Assess the patient for chronic constipation as well as laxative abuse.
- Check the patient's medication regimen for drugs that affect bowel activity, such as aspirin, some anticholinergic and antiparkinson agents, aluminum hydroxide, calcium carbonate antacids, diuretics, iron preparations, opiates, tranquilizers, tricyclic antidepressants, and phenothiazines.
- Assess the availability of the toilet, the amount of time needed to reach the toilet, the patient's mobility status, and his manual dexterity in removing clothing.
- Note the frequency, consistency, and volume of stool passed within the past 24 hours.
- For the examination, protect the patient's bed with an incontinence pad.
- Inspect the abdomen for distention, and auscultate for bowel sounds. If not contraindicated, check for fecal impaction (which can also be a factor in overflow incontinence).
- Obtain a stool specimen, if ordered.

Treatment

Patients with fecal incontinence should be carefully assessed for underlying causes. Retraining strategies similar to those used for urinary incontinence can also be used to manage fecal incontinence. Bowel retraining is the treatment of choice.

If the problem is poor anal sphincter tone, pelvic muscle exercises can help correct it. A person can be taught to contract and relax the anal sphincter in a regular program of exercise to strengthen the muscle.

If fecal incontinence is caused by impaction, the blockage can be removed with an enema or manually. Enemas and suppositories may be used concurrently to obtain complete bowel evacuation. In rare cases, fecal incontinence requires surgery (colostomy) and daily irrigations.

Complications

● Be alert for physiologic complications, such as skin breakdown and infection, especially in dual (urinary and fecal) incontinence.
● Also watch for psychological problems, including social isolation, loss of independence, decreased self-esteem, and depression.

Nursing interventions

Whether the patient reports urinary or fecal incontinence or both, you need to perform careful and continuing assessment to plan effective interventions.
● Be sure to schedule extra time to encourage and provide support for the patient and to mitigate any feelings of shame, embarrassment, or powerlessness from loss of control.
● Praise the patient's successful efforts.

For urinary incontinence

● Begin by implementing an appropriate bladder retraining program (see *Correcting urinary incontinence with bladder retraining,* page 336).
● To ensure healthful hydration and to prevent UTI, be sure the patient maintains adequate daily fluid intake (six to eight 8-oz glasses of fluid). Restrict fluid intake after 6 p.m., except in warm weather.
● To manage stress and urge incontinence, implement an exercise program to help strengthen the pelvic floor muscles.
● To manage functional incontinence, frequently assess the patient's mental and functional status. Regularly remind the patient to void. Respond to his calls promptly, and help him get to the bathroom as quickly as possible.

For fecal incontinence

● Begin a bowel retraining program (see *Correcting fecal incontinence with bowel retraining,* page 337).
● As appropriate, begin a scheduled toileting program. This involves assessing the patient to determine the usual time of day when a bowel movement occurs, often after breakfast or after a morning cup of coffee or other warm beverage. To promote continence, you can then remind or help the patient to use the toilet or commode 15 to 20 minutes before that time. At toileting time, ensure that your patient knows where the toilet is. You might have to stay with him to make sure that he has a complete bowel movement. Having him sway back and forth while on the toilet can help promote peristalsis. You also might have to stay with a patient who has Alzheimer's disease to make sure he remembers why he's on the toilet.
● Maintain effective hygienic care to increase the patient's comfort and prevent skin breakdown and infection. Clean the perineal area frequently, and apply a moisture barrier cream. Control foul odors as well.
● Advise the patient to consume a fiber-rich diet, with raw, leafy vegetables (such as carrots and lettuce), unpeeled fruits (such as apples), and whole grains (such as wheat or rye breads and cereals). Bran cereals provide the best source of fiber. If the patient has a lactase deficiency, suggest calcium supplements to replace calcium lost by eliminating dairy products from the diet.
● Encourage adequate fluid intake.
● Promote regular exercise by explaining how it helps to regulate bowel motility. Even a nonambulatory patient can perform some exercises while sitting or lying in bed.

Patient teaching

Your teaching can help many patients regain control.

For urinary incontinence

● To rid the bladder of residual urine, teach the

Correcting urinary incontinence with bladder retraining

An incontinent adult typically feels frustrated, embarrassed, and sometimes hopeless. Fortunately, though, incontinence usually can be corrected by bladder retraining, a program that establishes a regular voiding pattern. To implement such a program, follow these guidelines.

Assess elimination patterns
First assess your patient's intake pattern, voiding pattern, and reason for each accidental voiding (for example, a coughing spell). Use an incontinence monitoring record.

Establish a voiding schedule
Encourage the patient to void regularly; every 2 hours, for example. Once he can stay dry for 2 hours, increase the time between voidings by 30 minutes each day until he achieves a 3- to 4-hour voiding schedule (may not be enforced during the night).

Teach the patient to practice relaxation techniques, such as deep breathing, which helps decrease his sense of urgency.

Record the results and provide positive reinforcement. Keep a record of continence and incontinence for about 5 days; this might reinforce your patient's efforts to remain continent.

Promote health
Here are some additional tips to help boost the patient's success:
- Instruct the patient in measures to prevent urinary tract infections, such as adequate fluid intake (at least 1500 to 2000 ml/day unless contraindicated), drinking cranberry juice to help acidify the urine, using cotton panties, and bathing with nonirritating soaps.
- Be sure to provide access to toilet facilities and use assistive devices, such as grab bars and safety bars, as needed. Ensure patient safety with night light and railings if necessary.
- Encourage the patient to empty the bladder completely before and after meals and at bedtime.
- Advise the patient to urinate whenever the urge arises and never to ignore it.
- Instruct the patient to take prescribed diuretics upon rising in the morning.
- Advise the patient to limit the use of sleeping aids, sedatives, and alcohol; they decrease the sensation to urinate and can increase incontinence, especially at night.
- If the patient is overweight, encourage him to lose weight.
- Suggest exercises to strengthen pelvic muscles.
- Instruct the patient to increase dietary fiber or other bulk to decrease constipation and incontinence.
- Monitor the patient for signs of anxiety and depression and treat them promptly.
- Leave a light on at night. If the patient needs assistance getting out of a bed or a chair, promptly answer the call for help.
- Reassure your patient that periodic incontinent episodes don't mean the program has failed. Encourage persistence, tolerance, and a positive attitude. Remember, both your positive attitude and your patient's are crucial to successful bladder retraining.

---

patient to perform clean intermittent catheterization. Use an indwelling urinary catheter only as a last resort because of the risk of UTI.
- To aid bladder training at home, provide the teaching handouts, *Retraining your bladder,* page 338, and *Exercising your pelvic muscles,* page 339.

For fecal incontinence
- Teach the patient to gradually eliminate laxative use, if necessary. Point out, as needed, that using over-the-counter laxatives to promote regular bowel movement can have the opposite effect and cause either constipation or incontinence over time. Suggest using natural laxatives, such as prunes or prune juice, instead.

Documentation
Record all bladder and bowel retraining efforts, noting scheduled bathroom times, food and fluid intake, and elimination amounts, as appropriate. Record duration of continent periods. Note any complications, including emotional problems, and signs of skin breakdown and infection. Document treatment given for complications.

Correcting fecal incontinence with bowel retraining

Numerous regimens can be used to promote successful bowel elimination and control fecal incontinence. The key to any program is time and patience. Some examples of bowel retraining programs are listed below.

For fecal incontinence caused by impaction
- Irrigate the lower bowel with daily enemas.
- Administer a suppository every morning or evening.
- Remove the impaction manually, if necessary.
- Prevent recurrence with the following: adequate fluid intake of 2 L/day; adequate dietary fiber; stool softeners or bulk laxatives (if necessary); respond to the urge to defecate; activity and exercise regimen.

For fecal incontinence caused by neurologic disorders
- Provide adequate fluid intake.
- Provide a high-fiber diet.
- Initiate an activity and exercise program.
- Institute habit training, including scheduled toileting such as after breakfast, increase awareness of defecation reflex, and give a suppository or enemas to stimulate the bowel if there is no bowel movement for 2 consecutive days.
- If neurologic impairment is severe, induce constipation with an antidiarrheal, alternating with planned evacuation using enemas or suppositories.

PERFORMING BASIC CARE PROCEDURES

When performing any procedures on an older patient, especially those associated with elimination, be sensitive to the patient's feelings of embarrassment and self-consciousness. Take care to expose only the body areas necessary to accomplish the procedure.

When teaching older patients about performing a procedure to aid elimination, keep in mind that they might be reluctant to touch themselves, feeling that it's wrong. In addition, many older patients have little knowledge about the anatomy and physiology of their GU and GI tracts, making it difficult for them to comprehend some instructions. This, coupled with the possibility of decreased manual dexterity and fine motor ability, could make it necessary to include family members in the teaching program. However, keep in mind that the older patient's embarrassment and self-consciousness might be compounded if a family member — especially a son or daughter — must perform the procedure.

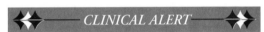

CLINICAL ALERT

Always maximize the patient's level of independence while minimizing the risks to his self-esteem.

Offering a bedpan or urinal

Using a bedpan or urinal permits elimination by the bedridden patient and accurate observation and measurement of urine and stools by staff. If possible, help your patient to use a bedside commode or regular commode, because these allow a more natural position for emptying the bladder and bowel.

A bedpan is used by a female patient for defecation and urination and by a male patient for defecation; a urinal is used by a male patient for urination. Offer either device frequently: before meals, visiting hours, morning and evening care, and any treatments or procedures. Whenever possible, allow the patient to use a bedpan or urinal in private.

Equipment
Bedpan or urinal with cover ■ toilet tissue ■ two washcloths ■ soap ■ gloves ■ towel ■ linen-saver pad ■ bath blanket ■ pillow. Optional: air freshener, talcum powder.

(Text continues on page 340.)

EACHING AID

Retraining your bladder

Dear Patient:

You can correct or manage incontinence by reestablishing a normal urination pattern.

You'll begin by keeping a careful record of your fluid intake and urination pattern. Then you'll schedule urination at regular intervals and increase the time between urinating gradually. Your goal will be to urinate no more than once every 3 to 4 hours.

Step 1: Keeping a record

Do your accidental urinations follow a pattern? You'll know at a glance by recording your fluid intake, how you urinated (intentionally or by accident), and why you think an accident occurred. Keep a chart like the one shown.

After a few days, your chart will show when

Date 10/17			
Time	**Fluid intake**	**Urinated in toilet**	**Small accid**
6 to 8 a.m.	Small glass of orange juice	✓	
8 to 10 a.m.	2 cups of coffee		small

you're most likely to become incontinent; for example, after meals or during the night. Your chart will also help your doctor evaluate your progress and adjust your treatment.

Step 2: Scheduling urination

Next, schedule specific times to urinate. Practice this technique at home, where you're relaxed and close to the bathroom. Start by

urinating every 1½ to 2 hours, whether or not you feel the need.

If you have to urinate sooner, practice "holding" it by relaxing, concentrating, and taking three slow, deep breaths until the urge decreases or goes away. Wait 5 minutes. Then go to the bathroom and urinate — even if the urge has passed. Otherwise, your next urge may be very strong and difficult to control.

If you have an accident before the 5 minutes have passed, shorten your next waiting time to 3 minutes. After a week of training, if waiting 5 minutes is easy, increase to 10 minutes.

Using the method above, gradually increase the intervals between urinations. Strive for 3- or 4-hour intervals. Don't get discouraged if you do have an accident.

Tips for success
● Set an alarm clock to remind you to use the toilet, including once or twice at night.
● Make sure you can reach the bathroom or portable toilet easily.
● Walk to the bathroom slowly.
● Always urinate just before bedtime.
● Learn Kegel exercises to tone the bladder.
● Avoid drinks that contain caffeine or alcohol.
● Drink eight to ten 8-ounce (240-milliliter) glasses of fluid every day. This helps to prevent urinary tract infection and constipation, which also can cause incontinence. To prevent nighttime accidents, drink most of your fluids before 6 p.m.

Remember to count foods containing mostly liquid (such as ice cream, soup, and gelatin) as fluids.

TEACHING AID

Exercising your pelvic muscles

Dear Patient:

Exercising your pelvic muscles every day can make them stronger and help to prevent incontinence. The following exercises, called Kegel exercises, are easy to learn and simple to do.

By exercising faithfully and correctly, you'll notice an improvement in about 4 weeks. In 3 months, you'll notice an even greater improvement.

If you have stress incontinence, try to do these exercises just before a sneeze or cough. Also try to do a few exercises before you lift something heavy or cumbersome.

Here's how to do the exercise.

Finding the right muscle

The muscle you want to strengthen is called the pubococcygeal (PC) muscle. This is the muscle that controls the flow of urine. You can find this muscle in two ways:
- by voluntarily stopping your urine stream
- by pulling in on your rectal muscle as you would to retain gas.

Once you've mastered these motions, you've mastered the exercise.

Practicing the exercise

Strengthen and tone your PC muscle by performing one of the two motions described above. Hold the muscle tight, working up to 10 seconds. Then relax the muscle for 10 seconds. Do 15 exercises in the morning, 15 in the afternoon, and 20 at night. Or exercise for about 10 minutes, three times a day.

When to exercise

You can do Kegel exercises almost anywhere and at any time. Most people sit in a chair or lie on a bed to do them. You can also do them standing up.

How can you remember to do these exercises? One way is to combine them with an activity you do regularly. For example, if you spend a lot of time in the car, do an exercise at every red light. Or exercise while watching the evening news.

Avoiding mistakes

Take time to think about which muscles you're using. If you find yourself using your abdominal, leg, or buttocks muscles, you're not performing the exercises correctly.

Here's an easy way to check yourself: Place one hand on your abdomen while you perform the exercise. Can you feel your abdomen move? If you can, then you're using the wrong muscles. Or, if your abdomen or back hurts after exercising, you're probably trying too hard or using abdominal or back muscles that you shouldn't be using.

If you get headaches after exercising, be careful not to tense your chest muscles or hold your breath while doing the exercises.

Remember: These exercises should feel mild and easy, not strenuous.

Additional instructions:

Bedpans, which are available in adult and pediatric sizes, may be disposable or reusable (sterilizable). A type of bedpan called a fracture pan may be used if the patient can't be moved because of spinal injury, a body or leg cast, or other immobilizing condition, or if the patient is especially thin and frail.

Preparation of equipment

Obtain a bedpan or urinal. If the item is metal, warm it under running water to avoid startling the patient and stimulating muscle contraction, which hinders elimination. Dry the bedpan thoroughly and test its temperature because metal retains heat; the older patient has diminished ability to detect changes in temperature and is more susceptible to burns. If necessary, lightly sprinkle talcum powder on the edge of the bedpan to reduce friction on the older patient's thin, friable skin during placement and removal. For a thin patient, place a linen-saver pad at the edge of the bedpan to minimize pressure on the coccyx.

Implementation

● Provide privacy to minimize embarrassment. Put on gloves to prevent contact with body fluids and comply with standard precautions.

To place a bedpan. Follow these steps.
● If allowed, elevate the head of the bed slightly to prevent hyperextension of the spine when the patient raises the buttocks.
● Rest the bedpan on the edge of the bed. Then, turn down the corner of the top linens and draw up the patient's gown.
● Ask the patient to raise the buttocks by flexing his knees and pushing down on his heels. While supporting the patient's lower back with one hand, center the curved, smooth edge of the bedpan beneath the buttocks.
● If the patient can't raise his buttocks, lower the head of the bed to horizontal and help him roll onto one side with buttocks toward you. Position the bedpan properly against the buttocks, and then help the patient roll back onto the bedpan.
● After positioning the bedpan, elevate the head of the bed further, if allowed, until the patient is sitting

erect. Because this position resembles the normal elimination posture, it aids defecation and urination. If possible, and the patient's condition permits it, use a commode instead of a bedpan (see *Using a commode*).
● If elevating the head of the bed is contraindicated, tuck a small pillow or folded bath blanket under the patient's back to cushion the sacrum against the edge of the bedpan and support the lumbar region.
● If the patient feels pain during turning or feels uncomfortable on a standard bedpan, use a fracture pan. Unlike the standard bedpan, the fracture pan is slipped under the buttocks from the front rather than the side. Because it's shallower than the standard bedpan, you need only lift the patient slightly to position it. If the patient is obese or otherwise difficult to lift, ask a coworker to help you.
● If the patient can be left alone, place the bed in a low position and raise the side rails to ensure his safety. Place toilet tissue and the call button within the patient's reach, and instruct him to push the button after elimination. If the patient is weak or disoriented, remain with him.
● Before removing the bedpan, lower the head of the bed slightly. Then ask the patient to raise his buttocks off the bed. Support his lower back with one hand, and gently remove the bedpan with the other to avoid skin injury caused by friction. If the patient cannot raise his buttocks, ask him to roll off the pan while you assist with one hand. Hold the pan firmly with the other hand to avoid spills. Cover the bedpan and place it on the chair.
● Assist with cleaning the anal and perineal area to prevent irritation and infection. Turn the patient on his side, wipe carefully with toilet tissue, clean the area with a damp washcloth and soap, and dry well with a towel. For the female patient, clean from front to back to avoid introducing rectal contaminants into the vagina or urethra.

To place a urinal. Follow these steps.
● Lift the corner of the top linens, hand the urinal to the patient, and allow him to position it.
● If the patient can't position the urinal himself, spread his legs slightly and hold the urinal in place to prevent spills.

Using a commode

Unlike a bedpan, a commode allows the patient to assume his normal elimination posture, which aids in defecation. The commode is a portable chair made of wood, plastic, or metal, with a large opening in the center of the seat. It has a bedpan or bucket that slides underneath the opening, or it slides directly over the toilet, adding height to the standard toilet seat. Here are some guidelines for using a commode.
● Before use, inspect the commode and make sure it's clean. Place it parallel and as close as possible to the patient's bed, and secure its brakes or wheel locks. If necessary, block its wheels with sandbags.
● Assist the patient onto the commode, provide toilet tissue, and place the call button within his reach.

Close the curtain to ensure privacy. Remain nearby if the person is unsteady, weak, or might need assistance. Instruct him to push the call button or call you when he has finished.
● If necessary, assist the patient with cleaning. Help him into bed and make him comfortable. Offer the patient soap, water, and a towel to wash his hands.
● Then close the lid of the commode or cover the bucket. Roll the commode or carry the bucket to the bathroom or hopper room. If ordered, observe and measure the contents before disposal. Rinse and clean the bucket, and then spray or wipe the bucket and commode seat with disinfectant. Use an air freshener if appropriate.

● After the patient voids, carefully withdraw the bedpan or urinal.
● Give the patient a clean, damp, warm washcloth for his hands. Check the bed linens for wetness or soiling, and straighten or change them, if needed. Make the patient comfortable. Place the bed in the low position and raise the side rails.
● Take the bedpan or urinal to the bathroom or hopper room. Observe the color, odor, amount, and consistency of urine and stools. If ordered, measure urine output or liquid stool, or obtain a specimen for laboratory analysis.
● Empty the bedpan or urinal into the toilet or hopper. Rinse the container with cold water and clean it thoroughly, using a disinfectant solution. Dry it and return it to the patient's bedside stand.
● Use an air freshener in the patient's room, if necessary, to eliminate offensive odors and reduce the patient's embarrassment.
● Remove the gloves and wash your hands.

Special considerations
Explain to the patient that any drug treatment and changes in his environment, diet, and activities may disrupt his usual elimination schedule. Try to anticipate elimination needs, and offer the bedpan or urinal frequently to help reduce embarrassment and

minimize the risk of incontinence.

Avoid placing a bedpan or urinal on top of the bedside stand or overbed table to avoid contamination of clean equipment and food trays. Similarly, avoid placing it on the floor to prevent the spread of microorganisms from the floor to the patient's bed linens when the device is used.

If the patient has an indwelling urinary catheter in place, carefully position and remove the bedpan to avoid tension on the catheter, which could dislodge it or irritate the urethra. After the patient defecates, wipe, clean, and dry the anal region, taking care to avoid catheter contamination. If necessary, clean the urinary meatus with povidone-iodine solution.

Documentation
Record the time, date, and type of elimination on the flowchart and the amount of urine output or liquid stool on the intake and output record, as needed. In your notes, document the presence of blood, pus, or other abnormal characteristics in urine or stool.

Administering an enema
This procedure involves instilling a solution into the rectum and the colon. In a retention enema, the

patient holds the solution within the rectum or colon for 30 minutes to 1 hour before finally expelling it. In an irrigating enema, the patient expels the solution almost completely within 15 minutes.

Both types of enema stimulate peristalsis by mechanically distending the colon and stimulating rectal wall nerves.

An enema may be used with a bowel retraining program for the older patient with incontinence. Enemas also are used to clean the lower bowel (called flush enemas) in preparation for diagnostic or surgical procedures; to relieve distention and promote the expulsion of flatus; to lubricate the rectum and colon; and to soften hardened stool for removal.

Enemas are contraindicated, however, after recent colon or rectal surgery or myocardial infarction, and in acute abdominal conditions of unknown origin, such as suspected appendicitis. Enemas should be administered cautiously to a patient with a cardiac arrhythmia.

Equipment
Prescribed solution ■ bath (utility) thermometer ■ enema administration bag with attached rectal tube and clamp ■ I.V. pole ■ gloves ■ linen-saver pads ■ bath blanket ■ two bedpans with covers, or bedside commode ■ water-soluble lubricant ■ toilet tissue ■ bulb syringe or funnel ■ plastic bag for equipment ■ water ■ gown ■ washcloth ■ soap and water. If you are observing enteric precautions: plastic trash bags ■ labels.

Optional (for patients who can't retain solution): plastic rectal tube guard, indwelling urinary catheter or Verden rectal catheter with 30-ml balloon and syringe.

Prepackaged disposable enema sets are available, as are small-volume enema solutions for both irrigating and retention types.

Preparation of equipment
Prepare the prescribed type and amount of enema solution, as indicated. Standard volumes for an irrigating enema are 750 to 1,000 ml for an adult; standard volumes for a retention enema are 50 to 250 ml or less for an adult.

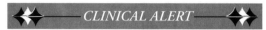

Use smaller fluid volumes for an older patient who is receiving an irrigating enema because using large volumes can cause colon distention and mild shock. Very thin or frail older patients may require smaller amounts of solution.

Because some ingredients can be mucosal irritants, be sure the proportions are correct and the agents are thoroughly mixed to avoid localized irritation.

Warm the solution to reduce the patient's discomfort. Test the temperature of the solution with a bath thermometer. Be sure to administer the enema at a temperature no higher than 100° to 105° F (37.7° to 40.5° C) to avoid burning rectal tissues. The older patient's ability to detect temperature changes is diminished, placing him at a high risk for burns.

Clamp the tubing and fill the solution bag with the prescribed solution. Unclamp the tubing, flush the solution through the tubing, then reclamp it. Flushing reveals leaks and removes air that could cause discomfort if introduced into the colon.

Hang the solution container on the I.V. pole and take all supplies to the patient's room. If you're using a Foley or Verden catheter, fill the syringe with 30 ml of water for inflating the catheter balloon.

Implementation
● Assess the patient's condition.
● Provide privacy and explain the procedure. Instruct the patient to breathe through the mouth to relax the anal sphincter, which will facilitate catheter insertion.
● Ask the patient if he's had previous difficulty retaining an enema to determine whether you need to use a rectal tube guard or a catheter.
● Wash your hands and put on gloves.
● Assist the patient, as necessary, in putting on a hospital gown. The gown makes enema administration easier, and the patient worries less about soiling it.
● Assist the patient into the left-lateral Sims' position. This will facilitate the solution's flow by gravity

into the descending colon. If this position is contraindicated or if the patient reports discomfort, reposition him on his back or the right side.

• Place linen-saver pads under the patient's buttocks to prevent soiling the linens. Replace the top bed linens with a bath blanket to provide privacy and warmth.

• Have a bedpan or commode nearby for the patient to use. If the patient can use the bathroom, be sure that it will be available when he needs it. Place toilet tissue within the patient's reach.

• Lubricate the distal tip of the rectal catheter liberally with water-soluble lubricant to facilitate insertion and reduce irritation and trauma.

• Separate the patient's buttocks and touch the anal sphincter with the rectal tube to stimulate contraction. Then, as the sphincter relaxes, tell the patient to breathe deeply through the mouth as you gently advance the tube.

• If the patient feels pain or the tube meets continued resistance, notify the doctor. This may signal an unknown stricture or abscess. If the patient has poor sphincter control, use a plastic rectal tube guard, or slip the tube through the cut end of a baby bottle nipple.

• You can also use a Foley or Verden catheter as a rectal tube if your facility's policy permits. Insert the lubricated catheter as you would a rectal tube. Then, gently inflate the catheter's balloon with 20 to 30 ml of water. Gently pull the catheter back against the patient's internal anal sphincter to seal off the rectum. If leakage still occurs with the balloon in place, add more water to the balloon in small amounts. When using either catheter, avoid inflating the balloon with more than 45 ml because overinflation can compromise blood flow to the rectal tissues and cause possible necrosis from pressure on the rectal mucosa.

• When you're using a rectal tube, hold it in place throughout the procedure because bowel contractions and the pressure of the tube against the anal sphincter can cause tube displacement.

• Hold the solution container slightly above bed level and release the tubing clamp. Then raise the container gradually to start the flow; usually at a rate of 75 to 100 ml/minute for an irrigating enema. For a retention enema, introduce fluid at the slowest possible rate to avoid stimulating peristalsis and to promote retention.

• Adjust the flow rate of an irrigating enema by raising or lowering the solution container according to the patient's retention ability and comfort. However, be sure not to raise it higher than 18" (46 cm) because excessive pressure can force colon bacteria into the small intestine or rupture the colon.

• Assess the patient's tolerance frequently during instillation. If he complains of discomfort, cramps, or the need to defecate, stop the flow by pinching or clamping the tubing. Then hold the patient's buttocks together or firmly press toilet tissue against the anus. Instruct the patient to gently massage his abdomen and breathe slowly and deeply through his mouth to help relax abdominal muscles and promote retention. Resume administration at a slower flow rate after a few minutes when discomfort passes, but interrupt the flow any time the patient feels uncomfortable.

• If the flow slows or stops, the catheter tip may be clogged with feces or pressed against the rectal wall. Gently turn the catheter slightly to free it without stimulating defecation. If the catheter tip remains clogged, withdraw the catheter, flush with solution, and reinsert.

• After administering most of the prescribed amount of solution, clamp the tubing. Stop the flow before the container empties completely to avoid introducing air into the bowel.

• To administer a commercially prepared, small-volume enema, first remove the cap from the rectal tube. If necessary, apply additional water-soluble lubricant to the tip to prevent trauma. Insert the rectal tube into the rectum and squeeze the bottle to deposit the contents in the rectum. Remove the rectal tube, replace the used enema unit in its original container, and discard.

• For a flush enema, stop the flow by lowering the solution container below bed level and allowing gravity to siphon the enema from the colon. Continue to raise and lower the container until gas bubbles cease to appear or the patient feels more comfortable and abdominal distention subsides. Don't allow the solution container to empty completely before lowering it because this could introduce air into the bowel.

● For an irrigating enema, instruct the patient to retain the solution for 15 minutes, if possible.

● For a retention enema, instruct the patient to avoid defecation for the prescribed time; 30 minutes or longer for oil retention. If you're using an indwelling catheter, leave the catheter in place to promote retention.

● If the patient is apprehensive, position him on the bedpan and allow him to hold toilet tissue or a rolled washcloth against his anus. Place the call button within his reach. If he will be using the bathroom or the commode, instruct him to call for help before attempting to get out of bed because the procedure can make the patient feel weak or faint. Also instruct him to call you if he feels weak at any time.

● When the solution has remained in the colon for the recommended time or for as long as the patient can tolerate it, assist the patient onto a bedpan or to the commode or bathroom, as required.

● If an indwelling catheter is in place, deflate the balloon and remove the catheter, if applicable.

● Provide privacy while the patient expels the solution. Instruct the patient not to flush the toilet.

● While the patient uses the bathroom, remove and discard any soiled linens and linen-saver pads.

● Assist the patient with cleaning, if necessary, and help him to bed. Make sure he feels clean and comfortable and can easily reach the call button. Place a clean linen-saver pad under him to absorb rectal drainage, and tell him that he may need to expel additional stool or flatus later. Encourage him to rest for a while because the procedure may be tiring.

● Cover the bedpan or commode and take it to the utility room for observation, or observe the contents of the toilet, as applicable. Carefully note fecal color, consistency, amount (minimal, moderate, or generous), and foreign matter, such as blood, rectal tissue, worms, pus, mucus, or other unusual matter.

● Send specimens to the laboratory, if ordered.

● Rinse the bedpan or commode with cold water, then wash it in hot soapy water. Return it to the patient's bedside.

● Properly dispose of the enema equipment. If additional enemas are scheduled, store clean, reusable equipment in a closed plastic bag in the patient's bathroom. Discard your gloves and wash your hands.

● Ventilate the room or use an air freshener, if necessary.

Special considerations

Don't give an enema to a patient who's in a sitting position, unless absolutely necessary, because the solution won't flow high enough into the colon and will only distend the rectum and trigger rapid expulsion. If the patient has hemorrhoids, instruct him to bear down gently during tube insertion. This causes the anus to open and facilitates insertion.

Because patients with salt-retention disorders, such as congestive heart failure, can absorb sodium from the saline enema solution, administer the solution to such patients cautiously and monitor electrolyte status.

Schedule a retention enema before meals because a full stomach could stimulate peristalsis and make retention difficult. Follow an oil-retention enema with a soap and water enema 1 hour later to help expel the softened feces completely.

Administer less solution when giving a hypertonic enema because osmotic pull moves fluid into the colon from body tissues, increasing the volume of colon contents. Alternative means of instilling the solution include using a bulb syringe or a funnel with the rectal tube.

For the patient who cannot tolerate a flat position (for example, a patient with shortness of breath), administer the enema with the head of the bed in the lowest position he can safely and comfortably maintain. For a bedridden patient who needs to expel the enema into a bedpan, raise the head of the bed to approximate a sitting or squatting position.

If the patient fails to expel the solution within 1 hour because of diminished neuromuscular response, you may need to remove the enema solution. First, review your facility's policy; you may need a doctor's order. Inform the doctor when a patient can't expel an enema spontaneously because of possible bowel perforation or electrolyte imbalance.

To siphon the enema solution from the patient's

rectum, assist him to a side-lying position on the bed. Place a bedpan on a bedside chair so it rests below mattress level. Disconnect the tubing from the solution container, place the distal end in the bedpan, and reinsert the rectal end into the patient's anus. If gravity fails to drain the solution into the bedpan, instill 30 to 50 ml of warm water (105° F [40.6° C]) through the tube. Then quickly direct the distal end of the tube into the bedpan. In both cases, measure the return to be sure all solution has drained.

In patients with fluid and electrolyte disturbances, measure the amount of expelled solution to assess for retention of enema fluid.

Double-bag all enema equipment and label it as isolation equipment if the patient is on enteric precautions.

If the doctor orders enemas until returns are clear, give no more than three to avoid excessive irritation of the rectal mucosa. Notify the doctor if the returned fluid isn't clear after three administrations.

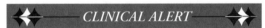

CLINICAL ALERT

Monitor the patient closely for signs of water intoxication, which can occur after repeated tap water enemas.

• For a person who's receiving treatment at home, describe the procedure to the patient and his family. Emphasize that administering an enema to a person in a sitting position or on the toilet could injure the rectal wall. Tell the patient how to prepare and care for the equipment. Discuss relaxation techniques, and review measures for preventing constipation, including regular exercise, dietary modifications, and adequate fluid intake.

Complications
Enemas can cause dizziness or faintness; excessive irritation of the colonic mucosa with repeated administration, or from sensitivity to the enema ingredients; hyponatremia or hypokalemia from repeated administration of hypotonic solutions; and cardiac arrhythmias from vasovagal reflex stimulation after inserting the rectal catheter. Colonic water absorption may result from prolonged retention of hypotonic solutions, which could, in turn, cause hyper-

volemia or water intoxication. The older patient is at high risk for these complications because of age-related physiologic changes.

Documentation
Record the date and time of enema administration; special equipment used; type and amount of solution; retention time; approximate amount returned; color, consistency, and amount of the return; abnormalities within the return; any complications that occurred; and the patient's tolerance of the treatment.

Removing a fecal impaction manually
Fecal impaction — a hard, dry mass of stool lodged in the folds of the rectum and, at times, in the sigmoid colon — results from prolonged retention and accumulation of stool. Fecal impaction is a common cause of fecal incontinence in older persons, and may result from poor bowel habits, inactivity, dehydration, improper diet (especially inadequate fluid intake), constipation-inducing drugs, and incomplete bowel cleaning after a barium enema or barium swallow. Manual removal, which is done only when oil retention and cleansing enemas, suppositories, and laxatives fail to clear the impaction, may require a doctor's order.

This procedure is contraindicated after rectal, GU, abdominal, perineal, or gynecologic reconstructive surgery; in patients with myocardial infarction, coronary insufficiency, pulmonary embolus, congestive heart failure, heart block, and Stokes-Adams syndrome (without pacemaker treatment); and in patients with GI or vaginal bleeding, hemorrhoids, rectal polyps, or blood dyscrasia.

Equipment
Gloves (2 pairs) ■ linen-saver pad ■ bedpan ■ plastic disposal bag ■ soap ■ water-filled basin ■ towel ■ water-soluble lubricant ■ washcloth.

Implementation
• Explain the procedure to the patient and provide privacy.
• Position the patient on his left side and flex his knees to allow easier access to the sigmoid colon and

rectum. Drape the patient, and place a linen-saver pad beneath the buttocks to prevent soiling the bed linens.

• Put on gloves, and liberally moisten an index finger with water-soluble lubricant to reduce friction during insertion, thereby avoiding injury to sensitive tissue.

• Instruct the patient to breathe deeply to promote relaxation. Then gently insert the lubricated index finger beyond the anal sphincter until you touch the impaction. Rotate the finger gently around the stool to dislodge and break it into small fragments. Then work the fragments downward to the end of the rectum, and remove each one separately.

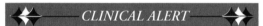
CLINICAL ALERT

Manipulate the blockage gently to avoid injuring the rectal lining, which is fragile in older patients.

• Before removing your finger, gently stimulate the anal sphincter with a circular motion two or three times to increase peristalsis and encourage further evacuation.

• Remove the finger and change your gloves. Then clean the anal area with soap and a basin of water and lightly pat dry with a towel.

• Offer the patient the bedpan or commode because digital manipulation stimulates the urge to defecate. Assist the patient to the commode to prevent injury.

• Place disposable items in the plastic bag and discard properly. If necessary, clean the bedpan and return it to the bedside stand.

• Wash your hands.

Special considerations

It may be impossible to remove an impaction all at once. Allow the patient to rest between attempts. Manual removal should be followed by a small irrigating enema.

If the patient experiences pain, nausea, rectal bleeding, changes in pulse rate or skin color, diaphoresis, or syncope, stop immediately and notify the doctor.

Complications

Manual removal of fecal impaction can stimulate

the vagus nerve and may decrease heart rate and cause syncope.

Documentation

Record the time and date of the procedure, the patient's response, and stool color, consistency, and odor.

Inserting an indwelling urinary catheter

Also known as a Foley or retention catheter, an indwelling catheter remains in the bladder to provide continuous urine drainage. A balloon inflated at the catheter's distal end prevents it from slipping out of the bladder after insertion. Indwelling catheters are used primarily to relieve bladder distention caused by urine retention and to allow continuous urine drainage when the urinary meatus is swollen from surgery or local trauma. They may also be used for urinary tract obstruction (by a tumor or enlarged prostate), urine retention or infection from neurogenic bladder paralysis caused by spinal cord injury or disease, and any illness in which the patient's urine output must be monitored closely.

An indwelling catheter is inserted using sterile technique and only when absolutely necessary. It is not recommended for treating urinary incontinence because of the risk of infection. However, it can be used if urinary incontinence delays the healing of a pressure ulcer. Perform insertion with extreme care to prevent injury and infection.

Equipment

Sterile indwelling catheter #10 to #22 French (average adult sizes are #16 to #18 French; the smallest catheter minimizes trauma to the urethra) ▪ syringe filled with 5 to 8 ml of normal saline solution ▪ washcloth ▪ towel ▪ soap and water ▪ two linen-saver pads ▪ sterile gloves ▪ sterile drape ▪ sterile fenestrated drape ▪ sterile cotton-tipped applicators (or cotton balls and plastic forceps) ▪ povidone-iodine or other antiseptic cleaning agent ▪ urine receptacle ▪ sterile water-soluble lubricant ▪ sterile drainage collection bag ▪ intake and output sheet ▪ adhesive tape. Optional: urine-specimen container and laboratory request form, leg band with Velcro closure, gooseneck lamp.

Prepackaged sterile disposable kits are available and usually contain all the necessary equipment. The syringes in these kits are prefilled with normal saline solution.

Preparation of equipment

Check the order on the patient's chart to determine if a catheter size or type is specified. Then wash your hands, select the appropriate equipment, and assemble it at the patient's bedside.

Implementation

- Explain the procedure to the patient and provide privacy. Check his chart and ask when he voided last. Percuss and palpate the bladder to establish baseline data. Ask if he feels the urge to void.
- So that you can see the urinary meatus clearly in poor lighting, place a gooseneck lamp next to the patient's bed.
- Place the female patient in the supine position, with her knees flexed and separated and her feet flat on the bed, about 2' (61 cm) apart. If she finds this position uncomfortable, have her flex one knee and keep the other leg flat on the bed. You may need an assistant to help the patient stay in position or to direct the light, especially if the older patient has mobility problems or decreased muscle strength. Place the male patient in the supine position with his legs extended and flat on the bed. Ask the patient to hold the position to give you a clear view of the urinary meatus and to prevent contamination of the sterile field.
- Use the washcloth to clean the patient's genital area and perineum thoroughly with soap and water. Dry the area with the towel. Then, wash your hands.
- Place the linen-saver pads on the bed between the patient's legs and under the hips. To create the sterile field, open the prepackaged kit or equipment tray and place it between the female patient's legs or next to the male patient's hip. If the sterile gloves are the first item on the top of the tray, put them on. Place the sterile drape under the patient's hips. Then drape the patient's lower abdomen with the sterile fenestrated drape so that only the genital area re-

mains exposed. Take care not to contaminate your gloves.
- Open the rest of the kit or tray. Put on the sterile gloves if you haven't already done so.
- Tear open the packet of povidone-iodine or other antiseptic cleaning agent, and use it to saturate the sterile cotton balls or applicators. Be careful not to spill the solution on the equipment.
- Open the packet of water-soluble lubricant and liberally apply it to the catheter tip; attach the drainage bag to the other end of the catheter. (If you're using a commercial kit, the drainage bag may be attached.) Make sure all tubing ends remain sterile, and be sure the clamp at the emptying port of the drainage bag is closed to prevent urine leakage from the bag. Some drainage systems have an air-lock chamber to prevent bacteria from traveling to the bladder from urine in the drainage bag.
- Before inserting the catheter, inflate the balloon with normal saline solution to inspect it for leaks. To do this, attach the saline-filled syringe to the luer lock, then push the plunger and check for seepage as the balloon expands. Aspirate the saline to deflate the balloon. Also inspect the catheter for resiliency. Rough, cracked catheters can injure the urethral mucosa during insertion, which can lead to infection.
- For the female patient, separate the labia majora and labia minora as widely as possible with the thumb, middle, and index fingers of your nondominant hand so you have a full view of the urinary meatus. Keep the labia well separated throughout the procedure, so they don't obscure the urinary meatus or contaminate the area once it's cleaned. Keep in mind that the older female's labia may be less elastic with a decrease in subcutaneous tissue in the vulvar area.
- With your dominant hand, use a sterile, cotton-tipped applicator (or pick up a sterile cotton ball with the plastic forceps) and wipe one side of the urinary meatus with a single downward motion. Wipe the other side with another sterile applicator or cotton ball in the same way. Then wipe directly over the meatus with another sterile applicator or cotton ball. Take care not to contaminate your sterile glove.

● For the male patient, hold the penis with your nondominant hand. If he's uncircumcised, retract the foreskin. Then gently lift and stretch the penis to a 60- to 90-degree angle. Hold the penis in this way throughout the procedure to straighten the urethra and maintain a sterile field.

● Use your dominant hand to clean the glans with a sterile cotton-tipped applicator or a sterile cotton ball held in forceps. Clean in a circular motion, starting at the urinary meatus and working outward.

● Repeat the procedure using another sterile applicator or cotton ball, taking care not to contaminate your sterile glove.

● Pick up the catheter with your dominant hand and prepare to insert the lubricated tip into the urinary meatus. To facilitate insertion by relaxing the sphincter, ask the patient to cough as you insert the catheter. Tell the patient to breathe deeply and slowly to further relax the sphincter and prevent spasms. Hold the catheter close to its tip to ease insertion and control its direction.

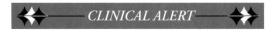

CLINICAL ALERT

Never force a catheter during insertion. Maneuver it gently as the patient bears down or coughs. If you still meet resistance, stop the procedure and notify the doctor. Strictures, sphincter spasms, misplacement in the vagina, or an enlarged prostate can cause resistance.

● For the female patient, advance the catheter about 2" to 3" (5 to 7.6 cm) — while continuing to hold the labia apart — until urine begins to flow.

● For the male patient, advance the catheter about 6" to 8" (15.2 to 20.3 cm) until urine begins to flow. If the foreskin was retracted, be sure to replace it to prevent compromised circulation and painful swelling.

● When urine stops flowing, attach the saline-filled syringe to the luer-lock.

● Push the plunger and inflate the balloon to keep the catheter in place in the bladder.

CLINICAL ALERT

Never inflate a balloon without first establishing urine flow, which assures you that the catheter is in the bladder, not in the urethral channel.

● Hang the collection bag below bladder level to prevent urine reflux into the bladder (which can cause infection), and to facilitate gravity drainage of the bladder. Make sure the tubing doesn't get tangled in the bed's side rails.

● Tape the catheter to the female patient's thigh to prevent possible tension on the urogenital trigone.

● Tape the catheter to the male patient's thigh or lower abdomen to prevent pressure on the urethra at the penoscrotal junction, which can cause urethrocutaneous fistulas. This also prevents traction on the bladder and preserves the normal direction of urine flow in males.

● As an alternative, secure the catheter to the patient's thigh using a leg band with a Velcro closure. This decreases skin irritation, especially in patients with long-term indwelling catheters.

● Dispose of all used supplies properly.

Special considerations

Several types of catheters are available with balloons of various sizes. Each type has its own method of inflation and closure. For example, in one type of catheter, sterile solution or air is injected through the inflation lumen; then the end of the injection port is folded over itself and fastened with a clamp or rubber band.

Note: Injecting a catheter with air makes identifying leaks difficult and doesn't guarantee deflation of the balloon for removal.

A similar catheter is inflated by penetrating a seal in the end of the inflation lumen with a needle or the tip of the solution-filled syringe. Another type of balloon catheter self-inflates when a prepositioned clamp is loosened. The balloon size determines the amount of solution needed for inflation, and the exact amount is usually printed on the distal extension of the catheter used for inflating the balloon.

The doctor may order an intermittent or straight catheter instead of an indwelling one. The procedure is the same except that the catheter doesn't have a balloon to inflate, the urine is drained into a collection device, and the catheter is removed after the bladder is drained. There is a high risk of infection.

If necessary, ask the female patient to lie on her side with her knees drawn up to her chest during the catheterization procedure. This position may be especially helpful for older or disabled patients, such as those with severe contractures. If necessary, provide the patient with detailed instructions for performing clean intermittent self-catheterization. (See "Teaching intermittent self-catheterization," in this chapter.)

If the doctor orders a urine specimen for laboratory analysis, obtain it from the urine receptacle with a specimen collection container at the time of catheterization, and send it to the laboratory with the appropriate laboratory request form. Reconnect the drainage bag when urine stops flowing.

Inspect the catheter and tubing periodically while they're in place to detect compression or kinking that could obstruct urine flow. Explain the principle of gravity drainage so that the patient realizes the importance of keeping the drainage tubing and collection bag lower than the bladder at all times.

For monitoring purposes, empty the collection bag at least every 8 hours. Excessive fluid volume may require more frequent emptying to prevent traction on the catheter, which would cause the patient discomfort, and to prevent injury to the urethra and bladder wall. Some hospitals encourage changing catheters at regular intervals, such as every 30 days, if the patient is to have long-term continuous drainage.

✦✦ CLINICAL ALERT ✦✦

Observe the patient carefully for adverse reactions, such as bladder contractions. Check the facility's policy beforehand to determine the maximum amount of urine that may be drained at one time (some facilities limit the amount to 700 to 1,000 ml). Whether or not to limit the amount of urine drained is currently controversial. Clamp the catheter at the first sign of an adverse reaction, and notify the doctor.

If the patient is ambulatory or will be going home with the catheter in place, instruct the patient and family members in how to use a leg bag for drainage.

✦✦ CLINICAL ALERT ✦✦

If the patient is to be discharged with a long-term indwelling catheter, teach him and his family all aspects of daily catheter maintenance, including care of the skin and urinary meatus, signs and symptoms of UTI or obstruction, and the importance of adequate fluid intake to maintain patency. Explain that a home care nurse should visit every 4 to 6 weeks, or more often if needed, to change the catheter. Provide the teaching handout, *Caring for your urinary catheter,* pages 350 and 351.

Complications

Urinary tract infection can result from the introduction of bacteria into the bladder. Improper insertion can cause traumatic injury to the urethral and bladder mucosa. Bladder atony or spasms can result from rapid decompression of a severely distended bladder.

Documentation

Record the date, time, and size and type of indwelling catheter used. Also describe the amount, color, and other characteristics of urine emptied from the bladder. Your facility may require only the intake and output sheet for fluid-balance data. If large volumes of urine were emptied, describe the patient's tolerance for the procedure. Note whether a urine specimen was sent for laboratory analysis.

Teaching intermittent self-catheterization

A patient with impaired or absent bladder function may perform self-catheterization for routine bladder drainage. Intermittent self-catheterization requires thorough and careful patient teaching. If your older patient lacks the ability or manual dexterity to do this, you can teach a family member or other caregiver how to do it. Provide the teaching handout, *Catheterizing yourself,* page 353, then guide your patient through the steps. The patient will probably use clean technique for self-catheterization at home, but sterile technique must be used in the

(Text continues on page 352.)

Caring for your urinary catheter

Dear Patient:

Your urinary catheter is a latex tube that permits continuous urine drainage so you don't need to use a bedpan or the toilet. A balloon on one end holds the tube inside your bladder.

Your catheter is connected to drainage tubing that leads to a drainage bag. Be sure to empty this bag every 3 to 4 hours. During the day, you may strap the bag to your leg at the thigh level. Don't strap it too tightly because this could cause skin irritation and decreased blood circulation. If your lower leg becomes discolored, check to make sure the bag is not attached too tightly.

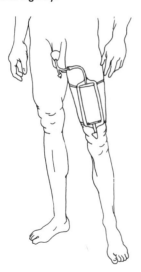

Emptying the leg bag
1. Wash your hands. Then remove the stopper and drain all the urine, either into the toilet or, if the doctor orders it, into a measuring container so you can record the amount, as shown . Don't touch the drain tip with your fingers or with the container.

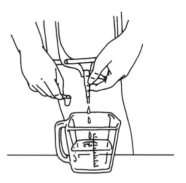

2. After the urine has drained completely, swab the drain tip and the stopper with an alcohol swab. Replace the stopper.

Attaching the bedside drainage bag
Before going to bed, replace the leg bag with a bedside drainage bag. This bag holds more urine, so you can sleep for 8 hours without emptying it.

1. To replace the leg bag, first empty it. Now clamp the catheter and swab the connection between the catheter and the leg bag with an alcohol swab.

Then disconnect the leg bag, and connect the catheter to the bedside drainage tubing and bag. Finally, unclamp the catheter.

2. Which side of the bed do you want the drainage bag to hang from? You'll tape the drainage tubing to your thigh on that side.

Shave your skin in that area, if needed. Leave some slack in the line so you won't pull on the catheter when you move your leg. Then tape the drainage tubing to your inner thigh below the groin.

3. When you get into bed, arrange the drain-

Caring for your urinary catheter (continued)

age tubing so it doesn't kink or loop. Then hang the drainage bag by its hook on the side of the bed. To ensure proper drainage and reduce the infection risk, keep the bag below your bladder level at all times, whether you're lying, sitting, or standing.

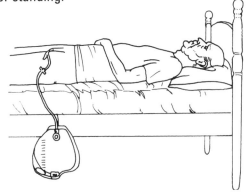

Reattaching the leg bag

1. When you're ready to reattach the leg bag in the morning, empty the bedside drainage bag. First unclamp the drainage tube and remove it from its sleeve, without touching its tip.

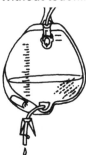

2. Then let the urine drain into the toilet or into a measuring container, if required. Don't let the drainage tube touch the toilet or container.

3. When the bag is completely empty, swab the end of the drainage tube with an alcohol swab. Reclamp the tube and reinsert it into the sleeve of the drainage bag.

Don't let anyone else empty your drainage bag, unless one member of your family performs your catheter care. If your doctor has requested it, record the amount of urine drained.

4. Now repeat the steps you took when connecting the bedside drainage bag, but use the leg bag instead: Clamp the catheter and swab the connection between the catheter and the bedside drainage bag with an alcohol swab, disconnect the bedside drainage bag, and connect the catheter to the drainage tubing and leg bag. Finally, unclamp the catheter.

Cleaning the drainage bags

When you're finished using either type of bag, wash it out with soap and water, and rinse it with a solution of 1 part white vinegar to 7 parts water to clean and deodorize it.

Soak the leg bag overnight in the vinegar-water solution. You can use either type of drainage bag for up to 1 month before replacing it.

Caring for your skin

● Use soap and water to wash the area around the catheter twice each day.
● Also, wash your rectal area twice each day and after each bowel movement.
● Periodically check the skin around the catheter for signs of irritation, such as redness, tenderness or swelling.

Avoiding problems

● Contact your doctor immediately if you have any problems, such as urine leakage around the catheter, pain and fullness in your abdomen, scanty urine flow, or blood in your urine.
● Above all, never pull on your catheter or try to remove it yourself.

health care facility because of the increased risk of infection.

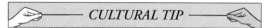

CULTURAL TIP

Be aware that the older patient may be very embarrassed and self-conscious about having to touch or look at "private parts" or having a family member do it.

Special considerations

Impress upon the patient that the timing of catheterization is critical to avoid overfilling the bladder. This can lead to infection or reflux of urine into the ureters and kidneys, resulting in kidney damage. Intermittent self-catheterization should be done every 4 to 6 hours around the clock (or more often at first).

Explain the difference between boiling and sterilization this way: Boiling kills bacteria, fungi, and viruses, but does not kill bacterial or fungal spores, whereas sterilization does. However, because the patient will be doing catheter cleaning in his own home, where risk of infection is lower, boiling provides sufficient protection against spreading infections.

Advise the patient to store cleaned catheters only after they're completely dry, to prevent growth of gram-negative organisms.

Stress the importance of regulating fluid intake, as ordered, to prevent incontinence while maintaining adequate hydration. However, explain that incontinent episodes could occur occasionally. For managing incontinence, the doctor or a home health care nurse can help develop a plan, such as more frequent catheterizations. After an incontinent episode, tell the patient to wash with soap and water, pat himself dry with a towel, and expose the skin to the air for as long as possible. He can reduce urine odor by putting methylbenzethonium chloride (Diaparene) or cornstarch on his skin. Bedding and furniture can be protected by covering them with rubber or plastic sheets and then covering the rubber or plastic with fabric.

Also stress the importance of taking medications as ordered to increase urine retention and help pre-

vent incontinence. Tell the patient to avoid calcium-rich and phosphorus-rich foods, as ordered, to reduce the chance of renal calculus formation.

Complications

Overdistention of the bladder can lead to urine leakage and UTI. Improper hand washing or equipment cleaning can also cause UTI. Incorrect catheter insertion can injure the urethral or bladder mucosa.

Documentation

Record the date and times of catheterization, character of the urine (color, odor, clarity, presence of particles or blood), the amount of urine (increase, decrease, no change), and any problems encountered during the procedure. Note whether the patient has difficulty performing a return demonstration.

Applying a condom catheter

Many patients don't require an indwelling urinary catheter to manage their incontinence. For male patients, a male incontinence device consisting of a condom catheter secured to the shaft of the penis and connected to a leg bag or drainage bag reduces the risk of UTI from catheterization, promotes bladder retraining when possible, helps prevent skin breakdown, and improves the patient's self-image.

Equipment

Condom catheter ■ drainage bag ■ extension tubing ■ nonallergenic tape or incontinence sheath holder ■ commercial adhesive strip or skin-bond cement ■ elastic adhesive or Velcro, if needed ■ gloves ■ razor, if needed ■ basin ■ soap and water ■ washcloth ■ towel.

Preparation of equipment

Fill the basin with lukewarm water. Then, bring the basin and the remaining equipment to the patient's bedside.

Implementation

● Explain the procedure to the patient, wash your hands thoroughly, put on gloves, and provide privacy.

TEACHING AID

Catheterizing yourself

Dear Patient:

Follow these instructions to perform self-catheterization.

To begin, gather the required equipment: catheter, water-soluble lubricant, clean washcloth, soap and water, paper towels, and a clean plastic bag. Then wash your hands.

For women

1. Separate the folds of your vulva with one hand and, using the washcloth, thoroughly clean the area between your legs with warm water and mild soap. Use downward strokes (front to back) to avoid contaminating the area with feces. Then pat the area dry with a towel.

2. Open the lubricant and squeeze a generous amount onto a paper towel. Then roll the first 3" (7.5 cm) of the catheter in it.

3. Spread the lips of the vulva with one hand and, using the other hand, insert the catheter in an upward and backward direction about 3" into the urethra (located above the vagina). If you meet resistance, breathe deeply. As you inhale, advance the catheter, angling it slightly upward. Stop when urine begins to drain from it. Allow all urine to drain into the toilet.

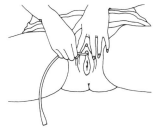

4. Pinch the catheter closed and slowly remove it. Wash it in warm, soapy water; then rinse and dry it. Place it in the plastic bag until the next use. (After you've used the catheter a few times, boil it in water for 20 minutes to keep it germ-free.)

For men

1. Wash your penis and the surrounding area with soap and water. Then pat dry.

2. Open the tube of lubricant and squeeze a generous amount onto a paper towel. Then roll the first 7" to 10" (17.5 to 25 cm) of the catheter in the lubricant.

3. Put the nonlubricated end of the catheter in the basin or toilet. Hold your penis at a right angle to your body, grasp the catheter as you would a pencil, and slowly insert the lubricated end into the urethra. If you meet resistance, breathe deeply.

As you inhale, continue advancing the catheter 7" to 10" until urine begins to flow. Allow all urine to drain into the basin or toilet.

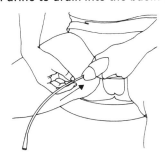

4. When the catheter stops draining, pinch it closed and slowly remove it. Empty the basin, if used; then rinse and dry it. Wash the catheter in warm, soapy water. Then rinse and dry it. Place it in a plastic bag until the next use. (After you've used the catheter a few times, boil it in water for 20 minutes to keep it germ-free.)

- If the patient is circumcised, wash the penis with soap and water, rinse well, and pat dry with a towel. If the patient is uncircumcised, gently retract the foreskin and clean beneath it. Rinse well but don't dry because moisture provides lubrication and prevents friction during foreskin replacement. Replace the foreskin to avoid penile constriction. Then, if necessary, shave the base and shaft of the penis to prevent the adhesive strip or skin-bond cement from pulling pubic hair. Be careful not to nick the patient when shaving to avoid creating a possible site for infection.
- If you're using a precut commercial adhesive strip, insert the glans penis through its opening, and position the strip 1" (2.5 cm) from the scrotal area. If you're using uncut adhesive, cut a strip to fit around the shaft of the penis. Remove the protective covering from one side of the adhesive strip and press this side firmly to the penis to enhance adhesion. Apply the adhesive strip in a spiral fashion around the penis. Then remove the covering from the other side of the strip. If a commercial adhesive strip isn't available, apply skin-bond cement and let it dry for a few minutes. Use care when applying the adhesive to prevent pulling on the patient's skin. Keep in mind that the patient's skin is thin, loose, and very friable.
- Position the rolled condom catheter at the tip of the penis, with its drainage opening at the urinary meatus.
- Unroll the catheter upward, past the adhesive strip on the shaft of the penis. Then gently press the sheath against the strip until it adheres.
- After the condom catheter is in place, secure it with hypoallergenic tape or an incontinence sheath holder.
- Using extension tubing, connect the condom catheter to the leg bag or drainage bag. Remove and discard your gloves.
- To remove the device, first put on gloves. Then simultaneously roll the condom catheter and adhesive strip off the penis and discard them. If you've used skin-bond cement rather than an adhesive strip, remove it with solvent. Also remove and discard the nonallergenic tape or incontinence sheath holder.
- Clean the penis with lukewarm water, rinse thoroughly, and dry. Check for swelling or signs of skin breakdown.
- Remove the leg bag by closing the drain clamp, unlatching the leg straps, and disconnecting the extension tubing at the top of the bag. Discard your gloves.

Complications
The condom catheter can cause skin irritation and edema, infection, and penile circulatory impairment.

Special considerations
If nonallergenic tape or an incontinence sheath holder isn't available, secure the condom with a strip of elastic adhesive or Velcro. Apply the strip snugly but not too tightly, to prevent circulatory constriction.

Inspect the condom catheter for twists and the extension tubing for kinks to prevent obstruction of urine flow, which could cause the condom to balloon, eventually dislodging it.

If the patient is to use the condom catheter at home, be sure to instruct him or a family member in how to apply it correctly. Provide the teaching handout, *Using a condom catheter,* pages 355 and 356.

Documentation
Record the date and time of application and removal of the catheter. Note urine characteristics, patient's skin condition, and his response to the device, including voiding pattern, to assist with bladder retraining.

*T*EACHING AID

Using a condom catheter

Dear Patient:

Here are some guidelines for wearing a condom catheter temporarily for urinary incontinence. This catheter fits over the penis and connects to a drainage bag that you strap onto your leg. You'll need to clean the bag about twice a day.

Follow these steps to apply the catheter, connect the drainage bag, remove the catheter and bag, and solve problems.

Getting started

● Wash your hands. Then gather your equipment: correct-sized condom catheter, double-sided elastic stomal tape, leg drainage bag with tubing, clamp, manicure scissors, soap, washcloth, and towel.

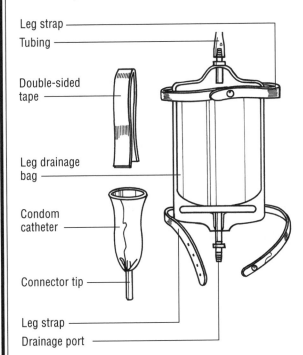

● Trim the hairs on the shaft and base of your penis so they won't stick to the stomal tape. Before each catheter change, wash, rinse, and dry your penis.
● If the condom isn't self-adhering, remove the backing from both sides of the tape. Place the side marked "skin side" against your penis. Starting at the penis base, spiral the tape.

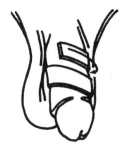

Caution: Don't let the edges of the tape overlap. Don't stretch the tape or you'll wind it too tightly. And never wrap the tape in a circle around your penis; you could cut off circulation.

Applying the catheter

First, tightly roll the condom sheath (balloonlike part) to the edge of the connector tip.

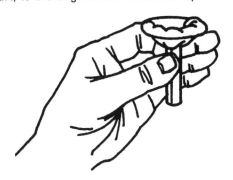

(continued)

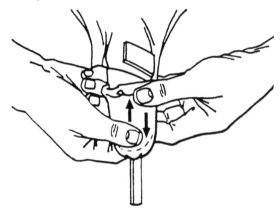

Using a condom catheter *(continued)*

Next, place the catheter sheath on the end of your penis, leaving about half an inch of space between the tip of your penis and the connector tip.

Gently stretch your penis as you unroll the condom. When the condom is unrolled, gently press it against your penis so that it sticks to the tape.

Connecting the drainage bag
Connect one end of the tubing to the connector tip and the other end to the drainage bag. Strap the drainage bag to your thigh.

Removing the equipment
To remove the drainage bag, clamp the tube closed. Release the leg straps, and disconnect the extension tubing at the top of the bag. Remove the condom catheter and the tape by rolling them forward.

Special instructions
● If the tape doesn't stick to your skin, make sure that your penis is completely dry.
● If urine leaks when you're wearing the catheter, squeeze the sheath to get a better seal.
● If the catheter sheath wrinkles when contacting the tape, the sheath might be too large. If so, select a smaller size sheath.
● Empty the drainage bag every 3 to 4 hours. Never let it fill completely to the top.
● Wash the drainage bag twice a day with soap and water. Rinse it with a solution of one part vinegar to seven parts water.
● Don't use the same drainage bag any longer than 1 month.
● Use only adhesives that are prescribed by your doctor.
● Don't wash with povidone-iodine (Betadine), which can irritate your skin.
● Remember to change the condom catheter every 24 hours. Be sure to thoroughly wash and dry your penis between changes. If you're not circumcised, pull the foreskin over the head of the penis as you wash to prevent swelling.
● Check your penis every 2 hours for swelling or unusual color. If it feels uncomfortable or doesn't look normal, take off the condom catheter and call your doctor.
● Call your doctor if you feel pain or burning when you urinate, have the urge to urinate very frequently, smell an unpleasant odor from your urine, or see blood or pus in your urine.

Additional instructions

_____

_____

_____

❧ 18 ❧

Providing skin and wound care

Maintaining skin integrity and managing skin injuries constitute a large part of nursing practice, especially in geriatric nursing. As you change a dressing on a surgical wound, apply a topical medication to relieve itching, or assess a patient for the risk of pressure ulcers, you need to be aware of the older person's special needs. The skin undergoes numerous changes with advancing age, and these changes affect its ability to recover from injuries and infections. Meticulous skin care is essential in maintaining the older person's overall health.

After briefly considering the skin as an organ and how it responds to injury, this chapter presents nursing care measures related to prevention and treatment of dryness, itching, and pressure ulcers, and then focuses on specific procedures.

UNDERSTANDING SKIN STRUCTURE AND FUNCTION

The skin consists of three major components: the epidermis, dermis, and subcutaneous tissue. Though interrelated, each layer of the skin has different structures, cell types, and functions.

Epidermis
The epidermis, the outermost layer of the skin, contains three major cell types. *Keratinocytes,* which occur chiefly in the uppermost layer of the epidermis, produce keratin, a protein that provides the waterproof covering for the body. As they are shed or worn from the skin surface, keratinocytes are continually replaced by new cells from deeper skin layers; the epidermis renews itself every 4 to 6 weeks. *Melanocytes* release melanin, a dark pigment that provides color tone to the skin and filters ultraviolet rays (sunlight). Exposure to ultraviolet light can stimulate melanin formation. Finally, *Langerhans' cells,* a part of the body's immune system, assist in initial processing of antigens that enter the epidermis, thereby protecting the skin from allergic reactions. These cells are gradually destroyed by prolonged exposure to ultraviolet radiation.

Dermis
The dermis lies directly beneath the epidermis and is joined to it by a membrane known as the *basement layer.* The dermis supports and nourishes the epidermis. It's composed of two layers of elastic connective tissue containing blood vessels, lymph vessels, nerves, sweat glands, and hair follicles. Fibroblast cells in the dermis produce collagen, the protein that gives skin its strength. Elastin, another dermal protein, forms fibers that help the skin retain its elastic qualities. The fibroelastic structure of the dermis allows the skin to resist external injury.

Subcutaneous tissue
The subcutaneous tissue is made up of dense connective and adipose (fatty) tissue and contains major

blood vessels, lymphatics, and nerves. It acts as a heat insulator and provides nutritional reserve for use during illness or starvation. This layer also acts as a mechanical shock absorber.

Besides helping to shape a patient's self-image, the skin performs many physiologic functions. For example, it protects internal body structures from the environment and from potential pathogens. It also regulates body temperature, maintains fluid and electrolyte balance, excretes metabolic wastes, and serves as an organ of sensation (pain, pressure, temperature, and vibration). The skin also facilitates communication (through facial expressions) and is an indicator of age, ethnic group, gender, and other personal characteristics.

AGE-RELATED SKIN CHANGES

Dramatic changes occur in all skin layers as a person ages. In the younger adult, skin cells turn over approximately every 3 weeks; in the normal older adult, this turnover slows to once every 2 months. Skin elasticity declines due to progressive degeneration of collagen and elastin. Photosensitivity increases as the number of melanocytes declines. Loss of melanocytes also results in graying of the hair and, coupled with reduced capillary blood supply, fading normal skin color.

Diminished adhesion between the dermis and epidermis causes increased wrinkling and slackness, especially in the extremities, neck, and face. Wrinkling is exacerbated by prolonged sun exposure.

A diminishing blood supply reduces the skin's thermoregulatory function, causing older people to feel colder in the extremities. The blood vessels themselves become more fragile, leading to easy bruising and formation of senile purpura.

Loss of fat from the subcutaneous tissue (as well as at other body sites) predisposes the older patient to pressure ulcer formation, especially at the scapulae, trochanters, knees, and other bony prominences.

Older people are also more likely to complain of dry skin and itching, which stems partly from diminished sweat gland secretions.

WOUNDS AND THE HEALING PROCESS

Regardless of their origin, wounds physically disrupt the normal structure and function of the skin and underlying tissues.

Wounds are classified according to their depth (the number of skin layers involved). *Partial-thickness wounds* affect only the epidermis and dermis. In *full-thickness wounds,* the epidermis and dermis are lost and deeper structures, such as subcutaneous tissue and even muscle and bone, may be involved.

The wound healing process is classified according to how the wound closes. Wounds with minimal tissue loss and well-approximated edges may be surgically closed by suturing and heal by *primary intention* (also known as direct union). Such wounds have a lower risk of infection and heal with minimal scarring. Wounds with substantial tissue loss that cannot be closed surgically heal by *secondary intention* (also known as indirect union). In such wounds, closure is achieved through contractions (formation of connective tissues, or scars). Connective tissue must completely fill the wound before skin cells can advance from the wound margins to cover the entire wound surface. Pressure sores are an example of this type of wound. Surgical wounds left open for 3 to 5 days to allow edema or infection to resolve or exudate to drain are closed with sutures, staples, or adhesive skin closures and heal by *tertiary intention* (also called delayed primary intention).

Phases of wound healing
The healing process begins at the instant of injury and proceeds through a repair "cascade." Partial-thickness wound healing proceeds in two phases: inflammation and proliferation. In full-thickness wounds, these phases are followed by a third — differentiation.

Inflammatory phase

Tissue trauma stimulates an acute inflammatory response characterized by local erythema, edema, and tenderness of the affected tissues as well as a serous exudate. The inflammatory changes serve to initiate clotting, fight bacterial invasion, remove wound debris, and encourage new epithelial cells to grow.

Proliferative phase

During this phase, the wound is filled with new connective tissue and capillary networks (granulation), and new epithelial cells migrate across the moist wound surface to cover the wound (epithelialization). In wounds that heal by secondary intention, contraction (scar formation) also occurs and helps reduce the size of the wound. Proliferation occurs 3 to 4 days after the initial injury and lasts for up to 16 days.

Differentiation phase

In this phase (also known as remodeling), the closed wound matures as the collagen scar undergoes repeated degradation and resynthesis by macrophages and other tissue-repairing cells. If the concurrent processes of collagen synthesis and breakdown are not balanced, scar tissue may be either weakened or overdeveloped. This balance is adversely affected by such factors as reduced capillary oxygen levels and nutritional deficiencies (especially of vitamins, needed for cellular activity, and amino acids, needed for tissue regeneration).

Effects of aging on wound healing

In older adults, the following factors impede wound healing: decreased epidermal cell turnover, increased capillary fragility coupled with reduced vascularization (which reduces the oxygen supply to newly formed skin cells), altered nutrition and fluid intake, impaired respiratory or immune system function, and reduced dermal and subcutaneous mass (which increases the risk of pressure ulcers).

PATIENT CARE MEASURES

As a health care provider, you play a key role in maintaining the older patient's skin integrity, promoting comfort by averting dryness and itching, and preventing pressure ulcers, a major complication.

Promoting healthy skin

Because your patient's skin condition largely depends on his overall health, you'll need to help him maintain optimal nutrition and hydration. You may also need to provide additional guidance in personal hygiene and in protecting the skin from harsh environmental conditions. (See *Keeping your skin healthy,* page 360.)

Treating dry skin

Dry skin (xerosis) is perhaps the most common skin problem among older people. Exposure to drying winds and sun, low indoor humidity levels, and inadequate diet contribute to skin dryness and dehydration. Hospital care procedures, such as routine bathing with harsh soaps, repeated wetting and drying, and prolonged bed rest, can exacerbate dry skin. Assess the patient for signs of dry skin: rash, scaling, and flaking of skin on the face, neck, hands, forearms, sides of the lower trunk, and exterior and lateral aspects of the thighs. Itching, which commonly accompanies dry skin, may be seen as skin irritation or scratch marks in the affected areas.

Dry skin (with or without itching) may be merely a nuisance or it may herald a more serious problem.

Dry skin treatments aim to rehydrate the epidermis. Superfatted soaps help restore protective lipids, and bath oils and other hydrophobic preparations help preserve skin moisture. Applying lotion or emollients to the body several times a day helps to keep the skin lubricated and hydrated. Vegetable and light mineral oils are as effective as commercial preparations but are less costly.

Treating itchy skin

Pruritus (itchiness), another common threat to skin

EACHING AID

Keeping your skin healthy

Dear Patient:

Skin care is important for older adults. The following steps can help you maintain healthy skin:

● Drink adequate amounts of fluid, and eat foods high in vitamins A and C.

Note: Apply emollients containing petroleum jelly, such as Keri and Eucerin lotions, twice a day; use them immediately after bathing while your skin is still wet.

Apply emollients directly to the skin rather than placing them in bath water, to reduce your risk of slipping and falling. If you use bath oils, take extra measures to prevent slipping, such as grab bars or safety strips.

● If you use an emollient on your feet, put on nonskid slippers or socks before walking.

● Use a superfatted soap, such as Dove or Basis, when bathing. Avoid bathing more than three times a week.

● Keep the bath temperature between 90° and 100° F (32.2° and 37.7° C). Check the temperature setting on the water heater to make sure it's not too high.

● After bathing, blot your skin dry with a soft cotton towel. Don't rub the skin vigorously; doing so removes skin moisture and intensifies itching. Don't forget to thoroughly dry the skin between your toes and other areas where the skin rubs together.

● To prevent irritation from friction, apply small amounts of powder or cornstarch on areas that rub together, such as the toes.

● Avoid using rubbing alcohol or products that contain alcohol, which further dehydrate the skin.

● To avoid damage from the sun, wear large-brimmed hats, sunglasses, and long-sleeved cotton clothing when outside; use a sunscreen with a sun protection factor (SPF) greater than 15, even on cloudy or rainy days, and apply it about 1 hour before going outside. Try to avoid going out in the sun between the hours of 10 a.m. and 3 p.m., when the sun's rays are the strongest.

● To prevent skin irritation from clothing, avoid washing clothes with strong detergents and bleach.

● Maintain indoor humidity between 40% and 60%.

Additional instructions:

_____

_____

_____

_____

_____

_____

_____

integrity, is aggravated by heat, sudden temperature changes, sweating, fatigue, contact with articles of clothing, and emotional upset. Pruritus also may accompany systemic disorders, such as chronic renal failure, biliary or hepatic disease, and iron deficiency anemia.

Although the urge to scratch is instinctive, you should discourage your patient from doing so because scratching is ineffective and may damage the skin. When rehydration is not sufficient to control itching, cool compresses with such additives as saline solution or oatmeal or lotions, such as Lubriderm, may be helpful. If itching interferes with sleep, you may give the patient a mild antihistamine, but discourage drug use during daytime hours.

Preventing pressure ulcers

As their name implies, pressure ulcers result when pressure — applied with great force for a short period or with less force over a longer period — impairs circulation, depriving tissues of oxygen and nutrients. Left untreated, ischemic areas can progress to tissue breakdown and infection.

Most pressure ulcers develop over bony prominences, where friction and shearing force combine with pressure to break down skin and underlying tissues. Common sites include the sacrum, coccyx, ischial tuberosities, and greater trochanters. Other sites include the skin over the vertebrae, scapulae, elbows, knees, and heels in bedridden and relatively immobile patients. (See *Pressure ulcers: Who's at risk?*)

Preventing pressure ulcers is crucial in older adults because the ulcers take longer to heal, thereby increasing the patient's risk of infection and other complications. Follow these guidelines to help prevent pressure ulcers:

● Assess the older person closely for risk factors; use an appropriate assessment tool to determine his risk of developing pressure ulcers (see *Braden scale: Predicting pressure ulcer risk*, pages 362 and 363).

● Turn and reposition the patient every 1 to 2 hours unless contraindicated. For older persons who can't turn themselves or who are turned on a schedule, use pressure-reducing devices, such as a special mat-

Pressure ulcers: Who's at risk?

Those at greatest risk of developing pressure ulcers are older persons, especially those with the following conditions:
● poor circulation
● diabetes mellitus
● malnutrition
● immunosuppression
● dehydration
● incontinence
● significant obesity or thinness
● paralysis
● diminished pain awareness
● history of corticosteroid therapy
● previous pressure ulcers
● chronic illness that requires bed rest
● mental impairment, possibly related to coma, altered level of consciousness, sedation, confusion, or use of restraints.

tress or mattress overlay made of air, gel, foam, or water.

● Post a turning schedule at the patient's bedside. Adapt position changes to the patient's situation. Emphasize the importance of regular position changes to the patient and family members, and encourage their participation by having them perform a position change correctly after you've demonstrated how.

● When turning the patient, lift him rather than slide him because sliding increases friction and shear. Use a turning sheet and get help from coworkers if necessary.

● Use pillows to position your patient and increase his comfort. Try to keep sheets free of wrinkles, which can increase pressure and cause discomfort.

● Avoid placing the patient directly on the trochanter. Instead, position him on his side, at an angle of about 30 degrees.

● Except for brief periods, avoid raising the head of the bed more than 30 degrees to prevent shearing pressure.

● As appropriate, perform active or passive range-of-motion exercises to relieve pressure and promote

(Text continues on page 364.)

HARTING GUIDE

Braden scale: Predicting pressure ulcer risk

The Braden scale, shown below, is the most reliable of **several existing** instruments for assessing the older patient's risk of developing pressure ulcers. The lower the score, the greater the risk.

Patient's name_ *Kevin Lawson* ___   Evaluator's name_ *Joan Morris, RN* ___

SENSORY PERCEPTION Ability to respond meaningfully to pressure-related discomfort	**1. Completely limited:** Unresponsive (does not moan, flinch, or grasp) to painful stimuli because of diminished level of consciousness or sedation OR Limited ability to feel pain over most of body surface	**2. Very limited:** Responds only to painful stimuli; cannot communicate discomfort except by moaning or restlessness OR Has a sensory impairment that limits the ability to feel pain or discomfort over half of body
MOISTURE Degree to which skin is exposed to moisture	**1. Constantly moist:** Skin is kept moist almost constantly by perspiration, urine, etc.; dampness is detected every time patient is moved or turned	**2. Very moist:** Skin is often but not always moist; linen must be changed at least once a shift
ACTIVITY Degree of physical activity	**1. Bedfast:** Confined to bed	**2. Chairfast:** Ability to walk severely limited or nonexistent; cannot bear own weight and/or must be assisted into chair or wheelchair
MOBILITY Ability to change and control body position	**1. Completely immobile:** Does not make even slight changes in body or extremity position without assistance	**2. Very limited:** Makes occasional slight changes in body or extremity position but unable to make frequent or significant changes independently
NUTRITION Usual food intake pattern	**1. Very poor:** Never eats a complete meal; rarely eats more than one-third of any food offered; eats two servings or less of protein (meat or dairy products) per day; takes fluids poorly; does not take a liquid dietary supplement OR Is NPO and/or maintained on clear liquids or I.V. fluids for more than 5 days	**2. Probably inadequate:** Rarely eats a complete meal and generally eats only about half of any food offered; protein intake includes only three servings of meat or dairy products per day; occasionally will take a dietary supplement OR Receives less than optimum amount of liquid diet or tube feeding
FRICTION AND SHEAR	**1. Problem:** Requires moderate to maximum assistance in moving; complete lifting without sliding against sheets is impossible; frequently slides down in bed or chair, requiring frequent repositioning with maximum assistance; spasticity, contractures, or agitation leads to almost constant friction	**2. Potential problem:** Moves feebly or requires minimum assistance; during a move, skin probably slides to some extent against sheets, chair restraints, or other devices; maintains relatively good position in chair or bed most of the time but occasionally slides down

Adapted with permission from Bergstrom, N., et al. "The Braden Scale for Predicting Pressure Sore Risk," *Nursing Research* 36(4):205-10, 1987.

Date of assessment _10/30/96_

3. Slightly limited: Responds to verbal commands but cannot always communicate discomfort or need to be turned OR Has some sensory impairment that limits ability to feel pain or discomfort in one or two extremities	**4. No impairment:** Responds to verbal commands; has no sensory deficit that would limit ability to feel or voice pain or discomfort	3
3. Occasionally moist: Skin is occasionally moist, requiring an extra linen change approximately once a day	**4. Rarely moist:** Skin is usually dry; linen only requires changing at routine intervals	3
3. Walks occasionally: Walks occasionally during day, but for very short distances, with or without assistance; spends majority of each shift in bed or chair	**4. Walks frequently:** Walks outside the room at least twice a day and inside room at least once every 2 hours during waking hours	4
3. Slightly limited: Makes frequent though slight changes in body or extremity position independently	**4. No limitations:** Makes major and frequent changes in position without assistance	4
3. Adequate: Eats over half of most meals; eats four servings of protein (meat, dairy products) each day; occasionally will refuse a meal, but will usually take a supplement if offered OR Is on a tube feeding or TPN regimen that probably meets most nutritional needs	**4. Excellent:** Eats most of every meal and never refuses a meal; usually eats four or more servings of meat and dairy products; occasionally eats between meals; does not require supplementation	4
3. No apparent problem: Moves in bed and in chair independently and has sufficient muscle strength to lift up completely during move; maintains good position in bed or chair at all times		3
	TOTAL SCORE	21

circulation. To save time, combine these exercises with bathing if possible.

● Instruct the patient confined to a chair or wheelchair to shift his weight every 30 minutes to promote blood flow to compressed tissues. Show a paraplegic patient how to shift his weight by doing push-ups in the wheelchair. If the patient needs your help, sit next to him and help him shift his weight to one buttock for 60 seconds; then repeat the procedure on the other side. Provide him with pressure-relieving cushions, as appropriate. However, avoid seating the patient on a rubber or plastic doughnut, which can increase localized pressure at vulnerable points.

● Adjust or pad appliances, casts, or splints, as needed, to ensure proper fit and to prevent increased pressure and impaired circulation.

● Tell the older person to avoid heat lamps and harsh soaps because they dry the skin. Advise him to apply lotion after bathing to help keep his skin moist. Also tell him to avoid vigorous massage because it can damage capillaries.

● If the older adult's condition permits, recommend a diet that includes adequate calories, protein, and vitamins. Dietary therapy may involve a consultation with a dietitian, food supplements, enteral feeding, or total parenteral nutrition.

● If the patient is incontinent or develops diarrhea, clean and dry his soiled skin. Then apply a protective moisture barrier to prevent skin maceration.

● Teach the patient and caregiver measures for preventing pressure ulcers (see *Preventing pressure ulcers*).

PERFORMING BASIC CARE PROCEDURES

This section explains how to perform specific procedures, such as applying heat or cold, administering therapeutic baths and soaks, applying pressure dressings, managing surgical and traumatic wounds, irrigating wounds, managing dehiscence and evisceration, managing pressure ulcers, and applying Unna's boot.

Applying direct heat

Heat applied directly to the patient's body enhances healing by causing vasodilation, which increases blood supply to the affected area, making more nutrients available for tissue growth, and by enhancing the inflammatory process (leukocytosis, suppuration, and drainage). Heat also reduces pain caused by muscular spasm and decreases congestion in deep visceral organs.

Direct heat may be dry or moist. Dry heat can be delivered at a higher temperature and for a longer time. Devices for applying dry heat include hot-water bottles, electric heating pads, K pads, and chemical hot packs. Moist heat softens crusts and exudates, penetrates deeper than dry heat, doesn't dry the skin, produces less perspiration, and usually is more comfortable for the patient. Devices for applying moist heat include warm compresses for small body areas and warm packs for large areas.

Direct heat treatment is contraindicated for patients at risk for hemorrhage, for those with a sprained limb in the acute stage (because vasodilation would increase pain and swelling), and for those with a condition associated with acute inflammation, such as appendicitis.

Use direct heat cautiously on older people because their decreased ability to detect changes in temperature places them at high risk for burns. Use direct heat judiciously, as well, on people with impaired renal, cardiac, or respiratory function; arteriosclerosis or atherosclerosis; and impaired sensation, all of which are common in older people. Use it with extreme caution on heat-sensitive areas, such as scar tissue or stomas.

Equipment

Patient thermometer ■ towel ■ adhesive tape or roller gauze ■ gloves (if the patient has an open lesion).

For a hot-water bottle: hot tap water ■ pitcher ■ bath (utility) thermometer ■ absorbent, protective cloth covering.

For an electric heating pad: absorbent, protective cloth covering.

For a K pad: temperature-adjustment key ■ distilled water ■ absorbent, protective cloth covering.

*T*EACHING AID

Preventing pressure ulcers

Dear Patient:

Sitting or lying for too long in one position can damage your skin, causing pressure ulcers. These ulcers develop around areas of skin pressure, such as your buttocks if you're sitting in a wheelchair. But with good skin care and frequent position changes, you can keep your skin healthy. Here are some guidelines.

Do's
● Change your position every 2 hours while awake if you're recuperating in bed. Try to follow a schedule. For example, lie on your right side, then your left side, then your back, then your stomach (if possible). Support yourself with pillows and pads.
● Shift your position every 15 minutes if you use a wheelchair. Sit on a firm seat covered by a wheelchair cushion. Avoid sling-style seats or use a board to distribute your weight evenly.
● Check your skin for signs of pressure ulcers twice a day. Use a hand mirror or ask your caregiver to check areas prone to these ulcers: your shoulders, tailbone, hips, elbows, heels, and the back of your head. Call your doctor if you notice any breaks in your skin or unusual changes in your skin temperature.
● Wear cotton clothing next to your skin to absorb moisture, or wear silk to reduce friction.
● Bathe daily or more often in warm weather. Before you get into the tub, check to make sure the water is tepid, not hot. (If you can't sense the temperature, have your caregiver check it with a bath thermometer.)
● Use a footstool to keep your legs elevated, if appropriate. Also, wear antiembolism stock-

ings to reduce swelling and prevent blood clots from forming in your legs.
● Follow your prescribed exercise program. Try to do range-of-motion exercises every 8 hours or as often as recommended.
● Keep your nails clean and short, and cut them straight across. Check your feet for ingrown toenails.
● Eat a well-balanced diet, drink lots of fluids, and try to maintain your ideal weight.
● Apply a sunblock before going outdoors.

Don'ts
● Avoid using commercial soaps or skin products that dry or irritate your skin. Instead, use oil-free lotions.
● Don't sleep on wrinkled bedsheets or tuck your covers tightly into the foot of your bed.
● Avoid exposing your skin to extreme conditions, such as hot summer sun or wintry cold.
● Avoid using heating pads, electric blankets, or other electrical devices in bed.
● Avoid wearing tight clothing or shoes or applying tight dressings or adhesive tape to your skin.
● Don't smoke in bed. Try to stop smoking. If you can't, keep lit cigarettes away from your body.

Additional instructions:

_____

_____

_____

_____

_____

For a disposable chemical hot pack: absorbent, protective cloth covering.

For a warm compress or pack: basin of hot tap water or container of sterile water ■ normal saline solution or another solution, as ordered ■ hot-water bottle, K pad, or chemical hot pack ■ linen-saver pad.

The following items may be sterile or nonsterile, depending on the type of procedure: compress material (flannel or 4" x 4" gauze pads) or pack material (absorbent towels or ABD pads), petroleum jelly, cotton-tipped applicators, forceps, bowl or basin, bath (utility) thermometer, waterproof covering, towel, dressing.

Preparation of equipment

Hot-water bottle: Fill the bottle with hot tap water to detect leaks and warm the bottle, and then empty it. Run hot tap water into a pitcher, and measure the water temperature with the bath thermometer. Adjust the temperature as ordered, usually to 105° to 115° F (40.6° to 46.1° C) for older patients. Next, pour hot-water into the bottle, filling it one-half to two-thirds full. Partially filling the bottle keeps it lightweight and flexible enough to mold to the treatment area. Squeeze the bottle until the water reaches the neck to expel any air that would make the bottle inflexible and reduce heat conduction. Fasten the top, and cover the bag with an absorbent, protective cloth to provide insulation and absorb perspiration. Secure the cover with tape or roller gauze.

Electric heating pad: Check the pad's cord for frayed or damaged insulation. Then plug in the pad and adjust the control switch to the desired setting. Wrap the pad in a protective cloth covering, and secure the cover with tape or roller gauze.

K pad: Check the pad's cord for safety, as above, and fill the control unit two-thirds full with distilled water. Do not use tap water because it leaves mineral deposits in the unit. Check the pad for leaks, and then tilt the unit in several directions to clear the pad's tubing of air, which could interfere with even heat conduction. Tighten the cap, and then loosen it a quarter turn to allow heat expansion within the unit.

After making sure the hoses between the control unit and the pad are free of tangles, place the unit on the bedside table, slightly above the patient so gravity can assist water flow. If the central supply department has not preset the temperature on the control unit, use the key provided to make this adjustment. The usual temperature is 105° F (40.6° C). Then place the pad in a protective cloth covering, and secure the cover with tape or roller gauze. Plug in the unit, turn it on, and allow the pad to warm for 2 minutes.

Chemical hot pack: Select a pack of the correct size. Then follow the manufacturer's directions (strike, squeeze, or knead) to activate the heat-producing chemicals. Place the pack in a protective cloth covering, and secure the cover with tape or roller gauze.

Sterile warm compress or pack: Warm the container of sterile water or solution by setting it in a sink or basin of hot-water. Measure the solution's temperature with a sterile bath thermometer. If a sterile thermometer is unavailable, pour some heated sterile solution into a clean container, check the temperature with a regular bath thermometer, and then discard the tested solution. Adjust the temperature of the sterile solution by adding hot or cold water to the sink or basin until the solution reaches 105° F. Pour the heated solution into a sterile bowl or basin. Then, using sterile technique, soak the compress or pack in the heated solution. If necessary, prepare a hot-water bottle, K pad, or chemical hot pack to keep the compress or pack warm.

Nonsterile warm compress or pack: Fill a bowl or basin with hot tap water or another solution, and measure the temperature of the fluid with a bath thermometer. Adjust the temperature as ordered, usually to 105° F for older patients. Then soak the compress or pack in the hot liquid. If necessary, prepare a hot-water bottle, K pad, or chemical hot pack to keep the compress or pack warm.

Implementation

● Check the doctor's order and assess the patient's condition.

● Explain the procedure to the patient, and tell him not to lean or lie directly on the heating device because this reduces air space and increases the risk of burns. Warn the patient not to adjust the temperature of the heating device or add hot-water to a hot-water bottle. If necessary, keep the controls away from a confused or disoriented older patient so that he can't inadvertently touch the temperature setting. Advise him to report pain or discomfort immediately and to remove the device himself if necessary.

● Provide privacy and make sure the room is warm and free of drafts. Wash your hands thoroughly.

● Record the patient's temperature, pulse, and respirations to serve as a baseline. If heat is being applied to raise the patient's body temperature, monitor his temperature, pulse, and respirations throughout the procedure.

● Expose only the treatment area because vasodilation will make the patient feel chilly.

To apply a hot-water bottle, an electric heating pad, a K pad, or a chemical hot pack. Follow these steps.

● Before applying the heating device, press it against the inner aspect of your forearm to test its temperature and heat distribution. If it heats unevenly, obtain a new device.

● Apply the device to the treatment area and, if necessary, secure it with tape or roller gauze. Begin timing the application.

● Assess the patient's skin condition frequently, and remove the device if you observe increased swelling or excessive redness, blistering, maceration, or pronounced pallor or if the patient reports pain or discomfort. Refill the hot-water bottle as necessary to maintain the correct temperature.

◆◆ *CLINICAL ALERT* ◆◆

Always check the temperature of a heating device before reapplying it to avoid burning the patient's skin.

● Remove the device after 20 to 30 minutes or as ordered.

● Dry the patient's skin with a towel, and re-dress the site if necessary. Take the patient's temperature, pulse, and respirations for comparison with baseline values. Position him comfortably in bed.

● If the treatment is to be repeated, store the equip-

ment in the patient's room, out of his reach; otherwise, return the equipment to its proper place.

To apply a warm compress or pack. Follow these steps.

● Place a linen-saver pad under the treatment area. Spread petroleum jelly (sterile, if necessary) over the affected area. Avoid applying it directly to any areas of skin breakdown or to eye tissues. (You may use sterile cotton-tipped applicators for a sterile procedure.) The petroleum jelly reduces maceration and the risk of burns by decreasing the rate of heat penetration.

● Remove the warm compress or pack from the bowl or basin (using sterile forceps for a sterile procedure).

● Wring excess solution from the compress or pack (using sterile forceps for a sterile procedure). Excess moisture increases the risk of burns.

● Apply the compress gently to the affected site (using forceps, if warranted). After a few seconds, lift the compress (with forceps, if needed) and check the skin for excessive redness, maceration, or blistering. When you're sure the compress isn't causing a burn, mold it firmly to the skin to keep out air, which reduces the temperature and effectiveness of the compress. Work quickly so the compress retains its heat.

● Apply a waterproof covering (sterile, if warranted) to the compress. Secure the covering with tape or roller gauze to prevent it from slipping.

● Place a hot-water bottle, K pad, or chemical hot pack over the compress and waterproof covering to maintain the correct temperature. Begin timing the application.

● Check the patient's skin every 5 minutes for signs of tissue intolerance. Remove the device if the skin shows excessive redness, maceration, or blistering or if the patient feels pain or discomfort. Change the compress as necessary to maintain the correct temperature.

● After 15 or 20 minutes or as ordered, remove the compress (using forceps, if warranted). Discard the compress in a waterproof trash bag.

● Dry the patient's skin with a towel (sterile, if necessary). Note the condition of the skin and re-dress the area if necessary. Take the patient's temperature, pulse, and respirations for comparison with baseline values. Then make sure the patient is comfortable.

Special considerations

If the patient is unconscious, anesthetized, irrational, neurologically impaired, or insensitive to heat for any reason, stay with him throughout the treatment.

When direct heat is ordered to decrease congestion within internal organs, the application must cover a large enough area to increase blood volume at the skin's surface. For relief of pelvic organ congestion, for example, apply heat over the patient's lower abdomen, hips, and thighs. To achieve local relief, you may concentrate heat only over the specified area.

As an alternative method of applying sterile moist compresses, use a bedside sterilizer to sterilize the compresses. Saturate the compress with tap water or another solution and wring it dry. Then place it in the bedside sterilizer at 275° F (135° C) for 15 minutes. Remove the compress with sterile forceps or sterile gloves, and wring out the excess solution. Then place the compress in a sterile bowl and measure its temperature with a sterile thermometer.

Complications

Because tissue damage may result from direct heat application, monitor the temperature of the compress carefully. Frequently assess the patient's skin under the heat application device and intervene appropriately as necessary.

Documentation

Record the time and date of heat application; the type, temperature or heat setting, duration, and site of application; the patient's temperature, pulse, respirations, and skin condition before, during, and after treatment; signs of complications; and the patient's tolerance of and reaction to the treatment.

Applying cold

The application of cold constricts blood vessels; inhibits local circulation, suppuration, and tissue metabolism; relieves vascular congestion; slows bac-

terial activity in infections; reduces body temperature; and may act as a temporary anesthetic during brief, painful procedures. Because treatment with cold also relieves inflammation and slows bleeding, it may be effective in initial treatment of eye injuries, strains, sprains, bruises, muscle spasms, and burns. Cold does not reduce existing edema, however, because it inhibits reabsorption of excess fluid.

Cold may be applied in dry or moist forms.

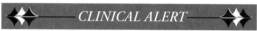

CLINICAL ALERT

Do not place ice directly on a patient's skin because it may further damage tissue.

Moist application of cold is more penetrating than dry because moisture aids conduction. Devices for applying dry cold include an ice bag or collar, a K pad (which can produce cold or heat), and chemical cold packs. Devices for applying moist cold include cold compresses for small body areas and cold packs for large areas.

Use cold treatments cautiously on older persons, especially those with impaired circulation or arthritis because of the risk of ischemic tissue damage.

Equipment

Patient thermometer ■ towel ■ adhesive tape or roller gauze ■ gloves (if necessary).

For an ice bag or collar: tap water ■ ice chips ■ absorbent, protective cloth covering.

For a K pad: distilled water ■ temperature-adjustment key ■ absorbent, protective cloth covering.

For a chemical cold pack: Single-use packs are available for applying dry cold. These lightweight plastic packs contain a chemical that turns cold when activated. Reusable, sealed cold packs, filled with an alcohol-based solution, are also available. These packs may be stored frozen until use and, after exterior disinfection, may be refrozen and used again. Other chemical packs are activated by striking, squeezing, or kneading them.

For a cold compress or pack: basin of ice chips ■ container of tap water ■ bath (utility) thermometer ■ compress material (4" x 4" gauze pads or washcloths) or pack material (towels or flannel) ■ linensaver pad ■ waterproof covering.

Preparation of equipment

Ice bag or collar: Select a device of the correct size, fill it with cold tap water, and check for leaks. Then empty the device and fill it about halfway with crushed ice. Using small pieces of ice keeps the device flexible enough to mold to the patient's body. Squeeze the device to expel air, which could interfere with conduction. Fasten the cap and wipe any moisture from the outside of the device. Wrap the bag or collar in a cloth covering, and secure the cover with tape or roller gauze. The protective cover prevents tissue trauma and absorbs condensation.

K pad: Check the cord for frayed or damaged insulation. Then fill the control unit two-thirds full with distilled water. Do not use tap water because it leaves mineral deposits in the unit. Check for leaks; then tilt the unit several times to clear the pad's tubing of air. Tighten the cap. After ensuring that the hoses between the control unit and pad are free of tangles, place the unit on the bedside table, slightly above the patient so gravity can assist water flow. If the central supply department has not preset the temperature on the control unit, use the key provided to adjust it to the lowest temperature. Cover the pad with an absorbent, protective cloth, and secure the cover with tape or roller gauze. Plug in the unit and turn it on. Allow the pad to cool for 2 minutes before placing it on the patient.

Chemical cold pack: Select a pack of the appropriate size, and follow the manufacturer's directions (strike, squeeze, or knead) to activate the cold-producing chemicals. Make certain that the container is not broken during activation; such damage could allow the chemicals to leak out. Wrap the pack in a cloth cover, and secure the cover with tape or roller gauze.

Cold compress or pack: Cool the tap water by placing the container of water in a basin of ice or by adding ice to the water. Using a bath thermometer for guidance, adjust the water temperature to 59° F (15° C) or as ordered. Immerse the compress or pack in the water.

Implementation

- Check the doctor's order and assess the patient's condition.

- Explain the procedure to the patient, provide privacy, and make sure the room is warm and free of drafts. Wash your hands thoroughly.
- Record the patient's temperature, pulse, and respirations to serve as a baseline.
- Expose only the treatment site to avoid chilling the patient.

To apply an ice bag or collar, K pad, or chemical cold pack. Follow these steps.
- Place the covered device on the treatment site, and begin timing the application.
- Observe the site frequently for signs of tissue intolerance: blanching, mottling, graying, cyanosis, maceration, or blisters. Because older adults have diminished sensation, they're at high risk for injury. Also, be alert for shivering and for complaints of burning or numbness. If any of these signs or symptoms develop, discontinue treatment and notify the doctor.
- Refill or replace the cold device as necessary to maintain the correct temperature. Change the protective cover if it becomes wet.
- Remove the device after the prescribed treatment period (usually 30 minutes).

To apply a cold compress or pack. Follow these steps.
- Place a linen-saver pad under the treatment area.
- Remove the compress or pack from the water, and wring it out to prevent dripping. Apply it to the treatment site, and begin timing the application.
- Cover the compress or pack with a waterproof covering to provide insulation and to keep the surrounding area dry. Secure the covering with paper tape or roller gauze to prevent it from slipping and injuring the older patient's friable skin.
- Check the application site frequently for signs of tissue intolerance. Also note any complaints of burning or numbness. If any of these signs or symptoms develop, discontinue treatment and notify the doctor.
- Change the compress or pack as necessary to maintain the correct temperature. Remove it after the prescribed treatment period (usually 20 minutes).

To conclude all cold applications. Follow these steps.

• Dry the patient's skin and re-dress the treatment site according to the doctor's orders. Then position the patient comfortably, and take his temperature, pulse, and respirations for comparison with baseline values.

• Dispose of liquids and soiled materials properly. If treatment will be repeated, clean and store the equipment in the patient's room, out of his reach; otherwise, return it to storage.

Special considerations

Apply cold immediately after an injury to minimize edema. Although colder temperatures can be tolerated for a longer time when the treatment site is small, don't continue any application for longer than 1 hour to prevent reflexive vasodilation. Application of temperatures below 59° F (15° C) will also cause local reflex vasodilation.

When applying cold to an open wound or to a lesion that may open during treatment, use sterile technique. Also maintain sterile technique during eye treatment, and use separate sterile equipment for each eye to prevent cross-contamination.

Avoid securing cooling devices with pins because an accidental puncture could allow extremely cold fluids to leak out and burn the patient's skin. If the patient is unconscious, anesthetized, neurologically impaired, irrational, or otherwise insensitive to cold, stay with him throughout the treatment and check the application site frequently for signs of complications.

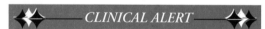

❖ ━━━ *CLINICAL ALERT* ━━━ ❖

Warn the patient not to place ice directly on his skin because the extreme cold can cause burns.

Complications

Thrombi may result from hemoconcentration. Pain, burning, or numbness may result from intense cold.

Documentation

Record the time, date, and duration of cold application; the type of device used (ice bag or collar, K pad, or chemical cold pack); the application site; the temperature or temperature setting; the patient's temperature, pulse, and respirations before and after application; the skin's appearance before, during, and after application; any signs of complications; and the patient's tolerance of the treatment.

Administering a therapeutic bath

Also referred to as balneotherapy, a therapeutic bath combines water and additives to soothe and relax the patient, clean the skin, relieve inflammation and pruritus, and soften and remove crusts, scales, debris, and old medications. Used primarily for their antipruritic and emollient effects, these baths coat irritated skin with a soothing, protective film. Because they constrict surface blood vessels, they also have an anti-inflammatory effect.

Antibacterial agents, such as acetic acid, potassium permanganate, or povidone-iodine, may be added to bath water to treat infected eczema, dirty ulcerations, furunculosis, and pemphigus. The addition of oatmeal powder, soluble cornstarch, or soybean complex to bath water creates a colloidal bath, which has a soothing effect and is used to treat generalized pruritus. Oil baths are useful for lubricating dry skin and easing eczematous eruptions. Sodium bicarbonate added to water produces an alkaline bath, which has a cooling effect and also helps relieve pruritus. A medicated tar bath may be used to treat psoriasis. The film of tar left on the skin works in combination with ultraviolet light to inhibit the rapid cell turnover characteristic of psoriasis.

A bedridden patient may benefit from a local soak with the therapeutic additive instead of a therapeutic tub bath.

Equipment

Bathtub ■ bath mat ■ rubber mat ■ bath (utility) thermometer ■ therapeutic additive ■ measuring device ■ colander or sieve for oatmeal powder ■ two washcloths and two towels ■ hospital gown or loose-fitting cotton pajamas ■ lubricating cream or ointment (if ordered).

Preparation of equipment

Assemble supplies and draw the bath before bringing the patient to the bath area to prevent chilling him. Make sure the tub is clean and disinfected because a patient with skin breakdown is particularly vulnerable to infection.

Use assistive devices such as grab bars to prevent falls and to help older people, especially those with limited mobility, get in and out of the tub. Place the bath mat next to the tub and the rubber mat on the bottom of the tub to prevent falls; the therapeutic additive may make the tub very slippery.

Fill the tub with 6" to 8" (15 to 20 cm) of water, usually measuring 95° to 100° F (35° to 37.8° C). The treatment's purpose and the type of additive used will determine the water temperature. Cool to lukewarm water is used to relieve pruritus and when adding tar or starch. Warm baths are soothing, but water warmer than 100° F causes vasodilation, which could aggravate pruritus.

Measure the correct amount of therapeutic additive, according to the doctor's order or package instructions. As the tub is filling, thoroughly mix the additive in the water. Add most substances directly to the water, but place oatmeal powder in a sieve or colander under the faucet to help it dissolve. Begin with 2 tablespoons of oatmeal powder; then add more powder or water as needed to regulate the thickness of the oatmeal bath.

When giving a tar bath, wear a plastic apron or protective gown because tar preparations stain clothing.

Implementation
● Check the doctor's order and assess the patient's condition.
● Explain the procedure to the patient and have him urinate. Wash your hands thoroughly and then escort the patient to the bath area. Close the door to provide privacy and eliminate drafts.
● Check the water temperature with a bath thermometer. Help the patient undress, and assist him into the tub if necessary. Advise him to use the safety rails to prevent falls.
● Tell him that the bath may feel unpleasant at first because his skin is irritated, but assure him that the medication will soon coat and soothe his skin.
● Ask the patient to stretch out in the tub and sub-

merge his body up to the chin. If he's capable, give him a washcloth to apply the bath solution gently to his face and other body areas that are not immersed.

◆◆ ——— *CLINICAL ALERT* ——— ◆◆
If the patient is taking a tar bath, tell him not to get the bath solution in his eyes because tar is an eye irritant.

● Warn the patient against scrubbing his skin to prevent further irritation.
● Add warm water to the bath as needed to maintain a comfortable temperature.
● Allow the patient to soak for 15 to 30 minutes. If you must stay with him, pull the bath curtain; this gives him some privacy and protects him from drafts. If you must leave the room, show the patient how to use the call button and ensure his privacy.
● After the bath, help the patient from the tub. Have him use the safety rails to prevent falls.
● Help him pat his skin dry with towels. Don't rub the skin because rubbing removes some solutes and oils clinging to the skin and produces friction, which increases pruritus and may injure the skin.
● Apply lubricating cream or ointment, if ordered, to help hold water in the newly hydrated skin.
● Provide a fresh hospital gown or loose-fitting cotton pajamas. Advise the patient to avoid wearing pajamas, underwear, or other clothing that isn't loose-fitting and made of cotton. Tight clothing and scratchy or synthetic materials can aggravate skin conditions by causing friction and increasing perspiration.
● Escort the patient to his room and make sure he's comfortable.
● Drain the bath water, clean and disinfect the tub, and dispose of soiled materials properly. If you have given an oatmeal powder bath, drain and rinse the tub immediately or the powder will cake, making later removal difficult.

Special considerations
Because pruritus seems worse at night, give a therapeutic bath before bedtime, unless ordered otherwise, to promote restful sleep. Don't use soap during a therapeutic bath because its drying effect counteracts the bath emollients.

Because the patient with a skin disorder may be self-conscious, maintain eye contact during conversation and avoid staring at his skin. Also avoid gestures and facial expressions that show revulsion. If the patient wishes, allow him to talk about his condition and how it affects his self-image.

Protect the patient from drafts because people with skin breakdown chill easily. But after the bath, don't cover or dress him too warmly because perspiration aggravates pruritus. Instruct him not to scratch his skin to prevent excoriation and infection.

If the patient is confined to bed, place the therapeutic additive in a basin of water at 95° to 100° F (35° to 37.8° C) and apply it with a washcloth, using light, gentle strokes.

Home care

● Instruct the older person to bathe only as often as prescribed. Excessive bathing can dry the skin.
● Suggest the patient purchase a commercial bath oil. Although salad or cooking oils are inexpensive alternatives, they may give clothes an unpleasant odor, and mineral oil mixes poorly with water.
● Tell the patient to follow the manufacturer's instructions for commercial colloidal preparations. Colloid for an oatmeal bath can be made at home by putting one-half cup of raw oatmeal into a blender, blending it at medium-high speed until the material has the consistency of flour, then sifting it to remove larger pieces.
● Suggest installing assistive devices for bathroom safety, such as grab bars and safety rails to prevent falls.

Documentation

Record the date, time, and duration of the bath. Note the water temperature, the type and amount of additive used, skin appearance before and after the bath, the patient's tolerance of the treatment, and the bath's effectiveness.

Administering soaks

A soak involves the immersion of a body part in warm water or a medicated solution. This treatment helps to soften exudates, facilitate debridement, enhance suppuration, clean wounds or burns, rehy-

drate wounds, apply medication to infected areas, and increase local blood supply and circulation.

Most soaks are applied with clean tap water and clean technique. Sterile solution and equipment are required for treating wounds, burns, or other breaks in the skin.

Equipment

Basin or arm or foot tub ■ bath (utility) thermometer ■ hot tap water or prescribed solution ■ cup and pitcher ■ linen-saver pad ■ overbed table or footstool ■ pillows ■ towels ■ gauze pads and other dressing materials ■ gloves (if necessary).

Preparation of equipment

Clean and disinfect the basin or tub. Run hot tap water into a pitcher or heat the prescribed solution, whichever applies. Measure the water or solution temperature with a bath thermometer. If the temperature is not within the prescribed range (usually 100° to 104° F [37.7° to 40° C]), add hot or cold water or reheat or cool the solution, as needed. If you're preparing the soak away from the patient's room, heat the liquid slightly above the correct temperature to allow for cooling during transport. If the solution for a medicated soak isn't premixed, prepare it yourself and heat it.

Implementation

● Check the doctor's order and assess the patient's condition.
● Explain the procedure to the patient and, if necessary, check his history for previous allergic reactions to the medicated solution. Provide privacy and wash your hands thoroughly.
● If the basin or tub will be placed in bed, make sure the bed is flat beneath it to prevent spills. For an arm soak, have the patient sit erect. For a leg or foot soak, ask him to lie down and bend the appropriate knee. For a foot soak in the sitting position, let him sit on the edge of the bed or transfer him to a chair.
● Place a linen-saver pad under the treatment site and, if necessary, cover the pad with a towel to absorb spillage.
● Expose the treatment site. Put on gloves before removing any dressing, and dispose of the soiled

dressing properly. If the dressing is encrusted and stuck to the wound, leave it in place and proceed with the soak. Remove the dressing several minutes later when it has begun to soak free.

• Position the basin under the treatment site on the bed, overbed table, footstool, or floor, as appropriate. Pour the heated liquid into the basin or tub. Then lower the patient's arm or leg into the basin gradually to allow him to adjust to the temperature change. Make sure the soak solution covers the treatment site.

• Stay with the patient if he's confused or restless or if he doesn't understand the treatment. If the patient becomes weak or can't remain in one position for a prolonged period, try dividing the treatment into several treatments of shorter duration given more frequently. Observe the older person for signs of discomfort or fatigue.

• Support other body parts and bony prominences with pillows or towels, as needed, to prevent discomfort and muscle strain. Make the patient comfortable and ensure proper body alignment.

• Check the temperature of the soak solution with the bath thermometer every 5 minutes. If the temperature drops below the prescribed range, remove some of the cooled solution with a cup. Then lift the patient's arm or leg from the basin to avoid burns, and add hot-water or solution to the basin. Mix the liquid thoroughly and then check its temperature. If the temperature is within the prescribed range, lower the patient's arm or leg back into the basin.

• Observe the patient for signs of tissue intolerance: extreme redness at the treatment site, excessive drainage or bleeding, or maceration. If such signs develop or the patient complains of pain, discontinue the treatment and notify the doctor.

◆✦ *CLINICAL ALERT* ✦◆

Because an older person may have decreased pain sensation, don't rely on him to inform you when he's in pain. Instead, look for more reliable signs of adverse reactions, such as increased pulse and respiratory rates or local tissue changes.

• After 15 to 20 minutes, or as ordered, lift the patient's arm or leg from the basin and remove the basin.

• Dry the arm or leg thoroughly with a towel using a patting motion to prevent injury. If the patient has a wound, dry the skin around it without touching the wound.

• While the skin is hydrated from the soak, use gauze pads to remove loose scales or crusts.

• Observe the treatment area for general appearance, degree of swelling, debridement, suppuration, and healing. Re-dress the wound if appropriate.

• Remove the towel and linen-saver pad, and make the patient comfortable in bed.

• Discard the soak solution, dispose of soiled materials properly, and clean and disinfect the basin. If the treatment is to be repeated, store the equipment in the patient's room, out of his reach; otherwise, return it to the central supply department.

Special considerations

To treat large areas, particularly burns, you may administer a soak in a whirlpool or Hubbard tank.

Documentation

Record the date, time, and duration of the soak; the treatment site; the type of solution and its temperature; the skin and wound appearance before, during, and after treatment; and the patient's tolerance of the treatment.

Applying a pressure dressing

Pressure dressings control capillary or small-vein bleeding by temporarily applying pressure directly over a wound. A bulk dressing may be held in place by a glove-protected hand, bound into place with a pressure bandage, or held under pressure by an inflated air splint. Pressure dressings must be checked frequently for wound drainage to determine their effectiveness in controlling bleeding. Patients who need a pressure dressing may have such diagnoses as fluid volume deficit, impaired skin integrity, impaired tissue integrity, or altered tissue perfusion. Remember that older people may already have compromised circulation, so check carefully for obstructed circulation.

Equipment

Two or more sterile gauze pads ▪ roller gauze ▪ tape ▪ clean disposable gloves ▪ metric ruler.

Preparation of equipment

Obtain the pressure dressing quickly to avoid excessive blood loss. Use clean cloth for the dressing if sterile gauze pads are unavailable.

Implementation

- Quickly explain the procedure to the patient to help decrease his anxiety, and put on gloves.
- Elevate the injured body part to help reduce bleeding.
- Place enough gauze pads over the wound to cover it. Don't clean the wound; you can do this when the bleeding stops.
- For an extremity or trunk wound, hold the dressing firmly over the wound and secure the bandage with adhesive tape.
- When applying a dressing to the neck, the shoulder, or another location that can't be tightly wrapped, apply tape directly over the dressings to provide the necessary pressure at the wound site. Use hypoallergenic tape to avoid injuring the patient's skin.
- Check pulse, temperature, and skin condition distal to the wound site because excessive pressure can obstruct normal circulation.
- Check the dressing frequently to monitor wound drainage. Use metric measurements to determine the amount of drainage, and document these serial measurements for later reference. Do not circle a potentially wet dressing with ink because this provides no permanent documentation in the medical record and also risks contaminating the dressing.
- If the dressing becomes saturated, do not remove it because this will interfere with the pressure. Instead, apply an additional dressing over the saturated one and continue to monitor and record drainage.
- Obtain additional medical care as soon as possible.

Special considerations

Apply pressure directly to the wound with your gloved hand if sterile gauze pads and clean cloth are unavailable. Avoid using an elastic bandage to bind the dressing because it can't be wrapped tightly enough to create pressure on the wound site.

Complications

Applying a pressure dressing too tightly can impair circulation.

Documentation

Once the bleeding is controlled, record the date and time of dressing application, the presence or absence of distal pulses, the integrity of distal skin, the amount of wound drainage, and any complications.

Managing a surgical wound

The procedures involved in caring for a surgical wound help prevent infection by stopping pathogens from entering the wound. Besides promoting patient comfort, they also protect the skin surface from maceration and excoriation caused by contact with irritating drainage. They also allow you to measure wound drainage to monitor fluid and electrolyte balance.

The two primary methods of managing a draining surgical wound are *dressing* and *pouching*. Dressing is preferred unless caustic or excessive drainage is compromising your patient's skin integrity. If your patient has a surgical wound, you must monitor him and choose the appropriate dressing. Usually, lightly seeping wounds with drains and wounds with minimal purulent drainage can be managed with packing and gauze dressings. Some wounds, such as those that become chronic, may require an occlusive dressing. A wound with copious, excoriating drainage calls for pouching to protect the surrounding skin.

Dressing a wound calls for sterile technique and sterile supplies to prevent contamination. You may use the color of the wound to help determine which type of dressing to apply. Be sure to change the dressing often enough to keep the skin dry. However, changing the dressing too often also can retard healing because the wound can only heal at body temperature. Changing the dressing lowers the wound's body temperature and delays healing until body temperature returns to normal. Be aware that older patients may require frequent dressing changes because their healing process is delayed.

Equipment

Waterproof trash bag ■ clean gloves or sterile gloves ■ gown and face shield or goggles (if indicated) ■ sterile 4" x 4" gauze pads ■ ABD pads (if indicated) ■ sterile cotton-tipped applicators ■ sterile dressing set ■ topical medication (if ordered) ■ tape ■ soap and water. Optional: skin protectant; nonadherent pads; collodion spray, acetone-free adhesive remover, or baby oil; sterile normal saline solution; graduated container; and Montgomery straps, a fishnet tube elasticized dressing support, or a T-binder.

For a wound with a drain: sterile scissors ■ sterile 4" x 4" gauze pads without cotton lining ■ sump drain ■ ostomy pouch or another collection bag ■ precut tracheostomy pads or drain dressings ■ tape (paper or silk tape if the patient is hypersensitive) ■ surgical mask.

For pouching a wound: collection pouch with drainage port ■ sterile gloves ■ skin protectant ■ sterile gauze pads.

Preparation of equipment

● Assemble all equipment in the patient's room.
● Check the expiration date on each sterile package, and inspect for tears.
● Open the waterproof trash bag, and place it near the patient's bed.
● Position the bag to avoid reaching across the sterile field or the wound when disposing of soiled articles.
● Form a cuff by turning down the top of the trash bag to provide a wide opening and to prevent contamination of instruments or gloves by touching the bag's edge.

Implementation

Explain the procedure to the patient to allay his fears and ensure his cooperation.

To remove the old dressing. Follow these steps.
● Check the doctor's order for specific wound care and medication instructions. Be sure to note the location of surgical drains to avoid dislodging them during the procedure.

● Assess the patient's condition.
● Identify the patient's allergies, especially to adhesive tape, other topical solutions, or medications.
● Provide the patient with privacy, and position him as necessary. To avoid chilling him, expose only the wound site.
● Wash your hands thoroughly. Put on a gown and a face shield, if necessary. Then put on clean gloves.
● Loosen the soiled dressing by holding the patient's skin and pulling the tape or dressing toward the wound. This protects the newly formed tissue, prevents stress on the incision, and minimizes the risk of injuring the patient's skin. Moisten the tape with acetone-free adhesive remover or baby oil, if necessary, to make the tape removal less painful (particularly if the skin is hairy). Don't apply solvents to the incision because they could contaminate the wound.
● Slowly remove the soiled dressing. If the gauze adheres to the wound, loosen it by moistening it with sterile normal saline solution.
● Observe the dressing for the amount, type, color, and odor of drainage.
● Discard the dressing and gloves in the waterproof trash bag.

To care for the wound. Follow these steps.
● Wash your hands. Establish a sterile field with all the equipment and supplies you'll need for suture-line care and the dressing change, including a sterile dressing set. If the doctor has ordered ointment, squeeze the needed amount onto the sterile field. If you're using an antiseptic from an unsterile bottle, pour it into a sterile container so you won't contaminate your gloves. Then put on sterile gloves.
● Saturate the sterile gauze pads with the prescribed cleaning agent. Avoid using cotton balls because they may shed fibers in the wound, causing irritation, infection, or adhesion.
● If ordered, obtain a wound culture; then proceed to clean the wound.
● Pick up the moistened gauze pad or swab, and squeeze out the excess solution.
● Working from the top of the incision, wipe once to the bottom and then discard the gauze pad. With a second moistened pad, wipe from top to bottom in a vertical path next to the incision.

● Continue to work outward from the incision in lines running parallel to it. Always wipe from the clean area toward the less clean area (usually from top to bottom). Use each gauze pad or swab for only one stroke to avoid tracking wound exudate and normal body flora from surrounding skin to the clean areas. Remember that the suture line is cleaner than the adjacent skin and that the top of the suture line is usually cleaner than the bottom because more drainage collects at the bottom of the wound.

● Use sterile cotton-tipped applicators to clean tight-fitting wire sutures, deep and narrow wounds, or wounds with pockets. Because the cotton on the swab is tightly wrapped, it's less likely than a cotton ball to leave fibers in the wound. Remember to wipe only once with each applicator.

● If the patient has a surgical drain, clean the drain's surface last. Because moist drainage promotes bacterial growth, the drain is considered the most contaminated area. Clean the skin around the drain by wiping in half or full circles from the drain site outward.

● Clean all areas of the wound to wash away debris, pus, blood, and necrotic material. Try not to disturb sutures or irritate the incision. Clean to at least 1" (2.5 cm) beyond the end of the new dressing. If you aren't applying a new dressing, clean to at least 2" (5 cm) beyond the incision.

● Check to see that the edges of the incision are lined up properly, and check for signs of infection (heat, redness, swelling, and odor), dehiscence, or evisceration. If you observe such signs or if the patient reports pain at the wound site, notify the doctor.

Observe the area around the wound where the tape adheres for signs of irritation and breakdown.

● Irrigate the wound as ordered.

● Wash skin surrounding the wound with soap and water, and pat it dry with a sterile 4" x 4" gauze pad. Avoid oil-based soap because it may interfere with pouch adherence. Apply any prescribed topical medication.

● Apply a skin protectant if needed.

● If ordered, pack the wound with gauze pads or strips folded to fit. Avoid using cotton-lined gauze pads because cotton fibers can adhere to the wound surface and cause complications. Pack the wound using the wet-to-damp method. Soaking the packing material in solution and wringing it out so it's slightly moist provides a moist environment that absorbs debris and drainage. But removing the packing won't disrupt new tissue.

To apply a fresh gauze dressing. Follow these steps.

● Gently place sterile 4" x 4" gauze pads at the center of the wound, and move progressively outward to the edges of the wound site. Extend the gauze at least 1" (2.5 cm) beyond the incision in each direction, and cover the wound evenly with enough sterile dressings (usually two or three layers) to absorb all drainage until the next dressing change. Use ABD pads to form outer layers, if needed, to provide greater absorbency.

● Secure the dressing's edges to the patient's skin with strips of tape to maintain the sterility of the wound site. For an older person who requires frequent dressing changes, secure the dressing with a T-binder or Montgomery straps to prevent skin excoriation, which may occur with repeated tape removal (see *How to make Montgomery straps*).

● Make sure that the patient is comfortable.

● Properly dispose of the solutions and trash bag, and clean or discard soiled equipment and supplies according to your facility's policy. If your patient's wound has purulent drainage, don't return unopened sterile supplies to the sterile supply cabinet because this could cause cross-contamination of other equipment.

To dress a wound with a drain. Follow these steps.

● Prepare a drain dressing by using sterile scissors to cut a slit in a sterile 4" x 4" gauze pad. Fold the pad in half; then cut inward from the center of the folded edge. Don't use a cotton-lined gauze pad because cutting the gauze opens the lining and releases cotton fibers into the wound. Prepare a second pad the same way.

● Gently press one folded pad close to the skin around the drain so that the tubing fits into the slit. Press the second folded pad around the drain from the opposite direction so that the two pads encircle the tubing.

How to make Montgomery straps

An abdominal dressing requiring frequent changes can be secured with Montgomery straps to promote the patient's comfort. If ready-made straps aren't available, follow these steps to make your own:
• Cut four to six strips of 2" or 3" (5- to 7.6-cm) wide hypoallergenic tape of sufficient length to allow the tape to extend about 6" (15cm) beyond the wound on each side. (The length of the tape varies, depending on the patient's size and the type and amount of dressing.)
• Fold one end of each strip 2" or 3" back on itself (sticky sides together) to form a nonadhesive tab. Then cut a small hole in the folded tab's center, close to its top edge. Make as many pairs of straps as you'll need to snugly secure the dressing.
• Clean the patient's skin to prevent irritation.
• After the skin dries, apply a skin protectant. Then apply the sticky side of each tape to a skin barrier sheet composed of opaque hydrocolloidal or nonhydrocolloidal materials, and apply the sheet directly to the skin near the dressing. Next, thread a separate piece of gauze tie, umbilical tape, or twill tape (about 12" [30.5 cm]) through each pair of holes in the straps, and fasten each tie as you would a shoelace. Don't stress the surrounding skin by securing the ties too tightly.
• Repeat this procedure according to the number of Montgomery straps needed.
• Replace Montgomery straps whenever they become soiled (every 2 or 3 days). If skin maceration occurs, place new tapes about 1" (2.5 cm) away from any irritation.

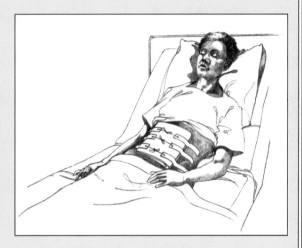

• Layer as many uncut sterile 4" x 4" gauze pads or ABD pads around the tubing as needed to absorb expected drainage. Tape the dressing in place, or use a T-binder or Montgomery straps.

To pouch a wound. Follow these steps.
• If your patient's wound is draining heavily or if drainage may damage surrounding skin, you'll need to apply a pouch.
• Measure the wound. Cut an opening ⅛" (0.3 cm) larger than the wound in the facing of the collection pouch.
• Apply a skin protectant as needed. (Some protectants are incorporated within the collection pouch and also provide adhesion.)
• Make sure that the drainage port at the bottom of the pouch is closed firmly to prevent leaks. Then gently press the contoured pouch opening around the wound, starting at its lower edge, to catch any drainage.
• To empty the pouch, put on gloves, insert the pouch's bottom half into a graduated biohazard container, and open the drainage port. Note the color, consistency, odor, and amount of drainage. If ordered, obtain a culture specimen and send it to the laboratory immediately. Remember to follow isolation precautions when handling infectious drainage.
• Wipe the bottom of the pouch and the drainage port with a gauze pad to remove any drainage that could irritate the patient's skin or cause an odor. Then reseal the port. Change the pouch only if it leaks or fails to adhere to the skin. More frequent changes are unnecessary and only irritate the patient's skin.

Special considerations

If the patient has two wounds in the same area, cover each wound separately with layers of sterile 4" x 4" gauze pads. Then cover both sites with an ABD pad secured to the patient's skin with tape. Don't use only one ABD pad to cover both sites because drainage quickly saturates a single pad, promoting cross-contamination.

Don't pack a wound too tightly; doing so would compress adjacent capillaries and could prevent the wound edges from contracting. Avoid using overly damp packing because it slows wound closure from within and increases the risk of infection.

To save time when dressing a wound with a drain, use precut tracheostomy pads or drain dressings instead of custom-cutting gauze pads to fit around the drain. Use paper or silk tape. It is less likely to cause a skin reaction, will peel off more easily than adhesive tape, and will minimize the risk of skin trauma. Use a surgical mask to cradle a chin or jawline dressing; this provides a secure dressing and avoids the need to shave the patient's hair.

If ordered, use a collodion spray or a similar topical protectant instead of a gauze dressing. Moisture- and contaminant-proof, this type of covering dries in a clear, impermeable film that leaves the wound visible for observation and avoids the friction caused by a dressing.

If a sump drain isn't adequately collecting wound secretions, reinforce it with an ostomy pouch or another collection bag. Use waterproof tape to strengthen a spot on the front of the pouch near the adhesive opening; then cut a small "X" in the tape. Feed the drain catheter into the pouch through the "X" cut. Seal the cut around the tubing with more waterproof tape; then connect the tubing to the suction pump. This method frees the drainage port at the bottom of the pouch so you don't have to remove the tubing to empty the pouch. If you use more than one collection pouch for a wound or wounds, record the drainage volume separately for each pouch. Avoid using waterproof material over the dressing because it reduces air circulation and promotes infection from accumulated heat and moisture.

Because many doctors prefer to change the first postoperative dressing themselves to check the incision, don't change the first dressing unless you've been instructed to do so. If you have no such order and drainage comes through the dressing, reinforce the dressing with fresh sterile gauze. Request an order to change the dressing, or ask the doctor to change it as soon as possible. A reinforced dressing should not remain in place longer than 24 hours because it's an excellent medium for bacterial growth.

For a recent postoperative patient or a patient with complications, check the dressing every 30 minutes or as ordered. For a patient with a properly healing wound, check the dressing at least once every 8 hours.

If the dressing becomes wet from the outside (for example, from spilled drinking water), replace it as soon as possible to prevent wound contamination.

If your patient will need wound care after discharge, provide appropriate teaching. If he'll be caring for the wound himself, stress the importance of using aseptic technique and teach him how to examine the wound for signs of infection and other complications. Also show him how to change dressings, and give him written instructions for all procedures to be performed at home. (See *Changing a dry dressing,* pages 379 and 380.)

Complications

A major complication of dressing changes is hypersensitivity to the antiseptic cleaning agent, the prescribed topical medication, or the tape, which may lead to skin redness, rash, excoriation, or infection.

Documentation

Document the date, time, and type of wound management procedure; the amount of soiled dressing and packing removed; the wound's appearance (size, condition of margins, presence of necrotic tissue) and odor (if present); the type, color, consistency, and amount of drainage (for each wound); the presence and location of drains; any additional procedures, such as irrigation, packing, or application of a topical medication; the type and amount of new dressing or pouch applied; and the patient's tolerance of the procedure.

EACHING AID

Changing a dry dressing

Dear Caregiver:

Changing a dry dressing at least once a day keeps the surgical wound clean, allows you to see how well the wound is healing, and lets you apply medication. If the surgeon recommends dressing changes, here's how to proceed.

Gather your supplies
You'll need:
- a new dressing
- several 4" x 4" gauze pads
- scissors
- cleansing solution, such as povidone-iodine (Betadine)
- normal saline solution
- special ointment or powder, if ordered
- baby oil
- surgical tape
- waterproof disposal bag for soiled supplies
- rubber gloves (optional).

Remove the old tape
Wash your hands before exposing the old dressing. To remove the tape, hold the skin taut and pull the old tape strips toward the wound. Be sure to remove *all* of the old tape. If the tape sticks, use a little baby oil to soften it and make removal easier.

Remove the old dressing
Next, slowly remove the old dressing. If it sticks to the wound, stop and moisten it with normal saline solution. Remove the dressing when it's loose.

Clean the wound
Before you clean the wound, check it for signs of infection: puffiness or swelling, redness, yellow or green drainage or pus, or a foul odor. If it looks infected, call the doctor immediately and follow his instructions.

Note: You may want to put on rubber gloves for your protection.

Next, saturate one of the gauze pads with cleansing solution. Then fold the pad into quarters. Pinching the pad between your thumb and first two fingers, gently wipe from the top of the wound to the bottom in one motion. Then discard the pad.

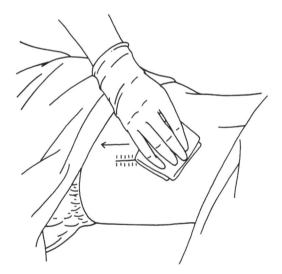

Then saturate another gauze pad; fold it in half and then into quarters. Wipe the wound again, this time on one side and then on the other. Do

(continued)

Changing a dry dressing (continued)

this several times to clean the entire wound area that the dressing will cover.

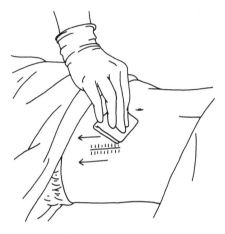

Finally, use another clean gauze pad to pat the wound dry.

Apply ointment or powder

Remove the cap from the ointment or powder container. If you're using special ointment, squeeze a generous strip of it along the wound's outline. Don't let the tube touch the wound. This helps to prevent infection from germs on the tube.

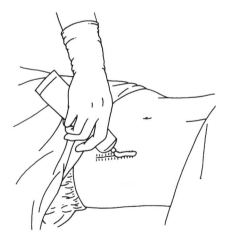

If you're using a special powder, dust the wound with a fine layer of it.

Apply the new dressing

Open the new dressing carefully, making sure it touches only the wound. Center and apply it over the wound. Next, secure the edges of the dressing to the skin around the wound with strips of surgical tape. Make sure the strips overlap and create a tight seal against germs.

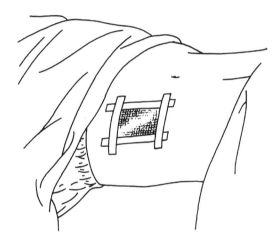

When you're finished, remember to wash your hands. Dispose of used items in a tightly sealed plastic trash bag.

Additional instructions:

_____

_____

_____

_____

_____

Document special or detailed wound care instructions and pain management steps on the nursing care plan. Record the color and amount of measurable drainage on the intake and output sheet.

Managing a traumatic wound

Traumatic wounds include abrasions, lacerations, puncture wounds, and amputations. In an abrasion, the skin is scraped and part of the skin surface is lost. In a laceration, the skin is torn, causing jagged, irregular edges; the severity of a laceration depends on its size, depth, and location. A puncture wound occurs when a pointed object, such as a knife or glass fragment, penetrates the skin. Traumatic amputation refers to removal of a part of the body, such as a limb or part of a limb.

When caring for a patient with a traumatic wound, first assess his ABCs: airway, breathing, and circulation. It may seem natural to focus first on a gruesome injury, but a patent airway and pumping heart take priority. An older person is less able to withstand physical trauma, so be especially alert for problems, such as shock or impending heart attack. Once the patient's ABCs are stabilized, you can turn your attention to the traumatic wound. Initial management focuses on controlling bleeding — usually by applying firm, direct pressure and elevating the extremity. If bleeding continues, you may need to compress a pressure point. Assess the condition of the wound. Management and cleaning technique usually depend on the specific type of wound and the degree of contamination.

Be aware that, besides having less physical stamina, the older person may have decreased pain sensation and therefore may underestimate the severity of his injury. Resistance to infection and healing rate are also slowed, so take care to reduce perioperative tissue damage as much as possible.

Equipment

Sterile basin ■ normal saline solution ■ sterile 4" x 4" gauze pads ■ sterile gloves or clean gloves ■ sterile cotton-tipped applicators ■ dry sterile dressing, nonadherent pad, or petroleum gauze ■ linen-saver pad. Optional: scissors, towel, goggles, mask, gown, 50-ml catheter-tip syringe, surgical scrub brush, antibacterial ointment, porous tape, sterile forceps, sutures and suture set, hydrogen peroxide.

Preparation of equipment

Place a linen-saver pad under the area to be cleaned, and remove any clothing covering the wound. If necessary, cut hair around the wound with scissors to promote cleaning.

Assemble needed equipment at the patient's bedside. Fill a sterile basin with normal saline solution. Make sure the treatment area has enough light to allow close observation of the wound.

Depending on the nature and location of the wound, wear sterile or clean gloves to avoid spreading infection.

Implementation

● Check the patient's medical history for previous tetanus immunization and, if needed and ordered, arrange for immunization.
● Administer pain medication if ordered.
● Wash your hands.
● Use appropriate protective equipment, such as a gown, mask, and goggles, if spraying or splashing of body fluids is possible.

For an abrasion. Follow these steps.
● Flush the scraped skin with normal saline solution.
● Remove dirt or gravel with a sterile 4" x 4" gauze pad moistened with normal saline solution. Gently rub in the opposite direction from which the dirt or gravel became embedded.
● If the wound is extremely dirty, you may use a surgical brush to scrub it.
● Allow a small wound to dry and form a scab. A larger wound may need to be covered with a nonadherent pad or petroleum gauze and a light dressing. Apply antibacterial ointment if ordered.

For a laceration. Follow these steps.
● Moisten a sterile 4" x 4" gauze pad with normal saline solution. Clean the wound gently, working outward from its center to approximately 2" (5 cm) beyond its edges. Discard the soiled gauze pad and use a fresh one for each wipe, as necessary. Continue

until the wound appears clean.

- If the wound is dirty, you may irrigate it with a 50-ml catheter-tip syringe and normal saline solution.
- Assist the doctor in suturing the wound edges using the suture kit, or apply sterile strips of porous tape.
- Apply the ordered antibacterial ointment to help prevent infection.
- Apply a dry sterile dressing over the wound to absorb drainage and help prevent bacterial contamination.

For a puncture wound. Follow these steps.
- If the wound is minor, allow it to bleed for a few minutes before cleaning it.
- A larger puncture wound may require irrigation before covering it with a dry dressing.
- Stabilize any embedded foreign object until the doctor can remove it. After he removes the object and bleeding is stabilized, clean the wound as you would clean a laceration or deep puncture wound.

Special considerations
When irrigating a traumatic wound, avoid using more than 8 pounds per square inch (psi) of pressure. High-pressure irrigation can seriously interfere with healing, kill cells, and allow bacteria to infiltrate the tissue.

To clean the wound, you may use sterile normal saline solution for debris removal. Hydrogen peroxide should never be instilled into a deep wound because of the risk of embolism from the evolving gases. Be sure to rinse your hands well after using hydrogen peroxide.

Avoid cleaning a traumatic wound with alcohol, which causes pain and tissue dehydration, or with antiseptics, which can impede healing. In addition, never use a cotton ball or a cotton-filled gauze pad to clean a wound because cotton fibers left in the wound may cause contamination.

After a wound has been cleaned, the doctor may want to debride it to remove dead tissue and reduce the risk of infection and scarring. If this is necessary, pack the wound with gauze pads soaked in normal saline solution until debridement.

Observe for signs and symptoms of infection, such as warm red skin or purulent discharge at the wound site. Be aware that infection of a traumatic wound can delay healing, increase scar formation, and trigger systemic infection, such as septicemia.

Observe all dressings. If edema is present, adjust the dressing to avoid impairing circulation to the area.

Complications
Cleaning and care of traumatic wounds may temporarily increase the patient's pain. Use a gentle, firm motion when cleaning these wounds because excessive vigorous cleaning may further disrupt tissue integrity.

Documentation
Document the date and time of the procedure, the wound size and condition, any medication administered, specific wound care measures, and patient teaching.

Irrigating a wound
Irrigation cleans tissues and flushes cell debris and drainage from an open wound. Irrigation with an antiseptic or antibiotic solution helps the wound heal properly from the inside tissue layers outward to the skin surface; it also helps prevent premature surface healing over an abscess pocket or infected tract.

Wound irrigation requires strict sterile technique. After irrigation, open wounds usually are packed to absorb additional drainage. Take care not to damage healthy tissue and be aware that, in older adults, healing takes place slowly, and older people fight infection more poorly than younger people. Also, be sure to guard the patient's privacy and protect him from hypothermia by exposing only the involved body part.

Equipment
Waterproof trash bag ■ linen-saver pad ■ emesis basin ■ clean gloves or sterile gloves ■ gown and goggles (if splashing is possible) ■ prescribed irrigant (such as sterile normal saline solution or commercial wound cleansing solution) ■ sterile water or normal

saline solution ■ soft rubber or plastic catheter ■ 50- to 60-ml piston syringe ■ sterile container ■ materials needed for wound care ■ sterile irrigation and dressing set ■ sterile petroleum jelly.

Preparation of equipment
Assemble all equipment in the patient's room. Check the expiration date on each sterile package, and inspect each one for tears. Check the sterilization date and the date that each bottle of irrigating solution was opened; don't use any solution that has been open longer than 24 hours.

Using aseptic technique, dilute the prescribed irrigant to the correct proportions with sterile water or normal saline solution, if necessary. Let the solution stand until it reaches room temperature, or warm it to 90° to 95° F (32.2° to 35° C).

Open the waterproof trash bag and place it near the patient's bed to avoid reaching across the sterile field or the wound when disposing of soiled articles. Form a cuff by turning down the top of the trash bag to provide a wide opening and prevent contamination by touching the bag's edge.

Implementation
● Check the doctor's order, and assess the patient's condition. Identify any allergies, especially to topical solutions or medications.
● Explain the procedure to the patient, provide privacy, and position him correctly for the procedure. Place the linen-saver pad under the patient to catch any spills and avoid linen changes. Place the emesis basin below the wound so the irrigating solution flows from the wound into the basin.
● Wash your hands thoroughly. If necessary, put on a gown to protect your clothing from wound drainage and contamination. Put on clean gloves.
● Remove the soiled dressing; then discard the dressing and gloves in the trash bag.
● Establish a sterile field with all the equipment and supplies you'll need for irrigation and wound care. Pour the prescribed amount of irrigating solution into a sterile container so you won't contaminate your sterile gloves later by picking up unsterile containers. Put on sterile gloves, gown, and goggles if splashing is possible.

● Fill the syringe with the irrigating solution; then connect the catheter to the syringe. Gently instill a slow, steady stream of irrigating solution into the wound until the syringe empties. Another method of cleaning the wound is to use a commercial product in a spray bottle that delivers the product at 8 psi. Avoid exceeding this force to prevent damage to healing tissues.

Make sure the solution flows from the clean to the dirty area of the wound to prevent contamination of clean tissue by exudate. Also make sure the solution reaches all areas of the wound.
● Refill the syringe, reconnect it to the catheter, and repeat the irrigation.
● Continue to irrigate the wound until you've administered the prescribed amount of solution or until the solution returns clear. Note the amount of solution administered. Then remove and discard the catheter and syringe in the waterproof trash bag.
● Keep the patient positioned to allow further wound drainage into the basin.
● Clean the area around the wound with a cleaning agent to help prevent skin breakdown and infection.
● Pack the wound, if ordered, and apply a sterile dressing. Discard your gloves, gown, and goggles.
● Make sure the patient is comfortable.
● Properly dispose of drainage, solutions, and trash bag, and clean or dispose of soiled equipment and supplies according to your facility's policy. To prevent contamination of other equipment, don't return unopened sterile supplies to the sterile supply cabinet.

Special considerations
Try to coordinate wound irrigation with the doctor's visit so he can inspect the wound. Use only the irrigant specified by the doctor because others may be erosive or otherwise harmful. Remember to follow your facility's policy concerning wound and skin precautions when appropriate.

Irrigate with a bulb syringe only if a piston syringe is unavailable; the piston syringe reduces the risk of aspirating drainage. If the wound is small or not very deep, you may want to use just the syringe for irrigation. A syringe with a 30-gauge over-the-needle catheter delivers irrigating solutions at 8 psi.

Home care

If the wound must be irrigated at home, teach the patient or a family member how to irrigate using strict aseptic technique. Ask for a return demonstration of the proper technique. Provide written instructions. Arrange for visiting nurses and delivery of home health supplies, as appropriate. Urge the patient to call his doctor if he detects signs of infection.

Complications

Wound irrigation increases the risk of infection. Excoriation and increased pain may also occur.

Documentation

Record the date and time of irrigation, the amount and type of irrigant, the appearance of the wound, any sloughing tissue or exudate, the amount of solution returned, any skin care performed around the wound, any dressings applied, and the patient's tolerance of the treatment.

Managing wound dehiscence and evisceration

Although the typical surgical wound heals without incident, occasionally the edges of a wound may fail to join, or they may separate even after they appear to be healing normally. This development, called wound dehiscence, may lead to evisceration, an even more serious complication, in which a portion of the viscera (usually a bowel loop) protrudes through the incision. Evisceration, in turn, can lead to peritonitis and septic shock. Dehiscence and evisceration are most likely to occur 6 or 7 days after surgery. By then, sutures may have been removed and the patient can cough easily and breathe deeply — both of which strain the incision.

Older people are at increased risk for this condition because of age-related changes that delay wound healing. Several other factors can contribute to these complications. Poor nutrition — whether from inadequate intake or a condition such as diabetes mellitus — may hinder wound healing, as may chronic pulmonary or cardiac disease, which deprives the injured tissue of sufficient nutrients and oxygen. Localized wound infection may limit clo-

sure, delay healing, and weaken the incision. And stress on the incision from coughing or vomiting may cause abdominal distention or severe stretching; for example, a patient with a midline abdominal incision has a high risk of developing wound dehiscence.

Equipment

Two sterile towels ▪ 1 L sterile normal saline solution ▪ sterile irrigation set, including a basin, a solution container, and a 50-ml catheter-tip syringe ▪ several large abdominal dressings ▪ sterile, waterproof drape ▪ linen-saver pads ▪ sterile gloves.

If the patient will return to the operating room, make sure you also gather the following equipment: I.V. administration set and I.V. fluids, equipment for nasogastric intubation, prescribed sedative, and suction apparatus.

Implementation

● Provide reassurance and support to ease the patient's anxiety. Tell him to stay in bed. If possible, stay with him while someone else notifies the doctor and collects the necessary equipment.

● Place a linen-saver pad under the patient to keep the sheets dry when you moisten the exposed viscera.

● Using sterile technique, unfold a sterile towel to create a sterile field. Open the package containing the irrigation set, and place the basin, solution container, and 50-ml syringe on the sterile field.

● Open the bottle of normal saline solution and pour about 400 ml into the solution container. Also pour about 200 ml into the sterile basin.

● Open several packages containing large abdominal dressings, and place the dressings on the sterile field.

● Put on the sterile gloves and place one or two of the large abdominal dressings in the basin to saturate them with saline solution.

● Place the moistened dressings over the exposed viscera. Then place a sterile, waterproof drape over the dressings to prevent the sheets from getting wet.

● Moisten the dressings every hour by withdrawing saline solution from the container through the syringe and then gently squirting the solution onto the dressings.

- When you moisten the dressings, inspect the color of the viscera. If it appears dusky or black, notify the doctor immediately. A protruding organ may become ischemic and necrotic if its blood supply is interrupted.
- Keep the patient on absolute bed rest in low Fowler's position (no more than 20 degrees elevation) with his knees flexed. This prevents injury and reduces stress on an abdominal incision.
- Monitor the patient's vital signs every 15 minutes to detect shock.
- If necessary, prepare the patient to return to the operating room. Gather the necessary equipment and start an I.V. infusion as ordered.
- Insert a nasogastric tube and connect it to continuous or intermittent low suction, as ordered.
- Also administer preoperative medications to the patient as ordered.
- Depending on the circumstances, some of these procedures may not be done at the bedside. For instance, nasogastric intubation may make the patient gag or vomit, causing further evisceration. For this reason, the doctor may choose to have the tube inserted in the operating room with the patient under anesthesia.
- Continue to reassure the patient while you prepare him for surgery. Be sure he has signed a consent form and the operating room staff has been informed about the procedure.

Special considerations

As always, the best treatment is prevention. If you're caring for an older postoperative patient, make sure he gets an adequate supply of protein, vitamins, and calories. Monitor him for dietary deficiencies, and discuss any problems with the doctor and a dietitian.

When changing wound dressings, always use sterile technique. Inspect the incision with each dressing change; if you recognize the early signs of infection, start treatment before dehiscence or evisceration can occur. If local infection develops, clean the wound as necessary to eliminate a buildup of purulent drainage. Always make sure bandages aren't so tight that they limit blood supply to the wound.

Complications

Infection, which can lead to peritonitis and possibly septic shock, is the most serious and most common complication of wound dehiscence and evisceration. Caused by bacterial contamination or by drying of normally moist abdominal contents, infection can impair circulation and lead to necrosis of the affected organ.

Documentation

Note when the problem occurred, the patient's activity preceding the problem, his condition, and the time the doctor was notified. Describe the appearance of the wound or eviscerated organ; the amount, color, consistency, and odor of any drainage; and any nursing actions taken. Record the patient's vital signs, his response to the incident, and the doctor's actions.

Finally, make sure you change the patient's care plan to reflect nursing actions needed to promote proper healing.

Caring for pressure ulcers

Successful pressure ulcer treatment involves relieving pressure, restoring circulation, and — if possible — resolving or managing related disorders, including poor nutrition. Typically, the effectiveness and duration of treatment depend on the pressure ulcer's characteristics. (See *Pressure ulcer stages,* page 386.)

Ideally, prevention is the key to avoiding extensive therapy. Preventive measures include ensuring adequate nourishment and mobility to relieve pressure and promote circulation.

When a pressure ulcer develops despite preventive efforts, treatment consists of methods to decrease pressure, including frequent repositioning to shorten pressure duration and use of special pressure-reducing devices, such as beds, mattresses, mattress overlays, and chair cushions. Other therapeutic measures include use of topical treatments, wound cleansing, debridement, and dressings to support moist wound healing. (See *Guide to topical agents for pressure ulcers,* page 387, and *Choosing an ulcer dressing,* page 388.)

You'll usually perform or coordinate treatments according to your facility's policy. The procedures

Pressure ulcer stages

To select the most effective treatment for a pressure ulcer, you first need to assess its characteristics. The pressure ulcer stages described below, used by the National Pressure Ulcer Advisory Panel and the Agency for Health Care Policy and Research, reflect the anatomic depth of exposed tissue. Keep in mind that if the wound contains necrotic tissue, you won't be able to determine the stage until you can see the wound base.

Stage 1

The first sign of a pressure ulcer is a reddened area of intact skin that does not blanch. In individuals with darker skin, discoloration, warmth, edema, induration, or hardness may be present.

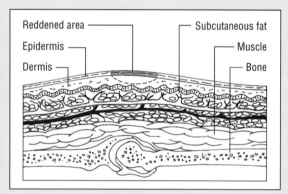

Stage 2

This stage is marked by partial-thickness skin loss involving the epidermis, dermis, or both. The ulcer is superficial and appears as an abrasion, a blister, or a shallow crater.

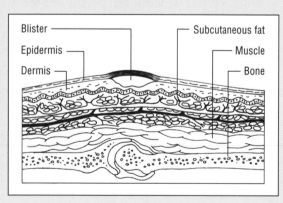

Stage 3

The ulcer constitutes a full-thickness wound penetrating the subcutaneous tissue, which may extend to — but not through — underlying fascia. It looks like a deep crater and may or may not undermine adjacent tissue.

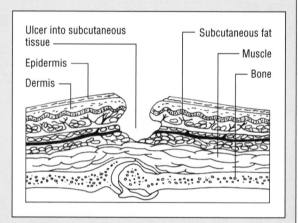

Stage 4

The ulcer extends through the skin, accompanied by extensive destruction, tissue necrosis, or damage to muscle, bone, or supporting structures (such as tendons and joint capsules). Adjacent tissue and sinus tracts may also be undermined.

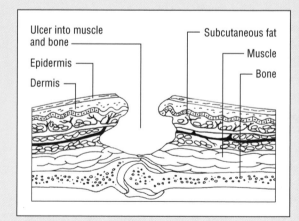

Guide to topical agents for pressure ulcers

Various agents can be used for pressure ulcer care. The chart below highlights some of the commonly used topical agents.

TOPICAL AGENTS	NURSING CONSIDERATIONS
Antibiotics Neomycin, polymyxin B, and bacitracin (Neosporin Ointment)	• Use only for early ulcers because these agents may not penetrate sufficiently to kill deeper bacterial colonies.
Circulatory stimulants Granulex	• Use these agents to promote blood flow. Both contain balsam of Peru and castor oil, but Granulex also contains trypsin, an enzyme that facilitates debridement.
Enzymes Collagenase (Santyl), fibrinolysin and desoxyribonuclease (Elase), sutilains (Travase)	• Apply collagenase in thin layers after cleaning the wound with normal saline solution. • To improve this treatment's effectiveness, avoid concurrent use of collagenase with agents that decrease enzymatic activity, including detergents, hexachlorophene, antiseptics with heavy-metal ions, iodine, or acid solutions such as Burow's solution. • Use collagenase cautiously near the patient's eyes. If contact occurs, flush the eyes repeatedly with normal saline solution or sterile water. • Use fibrinolysin and desoxyribonuclease only after surgical removal of dry eschar. • If you're using sutilains and topical antibiotics, apply sutilains ointment first. • Avoid applying sutilains to ulcers in major body cavities, to areas with exposed nerve tissue, or to fungating neoplastic lesions. Don't use sutilains on women of childbearing age or on patients with limited cardiopulmonary reserve. • Store sutilains at a cool temperature: 35.6° to 50° F (2° to 10° C). • Use sutilains cautiously near the patient's eyes. If contact occurs, flush the eyes repeatedly with normal saline solution or sterile water.
Exudate absorbers Dextranomer beads (Debrisan)	• Use dextranomer beads on secreting ulcers. Discontinue use when secretions stop. • Clean, but don't dry, the ulcer before applying dextranomer beads. Don't use these beads in tunneling ulcers. • Remove gray-yellow beads (which indicate saturation) by irrigating with sterile water or normal saline solution. • Use cautiously near the eyes. If contact occurs, flush the eyes repeatedly with normal saline solution or sterile water.
Isotonic solutions Normal saline solution	• This agent moisturizes tissue without injuring cells.

detailed below address cleaning and dressing of the pressure ulcer.

Equipment

Hypoallergenic tape or elastic netting ■ overbed table ■ piston-type irrigating system ■ two pairs of gloves ■ normal saline solution as ordered ■ sterile 4" x 4" gauze pads ■ selected topical dressing ■ linen-saver pads ■ impervious plastic trash bag ■ disposable wound-measuring device.

Choosing an ulcer dressing

The type of dressing used on a pressure ulcer depends on the ulcer's characteristics and on the patient's individual needs. The six major dressing types are reviewed below.

Gauze dressings
Made of absorptive cotton or synthetic fabric, these dressings are permeable to water, water vapor, and oxygen and may be impregnated with petroleum jelly or another agent. When uncertain about which dressing to use, you may apply a gauze dressing moistened in saline solution until a wound specialist recommends definitive treatment.

Hydrocolloid dressings
These adhesive, moldable wafers are made of a carbohydrate-based material and usually have waterproof backings. They are impermeable to oxygen, water, and water vapor, and most have some absorptive properties.

Transparent film dressings
Clear, adherent, and nonabsorptive, these polymer-based dressings are permeable to oxygen and water vapor but not to water. Their transparency allows visual inspection. Because they can't absorb drainage, transparent film dressings are used on partial-thickness wounds with minimal exudate.

Alginate dressings
Made from seaweed, these nonwoven, absorptive dressings are available as soft, white sterile pads or ropes. They absorb excessive exudate and may be used on infected wounds. As the dressing absorbs exudate, it turns into a gel that keeps the wound bed moist and promotes healing. When exudate is no longer excessive, switch to another type of dressing.

Foam dressings
These spongelike polymer dressings may be impregnated or coated with other materials. Somewhat absorptive, they may or may not be adherent. Foam dressings promote moist wound healing and are useful when a nonadherent surface is desired.

Hydrogel dressings
Water-based and nonadherent, these polymer-based dressings have some absorptive properties. They are available as a gel in a tube or in flexible sheets, and may have a cooling effect that eases pain.

Preparation of equipment
Assemble equipment at the patient's bedside. Cut tape into strips for securing dressings. Loosen lids on cleaning solutions and medications for easy removal. Loosen existing dressing edges and tapes before putting on gloves. Attach an impervious plastic trash bag to the overbed table to hold used dressings and refuse.

Implementation
● Before any dressing change, wash your hands and review the principles of standard precautions.

To clean a pressure ulcer. Follow these steps.
● Provide privacy and explain the procedure to the patient to allay his fears and promote cooperation.
● Position the patient so that he's comfortable, but make sure his position allows you easy access to the ulcer site.
● Cover the bed linens with a linen-saver pad to prevent soiling.
● Open the container of normal saline solution and the piston syringe package. Carefully pour normal saline solution into an irrigation container to avoid splashing. (This container may be clean or sterile, depending on your facility's policy.) Put the piston syringe into the opening provided in the irrigation container.
● Open packages of supplies.
● Put on gloves to remove the old dressing and expose the pressure ulcer. Discard the soiled dressing in the impervious trash bag to avoid contaminating the sterile field and spreading infection.
● Inspect the wound. Note the color, amount, and

Understanding pressure ulcer debridement

Because moist, necrotic tissue promotes the growth of pathologic organisms, removing such tissue aids pressure ulcer healing. A pressure ulcer can be debrided using various methods, which are reviewed below. The patient's condition and the goals of care determine which method to use. Sharp debridement is indicated for patients with an urgent need for debridement, such as those with sepsis or cellulitis. Otherwise, another method, such as mechanical, enzymatic, or autolytic debridement, may be used. Sometimes, several methods may be used together.

Sharp debridement
The most rapid method, sharp debridement removes thick, adherent eschar and devitalized tissue with a scalpel, scissors, or another sharp instrument. Small amounts of necrotic tissue can be debrided at the bedside; extensive amounts must be debrided in the operating room.

Mechanical debridement
Typically, this method involves the use of wet-to-dry dressings. Gauze moistened with normal saline

solution is applied to the wound and then removed after it dries and adheres to the wound bed. The goal is to debride the wound as the dressing is removed. Mechanical debridement has certain disadvantages; for example, it is often painful and it may take a long time to completely debride the ulcer. It is also nonselective and may damage healthy tissue.

Enzymatic debridement
This method removes necrotic tissue by breaking down tissue elements. Topical enzymatic debriding agents are placed on the necrotic tissue. If eschar is present, it must be cross-hatched to allow the enzyme to penetrate the tissue.

Autolytic debridement
This technique involves covering the wound bed with moisture-retentive dressings. Necrotic tissue is then removed through self-digestion by enzymes in the wound fluid. Although autolytic debridement takes longer than other debridement methods, it's appropriate for patients who can't tolerate any other method.

odor of any drainage and necrotic debris. Measure the wound perimeter with the disposable wound-measuring device (a square, transparent card with concentric circles arranged in bull's-eye fashion and bordered with a straight-edge ruler).

● Using the piston syringe, apply full force to irrigate the pressure ulcer to remove necrotic debris and help decrease bacteria in the wound.

● Remove and discard your soiled gloves and put on a fresh pair.

● Insert a gloved finger or a sterile cotton-tipped applicator into the wound to assess wound tunneling or undermining. Tunneling usually signals wound extension along fascial planes. Gauge tunnel depth by determining how far you can insert your finger.

● Next, reassess the condition of the skin and the ulcer. Note the character of the clean wound bed and the surrounding skin.

● If you observe adherent necrotic material, notify a wound care specialist or a doctor to ensure appropriate debridement (see *Understanding pressure ulcer debridement*).

● Prepare to apply the appropriate topical dressing. Directions for typical moist saline gauze, hydrocolloid, transparent, alginate, foam, and hydrogel dressings follow. For other dressings or topical agents, follow your facility's protocol or the manufacturer's instructions.

To apply a moist saline gauze dressing. Follow these steps.

● Irrigate the pressure ulcer with normal saline solution. Blot the surrounding skin dry.

● Moisten the gauze dressing with saline solution.

● Gently place the dressing over the surface of the ulcer. To separate surfaces within the wound, gently place a dressing between opposing wound surfaces.

Don't pack the gauze tightly to avoid damage to tissues.
- Change the dressing often enough to keep the wound moist.

To apply a hydrocolloid dressing. Follow these steps.
- Irrigate the pressure ulcer with normal saline solution. Blot the surrounding skin dry.
- Choose a clean, dry, presized dressing, or cut one to overlap the pressure ulcer by about 1" (2.5 cm). Remove the dressing from its package, pull the release paper from the adherent side of the dressing, and apply the dressing to the wound. To minimize irritation, carefully smooth out wrinkles as you apply the dressing.
- If the dressing's edges need to be secured with tape, apply a skin sealant to the intact skin around the ulcer. After the area dries, tape the dressing to the skin. The sealant protects the skin and promotes tape adherence. Avoid using tension or pressure when applying the tape.
- Remove your gloves and discard them in the impervious trash bag. Dispose of refuse according to your facility's policy and wash your hands.
- Change a hydrocolloid dressing every 2 to 7 days, as needed — for example, if the patient complains of pain, if the dressing no longer adheres, or if leakage occurs.

To apply a transparent dressing. Follow these steps.
- Irrigate the pressure ulcer with normal saline solution. Blot the surrounding skin dry.
- Select a dressing to overlap the ulcer by 2" (5 cm).
- Gently lay the dressing over the ulcer. To prevent shearing force, do not stretch the dressing. Press firmly on the edges of the dressing to promote adherence. Though these dressings are self-adhesive, you may have to tape the edges to prevent them from curling.
- Change the dressing every 3 to 7 days, depending on the amount of drainage.

To apply an alginate dressing. Follow these steps.
- Irrigate the pressure ulcer with normal saline solution. Blot the surrounding skin dry.

- Apply the alginate to the ulcer surface. Cover the area with a second dressing, such as gauze pads, as ordered. Secure the dressing with tape or elastic netting.
- If the wound is draining heavily, change the dressing once or twice daily for the first 3 to 5 days. As drainage decreases, change the dressing less frequently — every 2 to 4 days or as ordered. When the drainage stops or the wound bed looks dry, stop using the alginate dressing.

To apply a foam dressing. Follow these steps.
- Irrigate the pressure ulcer with normal saline solution. Blot the surrounding skin dry.
- Gently lay the foam dressing over the ulcer.
- Use tape, elastic netting, or gauze to hold the dressing in place.
- Change the dressing when the foam no longer absorbs the exudate.

To apply a hydrogel dressing. Follow these steps.
- Irrigate the pressure ulcer with normal saline solution. Blot the surrounding skin dry.
- Apply gel to the wound bed.
- Cover with a secondary dressing.
- Change the dressing daily or as often as needed to keep the wound bed moist.

Special considerations
Avoid using elbow and heel protectors that fasten with a single narrow strap because the strap could impair neurovascular function in the involved hand or foot. Also avoid using artificial sheepskin, which doesn't reduce pressure and may create a false sense of security.

Teach the caregiver how to change dressings if the patient is to be discharged home (see *Applying a dressing,* pages 391 and 392). Also teach measures to prevent further skin breakdown.

Complications
Infection may cause foul-smelling drainage, persistent pain, severe erythema, induration, and elevated skin and body temperatures. Advancing infection or cellulitis can lead to septicemia. Severe erythema may signal worsening cellulitis, which indicates that

EACHING AID

Applying a dressing

Dear Caregiver:

Follow this guide to cleaning, treating, and dressing a pressure ulcer (bed sore).

Assemble the equipment

Gather the equipment: sterile dressings (usually gauze pads or transparent adhesive dressings), scissors, hypoallergenic tape, cleaning solution (such as sterile normal saline solution), antibacterial ointment (if prescribed), a bowl in which to pour the cleaning solution, clean gloves, sterile gloves, and plastic disposable bags.

Have the new dressing ready before you take off the old one. Also cut strips of hypoallergenic tape in advance. Pour boiling water in the bowl to sterilize it, and discard the water. Then pour the cleaning solution into the bowl.

Position the person so you can reach the pressure ulcer easily.

Remove the old dressing

Remove all hand jewelry, wash your hands thoroughly, and put on clean gloves. Carefully remove the tape from the person's skin. If the skin under the tape is inflamed, don't apply the new tape there. Remove the old dressing, but don't touch any part of it that touched the ulcer. (If the dressing sticks, moisten it with sterile saline solution to help remove it.) Check the amount and color of any drainage on the dressing. Fold its edges together, place it in a disposable bag, and close the bag.

Check the ulcer

Inspect for signs of infection: swelling, redness, drainage, or pus. Is the ulcer healing?

Whether the ulcer appears to be infected, healing, or unchanged since the last dressing change, write down what you see; do this every time you change the dressing. *Do not touch the ulcer.*

Put on sterile gloves

Open the packages containing the sterile gauze pads or transparent dressings. Then remove the first pair of gloves, and wash your hands thoroughly before handling the sterile gloves.

Start with the glove for the hand you use most often. Grasp it by its cuff with your thumb and forefinger, and lift it from its wrapper. Be careful to touch only the inside of the glove (to keep the outside sterile). Now slip it on.

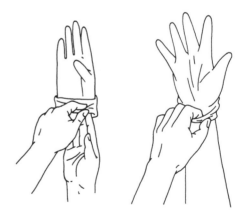

(continued)

Applying a dressing (continued)

Now pick up the second glove by slipping your gloved fingers under its cuff.

Pull on the second glove.

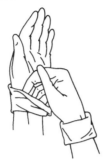

Clean the ulcer

Saturate a gauze pad with sterile saline solution. Now lightly clean both the ulcer and the area around it.

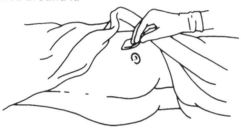

Saturate a second gauze pad in the sterile saline solution. Wring it out over the ulcer.

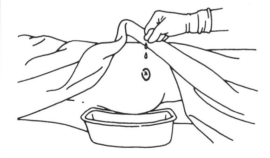

Use another gauze pad to gently blot dry the ulcer and the skin around it. Dispose of all pads in a disposable bag.

Put on the new dressing

If you're applying a *gauze dressing,* be careful not to touch any part of it that will touch the sore. If the doctor has ordered an antibacterial ointment, squeeze it onto the dressing before applying it. Tape around the edges of the dressing to keep it securely in place. If the person has sensitive skin, use a protective-barrier wipe or a skin preparation before applying the tape.

If you're applying a transparent adhesive dressing, remove part of the protective paper; then use your thumb to press the adhesive part of the dressing onto the skin near the ulcer. Peel the remaining paper off the dressing, and smooth it over the ulcer and surrounding skin.

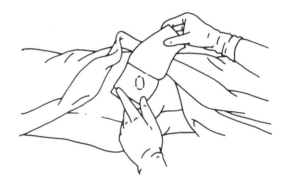

Press down on all four sides of the dressing to prevent leakage.

After you've finished applying the dressing, take off your gloves, throw them away in a disposable bag, seal the bag, and wash your hands thoroughly.

Additional instructions:

_____

_____

_____

the offending organisms have invaded the tissue and are no longer localized.

Documentation

Record the date and time of initial and subsequent treatments. Note the specific treatment given. Detail preventive strategies performed. Document the pressure ulcer's location and size (length, width, and depth); the color and appearance of the wound bed; the amount, odor, color, and consistency of drainage; and the condition of surrounding skin.

Update the care plan as required. Document any change in the condition or size of the pressure ulcer and any elevation of skin temperature. Also note when the doctor was notified of any pertinent abnormal observations. Record the patient's temperature daily on the graphic sheet to allow easy assessment of body temperature patterns.

Applying Unna's boot

Named for dermatologist Paul Gerson Unna, this bootlike dressing can be used to treat uninfected, nonnecrotic leg and foot ulcers that result from such conditions as venous insufficiency and stasis dermatitis, which are common in older people. A commercially prepared, medicated gauze compression dressing, Unna's boot wraps around the affected foot and leg. Alternatively, a preparation known as Unna's paste (gelatin, zinc oxide, calamine lotion, and glycerin) may be applied to the ulcer and covered with lightweight gauze. The boot's effectiveness results from compression applied by the bandage combined with moisture supplied by the paste. The boot is applied with greater pressure (compression) at the ankle and less at the knee.

Unna's boot is contraindicated for patients who are allergic to any ingredient used in the paste and for patients with arterial ulcers, weeping eczema, or cellulitis. Because the boot may affect the patient's balance and decrease his mobility, maintaining safety is crucial.

Equipment

Scrub sponge with ordered cleaning agent ■ normal saline solution ■ commercially prepared gauze bandage saturated with Unna's paste (or Unna's paste and lightweight gauze) ■ bandage scissors ■ gloves ■ elastic bandage to cover Unna's boot. Optional: extra gauze for excessive drainage.

Implementation

● Explain the procedure to the patient and provide privacy.
● Wash your hands and put on gloves.
● Assess the ulcer and the surrounding skin. Evaluate ulcer size, drainage, and appearance. Perform a neurovascular assessment of the affected foot to ensure adequate circulation. If you don't detect a pulse in the foot, check with the ordering doctor before applying Unna's boot.
● Clean the affected area gently with the sponge and cleaning agent to retard bacterial growth and to remove dirt and wound debris, which may create pressure points after you apply the bandage. Rinse with normal saline solution.
● Position the patient's leg in a slightly flexed position to ease application. Put on clean gloves.
● If a commercially prepared gauze bandage isn't available, spread Unna's paste evenly on the leg and foot. Then cover the leg and foot with the lightweight gauze. Apply three to four layers of paste interspersed with layers of gauze. (In a prepared bandage, the paste is impregnated into the bandage.)
● Apply gauze or the prepared bandage in a spiral motion, from just above the toes to the knee. Be sure to cover the heel. The wrap should be snug but not tight. To cover the area completely, make sure each turn overlaps the previous one by half the bandage width.
● Continue wrapping the patient's leg up to the knee, using firm, even pressure. Stop the dressing about 1" (2.5 cm) below the popliteal fossa to prevent irritation when the patient bends his knee. Mold the boot with your free hand as you apply the bandage to make it smooth and even.
● Cover the boot with an elastic bandage to provide external compression.
● Instruct the patient to remain in bed with his leg outstretched and elevated on a pillow until the paste dries (approximately 30 minutes). Observe the foot for cyanosis, loss of feeling, or swelling, any of

which indicates that the bandage is too tight and must be removed.

● Leave the boot on for 5 to 7 days or as ordered. Instruct the patient to walk on and handle the boot carefully to avoid damaging it. Tell him the boot will stiffen, but it won't be as hard as a cast.

● Change the boot weekly or as ordered to assess underlying skin and ulcer healing. Remove the boot by unwrapping the bandage from the knee back to the foot.

Special considerations

If the boot is applied over a swollen leg, it must be changed as edema subsides — if necessary, more often than every 5 days.

Don't make reverse turns while wrapping the bandage. This could create excessive pressure areas that may cause discomfort as the bandage hardens.

For bathing, instruct the patient to cover the boot with a plastic kitchen trash bag sealed at the knee with an elastic bandage to avoid wetting the boot. A wet boot softens and loses its effectiveness. If the patient's safety is a concern, instruct him to take a sponge bath.

Instruct the patient to call a nurse if he experiences increased swelling, pain, pallor, coldness, loss of function, or a change in color in the extremity. Remind him that the treatment takes a long time.

Complications

Contact dermatitis may result from hypersensitivity to Unna's paste.

Documentation

Record the date and time of application and the presence of a pulse in the affected foot. Specify which leg you bandaged. Describe the appearance of the older person's skin and ulcer before and after boot application. List the equipment used (commercially prepared bandage or Unna's paste and lightweight gauze). Describe any allergic reactions.

19

Controlling chronic pain

*P*ain is a complex phenomenon. It's a challenge to correctly diagnose and treat anyone whose chief complaint is pain; more so when the patient is older, frail, or in otherwise poor health. Pain assessment and management can be difficult in older patients because of cognitive impairment (including dementia), impaired communication, multiple medical diagnoses and pain problems, and increased sensitivity to adverse drug effects.

Older adults are at risk for undertreatment of pain. Paradoxically, pain is commonly assumed — by patients and caregivers alike — to be a normal part of aging, so appropriate pain management may not be viewed as an urgent geriatric care need. An older adult may be reluctant to complain of pain, fearing avoidance by a caregiver. In many instances, the primary caregiver for a person with chronic pain is an older spouse who is also burdened with chronic medical problems.

Ironically, many older adults undergo measures that are meant to prolong life, yet often fail to receive supportive care to improve the quality of life. We know that effective pain management can markedly improve the older person's functioning and quality of life and reduce the family members' caregiving burden as well. Yet older people have often been excluded from pain research and clinical service design.

Many pain problems can be successfully managed through more careful use of analgesic drugs combined with common nonpharmacologic strategies, including exercise programs and other physical therapies. Caregiver education, interdisciplinary staff involvement in pain management, and systematic, routine pain assessment of older patients can improve the success of pain management efforts.

Your efforts count

As a health care professional, you're responsible for assisting with or performing many pain-control measures. For example, in traditional pharmacologic and surgical treatments, you provide patient education, supply emotional support, and monitor therapeutic effects. In psychological pain-control techniques such as relaxation, you teach the patient how to perform the technique and help him overcome obstacles. Whatever the treatment, there's no substitute for your understanding of the patient's needs and condition. You can't feel your patient's pain, of course, but you can let him know that you recognize his suffering and will provide the best possible care.

UNDERSTANDING PAIN

Despite years of research, the exact mechanisms and routes that relay pain messages to the brain remain mysteries. In nursing, perhaps the most widely accepted and useful definition of pain is that proposed by Margo McCaffery (1979): "Pain is whatever the experiencing person says it is, existing whenever he

Comparing theories of pain

Because no one completely understands pain, theories abound. The four most significant ones are summarized below.

THEORY	DESCRIPTION
Specificity theory	● Single, specialized peripheral nerve fibers are responsible for pain transmission.
Pattern theory	● Excessive stimulation of all nerve endings produces a pattern interpreted by cerebral cortex as "pain."
Gate theory	● An anatomic gate regulates pain experience. ● Small-diameter nerve fibers conduct excitatory pain stimuli; large-diameter nerve fibers inhibit this transmission. ● The gate closes if too much information is sent through. ● Discovery of delta A and C fibers provided scientific basis for theory.
Affect theory	● Fear, anxiety, and other negative emotions exacerbate pain. ● Relief from these emotions eases it.

says it does." This is based on the concept that only the person who experiences the pain is a true authority on that pain. Therefore, caregivers must rely on a patient's descriptions of pain because only the patient can identify and describe this subjective symptom.

Theories of pain

Several theories have been proposed to explain pain and provide a basis for specific interventions. These include specificity, pattern, affect, and gate theories (see *Comparing theories of pain*).

Acute versus chronic pain

Pain is often classified as acute or chronic. Acute pain, usually caused by tissue damage from an injury or a disease, varies from mild to severe and lasts for a brief period (up to 6 months). Acute pain is considered a protective mechanism, warning of tissue damage or organ disease. Relief for acute pain is generally attainable; once the underlying problem is resolved, acute pain disappears. Therefore, treatment goals for acute pain include curing or healing the causative disease or injury. Palliative treatment

could include surgery, drug therapy, applications of heat or cold, or psychological techniques for controlling pain.

Chronic pain can stem from prolonged disease or dysfunction, as occurs in cancer or arthritis, or it can be associated with a mental disorder, such as posttraumatic stress syndrome. Chronic pain can be intermittent, limited, or persistent and usually lasts 6 months or longer. It's strongly colored by the patient's emotions and environment.

Chronic pain is further categorized as chronic nonmalignant pain (as with nonprogressive or healed tissue injury), chronic malignant pain (as with cancer or other progressive disorders), or chronic intractable pain (as with deterioration of an individual's coping ability).

Patients with chronic pain sometimes have difficulty describing it because it's not always localized. Health care professionals sometimes have difficulty assessing chronic pain because of the patient's unique way of responding to it. Every person's response to pain is unique. Some may cry our, some withdraw, others may moan and groan.

Treatment methods are meant to decrease or

eliminate chronic pain, maintain or improve the patient's ability to conduct daily activities, and reduce his need for medications. In mild chronic pain, treatment might simply involve ice massage and exercise. In severe chronic pain, though, a multidisciplinary program could be needed to address the physiologic, psychological, and social components of the patient's condition.

Pain and older people

Pain is usually initiated by sensory stimuli, then individualized by a person's memory, expectations, emotions, and behavior. The individual's perception of and psychological response to pain is complex. The widespread belief that aging brings decreased pain sensitivity or increased pain tolerance lacks scientific support, yet older people have been known to present with painless myocardial infarctions and intra-abdominal catastrophes. It's unclear whether these clinical observations result from deficient pain reporting or age-related changes in pain receptors, nerve transmission, or central nervous system (CNS) processing.

Incidence and causes of geriatric pain

Some studies indicate that 25% to 50% of community-dwelling older people suffer important pain problems, compared to 45% to 80% of nursing home residents. Most pain complaints from nursing home residents are due to arthritis and musculoskeletal problems, particularly degenerative arthritis and low back pain.

Cancer is also a source of severe pain in the older population. One-third to one-half of all cancer patients undergoing active treatment have pain, and among those with advanced disease, two-thirds have severe pain. Older patients also suffer disproportionately from painful peripheral vascular disease, herpes zoster, temporal arteritis, and polymyalgia rheumatica. Other common sources of pain in older people are leg cramps, headaches, and diabetic neuropathies.

Consequences of pain

Psychosocial and economic consequences of pain also strongly affect older people. Depression, de-

creased socialization, sleep disturbances, impaired ambulation, and increased health care needs and costs are all associated with pain. Deconditioning, gait disturbances, falls, slow rehabilitation, polypharmacy, cognitive dysfunction, and malnutrition are among the many geriatric problems that are exacerbated by pain. Pain is a complication that can disrupt treatment goals and diminish the quality of life for older people.

Assessing pain in older patients

Adequate pain assessment in older patients is a challenge. Multiple concurrent illnesses, underreporting of pain, and the prevalence of cognitive impairment make pain evaluation in older patients much more difficult than in younger adults. Moreover, the absence of diagnostic facilities in settings such as nursing homes often limits comprehensive pain evaluation.

An accurate assessment begins with asking about pain, believing the patient's responses, and taking pain complaints seriously (see *How to assess pain,* page 398). Begin the assessment of any pain complaint with a thorough history and physical examination. Because pain management often relies on the management of underlying disease, establishing a medical diagnosis cannot be overemphasized. For frail older patients, who are more likely to have occult fractures and other injuries, any history of trauma should be thoroughly evaluated.

Obtaining an accurate pain history from an older patient can entail special problems. Many older patients are afraid to report even severe pain that affects their mood and functional status. To obtain a more accurate history, consult other nursing staff members and family caregivers for additional observations and comments.

Approximately 3% to 15% of community-dwelling older people and 50% of nursing home residents have substantial cognitive impairment or dementia. Because of this, pain assessment instruments, such as visual analog scales, word descriptor scales, and numerical scales — while helpful among younger patients — have not been validated in older patients. Behavioral scales based on facial grimacing and posturing have been investigated in preverbal

How to assess pain

To assess pain properly, consider both the patient's descriptions and your own observations of his physical and behavioral responses. During your assessment, keep in mind the age-related changes in the older patient.

Start by asking the following series of key questions. Bear in mind that the older person's responses are shaped by his prior experiences, self-image, and beliefs about his condition. Allow him adequate time to process your questions and respond.
- Where is the pain located? How long does it last? How often does it occur?
- What does the pain feel like? (Have the patient describe it.)
- What relieves the pain or makes it worse?
- How do you usually get relief from it?

Ask the patient to rank his pain on a scale of 0 to 10, with 0 denoting lack of pain and 10 denoting the worst pain level. This helps the patient verbally evaluate pain therapies.

Observe the patient's behavioral and physiologic responses to pain. Physiologic responses may be sympathetic or parasympathetic.

Behavioral responses
These include altered body position, moaning, sighing, grimacing, withdrawal, crying, restlessness, muscle twitching, and immobility.

Sympathetic responses
These are commonly associated with mild to moderate pain and include pallor, elevated blood pressure, dilated pupils, skeletal muscle tension, dyspnea, tachycardia, and diaphoresis.

Parasympathetic responses
These are commonly associated with severe, deep pain and include pallor, decreased blood pressure, bradycardia, nausea and vomiting, weakness, dizziness, and loss of consciousness.

children but are not well established for clinical use in older patients who can't provide a verbal report of pain. However, ongoing research indicates that most patients with mild to moderate cognitive impairment can report pain intensity.

Psychological evaluation

Astute questioning and a comprehensive evaluation are vital to an accurate psychological evaluation. Most patients with chronic pain have substantial anxiety or depressive symptoms at some time and could benefit dramatically from psychological or psychiatric intervention. However, their pain might not result solely from depression or psychogenic causes. On the other hand, avoid attributing pain only to preexisting illness. Also, take care not to overlook pain that's associated with trauma or an acute disease. And remember, chronic pain is usually not constant; both the character and intensity of chronic pain fluctuate with time.

Physical findings and functional status

During the physical assessment of your patient, focus on the musculoskeletal and nervous system and palpate for trigger points and inflammation. Trigger points can result from tendinitis, muscle strain, or nerve irritation (any of which may improve through local injections of steroids or local anesthetics or through specific physical therapy). Maneuvers that reproduce the pain, such as straight leg raising and joint motion, can be useful in both the diagnosis and functional assessment of pain. Also perform a thorough neurologic examination to elicit signs of autonomic, sensory, and motor deficits that suggest neuropathic conditions and nerve injuries that might require specific treatments.

Evaluating the older patient's functional status provides an outcome measure for pain management so that mobility and independence can be maximized. A functional assessment could include information from the patient's history and physical examination and employ a functional assessment scale.

Scales frequently used in routine geriatric evaluation include the Katz Activities of Daily Living Scale and the Lawton Scale for Instrumental Activities of Daily Living. These scales are useful for predicting dependency needs, overall survival, and the need for alternative care.

State-of-the-art diagnostic procedures and expertise may be difficult to obtain for frail older patients. Laboratories and other diagnostic facilities are often not readily available to patients confined to home care or nursing homes. Many doctors and consultants don't make house calls or visit nursing homes or are unable to spend the time needed to assess and develop treatment plans for the complex problems of patients in these settings. Doctors tending cases in these settings often send patients to emergency rooms or distant facilities for examinations and procedures.

For some patients, short hospitalizations may be appropriate for risky or highly technical procedures related to severe pain problems; also, hospitalization may be necessary because some home care agencies and nursing homes are not equipped to manage acute illnesses. In other patients, however, transportation to other facilities can be physically exhausting and emotionally disruptive, increasing the risk of iatrogenic illness.

NURSING CARE MEASURES

Nurses play a key role in assessing and managing their patients' pain. Various strategies and interventions can be used, including pharmacologic measures; nonpharmacologic measures such as heat and cold therapy, transcutaneous electrical nerve stimulation (TENS), distraction, and imagery; and complementary therapies, including herbal remedies, aromatherapy, Swedish massage, acupuncture, therapeutic touch, biofeedback, and hypnosis.

Nurses also play a key role in educating patients and members of their families about pain and its management. When managing an older patient's pain, you can use certain principles to guide your

nursing care (see *Principles of pain management in older adults,* page 400).

Patient teaching

Increasingly, chronic pain — including the pain associated with cancer — is managed in a person's home on an outpatient basis. A structured pain education program includes three components: basic pain management principles and assessment, pharmacologic interventions, and nondrug treatments. Such a program begins with the patient's ongoing assessment of his pain — in a pain management log, for example. Through this type of program, you can improve your patient's understanding of the causes and effects of pain, elicit a more positive attitude about his ability to self-manage pain, and promote an understanding of how to use both drug and nondrug interventions to control pain.

Pharmacologic treatments

The control of most acute and postoperative pain begins with the diagnosis and treatment of the underlying condition and short-term administration of analgesic drugs. Chronic pain, on the other hand, often requires a multidimensional approach using a combination of nonpharmacologic interventions as well as analgesic and adjuvant drug therapies. Patients with malignant pain usually respond well to constant administration of opiate analgesics. However, long-term use of narcotic analgesics for chronic nonmalignant pain is controversial.

Neuropathic pain, such as herpes zoster and poststroke thalamic pain, may respond initially to traditional analgesic drugs but in the long run could require other adjuvant drugs, such as tricyclic antidepressants, anticonvulsants, or antiarrhythmics. In general, some combination of both pharmacologic and nonpharmacologic techniques provide more effective pain control with less reliance on drugs that have major adverse effects in older people.

The traditional approach to pain management is to use oral analgesics. Analgesic drugs are usually considered in two major categories: nonsteroidal anti-inflammatory drugs (NSAIDs) and opiate analgesic drugs. Acetaminophen has analgesic and antipyretic properties, but it exerts little anti-

Principles of pain management in older adults

Pain management involves the careful use of both pharmacologic and nonpharmacologic strategies. Use the following general principles as a guide when providing pain relief to older patients:

- Always ask the older person about pain. Many older people expect to have pain and don't want to complain.
- Accept the patient's report of the presence of pain and its intensity.
- Remember that pain is not normal with aging.
- Don't underestimate the impact of pain on quality of life in older people.
- Determine the underlying cause of the pain. Optimal treatment depends on an accurate diagnosis.
- Treat pain before starting diagnostic procedures. Unrelieved pain reduces the patient's tolerance for diagnostic tests.
- Use a combination of drug and nondrug interventions.
- Involve the patient in pain assessment and management.

- Remember that physical and psychosocial mobility (the ability to meet needs through socialization and other comfort measures) are important in treatment.
- Use analgesic drugs appropriately. Start with low doses and increase them gradually for older patients, as ordered.
- Ensure that the patient is receiving adequate doses of analgesics.
- Anticipate and treat adverse effects prophylactically.
- Treat anxiety and depression as common symptoms that influence pain in older patients.
- Evaluate the patient's response to treatment regularly.
- Address older patients' fears of addiction, tolerance, and respiratory depression.
- Involve family caregivers in the treatment plan.

inflammatory activity and has a site of action that differs from that of most NSAIDs. A variety of other drugs, such as tricyclic antidepressants and anticonvulsants, are useful for such specific pain problems as trigeminal neuralgia, herpes zoster neuralgia, and diabetic neuralgia. These drugs are called adjuvant analgesics because they have no inherent analgesic properties of their own; only partially effective when used alone, they're most effective as adjuncts to other pharmacologic or nonpharmacologic pain management strategies.

Pain management with NSAIDs

NSAIDs act primarily on the patient's peripheral nervous system, affecting pain receptors, nerve conduction, and inflammatory conditions that could stimulate pain. Individual drugs in this class vary widely in their analgesic properties, metabolism, excretion, and adverse effect profiles (see *Using NSAIDs in older adults*).

The analgesic activity of NSAIDs is limited by a low ceiling effect; they provide a certain level of analgesia at a given dosage, but increasing the drug dosage does not provide additional pain relief. NSAIDs often work well given alone or in combination with opiate analgesics for metastatic bone pain and inflammatory conditions. However, NSAIDs often cause a variety of adverse reactions in older patients, including peptic ulcer disease, renal insufficiency, and bleeding diathesis. Among frail older patients, they can cause constipation, cognitive impairment, and headaches.

Pain management with opiates

Opiate analgesics act primarily on the CNS (brain and spinal cord) to decrease the perception of pain. Some of these drugs (including morphine) also act as local anesthetics and have recently found widespread use in epidural administration.

Morphine and other opiates are also given by external and implantable infusion pumps that can supply continuous or intermittent infusions through subcutaneous (S.C.), I.V., or intraspinal routes. Some pumps are fully programmable; this feature —

Using NSAIDs in older adults

The chart below shows advantages and disadvantages that may accompany use of nonsteroidal anti-inflammatory drugs (NSAIDs).

DRUG	POTENTIAL ADVANTAGE	POTENTIAL PROBLEMS	POTENTIAL SOLUTIONS
Aspirin	Standard by which others are compared	Gastric bleeding; abnormal platelet function	Avoid high dose for prolonged periods of time.*
Acetaminophen	Analgesia similar to aspirin; no gastric or platelet toxicity	Hepatotoxic at high dose; little anti-inflammatory activity	Keep dose to < 4 g/24 hr.
Diflunisal (Dolobid)	May provide better analgesia than aspirin	Weak anti-inflammatory activity; adverse effects similar to other NSAIDs; requires loading dose	Requires continuous dosing for maximum effectiveness.
Ibuprofen (Motrin)	May be superior to aspirin	Gastric, renal, and platelet toxicity possibly dose- and time-dependent; constipation, confusion and headaches possibly more common in older patients	Avoid high dose for prolonged periods of time.*
Naproxen (Naprosyn)	Similar to ibuprofen	May require a loading dose; toxicity similar to ibuprofen	Avoid high dose for prolonged periods of time.*
Sulindac (Clinoril)	Similar to ibuprofen	Toxicity similar to ibuprofen	Avoid high dose for prolonged periods of time.*
Salsalate (Disalcid)	Perhaps less gastric toxicity	Prolonged half-life of 8 to 12 hr; toxicity similar to ibuprofen; high dose may cause classic salicylate toxicity	Monitoring of salicylate levels may be occasionally necessary to avoid toxicity.*
Trisalicylate (Trilisate)	Lowest adverse effect profile for gastric, renal, and platelet activity; prolonged half-life (12 to 24 hr)	May provide less analgesic and anti-inflammatory activity	Avoid drug accumulation with q 24 hr dosing.
Indomethacin (Indocin)	More anti-inflammatory activity	Highest incidence of gastric and other toxicities	Avoid entirely in older patients, or keep to minimum doses for very short periods of time.*
Ketorolac (Toradol)	The only NSAID approved for parenteral use	Adverse effects similar to other NSAIDs, including gastric and renal toxicity as well as anti-platelet activity	Avoid prolonged use (longer than 2 weeks).*

* Concomitant use of misoprostol (Cytotec) may at least partially prevent gastric toxicity.

Adapted with permission from Ferrell, B.A. "Pain," in *Ambulatory Geriatric Care*. Edited by Yoshikawa, T.T., et al. St. Louis: Mosby–Year Book, Inc., 1993.

patient-controlled analgesia (PCA) — allows patients to titrate medication. With appropriate supervision and patient education, this technology is feasible for selected patients. PCA using morphine infusions is safe and effective for postoperative pain management among selected older patients. However, continuous morphine infusions are expensive and can cost several thousand dollars a month. For more information about PCA and epidural analgesia, see the procedures later in this chapter.

Unlike NSAIDs, opiate drugs have no ceiling to their effects and relieve multiple types of pain. Advanced age is associated with a prolonged drug half-life and enhanced sensitivity for opiate drugs. Thus, older patients may achieve pain relief from smaller doses of opiate drugs than younger patients.

◆◆ —— CLINICAL ALERT —— ◆◆

Opiate drugs are more likely to cause cognitive disturbances, constipation, and respiratory depression among older people. Clinical experience suggests that opiates (like other psychoactive drugs) can also produce paradoxical excitement and agitation more commonly in older patients than in younger patients.

Morphine remains the standard by which all other opiate drugs are compared because its effects are the best understood and most predictable. Thus, morphine is the opiate of choice for severe pain in older people. Among patients taking morphine for both malignant and nonmalignant disease, drug tolerance is usually related to worsening disease, drug addiction is exceedingly rare, and when drug dependency does occur, it's easy to manage. This does not imply that morphine and other opiates can be used indiscriminately; only that dependency and other adverse effects do not justify withholding effective therapy from most older patients.

Tolerance to some of the adverse effects of opiate drugs does occur. This results in reduced manifestation of adverse effects following frequent exposure to a drug. This could reduce the risk for respiratory depression and drowsiness. Thus, opiates as well as other analgesic drugs should be administered on a continuous basis (around-the-clock as opposed to as-needed [p.r.n.]) whenever possible; this policy

results in reduced overall drug consumption, continuous analgesia, and improved tolerance to drowsiness and respiratory depression.

On the other hand, some adverse effects of opiates, such as constipation and perhaps nausea, do not diminish with time. Because these adverse effects make overall pain management more difficult, it's important to begin a bowel protocol when opiates are first started; provide increased fluids, bulk agents, lubricating agents, and bowel stimulants.

Nausea results from direct stimulation of a chemoreceptor trigger zone in the brain. Antiemetic drugs, such as antihistamines, phenothiazine, and others, are the mainstay for preventing opioid-related nausea and vomiting. But older patients are especially sensitive to the anticholinergic effects of these drugs, including bowel or bladder dysfunction, delirium, and movement disorders.

Precautions for opiate use. A variety of opiate drugs are available. They differ widely in analgesic potency and adverse effects among older patients (see *Using opiate analgesic drugs in older adults*). And, because of particular problems in older persons, certain opioid drugs should be avoided altogether in the elderly (see *Analgesics to avoid in older adults,* page 404).

Pain management with adjuvant analgesics
Adjuvant analgesic drugs may be helpful for some types of recalcitrant pain syndromes. These drugs are usually only partially successful and work best when used with opiates and other pharmacologic and nonpharmacologic pain management strategies. Tricyclic antidepressants, such as amitriptyline (Elavil, Enovil), may be helpful in the management of diabetic neuralgia and other neuropathic pain syndromes. Recently, desipramine (a tricyclic antidepressant from a different chemical class) was found to be as effective as amitriptyline for the management of diabetic neuralgia, thus offering an alternative for patients unable to tolerate the strong adverse effects of amitriptyline. And one study showed that fluoxetine (Prozac, a bicyclic antidepressant) was no more effective than a placebo.

As early as 1942, studies found that the anticon-

Using opiate analgesic drugs in older adults

The chart below shows advantages and disadvantages that may accompany use of opiate analgesics.

DRUG	POTENTIAL ADVANTAGE	POTENTIAL PROBLEMS	POTENTIAL SOLUTIONS
Morphine sulfate	Standard by which others are compared; opioid of choice for severe pain	Short half-life; older people more sensitive to adverse effects than younger people	Start low and titrate to comfort. Give continuously (q 3-4 hr); avoid "p.r.n." use. Anticipate and prevent opioid adverse effects.
Sustained-release morphine (MS Contin)	Appears to be well tolerated in majority of older people; no ceiling dose	Potential for drug accumulation; potency and toxicity similar to plain morphine sulfate; requires short-acting drugs for break-through pain	Use q 12 h doses (q 8 h rarely required); escalate dose slowly to avoid accumulation (daily or every other day).
Codeine, including combinations (Tylenol #3; Empirin #3)	Weak opioid for mild to moderate pain	Nonsteroidal anti-inflammatory drug (NSAID) or acetaminophen combinations limit maximum dose; constipation a major issue	Avoid high doses; anticipate and prevent NSAID adverse effects; begin bowel program early.
Oxycodone (Percodan [oxycodone/aspirin]; Tylox [oxycodone/acetaminophen])	More potent than plain codeine; adverse effect profile may be milder than codeine or other codeine derivatives	NSAID or acetaminophen combinations limit maximum dose	Now available uncompounded (Roxicodone); anticipate and prevent NSAID adverse effects; begin bowel program early.
Hydrocodone (Vicodin [hydrocodone/acetaminophen]; Lortab [hydrocodone/aspirin])	Potency similar to oxycodone	NSAID or acetaminophen combinations limit maximum dose; toxicity similar to codeine	Avoid high doses; anticipate and prevent NSAID adverse effects; begin bowel program early.
Hydromorphone (Dilaudid)	More potent than morphine	Short half-life (3 to 4 hr); toxicity similar to morphine	Similar to morphine; start low and titrate to comfort; give continuously (q 3–4 hr); avoid "p.r.n." use. Anticipate and prevent adverse effects.

Adapted with permission from Ferrell, B.A. "Pain," in *Ambulatory Geriatric Care,* Edited by Yoshikawa, T.T., et al. St. Louis: Mosby–Year Book, Inc., 1993.

vulsant drug phenytoin (Dilantin) could relieve the pain of trigeminal neuralgia. Diabetic neuralgia and other neuropathies have since been found to respond occasionally to other anticonvulsant drugs, including carbamazepine, valproate sodium, and clonazepam.

Intravenously administered local anesthetics, such as lidocaine and procaine, also possess anticonvulsant effects and have analgesic effects independent of nerve conduction blockade. Both oral tocainide and mexiletine (lidocaine analogs used as antiarrhythmics) are effective in trigeminal neuralgia and

Analgesics to avoid in older adults

The following analgesics have proven particularly dangerous for older adults.

DRUG	PRECAUTIONS	POTENTIAL SOLUTIONS
Meperidine (Demerol)	Extremely low oral potency and short duration of analgesia compared to morphine; metabolite normeperidine may accumulate and cause confusion, agitation, and seizure activity, especially among patients with renal impairment or those receiving MAO inhibitors	Choose a drug with higher oral potency. There are no advantages of either oral or parenteral meperidine over other opiates.
Pentazocine (Talwin)	Mixed opiate agonist-antagonist activity often leads to CNS excitement, agitation, confusion, and delirium in older patients	Avoid all use in frail older patients.
Propoxyphene (Darvon)	Controversial and probably overprescribed in older people; potency no better than aspirin or acetaminophen; significant potential for dependency and renal injury	Choose an NSAID, acetaminophen, or a more effective opiate.
Methadone (Dolophine)	Plasma half-life extremely prolonged in older people; analgesic effect relatively short	Sustained-release morphine appears to be a better alternative.
Transdermal fentanyl (Duragesic)	Extremely potent (perhaps 50 times as potent as morphine) with high potential for complications; tissue reservoir results in prolonged half-life (36 hr); may be expensive when high dosage is required	Avoid use in patients unfamiliar with opiates and in those unaccustomed to the respiratory depression of opioid drugs.

Adapted with permission from Ferrell, B.A. "Pain," in *Ambulatory Geriatric Care.* Edited by Yoshikawa, T.T., et al. St. Louis: Mosby–Year Book, Inc., 1993.

diabetic neuralgia. Although these drugs have serious adverse effect profiles, the dosage for mexiletine as an analgesic may be one-half the dosage traditionally used for cardiac indications. Thus, various adjuvant drugs can be useful for neuropathic pain syndromes that don't respond to other forms of therapy.

Capsaicin may be useful as a topical anesthetic for herpes zoster neuralgia, diabetic neuropathy, and postsurgical neuropathies. Although now available without a prescription, its overall efficacy for arthritis and other painful syndromes is controversial. A burning sensation normally caused by the drug is intolerable to some patients.

Guidelines for geriatric analgesia

Pain management for a frail older person is based on a plan of care that is reasonable for the available resources and skills. Use the following to guide your care:

● Administer short-acting analgesics for breakthrough pain or pain associated with physical therapy, bathing, or other potentially painful activities.

● When possible, simplify medication regimens.

● Anticipate using long-acting analgesics to provide a longer duration of comfort and simpler administration schedules.

● Prevent pain by administering routine analgesia and avoiding p.r.n. medications when possible.

● Simplify treatments so that nighttime monitoring requirements are minimized.

● Remember that pharmacy and formulary restrictions can delay obtaining prescriptions. Develop contingency plans for pain management so that delays don't occur during medication changes or dosage adjustments.

● Regulations governing prescriptions for analgesic medications (such as requirements for triplicate prescriptions and limited refills) might pose obstacles to effective pain management. Careful planning is the only solution.

Nonpharmacologic treatments

Physical treatments for pain include application of heat and cold, and massage. These measures relax tense muscles and are soothing for a variety of complaints. Some of these techniques can be performed by the patient, who thus obtains a sense of personal control over his symptoms and treatment. However, heat or cold treatments should be used cautiously in patients with cognitive impairment to avoid burns. (For additional information about applying heat and cold, see Chapter 18.)

Physical therapy to stretch and strengthen specific muscles and joints and maintenance exercise programs are available in most nursing homes. These improve muscle strength, reduce muscle spasms, and improve functional activity. Consultation and therapy by a skilled therapist (available in many nursing homes) is appropriate for many painful conditions.

Transcutaneous electrical nerve stimulation

Transcutaneous electrical nerve stimulation (TENS) therapy is successful for a variety of chronic pain conditions in older patients. Painful diabetic neuropathies, shoulder pain or bursitis, and fractured ribs respond to TENS therapy. Although some patients' pain has been relieved for years, the effectiveness of TENS usually diminishes with time and strong placebo effects have been associated with its use.

The success of TENS therapy depends on the appropriate placement of the electrodes and current adjustment. This involves meticulous searching, with the help of a trained physical therapist, to discover the best settings for an individual patient's optimum comfort. Also, care must be taken to prevent skin irritation and possible burns from the electrodes. (For more information, see the procedure later in this chapter.)

Complementary therapies

Complementary pain therapies (also called alternative medicine) are gaining popularity with both patients and health care professionals in the United States. Many people today are concerned with the overuse of drugs and surgery for conventional pain management and are unwilling to accept a painful condition when conventional therapy fails. Americans are turning toward more self-management of their health problems.

Nonprescription herbal and homeopathic remedies, once limited to health food stores, are now on the shelves of ordinary pharmacies and grocery stores. Many publications give lay people and health care professionals alike clear, concise, practical information on effective, medically sound alternative techniques for relief of chronic pain. Consumer organizations, such as the People's Medical Society, make medical information accessible so that people can make informed decisions about health care.

Complementary therapies are best administered, prescribed, or taught by licensed practitioners or experienced, credentialed lay people. Also, some of these therapies may require some adaptation before use with older patients.

Examples of complementary therapies include:
● nutritional therapy
● herbal remedies
● aromatherapy
● homeopathic remedies
● body manipulation
● massage
● trigger point therapy
● acupuncture
● acupressure
● therapeutic touch
● yoga
● mental and spiritual therapies, such as centering, relaxation, meditation, prayer, affirmation, and music
● hypnosis
● biofeedback.

Some psychological maneuvers can be effective in

controlling pain, just as biofeedback and relaxation can be helpful for some patients. However, these methods usually require high levels of cognitive function and therefore might not lend themselves to treating patients with significant impairment. A trained psychologist or therapist should be consulted for these techniques.

Finally, a variety of distractive techniques can decrease a person's perception of pain. Encourage your patient's involvement in activities, exercise, and recreation; inactivity and immobility can contribute extensively to depression and worsen pain.

PERFORMING BASIC CARE PROCEDURES

Managing a patient's pain

When a person feels severe pain, he often seeks medical help not only because he wants relief, but also because he believes the pain signals a serious problem. This perception produces anxiety, which in turn increases the patient's pain. To assess and manage pain properly, the nurse must depend on the patient's subjective description in addition to objective tools.

Many interventions are used successfully to manage pain. These may include pharmacologic measures, emotional support, comfort measures, and cognitive techniques to distract the patient. Severe pain usually requires an opiate analgesic. Invasive measures, such as PCA or epidural analgesia, may also be required (see procedures later on in this chapter).

When selecting interventions to help patients manage their pain, consider the following:

● Choose pharmacologic interventions that suit the patient's level of pain.

● Anticipate adverse effects from drug use, especially with an older patient, and treat them aggressively.

● Provide timely and thorough assessments of the patient's status to determine the optimal approach to achieving comfort.

● Acknowledge and address the impact of psychosocial variables on the perception of pain and its meaning.

● Use a multidisciplinary approach to manage the patient's pain.

● Communicate a sense of empathy and caring to the patient in pain.

Equipment

Patient's medication record and chart ■ Pain assessment tool or scale ■ oral hygiene supplies ■ water ■ nonnarcotic analgesic (such as aspirin or acetaminophen). Optional: PCA device, mild narcotic (such as oxycodone or codeine), strong narcotic (such as methadone, levorphanol, morphine, or hydromorphone).

Implementation

● Explain to the patient how pain medications work together with other pain management therapies to provide relief. Also explain that management aims to keep pain at the lowest acceptable level to permit optimal bodily function.

● Assess the patient's pain by asking key questions and noting his response to the pain. For instance, ask him to describe the duration, severity, and source of his pain. Look for physiologic or behavioral clues to the pain's severity. Tailor your questions to the patient's cognitive level, and allow sufficient time for the older patient to respond.

● Develop nursing diagnoses. Appropriate nursing diagnoses include pain, anxiety, activity intolerance, fear, risk for injury, knowledge deficit, powerlessness, and self-care deficit.

● Work with the patient and family to develop a care plan, choosing interventions appropriate to the patient's lifestyle. These may include prescription and nonprescription medications, emotional support, comfort measures, cognitive techniques, and education about pain and its management.

● Emphasize the importance of maintaining good bowel habits, respiratory function, and mobility because pain can exacerbate problems in these areas.

● Implement your care plan. Remember: Individuals respond to pain differently, so what works for one person might not work for another.

Give medications. Follow these steps.
● Administer medications orally whenever possible. Check the appropriate drug information for each medication you administer.
● Begin with a nonnarcotic analgesic, such as acetaminophen or aspirin, every 4 to 6 hours as ordered.
● If the patient needs more relief than a nonnarcotic analgesic provides, administer a mild narcotic (such as oxycodone or codeine) as ordered.
● If the patient needs still more pain relief, administer a stronger narcotic (such as morphine or hydromorphone) as prescribed.
● Administer the medication 30 minutes before any activity or procedure to ensure effectiveness.
● Monitor closely for adverse effects because of age-related changes affecting the pharmacokinetics and pharmacodynamics of the drug.
● If ordered, teach the patient to use a PCA device. Such a device can help the patient manage his pain and decrease his anxiety.

Provide emotional support. Follow these steps.
● Show your concern by spending time talking with the patient. Because of the pain and the patient's inability to manage it, he may be anxious and frustrated. Such feelings worsen the pain.
● Make sure that the patient understands the medication regimen.

Perform comfort measures. Follow these steps.
● Reposition the patient every 2 hours to reduce muscle spasms and tension and to relieve pressure on bony prominences. Use pillows and supports to provide support and cushioning. Sometimes, elevating the head of the bed helps. For example, it can reduce the pull on an abdominal incision, diminishing pain. If appropriate, elevate a limb to reduce swelling, inflammation, and pain.
● Give the patient a back massage to help relax tense muscles. Use lotion or emollients to lubricate the older patient's dry skin.
● Perform passive range-of-motion exercises to prevent stiffness and further loss of mobility, relax tense muscles, and provide comfort.
● Provide oral hygiene. Keep a fresh water glass or cup at the bedside. Offer your patient a favorite beverage, such as apple juice, because many medications tend to dry the mouth.
● Wash the patient's face and hands.

Use cognitive therapy. Follow these steps.
● Help the patient enhance the effect of analgesics by using such techniques as distraction, guided imagery, deep breathing, and relaxation. You can easily use these "mind-over-pain" techniques at the bedside. Choose whichever method the patient feels most comfortable with. If possible, start these techniques when the patient feels little or no pain. If pain persists, begin with short, simple exercises. Before beginning, dim the lights, remove the patient's restrictive clothing, and eliminate noise from the environment.
● When using distraction, have the patient recall an interesting or pleasant experience or focus his attention on an enjoyable activity. For instance, have him use music as a distraction by turning on the radio when the pain begins. Have him close his eyes and concentrate on listening, raising or lowering the volume as his pain increases or subsides. Note, however, that distraction is usually effective only against brief pain episodes lasting less than 5 minutes and that the effects last only as long as the distraction activity.
● When using guided imagery, help the patient concentrate on a peaceful, pleasant image. Encourage him to concentrate on the details of the image he's selected by asking about its sight, sound, smell, taste, and touch. The positive emotions evoked by this exercise minimize pain.
● When using deep breathing, have the patient stare at an object, then slowly inhale and exhale as he counts aloud to maintain a comfortable rate and rhythm. Have him concentrate on the rise and fall of his abdomen. Encourage him to feel more and more weightless with each breath while he concentrates on the rhythm of his breathing or on any restful image.
● When using muscle relaxation, have the patient focus on a particular muscle group. Then ask him to tense the muscles and note the sensation. After 5 to 7 seconds, tell him to relax the muscles and concentrate on the relaxed state. Have him note the differ-

ence between the tense and relaxed states. After he tenses and relaxes one muscle group, have him proceed to another and another until he's included his entire body.

• Provide the patient with instructions for performing these techniques at home (see the teaching handout, *Relieving your pain with relaxation techniques,* pages 409 and 410).

Special considerations

Evaluate your patient's response to pain management. If he's still in pain, reassess him and alter your care plan as appropriate. Use the pain management techniques that work best for the patient.

Remind the patient that results of cognitive therapy techniques improve with practice. Help the patient through the initial sessions. Monitor him closely for changes in level of consciousness, and institute safety measures to reduce the risk of injury.

During periods of intense pain, the patient's ability to concentrate diminishes. If your patient experiences such pain, help him to select a cognitive technique that's simple to use. Once he selects a technique, encourage him to use it consistently.

Complications

The most common adverse effects of analgesics include respiratory depression (the most serious), sedation, constipation, nausea, and vomiting. Monitor the patient closely.

Documentation

Document each step of the nursing process. Describe the subjective information you elicited from the patient, using his own words. Note the location, quality, and duration of the pain and any precipitating factors.

Record your nursing diagnoses, and include the pain relief method selected. Summarize your actions and the patient's response. If the patient's pain was not relieved, note alternative treatments to consider the next time pain occurs. Also record any complications of drug therapy.

Using TENS

TENS therapy is based on the gate theory of pain,

which proposes that painful impulses pass through a "gate" in the brain when they've reached a critical threshold. A portable, battery-powered TENS device transmits painless electrical current to peripheral nerves or directly to a painful area over relatively large nerve fibers. This treatment effectively alters the patient's perception of pain by blocking painful stimuli traveling over smaller fibers. Used for patients after surgery and those with chronic pain, TENS therapy reduces the need for analgesic drugs and may allow the patient to resume normal activities. (See *Positioning TENS electrodes,* page 411.)

Typically, a course of TENS treatments lasts 3 to 5 days. Some conditions, such as phantom limb pain, require continuous stimulation; other conditions, such as a painful arthritic joint, require shorter periods (3 to 4 hours).

TENS is contraindicated for patients with cardiac pacemakers because it can interfere with pacemaker function. It's also contraindicated in patients who are senile. TENS should be used cautiously in all patients with cardiac disorders. TENS electrodes should not be placed on the head or neck of patients with vascular disorders or seizure disorders.

Equipment

TENS device ■ alcohol sponges ■ electrodes ■ electrode gel ■ warm water and soap ■ lead wires ■ charged battery pack ■ battery recharger ■ adhesive patch or hypoallergenic tape.

Commercial TENS kits are available. They include the stimulator, lead wires, electrodes, spare battery pack, battery recharger, and sometimes the adhesive patch.

Before beginning the procedure, always test the battery pack to make sure it's fully charged.

Implementation

• Wash your hands. Provide privacy. If the patient has never seen a TENS unit before, show him the device and explain the procedure.

• With an alcohol sponge, thoroughly clean the skin where the electrode will be applied. Then dry the skin using a patting motion.

• Apply electrode gel to the bottom of each electrode.

Relieving your pain with relaxation techniques

Dear Patient:

Try each of these nondrug pain-relief techniques below and see which work for you.

Using distraction techniques
Use the following techniques to help distract you from your pain.

Listening to recordings
Get a tape recorder with headphones and cassettes of your favorite music, comedy routines, or stories. Then sit or lie down in a comfortable position, with legs and arms uncrossed and relaxed, while you listen to the cassette through the headphones. Close your eyes and concentrate on the recording or stare at a nearby object.

To make this technique more effective, try any of these ideas:
● Imagine yourself floating or drifting with the music. Or focus on a pleasant scene or on images suggested by the music. When listening to a story, try to imagine every detail the storyteller describes.
● Keep time with the music by slapping your thigh, tapping a finger or foot, or nodding your head.
● Keep your finger on the recorder's volume control. If the pain gets worse, turn up the volume; when it subsides, lower the volume.

Singing
Select a song you like. Then mouth the words while you sing it in your mind or aloud. Concentrate all your attention on the song's words and rhythm. (Closing your eyes may help). Sing faster or louder when the pain gets worse; sing slower when the pain diminishes.

Rhythmic breathing
Stare at an object or a person while you inhale slowly and deeply. Then exhale slowly. Continue breathing slowly (but not too deeply) while you count silently "In, 2, 3, 4; out, 2, 3, 4."

While performing this exercise, concentrate on how the breathing feels. You may want to close your eyes and imagine the air moving slowly in and out of your lungs. Continue to count silently to keep breathing comfortable and rhythmic. If you begin to feel breathless, breathe slower or take a deep breath.

If rhythmic breathing alone doesn't distract you enough to relieve pain, try lightly massaging the painful area with a stroking motion as you breathe or, if your condition permits, raising your arm as you inhale and lowering it as you exhale. Or try inhaling through your nose and exhaling through your mouth.

Using progressive muscle relaxation
This technique helps to relieve the muscle tension that accompanies pain. By learning to tense and relax your muscles one by one, you'll find that you can relax your entire body.
● Get comfortable and close your eyes. Now tense your forehead and face, and hold this tension for 5 to 10 seconds.
● Next, relax your forehead and face. Hold and enjoy this relaxation for 10 to 15 seconds.
● Now proceed downward toward your feet. First, tense and relax your jaw muscles. Pro-

(continued)

*T*EACHING AID

Relieving your pain with relaxation techniques (continued)

ceed to the muscles in each shoulder, arm, and hand; then to your stomach and buttocks; and, finally, to each thigh, lower leg, ankle, and foot.

If you have trouble relaxing some muscle or if the tension causes pain, gently massage that body part until the muscles feel comfortable.

● To complete the exercise, open your eyes, stretch, and then relax your entire body. Take a few deep breaths. Don't engage in any activity until you're alert.

Using breathing relaxation exercises

You can use these special breathing techniques anywhere and at any time. You can also combine them with other techniques to help control pain. Try to practice them daily.

● Close your eyes. Inhale slowly and deeply through your nose as you count silently "In, 2, 3, 4." Notice how the stomach expands first, then the rib cage and, finally, the upper chest. Now exhale slowly through your mouth as you count silently "Out, 2, 3, 4, 5, 6."

Pretend you're breathing out through a straw to lengthen exhalation. Let your shoulders drop slightly as your upper chest, rib cage, and stomach gently deflate. Repeat this exercise four or five times.

● Inhale for 4 seconds and hold your breath for the count of 4, but don't strain. Then exhale through your mouth for 6 to 8 seconds. Practice this exercise four or five times.

A few tips

Perform these breathing exercises as long as needed during painful periods. You may vary the rhythm, but always exhale 2 to 4 seconds longer than you inhale.

If you feel light-headed or your fingers tingle, you may be breathing too deeply or too fast. Reduce the depth and speed of your breathing, or breathe into a paper bag until the feeling goes away.

Using imagination

Following these steps will help you use your imagination to cope with stress and pain.

● Begin by focusing on your breathing. Spend a few minutes breathing slowly and smoothly.

● As you breathe, slowly count backward from 5, sinking deeper and deeper into a state of relaxation. Say to yourself, "I feel deeply relaxed."

● Next, imagine a pleasant place that you can return to whenever you need relaxation or pain relief — for example, a warm, quiet beach or a tranquil, fragrant garden. Close your eyes to help you concentrate.

● Experience the place with all your senses: sight, touch, smell, hearing, and taste. Remain there for about 5 minutes or longer, depending on the time needed for pain relief.

Let your imagination run free. Try to name the colors you see, or trace the shapes of the flowers blooming in the garden. Breathe in the sweet fragrance of the blossoms, listen to the birds chirping, and feel the sun warm your skin. Now, sip a cool beverage before you step along the garden path and greet a friend.

● Slowly let the image you've chosen fade from the center of your attention as you focus again on your breathing. Maintain a relaxed feeling. When you're ready, count slowly to 5 and open your eyes.

Positioning TENS electrodes

In transcutaneous electrical nerve stimulation (TENS), electrodes placed around peripheral nerves (or an incision site) transmit mild electrical pulses to the brain. The current is thought to block pain impulses. The patient can influence the level and frequency of his pain relief by adjusting the controls on the impulse generator.

Typically, electrode placement varies even though patients may have similar complaints. Electrodes can be placed in several ways:
- to cover the painful area or surround it, as with muscle tenderness or spasm or painful joints

- to "capture" the painful area between electrodes, as with incisional pain.

For the patient with peripheral nerve injury, place electrodes proximal to the injury (between the brain and the injury site) to avoid increasing pain. Placing electrodes in a hypersensitive area also increases pain. In an area lacking sensation, place electrodes on adjacent dermatomes.

The illustrations show combinations of electrode placement (black squares) and areas of nerve stimulation (shaded red) for low back and leg pain.

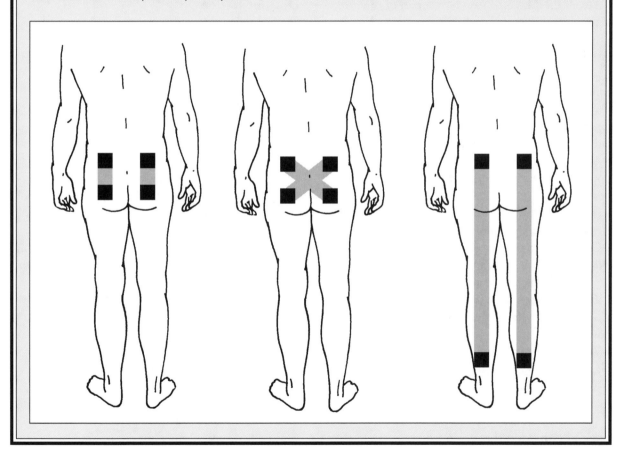

- Place the ordered number of electrodes on the proper skin area, leaving at least 2" (5 cm) between them. Then secure them with the adhesive patch or hypoallergenic tape. Because the older patient's skin is often loose and thin, tape all sides evenly so the electrodes are firmly attached to the skin while ensuring that the patient's skin isn't damaged by securing the electrodes.
- Plug the pin connectors into the electrode sockets. To protect the cords, hold the connectors — not the

cords themselves — during insertion.
• Turn the channel controls to the "off" position or to the position recommended in the operator's manual.
• Plug the lead wires into the jacks in the control box.
• Turn the amplitude and rate dials slowly, as the manual directs. (The patient should feel a tingling sensation.) Then adjust the controls on this device to the prescribed settings or to settings that are most comfortable. Most patients select stimulation frequencies of 60 to 100 Hz. If the patient requires excessive levels of stimulation, contact the doctor before continuing treatment.
• Attach the TENS control box to part of the patient's clothing, such as a belt, pocket, or bra.
• To make sure the device is working effectively, monitor the patient for signs of excessive stimulation, such as muscular twitches, or signs of inadequate stimulation, which are signaled by the patient's inability to feel any mild tingling sensation. Question the patient about his feelings since the older patient may have diminished sensation.
• After TENS treatment, turn off the controls and unplug the electrode lead wires from the control box.
• If another treatment will be given soon, leave the electrodes in place; if not, remove them.
• Clean the electrodes with soap and water, and clean the patient's skin with alcohol sponges and pat dry. (Don't soak the electrodes in alcohol because it will damage the rubber.)
• Monitor the site for signs of irritation and breakdown.
• Remove the battery pack from the unit and replace it with a charged battery pack.
• Recharge the used battery pack so it's always ready for use.

Special considerations
If you must move the electrodes during the procedure, first turn off the controls. Follow the doctor's orders regarding electrode placement and control settings. Incorrect placement of the electrodes will result in inappropriate pain control. Setting the controls too high can cause pain; setting them too

low will fail to relieve pain. Never place the electrodes near the patient's eyes or over the nerves that innervate the carotid sinus or laryngeal or pharyngeal muscles, to avoid interference with critical nerve function.

If TENS is used continuously for postoperative pain, remove the electrodes at least daily to check for skin irritation, and provide skin care. If the patient is at high risk for skin irritation and breakdown, check the skin more often.

If appropriate, let the patient study the operator's manual. Teach him how to place the electrodes properly and how to take care of the TENS unit.

Documentation
On the patient's medical record and the care plan, record the electrode sites and the control settings. Document the patient's tolerance to treatment. Also evaluate pain control.

Using PCA
PCA puts the patient in charge of relieving his own pain. Steadily improving technology in this area has increased the popularity of PCA, which is usually administered I.V. (See *Selecting a PCA pump.*)

An I.V. PCA pump can deliver small amounts of a narcotic at a slow, continuous rate, and it allows the patient to give himself boluses of the narcotic when pain increases. With I.V. administration, drug absorption is faster and more predictable than with I.M. administration.

When patients control their own analgesia, they use less narcotic and they're sedated for less time than when they receive prescribed doses of pain reliever through another route. Patients tend to experience less pain and return to normal activities sooner.

Morphine is the most commonly prescribed drug for PCA, but many other drugs are also given, including hydromorphone, buprenorphine, and methadone. The anesthesiologist determines the drug based on the patient's weight, age, and previous narcotics usage. He may establish a basal rate (the maximum amount the patient may receive hourly in continuous infusion). He'll also determine whether a bolus dose can be given and how often.

Selecting a PCA pump

Many types of patient-controlled analgesia (PCA) pumps are available. Although certain features are necessary, others simply add to the cost of the pump. Determining the type of pump to use depends on the needs of your patient. Here are some tips.
• In evaluating a pump, first consider its cost and the cost of its operation. Does it include expensive refill cassettes or syringes?
• Next, consider the pump's complexity. How easy is it to operate, both for you and the patient? Operating the pump should be a straightforward procedure but not so simple that anyone can manipulate the program.
• Evaluate the pump's size and portability. An ambulatory patient should have a small, portable PCA pump. Can the pump be used on an I.V. pole and carried or worn as well?
• Some pumps can provide both continuous infusion and bolus doses. Others provide only bolus doses. For many patients, bolus dosing is less desirable than

continuous infusion. If the patient doesn't receive a regular amount of the drug, he may suffer a rapid decline in relief followed by an excessive peak of medication effects. If the bolus dose is too low, he may need up to 10 doses an hour. And if he falls asleep, he might awaken in pain.
• Some pumps offer a wide range of volume settings for both bolus doses and continuous infusion. They may have a panel that displays the amount delivered or, if necessary, an alarm message. You can program some pumps to record the concentration in either milligrams (mg) or milliliters (ml), allowing greater flexibility in choosing rates. With some pumps you can vary the length of the lockout interval (how often a dose can be delivered) from 5 to 90 minutes. And some pumps can be programmed to store and retrieve information such as the total dose allowed in a specified length of time.

Within these limits, the patient controls the amount of drug he receives.

Patients receiving PCA therapy need to be mentally alert and able to understand and comply with instructions and procedures. PCA is contraindicated in patients with limited respiratory reserve, a history of drug abuse, or a psychiatric disorder.

Equipment

Patient's medication record and chart ▪ PCA device including specified concentration of drug in solution ▪ I.V. line or S.C. site (including 27G butterfly needle or commercial S.C. infusion needle) ▪ alcohol ▪ appropriate site dressing ▪ gloves.

Implementation

With PCA, the patient controls drug delivery by pressing a button on the pump. Before the device can be used, it must be programmed to deliver the specified doses at the correct time intervals. You can set up a pump to deliver PCA S.C. or I.V. (See *Initiating subcutaneous PCA therapy,* page 414.)

If the patient is using a pump that provides con-

tinuous infusion, he can control incidental pain (from coughing, for example) or breakthrough pain. If he's receiving continuous infusion therapy at home, the pump should allow him to stop and start the infusion.

If the patient is having steady pain that gradually increases or decreases or pain that's worse at one time or another, he should be able to regulate the hourly infusion rate. If he has sudden but brief increases in pain, he should be able to give himself bolus doses along with the infusion. But if his pain is intermittent, he might not need continuous infusion at all.

Programming the PCA pump. Follow these steps.
• Determine the initial trial bolus dose and a time interval between boluses in conjunction with the doctor. Program this information into the pump. Once these safety limits are set, the patient can push the button to receive a dose when he feels pain. You and the doctor may decide to change the dose or the lock-out interval after you see how the patient responds.

Initiating subcutaneous PCA therapy

Subcutaneous (S.C.) patient-controlled analgesia (PCA) therapy is often used to manage chronic pain. Therapy can be administered through a number of routes, such as the abdominal route shown below. If you're initiating PCA through this route, follow these steps:

● Insert a 27G butterfly needle or a commercial S.C. infusion needle into the patient's abdomen or into another area with accessible subcutaneous tissue.

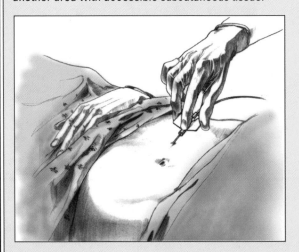

● Cover the site with a dressing.
● Calculate the hourly S.C. dose the same way you would an I.V. dose, considering both the hourly infusion rate and the bolus doses.
● S.C. absorption of a drug depends on the patient's condition. The maximum volume per hour that a well-nourished and well-hydrated patient can usually absorb is about 2 to 2.5 ml. If your patient can't absorb that much, you may need to increase the drug's concentration. The minimum volume per hour should be about 1 ml.
● Inspect the site twice a day for signs of irritation. If it becomes irritated, change to a new site as often as necessary and apply a corticosteroid cream two or three times a day. Otherwise, change the site weekly or according to your facility's policy.

● Follow these suggestions for determining bolus doses for bolus-only PCA pumps and lock-out intervals in bolus-only or bolus plus continuous-infusion devices.

● *To determine bolus doses:* If the patient has only intermittent pain, simply estimate a dose and increase or decrease it until you determine the amount that relieves pain. Calculate the number of milligrams per dose and the total dose (or number of boluses) that he may receive per hour.

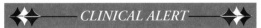

CLINICAL ALERT

When working with older patients, the rule of thumb is to start low and go slowly.

● *To determine lock-out intervals for bolus doses:* For I.V. boluses (bolus only or bolus plus continuous infusion), set the lock-out interval for 6 minutes or more. Typically, pain relief following an I.V. narcotic bolus takes 5 to 10 minutes.

For S.C. boluses (bolus only or bolus plus continuous infusion), set the lock-out interval for 30 minutes or more. Typically, pain relief following an S.C. bolus takes 15 to 60 minutes.

For spinal boluses (bolus only or bolus plus continuous infusion), set the lock-out interval for 60 minutes or more. Typically, pain relief following a spinal bolus takes 30 to 60 minutes.

● If the patient hasn't been receiving opiates, first give the drug until his pain is relieved (the loading dose). With morphine, for example, give 1 to 5 mg every 10 minutes until the patient's pain subsides. Then set the pump's hourly infusion rate to equal the total number of milligrams per hour needed to control the pain.

• If you set the pump so that the patient can give himself bolus doses, decrease the hourly infusion rate. Check his response every 15 to 30 minutes for 1 to 2 hours after changing the settings.

• If you can program the pump to deliver a continuous infusion plus bolus doses, remember this rule of thumb: The initial total hourly dose should not exceed the cumulative bolus doses per hour needed to relieve the patient's pain. For example, if the patient needs a total of 6 mg of morphine over 1 hour, you could begin therapy with a continuous infusion of 3 mg/hour, allowing bolus doses of 0.5 mg every 10 minutes (six boluses/hour). If the patient needs six or more boluses, check with the doctor about increasing the hourly infusion rate.

Special considerations

Before giving an opiate analgesic, review the patient's medication regimen. Because of age-related changes affecting pharmacokinetics and pharmacodynamics, the older patient is at risk for adverse effects and may require a smaller loading dose or bolus doses. Also, concurrent use of two CNS depressants can cause excessive drowsiness, oversedation, disorientation, and anxiety.

Use caution when programming the PCA pump. After changing the program, don't start the pump until another nurse has double-checked the new settings.

Monitor vital signs every 2 hours for the first 8 hours after starting PCA. Check the pump at least twice a day to ensure adequate dosing of the pain medication.

Because opiate analgesics can cause postural hypotension, guard against accidents. Keep the side rails raised on the patient's bed. If the patient is mobile, help him out of bed and assist him in walking. Encourage him to practice coughing and deep breathing to promote ventilation and to prevent pooling of secretions, which could lead to respiratory difficulty.

If anaphylaxis occurs, treat the symptoms and give another drug for pain relief, as ordered.

Watch for respiratory depression during administration. If the patient's respiratory rate declines to 10 or fewer breaths per minute, call his name and touch him. Tell him to breathe deeply. If he can't be roused or is confused or restless, notify the doctor and prepare to give oxygen. If ordered, give a narcotic antagonist such as naloxone. Respiratory depression during PCA isn't common because if a patient receives too much narcotic, he falls asleep and is unable to press the bolus button. Make sure family or staff members don't give extra doses of the narcotic when a patient hasn't requested them.

Evaluate the drug's effectiveness at regular intervals. Assess the patient's level of comfort and reaction to the pain frequently, according to your facility's policy. Is the patient getting relief? Is he developing a tolerance to the drug? Does the dosage need to be increased because of persistent or worsening pain? Although you should give the smallest effective dose over the shortest time period, opiate analgesics should not be withheld or given in ineffective doses. These drugs lead to psychological dependence in fewer than 1% of hospitalized patients.

If a patient has persistent nausea and vomiting during therapy, the doctor may change the medication. If ordered, give the patient an antiemetic such as chlorpromazine.

To prevent constipation, give the patient a stool softener and, if necessary, a senna derivative laxative. Provide a high-fiber diet and encourage the patient to drink fluids. Regular exercise might also help. In case of urine retention, monitor the patient's intake and output.

Complications

The primary complication of PCA is respiratory depression. Other complications include anaphylaxis, nausea, vomiting, constipation, postural hypotension, and drug tolerance. Infiltration into subcutaneous tissue and catheter occlusion also can occur, which can cause the drug to back up into the primary I.V. tubing.

Patient teaching

Your patient must understand how PCA works for therapy to succeed. In many cases, you're in the best position to teach him and members of his family about PCA. You might have to reinforce your teaching several times, especially with an older patient or one who's confused. Keep in mind that PCA isn't for everyone. A patient won't do well with this method if he can't understand it.

When teaching your patient the techniques involved in PCA, emphasize that he'll be able to control his pain. Reassure him that the method is safe and effective but that he could experience mild discomfort.

Home care patients must receive particularly good instructions. Include the patient's family in your teaching session, if possible, and instruct the family members to contact the doctor whenever they suspect a problem.

Documentation
Always document the drug given, the amount (including boluses), the effectiveness of the treatment, any adverse reactions the patient experiences, and the patient's vital signs.

Administering epidural analgesia
In this procedure, the doctor injects or infuses medication into the epidural space, which lies just outside the subarachnoid space where cerebrospinal fluid (CSF) flows. The drug diffuses slowly into the subarachnoid space of the spinal canal and then into the CSF, which carries it directly into the spinal area, bypassing the blood-brain barrier. In some cases, the doctor injects drugs directly into the subarachnoid space.

Epidural analgesia helps manage acute or chronic pain, including moderate to severe postoperative pain. It's especially useful in patients with cancer or degenerative joint disease. This procedure works well because opiate receptors are located along the entire spinal cord. Narcotic drugs act directly on the receptors of the dorsal horn to produce localized analgesia without motor blockade.

Narcotics, such as morphine, fentanyl, and hydromorphone, are administered as either an I.V. bolus dose or by continuous infusion, either alone or in combination with bupivacaine (a local anesthetic). The infusion, given through an epidural catheter, is preferred because it allows a smaller drug dosage to be given continuously. The epidural catheter, inserted near the spinal cord, eliminates the risks of multiple I.M. injections, minimizes adverse cerebral and systemic effects, and eliminates the analgesic peaks and valleys that usually occur with intermittent I.M. injections. (See *Placement of a permanent epidural catheter*.)

Typically, epidural catheter insertion is performed by an anesthesiologist using aseptic technique. Once the catheter has been inserted, the nurse is responsible for monitoring the infusion and assessing the patient.

Epidural analgesia is contraindicated in patients who have local or systemic infection, neurologic disease, anticoagulant therapy, coagulopathy, spinal arthritis or deformity, hypotension, marked hypertension, or an allergy to the prescribed drug.

Equipment
Patient's medication record and chart ■ volume infusion device and epidural infusion tubing (depending on facility policy) ■ prescribed epidural solutions ■ transparent dressing or sterile gauze pads ■ epidural tray ■ labels for epidural infusion line ■ silk tape. Optional: monitoring equipment for blood pressure and pulse, apnea monitor.

Have on hand the following drugs and equipment for emergency use: naloxone 0.4 mg I.V.; ephedrine 50 mg I.V.; oxygen; intubation set; handheld resuscitation bag.

Preparation of equipment
Prepare the infusion device according to the manufacturer's instructions and your facility's policy. Obtain an epidural tray. Be sure the pharmacy has been notified ahead of time regarding the medication order because epidural solutions require special preparation. Check the medication concentration and infusion rate and make sure they agree with the doctor's order.

Implementation
• Explain the procedure and its possible complications to the patient. Tell him he'll feel some pain as the catheter is inserted. Answer any questions he has. Make sure that a consent form has been properly signed and witnessed.
• Position the patient on his side in the knee-chest

Placement of a permanent epidural catheter

An epidural catheter is implanted beneath the patient's skin and inserted near the spinal cord at the first lumbar (L1) interspace.

For temporary analgesic therapy (less than 1 week), the catheter may exit directly over the spine and be taped up the patient's back to the shoulder. However, for prolonged therapy, the catheter may be tunneled subcutaneously to an exit site on his side or abdomen, or over his shoulder.

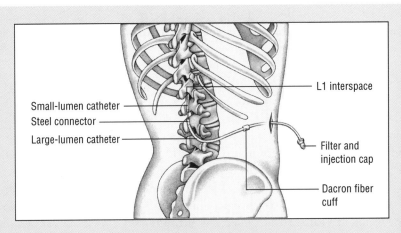

Small-lumen catheter
Steel connector
Large-lumen catheter

L1 interspace

Filter and injection cap

Dacron fiber cuff

position, or have him sit on the edge of the bed and lean over a bedside table. Assist the older patient to attain the correct position; use pillows to help maintain the position and promote comfort.

● After the catheter is in place, prime the infusion device, confirm the appropriate medication and infusion rate, and then adjust the device for the correct rate.

● Help the anesthesiologist connect the infusion tubing to the epidural catheter. Then connect the tubing to the infusion pump.

● Bridge-tape all connection sites and label the catheter, infusion tubing, and infusion pump with "EPIDURAL INFUSION" to prevent accidental infusion of other drugs into the epidural lines.

● Then start the infusion.

● Tell the patient to report any feeling of pain immediately. Instruct him to use a pain scale from 0 to 10, with 0 denoting no pain and 10 denoting the worst pain imaginable. A response of 3 or less typically indicates tolerable pain. If the patient reports a higher pain score, the infusion rate might need to be increased. Call the doctor or change the rate within prescribed limits.

● Monitor the patient closely for possible adverse reactions because older people are more susceptible to the effects of the medication.

● If ordered, place the patient on an apnea monitor for the first 24 hours after beginning the infusion.

● Change the dressing over the catheter's exit site every 24 to 48 hours or as needed. The dressing is usually transparent to allow inspection of drainage and commonly appears moist or slightly blood-tinged; the older patient's skin is thin and fragile and easily injured.

● Change the infusion tubing every 48 hours or as specified by your facility's policy.

● Typically, the anesthesiologist orders analgesics and removes the catheter. However, policy may allow a specially trained nurse to remove the catheter.

● If you feel resistance when removing the catheter, stop and call the doctor for further orders.

● The doctor examines the catheter tip to rule out any damage during removal, so be sure to save the catheter.

Special considerations

Assess the patient's respiratory rate and blood pressure every 2 hours for 8 hours, then every 4 hours for 8 hours, during the first 24 hours after starting the infusion. Then assess the patient once per shift, depending on his condition or unless ordered otherwise. Notify the doctor if the patient's respiratory rate is less than 10 breaths/minute or if his systolic blood pressure is less than 90 mm Hg.

Assess the patient's sedation level, mental status, and pain relief status every hour initially, then every 2 to 4 hours, until adequate pain control is achieved. Notify the doctor if the patient appears drowsy or experiences nausea and vomiting, refractory itching, or inability to void — which are adverse effects of certain narcotic analgesics — or if he complains of unrelieved pain.

Assess lower-extremity motor strength every 2 to 4 hours, comparing it with the patient's baseline data. Older patients often have some changes in motor strength and sensation. If sensory and motor loss occurs, large motor nerve fibers have been affected and the dosage may need to be decreased.

Keep in mind that drugs given epidurally diffuse slowly and can cause adverse effects — including excessive sedation — up to 12 hours after epidural infusion is discontinued. This time may be prolonged in older people because of age-related changes affecting the pharmodynamics of the drug.

The patient should always have a peripheral I.V. line (either continuous infusion or heparin lock) open to allow immediate administration of emergency drugs.

If CSF leaks into the dura mater during removal of an epidural catheter, the patient usually experiences headache that worsens with posture changes, such as standing or sitting. The headache can be treated with a "blood patch," in which the patient's own blood (about 10 ml) is withdrawn from a peripheral vein and then injected into the epidural space. When the epidural needle is withdrawn, the patient is instructed to sit up. Because the blood clots seal off the leaking area, the blood patch should relieve the patient's headache immediately. The patient need not restrict his activity after this procedure.

Complications

The most common complication of epidural infusion is numbness and leg weakness, which may occur after the first 24 hours and is drug- and concentration-dependent. Identifying the dosage level that provides adequate pain control without causing excessive numbness and weakness requires that the doctor titrate the dosage. Monitor the patient closely for neurologic changes from his baseline.

Other possible complications include respiratory depression, which usually occurs during the first 24 hours (treated with naloxone, 0.2 to 0.4 mg I.V.), pruritus (treated with nalbuphine, 5 mg I.V., or diphenhydramine, 25 mg I.V.), and nausea and vomiting (treated with prochlorperazine, 5 to 10 mg I.V., or metoclopramide, 10 mg I.V.).

Documentation

Record the patient's response to treatment, catheter patency, condition of the dressing and insertion site, vital signs, and assessment results. Also document the labeling of the epidural catheter, changing of the infusion bags, ordered analgesics, if any, and the patient's response.

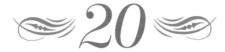

20

Legal and ethical concerns

Most people in the United States today are expected to live beyond age 75 and, as the number of older adults grows, an increasing number of patients in health care facilities will be elderly. Approximately 23% of people over age 65 have one or more self-care deficits, 40% over age 75 have multiple chronic illnesses, and 40% over age 75 reportedly suffer from dementia. And because the population of people age 85 and older is growing six times faster than the population as a whole, care of older people in the United States is an enormous issue now and will become even greater.

New technologies, differing philosophies about patients' rights, and financial concerns make the delivery of competent, high-quality nursing care to the aging adult a complex issue involving numerous legal and ethical concerns. Caring for older patients gives health care professionals the responsibility to support patients' preferences and serve as patient advocates for people with diminished capacity or those who are otherwise vulnerable. You have an obligation, therefore, to understand the challenging legal and ethical issues associated with caring for this aging population.

PATIENT RIGHTS

A fundamental legal and ethical issue is the concept of patient rights. Competent individuals have the right to make their own decisions about health care issues, including whether or not to be hospitalized or subjected to lifesaving devices and measures. Ethicists call this right *autonomy;* the legal profession refers to it as *informed consent* and *self-determination.* The right of autonomy and self-determination is not lost merely because a person is older or has diminished capacity, and there are several ways in which the patient's wishes can be honored.

To ensure that his wishes are known and respected, the patient should declare those wishes while he's still competent. One way to elicit this information is to have the patient prepare a document that encompasses his values and expectations. Several different forms are available. The values history form uses common terminology and covers a variety of important issues. (See *Values history form,* pages 420 to 423.)

The health care provider should ensure that a competent older person completes the values history form or a similar document when he enters any health care facility. Because of the valuable information it contains, this form becomes a permanent part of the patient's record and is referred to when assisting the patient and family members who choose care options.

Role of consent
Generally, the health care provider's right to treat a patient — except in emergencies and other unanticipated situations — is based on a contract that arises

(Text continues on page 423.)

Values history form

Name: _Joyce Nielsen_
Address: _301 N. Jerome St._
Erie, Pa.

The purpose of this form is to assist you in thinking about and writing down what is important to you about your health. If you should at some time become unable to make health care decisions for yourself, your thoughts as expressed on this form may help others make a decision for you in accordance with what you would have chosen. The first section of this form asks whether you have already expressed your wishes concerning medical treatment through either written or oral communications and if not, whether you would like to do so now. The second section provides an opportunity for you to discuss your values, wishes, and preferences in a number of different areas, such as your personal relationships, your overall attitude toward life, and your thoughts about illness.

SECTION 1

A. WRITTEN LEGAL DOCUMENTS

Have you written any of the following legal documents?
Yes

If so, please complete the requested information.

Living Will
Date written: _Yes 10/95_
Document location: _file folder@ home_
Comments (e.g., any limitations, special requests, etc.):

Durable Power of Attorney
Date written: _3/94_
Document location: _file folder @ home_
Comments (e.g., whom have you named to be your decision maker?): _husband, then daughter if husband unable to act_

Durable Power of Attorney for Health Care Decisions
Date written: _____
Document location: _____
Comments (e.g., whom have you named to be your decision maker?) _feel durable POA is sufficient & don't need a specific one for health care_

Organ Donation
Date written: _7/96_
Document location: _on driver's license_
Comments (e.g., whom have you named to be your decision maker?): _no one —_

B. WISHES CONCERNING SPECIFIC MEDICAL PROCEDURES

If you have ever expressed your wishes, either written or orally, concerning any of the following medical procedures, please complete the requested information. If you have not previously indicated your wishes on these procedures and would like to do so now, please complete this information.

Organ Donation
To whom expressed: _spouse_
if oral, when? _____
If written, when? _7/96_
Document location: _on drivers license_
Comments: _don't want body used for science, i.e. med school anatomy dissections_

Kidney Dialysis
To whom expressed: _no_
If oral, when? _____
If written, when? _____
Document location: _____
Comments: _____

Cardiopulmonary Resuscitation (CPR)
To whom expressed: _spouse_
If oral, when? _1995_
If written, when? _____
Document location: _____
Comments: _to be done only if not in a terminal situation_

Respirators
To whom expressed: _spouse_
If oral, when? _1995_
If written, when? _____
Document location: _____
Comments: _as above_

Artificial Nutrition
To whom expressed: _spouse_
If oral, when? _1995_
If written, when? _____
Document location: _____
Comments: _as above_

Artificial Hydration
To whom expressed: _spouse_
If oral, when? _1995_
If written, when? _____

Values history form (continued)

Document location: _____
Comments: *as above* _____
_____

C. GENERAL COMMENTS

Do you wish to make any general comments about the information you provided in this section? *no* _____
_____

SECTION 2
A. YOUR OVERALL ATTITUDE TOWARD YOUR HEALTH

1. How would you describe your current health status? If you currently have any medical problems, how would you describe them? *good except cholesterol is borderline. Slightly overweight* _____

2. If you have current medical problems, in what ways, if any, do they affect your ability to function? _____
weight problem causes fatigue _____

3. How do you feel about your current health status? *good except would like to lose 20 pounds* _____

4. How well are you able to meet the basic necessities of life, such as eating, food preparation, sleeping, personal hygiene, etc.? *no problems* _____

5. Do you wish to make any general comments about your overall health? *no* _____

B. YOUR PERCEPTION OF THE ROLE OF YOUR DOCTOR AND OTHER HEALTH CAREGIVERS

1. Do you like your doctors? *yes, we have an excellent physician* _____

2. Do you trust your doctors? *yes* _____

3. Do you think your doctors should make the final decision concerning any treatment you might need? *no—I want that decision along c̄ my family.* _____

4. How do you relate to your caregivers, including nurses, therapists, chaplains, social workers, etc.? *not applicable* _____

5. Do you wish to make any general comments about your doctor and other health caregivers? *have a very caring & concerned doctor* _____

C. YOUR THOUGHTS ABOUT INDEPENDENCE AND CONTROL

1. How important is independence and self-sufficiency in your life? *very important although I* _____

depend on my husband in many ways. _____

2. If you were to experience decreased physical and mental abilities, how would that affect your attitude toward independence and self-sufficiency? *I think I would become depressed & frustrated esp if I couldn't function mentally.* _____

3. Do you wish to make any general comments about the value of independence and control in your life? *I love to be independent & come & go as I please—I'm also best when I can control a situation or at least know what an outcome will be.* _____

D. YOUR PERSONAL RELATIONSHIPS

1. Do you expect that your friends, family, and/or others will support your decisions regarding medical treatment that you may need now or in the future? *Yes, they will be supportive* _____

2. Have you made any arrangements for your family or friends to make medical treatment decisions on your behalf? If so, who has agreed to make decisions for you and in what circumstances? *have told my husband about not using extraordinary measures of life support* _____

3. What, if any, unfinished business from the past are you concerned about (such as personal and family relationships, business and legal matters)? *none* _____

4. What role do your friends and family play in your life? *family is very important to me & is very supportive.* _____

5. Do you wish to make any general comments about the personal relationships in your life? *excellent relationships c̄ spouse & children* _____

E. YOUR OVERALL ATTITUDE TOWARD LIFE

1. What activities do you enjoy (e.g., hobbies, watching TV, etc.)? *love to swim, read, do computer work on internet, walk, be c̄ my husband*

2. Are you happy to be alive? *oh yes* _____

3. Do you feel that life is worth living? *of course—life is great except for an occasional bump along the way* _____

4. How satisfied are you with what you have achieved in your life? *have 4 great children—they are*

(continued)

Values history form (continued)

my legacy

5. What makes you laugh or cry? _my husband makes me laugh_

6. What do you fear most? What frightens or upsets you? _death; financial ruin_

7. What goals do you have for the future? _to enjoy our life together & prepare for retirement_

8. Do you wish to make any general comments about your attitude toward life? _no_

F. YOUR ATTITUDE TOWARD ILLNESS, DYING, AND DEATH

1. What will be important to you when you are dying (e.g., physical comfort, no pain, family members present, etc.)? _family c̄ me, no pain,_

2. Where would you prefer to die? _@ home_

3. What is your attitude toward death? _somewhat frightened_

4. How do you feel about the use of life-sustaining measures in the face of:
   terminal illness? _no_
   permanent coma? _no_
   irreversible chronic illness (such as Alzheimer's disease)? _depends on the individual situation; if a condition can be easily treated, then do it._

5. Do you wish to make any general comments about your attitude toward illness, dying, and death? _I don't want to suffer pain_

G. YOUR RELIGIOUS BACKGROUND AND BELIEFS

1. What is your religious background? _Strong — from early childhood — educated in Catholic schools & active in church_

2. How do your religious beliefs affect your attitude toward serious or terminal illness? _believe in an after-life, "heaven" & a loving God_

3. Does your attitude toward death find support in your religion? _absolutely._

4. How does your church, synagogue, or faith community view the role of prayer or religious sacraments in an illness? _prayer has a very real role, i.e. Sacrament of the Sick (anointing)_

5. Do you wish to make any general comments about your religious background and beliefs? _Strong reli-_

gious background c̄ a belief in God

H. YOUR LIVING ENVIRONMENT

1. What has been your living situation over the last 10 years (e.g., lived alone, lived with others, etc.)? _with husband & teenaged children; a stable & loving family_

2. How difficult is it for you to maintain the kind of environment for yourself that you find comfortable? Does any illness or medical problem you have now mean that it will be harder in the future? _not difficult; I'm very comfortable in my living situation. Am in good physical health c̄ no medical problems_

3. Do you wish to make any general comments about your living environment? _no_

I. YOUR ATTITUDE CONCERNING FINANCES

1. How much do you worry about having enough money to provide for your care? _occasionally think about it but we have a good savings setup — worry about a catastrophic illness taking all savings._

2. Would you prefer to spend less money on your care so that more money could be saved for the benefit of your relatives and friends? _no, I want to be cared for properly but I also want my husband to have enough for him to live comfortably_

3. Do you wish to make any general comments concerning your finances and the cost of health care? _see above_

J. YOUR WISHES CONCERNING YOUR FUNERAL

1. What are your wishes concerning your funeral and burial or cremation? _a traditional mass & burial — no cremation_

2. Have you made your funeral arrangements? If so, with whom? _no_

3. Do you wish to make any general comments about how you would like your funeral and burial or cremation to be arranged or conducted? _see question #1. Family shouldn't be too sad_

Optional Questions

1. How would you like your obituary (announcement of

Values history form (continued)

your death) to read? _that I was a good wife & mother who made some small contribution to others._

2. Write a brief eulogy (a statement about yourself to be read at your funeral). _"She was a good person who loved her family."_

Suggestions for Use

After you have completed this form, you may wish to provide copies to your doctors and other health care providers, your family, your friends, and your attorney. If you have a Living Will or a Durable Power of Attorney for Health Care Decisions, you may wish to attach a copy of this form to those documents.

Form courtesy of University of New Mexico, Center for Health Law and Ethics, Institute of Public Law, School of Law, Albuquerque, N. Mex.

through the mutual consent of the parties to the relationship. *Consent* is the voluntary authorization by a patient or the patient's legal representative to do something to the patient. The key to valid consent is the patient's comprehension.

Consent concerns the health care provider's right to treat an individual, not the manner in which treatment is delivered. Thus, one can deliver safe, competent care and still be sued for lack of consent. For example, a patient may sue for battery (unconsented touching) if he hasn't given consent for a procedure and a health care provider performs it anyway. The patient may bring a lawsuit and be awarded damages even if the therapy is performed correctly and the patient's health improves because of the procedure or treatment. The trend, though, in negligence or malpractice cases is to raise the issue of consent by arguing that the patient did not fully comprehend the information presented or that all pertinent information was not given.

A health care provider has a duty to obtain consent before treating a patient. Consent is not implied by a patient's request for information or clarification; it must be actively sought by the health care practitioner. The rights to consent and to refuse consent are based on a long-recognized, common-law right of people to be free from harmful or offensive touching of their bodies. In a landmark 1914 case, *Schloendorff v. Society of New York Hospitals,* the

court declared the reason for consent, which is still quoted today: "Every human being of adult years has a right to determine what shall be done with his own body, and a surgeon who performs an operation without his patient's consent commits an assault for which he is liable in damages."

Consent versus informed consent

Consent, technically, is an easy yes or no: "Yes, I will allow the surgery" or "No, I want to try medications first, and then maybe I'll allow the surgery." Yet the patient may not fully understand what he's allowing. The law concerning consent in health care situations is therefore based on informed consent. The doctrine of *informed consent* was developed from negligence law when courts realized that in some cases, though consent was given, not enough information was provided for the patient to make an informed decision.

Informed consent mandates that the health care practitioner disclose needed facts in terms that the patient can reasonably understand so that he can make an informed choice. The information should include descriptions of available alternatives to the proposed treatment and the risks and dangers of each.

Failure to disclose the needed facts in understandable terms does not negate consent that's been given, but it does make the practitioner potentially liable for negligence. In 1957, the California courts found a doctor negligent for failing to explain the potential risks of a vascular procedure to a patient who was paralyzed by the procedure *(Salgo v. Leland Stanford, Jr. University Board of Trustees).*

To sum up, if a practitioner fails to obtain any consent, he may be sued for battery; if he fails to obtain informed consent, he may be sued for negligence.

Some courts have extended the right to informed consent to what might be called "informed refusal." A practitioner may be liable for failure to inform a patient of the risks of *not* consenting to a therapy or diagnostic test. *Truman v. Thomas* (1980) was one of the first cases to recognize this important corollary to informed consent. In that case, the court awarded damages against a doctor for failure to tell the patient about the potential risks of not consenting to a recommended Papanicolaou (Pap) smear.

Inclusions in informed consent

To be informed, a patient must receive — in terms that he can understand — the following information:

● a brief but complete explanation of the treatment or procedure to be performed
● the name and qualifications of the person (and any assistants) who is to perform the procedure
● a description of any serious harm, pain, or discomforting adverse reactions that can occur during and after the procedure (including death if that's a realistic outcome)
● an explanation of alternative therapies to the procedure or treatment, including the risk associated with doing nothing
● an explanation that the patient can refuse the therapy or procedure without having alternative care or support discontinued
● the fact that the patient can still refuse even after a procedure or therapy has begun; for example, scheduled radiation treatments may be cancelled if a patient decides against completing a planned series.

Forms of informed consent

Consent may be given in several forms: expressed or implied, written or oral, complete or partial.

Expressed consent is authority given by direct words, written or oral — for example, after the nurse informs a patient that an I.V. infusion is going to be given, the patient says, "Okay, but could you put the needle in my left arm since I'm right-handed?" Expressed consent is the type health care providers most often seek and receive.

Implied consent is consent that's inferred by the patient's conduct or that's legally presumed in emergency situations. This principle has its foundation in the classic case of *O'Brien v. Cunard Steamship Company* (1899), in which a ship's female passenger joined a line of people receiving vaccinations. She neither questioned nor refused the injection; in fact, she willingly held out her arm for the vaccination. Later, she unsuccessfully brought suit for battery. A reasonable practitioner would infer that by extending her arm and saying nothing, the patient both understood the therapy and consented by action. Health care practitioners often use implied consent for minor procedures and routine care.

Implied consent is presumed in emergency situations — when a delay in providing care would result in the loss of life or limb, and the patient cannot make his wishes known. An important element in allowing emergency consent is that the health care provider has no reason to think that consent would not be given were the patient able to give or deny consent. For example, the health care provider is not permitted to wait until the patient loses consciousness to order treatment that the patient had previously refused, such as a blood transfusion for a known Jehovah's Witness patient.

Consent also may be implied by law, as when the patient is a minor and the parent or the state — standing in the place of a parent — consents to treatment. The law implies the minor's consent for the treatment.

Consent may be given orally or in writing. Unless state law mandates written consent, the law views oral and written consent as equally valid. As a precaution, health care providers should recognize that oral consent is much more difficult to prove in court. As a convenience and to prevent such court cases, most health care facilities require written consent.

Consent may be partial or complete. In other words, a patient may authorize the entire treatment or procedure or only part of the proposed therapy. For instance, if the patient authorizes a breast biopsy but refuses to sign the consent form for a mastectomy based on the biopsy results, only a biopsy may be performed. The health care practitioner would then need to have a separate consent form signed before performing a mastectomy.

Standards of informed consent

Various jurisdictions apply standards of disclosure for informed consent in one of three manners. These have evolved to ensure that patients are informed in their decisions and to allow a means for determining the adequacy of the disclosure.

The majority of states use a *medical community standard,* sometimes referred to as the reasonable medical practitioner standard. This standard evolved from the landmark *Karp v. Cooley* case (1974) and is based on a model of medical paternalism. It requires that a practitioner "disclose facts which a reasonable medical practitioner in a similar community and of the same school of medical thought would have disclosed regarding the proposed treatment." This standard is fluid and changing, based on the prevailing medical thought and community, and is established in court through expert medical witness testimony. Generally, the patient must be told of inherent risks, but not necessarily unexpected risks, that could occur after the treatment or procedure is initiated. Disclosure must include serious injuries that could occur. In general, courts favor more rather than fewer facts for full disclosure.

The other two tests are based on a reasonable patient standard. One is the *objective patient standard* (also known as the prudent patient standard or material risk standard) and is based on disclosure of the risks and benefits that a prudent person in the given patient's position would deem material. Material facts are those that can make a significant difference to the reasonable and prudent patient. In *Joswick v. Lenox Hill Hospital* (1986) and *Arato v. Avedon* (1993), the courts decided that a person must have enough information on which to base a decision, including material risks. In *Korman v.*

Mallin (1993), the court stated that determining materiality is a two-step process: first, defining the existence and nature of the risk and the likelihood of occurrence; and second, determining whether the probability of harm is a risk that a reasonable patient would consider.

The second reasonable patient standard is the *subjective patient standard* (or the individual patient standard). This requires full disclosure of the facts that a particular patient — rather than a reasonable person — would want to know. A judge and jury must determine what risks were or were not material to a particular patient's decision with respect to treatment that's accepted or refused. No expert testimony is required on the scope of disclosure, although such expert testimony may be required to establish risks and alternatives to therapy. Only a handful of states have adopted this standard.

Some states have attempted to bypass the three tests of disclosure by statutorily defining what must be disclosed to a patient before therapy or surgery. These medical disclosure laws mandate that certain risks and consequences be printed on the face of the consent form in language that the patient can be reasonably expected to understand.

Some states have not adopted one standard for disclosure, instead relying on a case-by-case analysis, and others restrict informed consent to certain types of procedures, such as operative or surgical procedures (*Jones v. Philadelphia College of Osteopathic Medicine,* 1993).

A newer collaborative model for informed consent has been proposed by Piper (1994). In this proposal, the patient and doctor would define jointly what informed consent means to them. Such a standard would assign at least four responsibilities to patients:
• to communicate their values and expectations of treatment to the doctor
• to ask questions and seek clarification in patient-doctor discussions
• to evaluate symptoms and report subjective impressions of how well treatment is satisfying their individual goals and values
• to make reasonable efforts to participate appropriately in treatment.

This model would ensure that patients' values and concerns about death and dying are communicated to the primary health care provider while the patient is competent or that they're communicated to the primary health care provider by the patient's surrogate.

Arguments for standards of full disclosure center on four key points:

• The patient assumes all potential risks, since it's his body and life that are affected.

• Informed consent mandates increased communication between the patient and the health care provider. More communication means, the caregiver is less apt to violate the informed consent standards and more likely to fully answer the patient's questions.

• Informed consent improves the consumer's health awareness and ultimately encourages better health care practices.

• Informed consent improves the quality of medical care because the health care provider explains all risks and benefits of the proposed procedure and outlines alternatives, thus aiding selection of the best type and quality of care.

To bring a successful malpractice suit based on informed consent, the plaintiff must be able to prove all of the following:

• the doctor's duty to know of a risk or alternative treatment

• the doctor's duty to disclose the risk or alternative treatment

• a breach of the duty to disclose

• if the case is in a reasonable patient standard jurisdiction, that a reasonable person in the plaintiff's position would not have consented to the treatment if the risk had been known

• that the undisclosed risk caused harm or that the harm would not have occurred if an alternative treatment plan was selected

• that the plaintiff suffered damages.

Exceptions to informed consent

The courts recognize four exceptions to the need for informed consent when consent is still required: emergency situations, therapeutic privilege, patient waiver, and prior patient knowledge. The practition-

er still needs consent to prevent charges of battery, but the informed consent requirements are relaxed.

Emergencies give rise to implied consent. Some courts recognize that if there's time to give information, limited disclosure may be valid. If no time exists or if the patient is incapable of understanding because of physical disability, then no information need be given. Note that it's not necessary to later request that the patient or his surrogate sign an informed consent form. Emergency consent negates the need for a completed informed consent form. In this case, the primary health care provider documents the reason for proceeding under an emergency consent doctrine.

Therapeutic privilege, which has its origins in the common law defense of necessity, allows primary health care providers to withhold information and any disclosures that they feel would be detrimental to the patient's health. The detriment must be more than a suspicion that the information would lead to the patient's refusal; it must be a recognized and documented increase of anxiety in the patient. In using this exception, doctors must be able to show that full disclosure of material facts would be likely to hinder or complicate necessary treatment, cause severe psychological harm, or be so upsetting as to render a rational decision by the patient impossible.

Therapeutic privilege typically comes into play only when the patient is severely and emotionally disturbed and his current medical status presents an imminent danger to his life. Some courts hold that a relative must concur with the patient's decision to consent and that the relative must be given full disclosure, whereas other courts hold that no relative need give concurrent consent. Once the risk to the patient has abated, the doctor or independent practitioner must fully disclose the previously withheld information to the patient.

The courts may be more tolerant of therapeutic privilege when it applies to an older patient who has periods of confusion alternating with competence or who is slower to realize the full intent of a proposed medical therapy. Courts insist that the patient's next-of-kin or another family member be consulted when using this exception to informed consent.

The patient may also waive the right to full disclosure and still consent to a procedure. The caveat is that the health care provider may not suggest such a waiver. To be valid, the waiver must be initiated by the patient.

Prior patient knowledge means that the risks and benefits were fully explained the first time the patient consented to a procedure. Liability does not exist for nondisclosure of risks that are public or common knowledge or that the patient had previously experienced.

Accountability for obtaining informed consent

The doctor or independent practitioner is responsible for obtaining informed consent. Health care facilities have no responsibility for obtaining informed consent unless the doctor or independent practitioner is an employee or agent of the facility or the facility knew or should have known about the lack of informed consent and took no action. Court cases and state statutes have repeatedly upheld this principle. In one case, the court concluded that the patient should discuss risks of procedures with the doctor, who "is the best person to inform the patient about the procedure and where to obtain proper services and facilities."

Attorneys argue both sides of the accountability issue as it relates to hospitals and other health care settings, but most medical professionals feel that to allow liability — and thus allow the hospital to monitor consulting procedures and the disclosure of material facts — would destroy the professional relationship with the patient.

Nurses who are not independent practitioners may be involved in obtaining informed consent. Because consent must be obtained for all procedures and treatments, not just medical procedures, the impact of this doctrine is vast. This does not mean that nurses must obtain written consent each time they give an injection or turn a patient. Most nursing interventions rely on oral expressed consent or implied consent that may be readily inferred through the patient's actions.

The doctrine of informed consent means that nurses must continually assess a patient's competence and communicate with him, explaining proce-

dures and obtaining his permission. It also means that they must respect a patient's refusal to allow a certain procedure. However, state laws vary on allowing patients to refuse life-sustaining treatment. Even if a patient refuses life-sustaining treatment, a nurse could face charges for honoring this request. If a patient is unable to communicate, permission may be derived from his admission to the hospital or obtained from his legal representative.

A major concern for nurses involves obtaining consent for nursing procedures when the primary procedure is performed by another practitioner. For example, who is responsible for teaching postoperative care — the primary practitioner or the nursing staff? Postoperative teaching is considered a nursing procedure, but a doctor performs the surgery (primary procedure). The answers from a legal perspective are far from clear.

The best way to handle this dilemma is probably for the nurse to give postoperative care information after the patient has consented to the surgical procedure. This approach prevents interference with the doctor-patient relationship and conflicting explanations.

Another approach is to provide postoperative teaching materials and films that orient the patient to the entire procedure *after* consent has been given and *before* the procedure. This approach may be augmented by having a nurse answer questions or provide clarification as needed. Many hospitals have implemented this approach for major procedures and operations, such as heart catheterization, vascular arteriography, and open-heart surgery.

Another concern for health care professionals is obtaining informed consent for medical procedures that are provided entirely by another practitioner. In the past, nurses obtained consent for surgical or medical therapies performed by doctors. Some facilities still permit nurses to obtain the patient's signature on a consent form, but most avoid potential liability by prohibiting nurses from doing this.

Still, doctors may legally delegate to a nurse the responsibility for obtaining a patient's informed consent. However, the doctor does so at some peril because most medical practice acts hold that the doctor is responsible for obtaining informed consent. Thus, any deficiencies in the informed consent obtained by the nurse may be imputed back to the doctor.

The general rule is that the responsibility for obtaining a patient's informed consent rests with the person who will carry out the procedure. This is usually the attending doctor. Any additional information that the patient requests should be supplied by the doctor, and the nurse should contact the doctor immediately rather than attempt to talk a reluctant patient into a proposed procedure.

Many hospitals and long-term care facilities prohibit doctors from delegating responsibility for obtaining informed consent to a nurse because once the nurse becomes an integral part of the informed consent process, the facility also assumes liability under the doctrine of *respondeat superior.*

The nurse also has an important role if the patient wishes to revoke consent that was previously given or if it becomes obvious that the patient's signed consent form does not meet the standards of informed consent. Most nurses have been faced with the problem of what to do when a patient doesn't understand a procedure or believes it poses no major risks or adverse consequences. If a patient changes his mind about consenting to a procedure or fails to understand the procedure and any risks it poses, the nurse should contact her immediate supervisor and the responsible doctor. Both need to be informed of a patient's change of mind or lack of comprehension. In general, the health care professional and the facility may incur liability if the standards of informed consent have not been met.

If the doctor performs a procedure without the patient's informed consent and the patient sues for battery, the courts might hold the nurse responsible if:

● the nurse took part in the battery by assisting with the procedure.

● the nurse knew the procedure was taking place and didn't try to stop it.

If the doctor fails to provide adequate information for consent and the patient sues the doctor for negligent nondisclosure, the courts might hold the nurse responsible if, knowing the doctor hadn't provided enough information to the patient, the nurse fails to try to stop the procedure by informing her superior.

Consent forms

Two types of consent forms are commonly used. A *blanket consent form* that a patient is required to sign before admission is sufficient for routine and customary care. Consent to perform routine and customary care may also be implied by the patient's voluntary admission to the facility, so the initial blanket consent form is only needed for insurance coverage and assignment of benefits.

A *specific consent form* provides specific information, such as the name and description of the procedure to be performed. It usually also states that the person who signed the form was told about the medical procedure, its risks and benefits, and any alternatives and that all questions have been answered. With this type of form, the doctor and facility can show that no battery occurred because consent was given. However, the plaintiff may still be able to convince a court that informed consent was not given.

A second type of specific consent form might prevent the latter possibility. This is a detailed consent form that lists the procedure, consequences, risks, and alternatives. Many states now mandate this type of form.

Most of these forms include the following elements:

● name and full description of the proposed procedure

● description of probable consequences of the proposed procedure

● description of risks and alternatives to the proposed procedure, including nontreatment

● signature of the competent patient or a legal representative

● signatures of one or two witnesses, depending on state law.

When using such detailed forms, three things are important. First, witnesses are not required for consent to be valid. Witnesses merely attest to the competence of the patient signing the form and to the genuineness of the signature, not to the fact that the patient had all the information needed to make an informed choice. Although a nurse need not be a witness to make the consent form valid, observing the signing and documenting that such information was given at the time of the signing would make the nurse an excellent witness if a medical malpractice case arose.

Second, consent may be withdrawn at any time. Nothing in the written form precludes a patient's right to withdraw consent at will. Third, consent forms are not conclusive evidence of informed consent. Several challenges to this notion have surfaced — for example, that technical language prevented the patient from understanding what was signed; that the signature was not voluntarily given, but was coerced or forced; and that the competence of the signer was impaired by medications.

A consent form is considered valid until the patient withdraws it or until his condition or treatments change significantly. Some facilities use a 30-day guideline, but most prefer to have none, particularly with patients who may require prolonged hospitalization or rehabilitation at a skilled nursing facility.

Who must consent?
Informed consent becomes a moot point if the wrong person consents to a procedure or therapy.

Competent adult. The basic rule is that if a patient is an adult according to state law, only that person can give or refuse consent. In most states, 18 is the age at which one is considered an adult, although some actions — for example, marriage — may qualify a younger person to act as an adult. The adult giving or refusing consent must be competent to sign or refuse to sign the necessary consent forms.

Competence legally means that the court has not declared a person to be incompetent and the person is generally able to understand the consequences of his actions. A person's legal competence is usually based on an assessment by a doctor or other health care professional, often at the time informed consent is requested. Other health care professionals should be consulted if the patient is mentally retarded or has an obvious mental disorder or a disease that affects mental functions. In the case of an older

patient, especially one who has alternating periods of confusion and competence, it's advisable to document how the health care provider assessed the patient for competence at the time of consent or refusal of consent. A simple entry clarifying the patient's competence may well prevent a lawsuit.

Courts generally hold that there is a strong presumption of continued competence. Exceptions may involve a person who is disoriented at times or confined to a mental institution. In these cases, the court is likely to seek evidence to show whether the person is capable of understanding the alternatives to a procedure as well as the consequences of refusing consent to it.

There are two exceptions to the legal adult's right to give or to refuse consent. The hospital must seek and abide by the decision of a court-appointed guardian or a person with a valid, written power of attorney. Such persons present themselves to the hospital administration if they have previously been appointed and if the adult patient is incapable of giving or refusing consent.

Legal guardian. A legal guardian or representative is a person who is legally responsible for giving or refusing consent for an incompetent adult. A guardian or representative has a narrower range of permissible choices than he would if deciding for himself. Some states insist that the known choices of a patient be considered first. Any expressed wishes concerning therapy or refusal of therapy made while the patient was still fully competent should be evaluated and followed if at all possible. A values history form completed by the patient while still competent may prevent treatment delays and needless questions about patient preferences.

To appoint a legal guardian or representative, the court must first declare an adult incompetent. The court then appoints either a temporary or permanent guardian. If the court has reason to believe the adult is only temporarily incapacitated, it appoints a guardian to act until the adult is able to resume managing personal affairs.

Three types of guardians may be appointed. A person may assume *guardianship of property*, which allows him to take care of financial matters but gives him no authority to make medical decisions for the incompetent patient. *Guardianship of person* permits medical decisions to be made, but the guardian has no financial responsibilities. A *plenary guardianship* allows the guardian to make all types of decisions about the incompetent person's medical and financial needs.

Because the language and requirements for guardianships vary from state to state, health care providers should ensure that their state requirements are met before relying on the guardianship papers as presented. A guardian is usually selected from a patient's family in the belief that such a person has the patient's best interests at heart and is in a position to best know the patient's desires. If the spouse of an incompetent adult is also elderly and ill, an adult child may be the appointed guardian.

In cases where a person has not been adjudicated as incompetent by a court of law, some states will ask family members to make decisions for the incompetent patient. The order of selection in cases involving older patients is usually: (1) spouse; (2) adult children or grandchildren; (3) adult brothers and sisters; and (4) adult nieces and nephews. Other states require durable power of attorney for valid, informed consent to health care or other formal procedures.

The provider should validate state laws and judicial decisions because family consent may not be valid in a handful of states. Lack of valid consent may lead to a court battle, especially if the provider acts on family consent and family members disagree about which course of action to take.

Right to refuse to consent

People have not only the right to consent, but also the right to refuse to consent. A person may refuse consent even after giving it initially. The patient or guardian need only notify the health care provider that the patient no longer wishes to continue with the therapy. In some circumstances, when the danger of stopping therapy poses too great a risk for the patient, the law allows the therapy to continue. For example, a postoperative patient cannot refuse procedures that ensure a safe transition from anesthesia. Likewise, a patient may not refuse immediate care

for life-threatening arrhythmias following a myocardial infarction if that refusal would worsen his condition. After the arrhythmias have abated, the patient may refuse further therapy.

The right of refusal does have potential consequences. The patient or guardian must be informed that refusing treatment will likely cause the patient's physical condition to deteriorate and may hasten death. The right of refusal can also cause third-party reimbursements to be denied because most insurance policies have a clause that denies or limits reimbursement for refusing procedures that would aid in diagnosing or reducing injury or illness.

Limitations on refusal of therapy. The state may deny a patient's right of refusal in several instances. These state rights exist to prevent crimes and protect the welfare of society as a whole. Limitations on refusal are designed to:
• preserve life if the patient does not have an incurable or terminal disease
• protect minor dependents
• prevent irrational self-destruction
• maintain the ethical integrity of health professionals by allowing the hospital to treat the patient
• protect the public's health.

In cases filed to enforce the right to refuse care, the courts have attempted to balance the rights of the individual against those of society at large. In *Leach v. Akron General Medical Center* (1984), the court found that a patient has the right to refuse therapy based on a right to privacy. In this case, the patient was incompetent and the issue was whether to allow him to forgo life-sustaining treatment.

Patient self-determination

The concept of self-determination — the right of a person to decide what will or will not happen to his body — has its origins in both constitutional (legal) rights and autonomy (ethical) rights. This concept is most often evoked in cases involving death and dying, but it applies to all aspects of consent and refusal.

Competent adults have the right to refuse medical treatment unless the state can show that its interests outweigh that right. Examples of overriding state interests include protecting third parties, especially minor children; preserving life, especially that of minors and incompetents; and protecting society from the spread of disease. Competent adults may decide which treatments they will receive and which they will refuse. In some states, oral wishes are upheld by the judiciary. The court examines documentation of the patient's wishes and then determines whether the patient knew of a terminal condition when expressing these wishes or was talking in general terms about future care in case of terminal illness. The courts are reluctant to enforce generalities: Vague talk about potential future events usually carries little weight in court.

Important court cases

For years, legal experts have concluded that competent adults have the right to refuse medical treatment even if the refusal is certain to cause death — a view that is consistent with the trend in a majority of states to decriminalize suicide. But it was not until 1984 that an appellate court directly confronted this issue, when a clearly competent patient — who had a serious illness that was probably incurable but not necessarily terminal — refused necessary life-sustaining treatment.

Bartling v. Superior Court (1984) concerned the rights of a competent adult to have life-support equipment disconnected (over the objections of his doctors and the hospital) even though this action would hasten his death. Bartling, a severely emphysemic patient, entered the hospital for depression. While hospitalized, a tumor was noted on his X-ray. During the subsequent biopsy, his lung collapsed and a tracheostomy tube was inserted. The patient was dependent on a ventilator when the case was heard in court. Although Bartling died during the course of the appeal, the appellate court held that the "right of a competent adult to refuse medical treatment is a constitutionally guaranteed right which must not be abridged."

In *Bouvia v. Superior Court* (1986), the court addressed many of the same issues. Bouvia, a 28-year-old patient with severe cerebral palsy, sought removal of a nasogastric tube, which was inserted and maintained against her will to allow forced

feedings. Here the court wrestled not only with the right of a competent adult to refuse medical treatment, but also with the facility's obligation to serve the autonomous interests of individual patients. In *Bouvia,* those autonomous interests included medical support to prevent further pain and suffering during the dying process, so the patient received appropriate medications. The court sided with Bouvia.

Incompetent patients present a totally different picture. The first court case to challenge the judiciary in this respect was the Karen Quinlan case (1976). In this case, Karen Quinlan's parents argued that unwanted life support violated their comatose daughter's constitutional right to privacy. The New Jersey Supreme Court allowed Quinlan's father to authorize the withdrawal of life support systems for her, arguing that: "The only practical way to prevent destruction of the (privacy) right is to permit the guardian and family of Karen to render their very best judgment...as to whether she would exercise it in these circumstances."

The decision was a difficult one to reach because Karen did not meet the Harvard criteria for brain death. Although she was dependent on a respirator at the time of the court case, she did have some brain activity and some reflex movements. The decision also conflicted significantly with a precedent-setting New Jersey case that held that one should always save a life, even if the patient's objection to lifesaving procedures was based on religious beliefs (*John F. Kennedy Memorial Hospital v. Heston,* 1971).

The next significant decision in this area of the law was *Superintendent of Belchertown State School v. Saikewicz* (1977). The case concerned the issue of whether Mr. Saikewicz, a 67-year-old profoundly retarded resident of a state facility, should receive therapy for his newly diagnosed leukemia. Here the Massachusetts Supreme Court used the doctrine of *substituted judgment* (subjective determination of how a person would have chosen to exercise his right to refuse treatment if he were capable of making his wishes and opinions known) to decide what the patient would have wanted. Unlike the Quinlan decision, the Saikewicz decision met with general disfavor because the court rejected the notion that decisions to refuse treatment should be made by patients' families and doctors with the aid of ethics committees. Instead, it held that the decision to discontinue therapy "must reside with the judicial process and the judicial process alone."

In *Eichner v. Dillon* (1980), the court restricted the decision to terminate extraordinary life-support treatments to the patient who was terminally ill or in a "vegetative coma characterized as permanent or irreversible with an extremely remote possibility of recovery." But it allowed the family or legal guardian of the incompetent patient to request the right to terminate life-support treatments. In this case, the patient's religious superior, Father Eichner, requested the right to terminate treatment. The Eichner case combined the substituted judgment doctrine applied in the Saikewicz decision with the best interest test derived from the Quinlan case. (Best interest refers to personal preferences that were made known while a now-incompetent patient was rational and capable of stating preferences in the event of a catastrophic event.) While not a perfect solution, the decision did soften the negative impact of the Saikewicz decision.

In *Cruzan v. Director, Missouri Department of Health* (1990), the court ruled that right-to-die issues should be decided by the states and that there should be little, if any, constitutional limit on what states may do. Since this decision, the states have given more latitude to family members, and the courts have struggled to find instances where patients expressed, however fleetingly, their desires about sustaining life with artificial or life-support measures.

Two recent cases illustrate this trend. In *re Fiori* (1995), a Pennsylvania court held that a hospital may terminate life-support treatment for a patient in a persistent vegetative state without a court order if the hospital obtained the consent of close family members and two doctors. The court limited this ruling to patients in a persistent vegetative state with no cognitive powers and no chance of recovery who never clearly expressed a preference for termination. In a 1993 case, *Grace Plaza of Great Neck, Inc. v. Elbaum,* the court held that where doubt exists as to

an incompetent patient's desired course of treatment, a judicial determination is necessary before life support can be terminated. The court further stated that proof of a patient's desires, as expressed in a living will or a prior statement, for example, should limit a health care provider's autonomy in denying termination of treatment.

Advance directives

To prevent needless worry by patients about relying on others to make decisions should they become unable to speak for themselves, most states and the District of Columbia have adopted some type of advance directive, a document that expresses the patient's wishes in writing while he is competent.

Many states recognize more than one form of advance directive, giving patients choices to suit their individual needs and circumstances. Experts estimate that the numbers of advance directives presented to health care providers will dramatically increase in the next 10 years as more and more people, particularly competent older people, decide to convey their wishes about future care should they become incompetent.

Living wills. A living will is a directive from a competent individual to medical personnel and family members regarding the treatment he is to receive if he becomes seriously ill and incompetent. It's not applicable while the patient is competent and capable of making his wishes known. Typically, the language of a living will is broad and vague. It gives little direction to the health care provider concerning the circumstances and actual time that the declarant wishes the living will to be honored.

Living wills are typically not legally enforceable; medical practitioners may choose to abide by the patient's wishes or to ignore them as they see fit. And because these documents do not protect practitioners from criminal or civil liability, many doctors have refused to follow a living will's direction for fear that family members or the state would file charges of wrongful death. (See *Living will.*)

Natural death acts. To protect medical practitioners from potential civil and criminal lawsuits and to

Living will

The living will is an advance care document that specifies a person's wishes with regard to medical care should he become terminally ill and incompetent or unable to communicate. All states and the District of Columbia have living will laws that outline documentation requirements. The sample living will below is from Nebraska.

Nebraska Declaration

If I should lapse into a persistent vegetative state or have an incurable and irreversible condition that, without the administration of life-sustaining treatment, will, in the opinion of my attending physician, cause my death within a relatively short time and I am no longer able to make decisions regarding my medical treatment, I direct my attending physician, pursuant to the Rights of the Terminally Ill Act, to withhold or withdraw life-sustaining treatment that is not necessary for my comfort or to alleviate pain.

Other directions:

none

Signed this *14th* day of *Sept. 1996*
Signature *Rosey R. Kramick*
Address *12700 Clearwater*
York, Neb.

The declarant voluntarily signed this writing in my presence.
Witness *Janice Mason*
Address *280 W. Queen Blvd.*
York, Neb.
Witness *Harry I. Hopkins*
Address *14-338 Euclid*
Lincoln, Neb.

OR

The declarant voluntarily signed this writing in my presence.
Adele A. Chu

Notary Public

Form courtesy of Choice in Dying, Inc.

ensure that the patient's wishes are followed when he is no longer able to express them, nearly all the states have enacted some form of natural death act. These documents are living wills that *are* legally enforceable. Recognizing that some doctors may be unwilling to follow the directive, several of these laws require the doctor to make a reasonable effort to transfer the patient to a doctor who will abide by the patient's wishes.

The provisions of natural death acts vary greatly from state to state. Generally, people over age 18 may sign a natural death act if they are of sound mind and capable of understanding the purpose of the document. The document usually calls for with-

holding or withdrawing life-sustaining treatment should the patient ever be in a terminal state. In most states, the natural death act must be in written form, signed by the patient, and witnessed by two people age 18 or older.

Some states also specify that the witnesses to the natural death act not be related to the patient by blood or marriage; not be entitled to any portion of the patient's estate by will or intestacy; not be directly financially responsible for the patient's medical care; not be the attending physician, his employee, or an employee of the facility in which the declarant is a patient; and not be the same person who signed the declaration because the patient was unable to do so. Other states incorporate some of these restrictions.

The forms of natural death acts also vary from state to state. For states that have no set form, private organizations have suggested formats for these special living wills.

Once signed and witnessed, most natural death acts are effective until revoked, although some states require that they be re-executed every 5 years or another stated time frame. It may be advisable for the declarant to review, redate, and re-sign the natural death act every year or so. This assures family members and health care providers that the directions contained in the document reflect the declarant's current wishes.

The natural death act may be revoked by physical destruction or defacement, by a written revocation, or by an oral statement indicating the declarant's wish to revoke it. Some states place fewer restrictions on revocation, for example, allowing the document to be revoked without regard to the patient's mental condition or making the revocation ineffective until the attending physician is notified.

Once a valid natural death act exists, it is effective only when the person becomes qualified; that is, when he is diagnosed with a terminal condition and the use of life-support systems would only prolong the death process. Most states require that two doctors certify in writing that any procedures and treatments will not prevent the ultimate death of the patient but will only serve to postpone death in a patient with no chance of recovery. Medications and procedures used to prevent the patient's suffering and to provide comfort are excluded from this definition.

Today, many states permit oral invocation by a patient of a natural death act or allow another person to invoke a natural death act for the patient.

Durable power of attorney for health care. *Power of attorney* is a common-law concept that allows one person (an agent) to speak for another (the principal). Earlier, the power of attorney ended with the death or incapacity of the principal. To prevent this limitation, legislatures adopted the Uniform Durable Power of Attorney Act. This act allows an individual the right to grant a durable power of attorney, which is valid even if the principal becomes incapacitated and legally incompetent.

The Durable Power of Attorney for Health Care (DPAHC), sometimes known as the Medical Durable Power of Attorney (MDPA), allows a competent person to appoint a surrogate or proxy to make health care decisions for him in case he becomes incompetent to do so. With these statutes, family members and health care providers need no longer guess whether the patient would have wanted his living will to be followed. (See *Durable power of attorney for health care,* pages 435 and 436.)

Under most DPAHC statutes, the agent whom an individual designates to make medical decisions for him has the right to ask questions, to select and remove doctors from the patient's care, to assess risks and complications, to select treatments and procedures from a variety of therapeutic options, and to refuse care or life-sustaining procedures.

Agents further have the authority to enforce the patient's treatment plans by filing lawsuits or legal actions against health care providers or family members. In short, they have the full authority to act as the principal would have acted. In addition, DPAHC statutes protect health care providers from liability if they abide, in good faith, by the agent's decisions.

Caution your patient to appoint agents who understand what he would want and are capable of making difficult decisions for him — typically, a spouse, relative, or friend. Most states allow the patient to appoint a second or third agent, who would assume authority in the event the first person named was unable or unwilling to serve in this capacity. Without this latter provision, the patient's wishes might not be honored.

◆◆ —— CLINICAL ALERT —— ◆◆

When presented with a DPAHC document, have your facility's legal counsel verify that the document meets state requirements. Competent older patients may be required to re-sign the document if the original form is deficient or doesn't fulfill state requirements.

Durable power of attorney for health care

I, *Josephine Kessler*   , appoint *Robert Kessler*

(Address) *709 Strahle St., Phila, PA*

(phone) *215-652-0610*

as my agent to make any and all health care decisions for me except to the extent I state otherwise in this document. This Durable Power of Attorney for Health Care takes effect if I become unable to make my own health care decisions and this fact is certified in writing by my physician.

LIMITATIONS ON THE DECISION-MAKING AUTHORITY OF MY AGENT ARE AS FOLLOWS:

DESIGNATION OF ALTERNATE AGENT

(You are not required to designate an alternate agent but you may do so. An alternate agent may make the same health care decisions as the designated agent if the designated agent is unable or unwilling to act as your agent. If the agent designated is your spouse, the designation is automatically revoked by law if your marriage is dissolved.)

If the person designated as my agent is unable or unwilling to make health care decisions for me, I designate the following persons to serve as my agent to make health care decisions for me as authorized by this document, who serve in the following order:

A. First Alternate Agent

Name: *Marion Kessler Davidoff*

Address: *1224 Ellis Circle, York, PA*

Phone: *717-925-3050*

B. Second Alternate Agent

Name: _____

Address: _____

Phone: _____

The original of this document is kept at   *safe deposit box*

The following individuals or institutions have signed copies

Name: _____

Address: _____

Name: _____

Address: _____

DURATION

I understand that this power of attorney exists indefinitely from the date I execute this document unless I establish a shorter time or revoke the power of attorney. If I am unable to make health care decisions for myself when this power of attorney expires, the authority I have granted my agent continues to exist until the time I become able to make health care decisions for myself.

(IF APPLICABLE) This power of attorney ends on the following date: _____

PRIOR DESIGNATIONS REVOKED

I revoke any prior durable power of attorney for health care.

ACKNOWLEDGMENT OF DISCLOSURE STATEMENT

I have been provided with a disclosure statement explaining the effect of this document. I have read and understand the information contained in the disclosure statement.

(continued)

Durable power of attorney for health care *(continued)*

(YOU MUST DATE AND SIGN THIS POWER OF ATTORNEY)

I sign my name to this durable power of attorney for health care on the _15th_ day of _November_ , 19_96_ at _my home_ .

Signature _Josephine Kessler_

Printed name _Josephine Kessler_

STATEMENT OF WITNESSES

I declare under penalty of perjury that the principal has identified himself or herself to me, that the principal signed or acknowledged this Durable Power of Attorney in my presence, that I believe the principal to be of sound mind, that the principal has affirmed that he or she requested that I serve as witness to the principal's execution of this document, that I am not the person appointed as agent by this document, and that I am not a provider of health or residential care, an employee of a provider of health or residential care, the operator of a community care facility, or an employee of an operator of a health care facility.

I declare that I am not related to the principal by blood, marriage, or adoption and that to the best of my knowledge I am not entitled to any part of the estate of the principal on the death of the principal under a will or by operation of law.

Witness Signature: _Ingrid Donahue_

Print Name: _Ingrid Donahue_

Date: _11/15/96_

Address: _1902 Englewood Rd., Phila., PA_

Witness Signature: _Alfred Ehrlich_

Print Name: _Alfred Ehrlich_

Date _11/15/96_

Address: _603 Kentwood Drive, York, PA_

Form courtesy of Choice in Dying, Inc.

Medical or physician directives. Some states allow for a medical or physician's directive that lists a variety of treatments and lets the patient decide which treatment he will want in the future, depending on his condition. For example, the patient can select life-sustaining therapy if the condition is not terminal or can refuse life-sustaining therapy if the condition is terminal and irreversible. This document is legally comparable to a living will.

Uniform Rights of the Terminally Ill Act

This act, adopted in 1989, is narrow in scope and limited to treatment that would prolong life in a patient whose condition is incurable and irreversible, whose death will occur soon, and who is unable to participate in treatment decisions. The act's pur-pose is to legally implement the patient's desires to withhold or withdraw life-support procedures.

Many provisions of the act are identical to some states' natural death act provisions. For example, the qualified patient must be diagnosed as terminal, whereby life-sustaining procedures would only prolong dying; a patient in a persistent vegetative state is not qualified (not judged terminal); and a physician who is unwilling to comply with the patient's requests is expected to transfer the patient to a physician who will.

Patient Self-Determination Act of 1990

The Patient Self-Determination Act of 1990 was enacted into law in direct response to the Nancy Cruzan case in Missouri. It mandates that patients be queried about advance directives and have advance directives made available if they so wish.

In 1983, Cruzan was involved in a one-car automobile accident. She was discovered lying face down in a ditch without cardiac or respiratory functioning and life support was started. She eventually was diagnosed as being in a persistent vegetative coma and her parents requested the removal of artificial hydration and nutritional support. The trial court allowed such removal because Cruzan reportedly "expressed thoughts at age 25 in a somewhat serious conversation with a friend that if sick or injured she would not wish to continue her life unless she could live at least halfway normal." The Supreme Court of Missouri (1990) reversed that decision, stating that such statements were unreliable for the purpose of determining her intent and further held that the family was not entitled to direct the termination of her treatment in the absence of a living will or "clear and convincing, inherently reliable evidence."

The United States Supreme Court then held that states had the authority to impose requirements on decisions to discontinue therapy for incompetent patients. The case was then remanded back to trial in Missouri and, on retrial, the court concluded that the friend's statement of Cruzan's desires was sufficient to allow removal of the feeding tube.

Justice Scalia, in a separate concurrence, praised states for grappling with the issue of terminating medical treatment through legislation. Almost every state recognizes some form of advance directive, from living wills to durable powers of attorney for health care. The problem, though, is that few people prepare advance directives. Thus, the Patient Self-Determination Act was passed to ensure that people be informed about advance directives and receive help in making them if they so desire. However, the legislation specifically states that providers may not discriminate against a patient in any way based on the absence or presence of an advance directive.

This act lets people know about existing rights but does not create any new rights for patients. Nor does it change state law, although it may have served as incentive for more states to pass durable powers of attorney for health care statutes. The act also does not legislate communication or conversation, although one of its purposes is to encourage communication and conversation about advance directives while the patient is competent to understand and to execute them. Ideally, this communication is between the patient and the primary health care provider, not between patients and admitting clerks in health care facilities.

Written information described in the act is to be provided to adult individuals at the following times:
- for a hospital admission, at the time of the individual's admission as an inpatient
- for a skilled nursing facility, at the time of the individual's admission as a resident
- for a home health agency, in advance of the individual coming under the care of the agency
- for a hospice program, at the time that the individual begins receiving hospice care
- for an eligible managed care program, at the time of that the individual enrolls in the organization.

Do-not-resuscitate directives

Some health care organizations have initiated do-not-resuscitate directives that patients may execute on admission to health care facilities. The doctor then follows the facility's policy in attaching such orders to the patient record. Most facilities require documentation that the patient's decision was made after consultation with the doctor regarding diagnosis and prognosis. The order is then reevaluated according to the facility's policy.

New York State has enacted a do-not-resuscitate statute that establishes the hierarchy of surrogates who may request do-not-resuscitate status for incompetent patients and has also mandated that all health care facilities inquire of patients as they are admitted their desires concerning resuscitation. The act was prompted by worry over the overuse of cardiopulmonary resuscitation. Cases involving do-not-resuscitate directives often focus on whether the patient was fully informed when a doctor ordered a do-not-resuscitate for the patient.

Nursing guidelines for advance directives

Use the following guidelines regarding advance directives:
- Review state statutes and provisions regarding

durable powers of attorney for health care, natural death acts, and living wills — which may vary greatly from state to state — and have the facility's attorney hold classes for health care professionals so that the staff is fully aware of statutory requirements and the means by which advance directives are enforced.

• Review your facility's policy and procedure manual for guidelines. If no policies exist, suggest to the committee or persons responsible for such policies the need for guidance in this area.

• If the patient or family members tell you that an advance directive was signed, document this information and make it known to the doctor and the administration immediately. Have the in-house legal consultant review the document before placing it in the medical record and ensure that subsequent health care providers know that the document has been reviewed and is valid.

• If the patient expresses a desire to revoke the declaration, document this in the record and immediately notify the attending doctor and the administration. Do this even if the patient's competence is questionable because some statutes allow for revocation even if the declarant is not of sound mind. The fact that the patient knows of its existence implies understanding of what invalidating the declaration means.

• Health care professionals should not be a witness to the living will or natural death act. Many natural death acts forbid a witness from being employed by the attending doctor or facility in which the patient is hospitalized. Usually a friend or someone unrelated to the patient serves as witness for this declaration.

• If the patient's medical record includes a copy of the living will or natural death act, read it carefully to ascertain the scope of its provisions. It's much easier to clarify the declaration while the patient is still competent than to speculate about the directives. Document in the medical record any clarification that the patient gives to you, and ensure that the attending doctor also understands the scope of the patient's declaration.

• In most states, the health care professional or another person may write and sign advance directives as proxy for a competent patient. Here you must be sure that the patient is of sound mind because competence is an important issue in the execution of such a directive. If you're in this position, document in the record what occurred and the circumstances that made it necessary for a second person to sign for the patient (for example, partial paralysis or another medical reason).

• Assist the family members in this time of crisis by being available and by answering as many of their questions as possible. Tell the family members of any existing ethics committee or other persons who are available to talk with them. Remember that they need time to internalize what is happening, especially if they are called on to concur with or to insist on implementation of the patient's directive.

Hospice care

A terminally ill patient can avoid the need for a natural death act and living will by entering a hospice. In a hospice, the patient receives required nursing and medical care and is kept comfortable, but he is not resuscitated or placed on life-support systems when death occurs. Some states allow similar home hospice care.

Congress recognized the need for such terminal care apart from the hospital setting and authorized Medicare reimbursement for hospice care in 1982. Medicare reimbursement is limited to 6 months.

ASSISTED SUICIDE

Although suicide as a crime has been abrogated in all states, most states still prohibit assisted suicide. Some states treat assisted suicide harshly; others only prohibit causing suicide, not assisting with it. Washington, Oregon, and California have tried, through legislation, to pass assisted suicide statutes. Although these measures have either failed or are being challenged in the courts, they seem likely to pass at some future date. The Supreme Court may be the judiciary body that finally attempts to come to terms with this issue.

The Oregon Death with Dignity Act, passed by the voters in November 1994 and now under judicial review, would allow a doctor to write a lethal drug prescription for a competent, terminally ill adult who is a resident of the state. Other provisions that must be met before the prescription is written include the following:

• Both the attending doctor and a consulting doctor must certify that the patient has no more than 6 months to live.

• The patient must make both an oral and written request for the prescription, followed by a second oral request 15 days or more after the first requests.

• The attending doctor must refer the patient for counseling if a psychological illness or depression is suspected.

• The doctor must wait at least 48 hours after a third request before prescribing the medication.

Michigan has dealt with the assisted suicide issue extensively because of the actions of Dr. Jack Kevorkian. Michigan originally filed murder charges against Kevorkian, who has assisted dozens of gravely or terminally ill patients in ending their lives, but the charges were dismissed. The state then passed a statute "prohibiting one who has knowledge that a person intends to commit suicide from intentionally providing the physical means or participating in the physical act by which the person attempts or commits suicide," but the prohibition does not apply to "withholding or withdrawing by a licensed health care professional." This law is currently being challenged.

The health care professional's role in this area is still developing. The American Nurses Association opposes assisted suicide as well as nurses' participation in either assisted or active euthanasia because it violates the ethical traditions embodied in the Code for Nurses (1994). However, the Michigan Nurses Association has come out in favor of legalizing assisted suicide for "competent persons whose suffering cannot be relieved or satisfactorily reduced with alternative strategies."

If a patient asks you directly to assist with suicide, you must clearly refuse. If this occurs, reassure the patient that you care about him and will provide assistance through appropriate nursing interven-

tions. Explore the possibility that the patient is expressing a need for greater pain control or for someone to talk to about fears of death. Also, ensure that a chaplain or representative of the patient's faith or a social worker speaks with the patient.

RESEARCH AND OLDER ADULTS

Using vulnerable groups of people for research is ethically controversial because of the ease with which some people can be coerced and because they may be unaware that they are subjects in a research study. This is especially true of older people, as more and more clinical research focuses on changes that occur with the aging process. Other major issues of concern are informed consent, patient autonomy, beneficence, and nonmaleficence.

Before conducting research, investigators must disclose the research to the subjects or the subjects' representatives and obtain valid informed consent. Federal guidelines specify the procedures used to review research and the disclosures that must be made to ensure valid informed consent. Since 1974, the Department of Health and Human Services (DHHS) has required that an institutional review board examine and approve the research study prior to any funding from DHHS. This board determines whether subjects will be placed at risk and, if so, ensures that the following criteria are met:

• that risks to the subjects are minimized

• that risks to the subjects are reasonable in relation to anticipated benefits to the subjects and to the importance of the knowledge that may reasonably be expected to result

• that selection of subjects is equitable

• that informed consent is sought from each prospective subject or the subject's legally authorized representative

• that informed consent is appropriately documented

• where appropriate, that the research plan provides for monitoring data collection to ensure the safety of the subjects

• where appropriate, that there are adequate provisions to protect the privacy of the subjects and to maintain the confidentiality of the data

• where the subjects are likely to be vulnerable to coercion or undue influence — such as persons with acute or severe physical or mental illness or persons who are economically or educationally disadvantaged — that appropriate additional safeguards are included in the study to protect the rights and welfare of the subjects.

The federal government has also mandated the basic elements of information that must be included to meet the standards of informed consent. These basic elements include the following:

• a statement that the study involves research, an explanation of the purposes of the research and the expected duration of the subject's participation, a description of the procedures to be followed, and identification of any experimental procedures

• a description of any reasonably foreseeable risks or discomforts to the subject

• a description of any benefits to the subjects or others that may reasonably be expected from the research

• a disclosure of appropriate alternative procedures or courses of treatment that may be advantageous to the subject

• a statement describing the extent to which confidentiality of records identifying the subject will be maintained

• for research involving more than minimal patient involvement, an explanation as to whether any compensation or medical treatments are available if injury occurs, and, if so, what they consist of or where further information may be obtained

• an explanation of whom to contact for answers to pertinent questions about the research and the research subject's rights and whom to contact in the event of a research-related injury to the subject

• a statement that participation is voluntary, refusal to participate will involve no penalty or loss of benefits to which the subject is otherwise entitled, and the subject may discontinue participation at any time without penalty or loss of benefits to which the subject is otherwise entitled.

The information given must be in language that is understandable by the subject or the subject's legal representative. No exculpatory wording may be included, such as a statement that the researcher incurs no liability for the outcome to the subject. Subjects must also be advised of:

• any additional costs that they may incur

• potential for any foreseeable risks

• rights to withdraw at will, with no questions asked or additional incentives given

• consequences, if any, of withdrawal before the study is completed

• a statement that any significant new findings will be disclosed

• the number of proposed subjects for the study.

Excluded from these strict requirements are studies that use existing data, documents, records, or pathological or diagnostic specimens, so long as these sources are publicly available or the information is recorded so that the subjects cannot be identified. Other studies that involve minimal risks, such as moderate exercise by healthy adults, may be expedited through the review process.

Before proceeding under these specific guidelines, state and local laws must be reviewed for laws regulating research on human subjects. Proposals involving new investigational medications or devices must also meet federal drug regulations.

Although the rights of older adults are no greater than the rights of others involved in research, the need to protect their rights is greater. Aging adults, as a group, are less likely to understand the nature of research or the fact that they can terminate their participation at will, and they are more easily coerced into becoming subjects for proposed studies. Health care professionals working with these individuals must guard against this and ensure that valid informed consent is obtained before a study begins.

FEDERAL STATUTES AFFECTING CARE

The most important federal laws affecting the care of older people are the Social Security Act of 1935, the Older Americans Act of 1965, and the Omnibus Budget Reconciliation Act of 1981.

Social Security Act of 1935

The Social Security Act of 1935 was signed into legislation by President Franklin D. Roosevelt following the Great Depression. Many of its roots can be traced back to early European laws to protect the poor. The original purpose of the act was to provide cash assistance to older adults to aid with their medical costs. It did not apply to institutionalized older adults, for whom the states were expected to provide support.

Over time, several states that had placed long-term residents in private homes filed lawsuits challenging the federal refusal to pay for institutionalized older people. These suits were generally successful, resulting in the creation of the nursing home industry and the expansion of government involvement in long-term geriatric health care.

The original act defined the program, established administrative guidelines, and authorized taxes for funding the program. In 1950, an addition to the act provided for matching federal monies to individual states to support funding for persons receiving public assistance. This was the forerunner of the Medicaid program.

Medicare

In 1965, the Medicare program was added to the act. Part A is automatically available to each recipient of Social Security benefits. This part covers primarily in-hospital coverage but also extends to nursing home costs and home health care costs for individuals who qualify. The requirements and benefits under this part change frequently, making it difficult for older people and health care providers to know the latest changes.

Many older people today believe that Medicare is an insurance program that will meet all of their health care needs. Working with older people, you should be aware of the latest changes and benefits because you may be expected to explain to patients the deductibles, exclusions, limitations, and restrictions as these apply to hospital and health care bills. Health care professionals in long-term care settings are frequently the first providers to explain that Medicare does not cover routine and ongoing nursing home services.

Participation in Part B of the program, which remains voluntary, calls for patients to contribute monthly payments for coverage. Part B covers selected services, such as outpatient services, laboratory fees, and durable medical equipment and supplies. It does not cover eye examinations and eyeglasses, dental examinations, hearing tests and hearing aids, or supportive and corrective devices for ambulation — services that would keep older people independent and able to remain in community settings. The amount of paid services is shrinking and deductibles are increasing, so patients are becoming more and more responsible for payment of their care. The number of services not covered currently exceeds the number of covered services.

Efforts to reduce the federal deficit have a direct impact on health care for older adults. Both the House and Senate Finance Committees are proposing greater cuts in the amount of money allocated to Medicare, and beneficiaries of Medicare are expected to absorb more of the cost of the overall program.

Medicaid

Enacted in 1965, Medicaid provides for medical care of people of all ages on welfare programs and of those who are medically indigent. Medicaid funds the states through grants from the federal government, covering 55% of the costs nationwide.

By 1991, hospitals and nursing homes in 13 states had filed lawsuits charging that payment rates were inadequate and requesting adequate reimbursement of reasonable costs. Many doctors and other independent practitioners are withholding services from Medicaid patients because of low reimbursement rates. Thus, many patients who are eligible for Medicaid cannot receive services.

Despite increasing costs at both state and federal levels for Medicare and Medicaid for older people, the out-of-pocket expense to the individual older patient was proportionately higher in 1994 than in 1965, when the program began. Today, about 25% of the patient's annual income is spent on health care costs.

Social Services Block Grant

In 1974, the Social Services Block Grant program was added to provide home-based services, employment, education, information and referral, legal services, day services, and home and congregate meals. Fees for services are charged to people whose income averages 80% or more of the state's median income. For older people, programs such as Meals on Wheels and homemaker services are available to provide support in their homes. Other services that may be available through the state include visiting volunteers, senior citizen centers, adult day care centers, and geriatric mental health services.

Amendments

The Social Security Act has been amended numerous times since its enactment, with Medicare and Medicaid being the most important health programs that affect nursing services. Through Medicare-reimbursable services, regulations specify which clients nurses see, what type of care they can provide, how they provide care, and how long they may provide care.

Medicare benefits have changed greatly since their enactment. For example, alcohol detoxification facility benefits were added in 1980, hospice reimbursements were added in 1983, and a 1990 amendment allows Medicare Part B premiums to be paid to eligible beneficiaries.

Older Americans Act of 1965

The Older Americans Act (OAA), signed by President Johnson in 1965, is an important piece of federal legislation that promotes care of older people. This act set forth congressional policies related to aging, defined responsibilities of state and local government agencies, and provided for demonstration projects, research, and training programs. The original act called for better coordination of resources and state assistance in developing programs for older adults, and established a network of state and local "area agencies on aging," known as AAAs. These agencies are responsible for planning, coordinating, and funding local services and programs for persons age 60 and older.

The OAA is the strongest governmental policy demonstrating a national commitment to older Americans. The act is designed to meet the needs of persons over age 60 who have low incomes, belong to minority groups, and are isolated from family members. It requires no financial means test before elders can access its programs. The act supports continuing financial assistance for older adults, regardless of age, race, or prior work service. It also directs that health care of older people should include preventive and restorative care as well as acute care. The OAA also provides for cost controls and encourages low-cost, optimum quality of care.

However lofty its intent, the OAA has never been fully implemented because of budget constraints. Nor is the act likely to be fully funded in the near future. A recent House appropriations subcommittee cut over $100,000,000 of funding for the act in the next fiscal year. While some of the monies are likely to be restored, full funding is not considered achievable, a fact that colors the intended outcome of all the following titles and amendments to the OAA.

Provisions

The original OAA contained five titles; it now has seven. Title I states that the goals of the program are open and are to be shared equally by every aging individual. These goals include full and free enjoyment of affordable housing; retirement in health; adequate income; optimal physical and mental health; employment opportunities; freedom of independence and self-determination in planning and managing one's life; efficient community services such as transportation; coordinated social services; access to civic, cultural, educational, and recreational activities; and full restorative services for older people who require institutionalization. Title II established the Administration on Aging, a division of DHHS.

Title III, covering major service provisions, directs AAAs to be responsible for needs assessments and planning at the local community level. Although the AAAs do not provide direct services except for information and referral, they do administer a variety of local services, including home delivery of meals, nutrition services, and social services.

They may also enter into contracts that cover health, educational, recreational, and transportation services and may contract for legal services, counseling, and physical exercise programs. The main purpose of their contracted services is to help older individuals avoid institutionalization.

The purposes of the Ombudsman Program, a 1978 amendment to Title III, is to:

• investigate and resolve complaints on behalf of nursing home residents
• monitor, develop, and ensure implementation of federal, state, and local laws governing long-term care facilities
• give public agencies information about problems for residents in long-term care facilities
• train volunteers for the program.

States are required to develop policies and procedures that allow ombudsmen access to residents' facilities and facility records without disclosing the identity of a person or group who files a complaint. States must develop and maintain a system of reporting and recording complaints while ensuring the security of the ombudsmen's records. While the ombudsman program has no legal authority over the long-term care facility, it does have the authority to communicate information to state licensing and certification agencies.

Title IV provides for mental health services. Although the preamble of the OAA identified such services as paramount, they were not given priority until 1981, when demonstration programs that targeted mental health services were funded. Alzheimer's patients and their family members were included in 1984. To date, though, mental health services have not been emphasized on local levels.

Titles V provides for community service employment opportunities for older people. Title VI provides grants to Native American tribes. Title VII was added in 1984 to promote health and health education for older Americans.

Omnibus Budget Reconciliation Act

The Omnibus Budget Reconciliation Act (OBRA) of 1981 brought significant changes to uninsured people in the United States, allowing individual states to alter eligibility requirements for Medicaid.

When added to Medicaid cutbacks of the late 1970s and early 1980s, the percentage of low-income people insured by the Medicaid program decreased from 63% to 46%. Most of those affected by the cutbacks were low-income older people, women under age 65, and children.

OBRA also affected older people with mental illnesses. It allowed states to set limits for community-based services and determine mandatory and optional services. As a result, mental health services vary greatly from state to state.

1987 amendments

Amendments to OBRA in 1987 led to significant changes in the nursing home industry. These changes required established criteria for quality of care and quality of life in nursing homes, including a provision allowing for freedom from physical and chemical restraints unless medically necessary. They ensured full access by ombudsmen to nursing facilities and allowed unannounced inspections that focused on care of residents. The amendments also set standards for nursing staffs, staff training and certification, and ongoing education. They provided for the following:

• full-time social workers in nursing homes with more than 120 beds
• resident participation in the planning of care
• resident rights in nursing homes
• assessment of residents for mental illness or mental retardation before admission
• interdisciplinary assessment and care plan development for individual residents within a specific time frame
• establishment of a facility-wide quality assessment and assurance committee.

State agencies that implement the Medicaid program were also affected by the 1987 amendments. Increased staffing to monitor nursing home complaints and increased enforcement capabilities are among the most significant changes. States were required to pay for implementing the 1987 provisions and to supply cost reports to the public showing how individual nursing homes spend Medicaid monies. Surveys of nursing homes for compliance with the provisions began in October 1990.

1990 amendment

A 1990 amendment provided for direct reimbursement to nurse practitioners and specialists in rural areas for services that they are authorized to perform under state law. Also, patients are to be given written information at the time of admission about their rights to accept or refuse treatment, their rights concerning advance directives, and their rights to refuse intra-facility transfer if the sole purpose of the transfer is to move the patient from an area of the facility reserved for Medicare-skilled nursing care.

A final provision of the act holds the Secretary of DHHS responsible for devising a plan to make reimbursement for nursing facilities a prospective type of payment system. This system would take into account the number of low-income older adults, case mix and volume, and individual patient characteristics.

RESTRAINTS AND OLDER PEOPLE

Restraints, both physical and chemical, are used daily in many health care settings. Physical restraints help prevent patient falls, discourage patients from disconnecting vital equipment and I.V. and feeding lines, and prevent patients from harming themselves and others. Chemical restraints may be added if physical restraints are ineffective or cause the patient to become more combative. (Research has shown that restraints can cause or aggravate behavioral symptoms such as confusion or agitation in older people.) They prevent patients from disconnecting life-sustaining equipment, help prevent hostile or impaired patients from harming themselves and others, and allow staff to care for all patients on a given unit.

Restraints, though, can cause serious adverse effects and harm. Physical restraints can result in skin breakdown, impaired respiratory status, strangulation, neurologic damage, and death. Chemical restraints may result in increased drowsiness, respiratory distress, hemodynamic instability, decreased competence and judgment, and confusion.

Physical and chemical restraints should be used only as a last resort. Their use is regulated by OBRA 1987, which states that nursing home residents have the right to be free from physical or chemical restraints that are not required to treat "specific medical symptoms." All health care facilities have policies and procedures indicating when restraints are to be used and the care that must be documented on restrained individuals. Because of the inappropriate use of restraints and the 1987 OBRA law, most health care settings insist on securing a doctor's order before applying restraints.

Case law has several examples of patients harmed because they were not properly restrained or informed. For example, in *Reifschneider v. Nebraska Methodist Hospital* (1986), a patient was allowed to fall because the side rails on a stretcher had been raised, but the patient was not belted or restrained in any other way and no hospital employee was in attendance. The cause of action was failure to restrain and negligent failure to provide adequate supervision of the patient.

Documentation requirements

◆◆ —— *CLINICAL ALERT* —— ◆◆

When using restraints, it is vital to follow your facility's policy and procedure and to document why and how the patient was restrained, how patient safety needs were met while restraints were in use, and why restraint was continued or discontinued.

Document what type of patient behavior necessitated the restraints, including ineffective means of restraint that may have been used and the exact type of restraint used, such as soft wrist restraints, a Posey belt, or gauze hand restraints. Also record the date and time of application as well as the patient's responses to the restraints. Patient safety needs, including skin integrity, circulation in the restrained extremities, respiratory status, nutrition and elimination needs, and elevation of the patient's head before feeding, should be documented. Include in the documentation the need for continued restraints and periodic assessments to ascertain when restraints may be removed or discontinued.

Bed occupancy monitors

A newer trend in restraints is to use a bed occupancy monitor to alert staff immediately when the patient is no longer in bed. Although this device may not prevent the patient from falling, it does ensure rapid assistance. (Because some patients can successfully free themselves from all restraints, courts look at how quickly and effectively the patient receives treatment after a fall.)

Alternatives to restraints

Four recommended alternatives to restraints include developing an ambulation program, providing frequent assistance to bathroom facilities, incorporating daily exercise into the plan of care, and encouraging staff and resident interaction. Other strategies include putting the call light within easy reach of the resident and implementing closer monitoring.

In a study done to evaluate the effect of recent OBRA laws on nursing homes, most nursing home directors said that they had not increased their staffing since OBRA addressed the use of restraints, and nearly 90% of the respondents reported a decrease in restraint use since October 1990.

Nearly all of the survey respondents noted that support from administration — including the facility owner, medical director, and director of nursing — was a major factor in decreasing restraint use. Other factors included education of all staff members, reassessment of residents to determine the need for restraints, cooperation of doctors, and involvement of residents' family members in the program.

Most alternatives to restraint usage — such as daily indoor or outdoor walks with residents, saddle-type seats to prevent sliding out of chairs, and volunteers to assist residents — aren't difficult to implement. The most effective interventions are those that reflect high-quality patient care.

Making the transition to decreased restraint use requires an organized, planned effort to change attitudes, beliefs, practices, and policies within a health care facility. Cooperative effort at all levels can ultimately improve the quality of life for residents.

ELDER ABUSE

Researchers estimate that 700,000 to 1.5 million cases of elder abuse — maltreatment of people age 65 and older — occur yearly in the United States and that 1 in 20 older Americans is physically abused. Aging adults risk abuse from health care providers, family members, and caregivers, with those in nursing homes or living with younger family members at greatest risk.

One of the most difficult problems is that older people are unlikely to report abuse, usually because they or their spouses fear retaliation from their caregivers, are ashamed of the problem, or have limited alternatives for living arrangements. Health professionals also fail to report abuse because of ignorance of the problem or of their legal responsibilities to report suspected cases, lack of knowledge about or failure to adequately assess at-risk situations, and concerns that an alternative living arrangement may be less tolerable than the current one.

Elder abuse occurs in all socioeconomic groups and at all educational levels. The most common type is abuse by the patient's spouse, followed by abuse by the children or other caregivers. Recent studies indicate that abusers may be either men or women, with men being slightly more abusive.

The single most important contributing factor in abuse is the older person's loss of physical or financial independence. Confusion, incontinence, frailty, and severe physical and mental disabilities demand enormous amounts of energy, time, and patience from caregivers. Many caregivers do not have the time and energy needed to cope with the care of an aging adult because of their own family and work responsibilities. Sometimes called "the sandwich generation," many middle-aged adults today find themselves responsible for caring for two generations — their parents and their children.

Legal responsibilities

Health care professionals must be able to recognize

the signs and symptoms of elder abuse so they can identify the problem early. Their legal responsibility varies from state to state. Most definitions of elder abuse don't include financial exploitation; some don't include neglect.

The specific agency to which you must report abuse also varies but is usually the state adult protective services or social service agency. As with child abuse, you must report all suspected cases of elder abuse in good faith to the correct agency. The report must include the reasons you suspect abuse, the patient's name and address, and caregiver's name if known. You may be held accountable for failure to report suspected abuse, particularly if the patient is further abused and harmed.

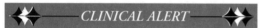

Caregivers and patients may view your investigation of suspected abuse as a threat rather than an advocate if the patient fears removal from his home. If so, they may be reluctant to answer questions or discuss the situation.

All health care providers must be guided by the principles of safety and well-being of the aging adult when confronted by possible abuse cases. For more information about detecting and intervening in elder abuse and neglect, see Chapter 15.

INCORPORATING ETHICAL PRINCIPLES

Remember the following eight ethical principles and apply them daily:
• *Autonomy* concerns personal freedom and self-determination — the right to choose what will happen to one's own person. The legal doctrine of informed consent is a direct reflection of this principle. You enforce this principle daily in allowing patients to make their own decisions and then by supporting those decisions, even when you don't agree.
• *Beneficence* requires that your actions promote

good. In geriatric care, good may be defined in various ways, including allowing a person to die without advanced life or nutritional support.
• *Nonmaleficence* requires you to do no harm. This principle is usually reserved for issues that affect more than one patient, such as deciding if it is ethical to allow patients to die slowly without providing some degree of comfort (as with a morphine drip for a patient with end-stage emphysema).
• *Veracity* involves always telling the truth. You follow this principle daily when giving information to patients and families and by answering all of their questions honestly so that they can make informed decisions about treatments.
• *Fidelity* refers to honoring your promises or commitments and not promising something you can't deliver — for example, that the patient will be pain-free and competent at all times.
• *Justice* requires that all persons be treated fairly and equally. This principle frequently arises when there is competition for supplies or resources, such as scarce beds in a skilled facility.
• *Paternalism*, the principle that allows one person to make decisions for another, is often considered undesirable. But you follow a modified, positive version of this principle when you help patients and family members to fully understand the impact that a decision may have and then assist them in areas in which they lack insight or information. When decision making is removed entirely from a patient, this principle is to be avoided. But when the health care provider can assist with the decision, the principle is desirable.
• *Respect* for others is the highest principle and incorporates all the other principles.

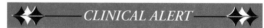

Respect for others requires acknowledgement of the rights of individuals to make decisions and then either live or die by those decisions. Respect for others transcends cultural, gender, religious, and racial differences. You have a chance to practice this principle daily in action with peers, interdisciplinary health care members, patients, and family members.

APPENDIX

Community services for the elderly

Whether they're official programs or volunteer efforts, community services provide a wealth of support for the community-dwelling older adult. These services may be social, economic, health-related, legal, advocacy, or spiritually focused in nature. Some programs have specific financial qualifications. Many community services are local, grassroots efforts initiated to meet a defined need within the particular community. The federal government laid the groundwork for many of these programs with the passage of the Older Americans Act of 1965.

Older Americans Act
This law and its subsequent amendments established a group of policy goals to benefit older Americans (age 60 and older) in the areas of income, health, restorative services, housing, retirement, employment, cultural and recreational opportunities, community services, and gerontologic research. It also laid the legislative foundation for the creation of the Administration on Aging within the Department of Health and Human Services (DHHS). State and local Area Agencies on Aging, the administrative vehicles for establishing programs for the elderly, are charged with identifying and supporting existing services and initiating new programs. One such program involves the designation of certain community sites as "focal points" where people can find information and access to all of the services available to older adults in that geographic area.

SURVEY OF SERVICES

The types of services furnished through the Area Agencies on Aging include the following:
- information and referrals
- legal assistance
- transportation
- chore services
- multipurpose senior centers
- recreational activities and nutritional support through congregate or home-based meal services.

In addition to the programs designated by the Older Americans Act, older people with financial limitations may also qualify for entitlement programs, such as food stamps, subsidized housing, and energy assistance.

A valuable resource number for all those who care for older people is the National Eldercare Locator at 1-800-677-1116. A call to this number will provide free information about the full range of services available to older adults according to zip code. This initiative is jointly supported by the U.S. Administration on Aging, the National Association of State Units on Aging, and the National Association of Area Agencies on Aging.

Health care providers who work with the elderly need to have an accurate picture of all available services in the geographic area where their patients live. You'll find many of the most useful programs —

along with a list of specific resources — discussed below.

Access

Access to services may be provided by families, home health agencies, Area Agencies on Aging, managed care agencies, social workers, nurse practitioners, or parish nurses. This process usually involves an in-home needs assessment, coordination of services and referral, and ongoing follow-up. Information and referral services may be located through:

- Eldercare Locator
- special pages in telephone directories
- advertisements in publications read by older adults
- American Association of Retired Persons (AARP)
- Area Agencies on Aging
- multipurpose senior centers
- home health agencies
- local "focal points"
- DHHS pamphlet "Where to Turn for Help for Older Persons."

Advocacy

Numerous advocacy groups represent older people who cannot speak for themselves. AARP is the leading organization for people over age 50 in the U.S.; it offers an extensive network of programs and services on a national, regional, and local basis. Health professionals working with older people can receive AARP publications. A good introductory reference guide is their "Education and Community Service Programs" pamphlet. For information on elder abuse and protective services, see Chapter 15.

Check-in services

Some senior centers, churches, and other community agencies offer telephone check-in services, in which a volunteer phones a client at a certain time each day to ascertain his status and to provide social contact. Some programs have a buddy system or backup should the client fail to answer.

Friendly visitors are volunteers who make periodic, scheduled visits to older people to provide social contact, assistance with correspondence, and possibly transportation to a community activity. The visitors may come from a senior center, retired senior volunteer program, or church group.

Community-based adult day care

Adult day care programs offer numerous services for frail or cognitively compromised older adults in a variety of settings. These include structured activities, personal care, recreation and socialization, nutritional support, and health care. Social services and caregiver support are frequently part of these programs, which typically operate 5 days a week and include transportation. Some centers also offer nursing services.

Adult day care centers, which usually charge a fee, are valuable because they allow caregivers and families to maintain their jobs and to postpone or avoid institutionalizing the older person.

Emergency response systems

Personal emergency response systems provide immediate access to emergency services through activation of a transmitter device worn by the older person. This device is connected to a central monitoring system, which dispatches help when the device is activated. Emergency response systems are expensive and require that the client sign an advance directive form.

Health screening

Health screening and wellness promotion services can be incorporated into a number of community settings, including senior centers, adult day care centers, congregate meal sites, churches, senior housing and retirement communities, and health fairs at malls. (See Chapter 3 for more information.)

Home health care

Medicare and Medicaid provide home health services to older adults who meet eligibility criteria for skilled care. These services may include a registered nurse; physical, occupational, or speech therapist; home health aide; or social worker on a short-term, episodic basis. Special "maintenance level" programs also have been initiated in recent years. These provide personal care services and periodic nursing assessments to support the frail elderly in the home setting.

Home maintenance and repair

Various programs can provide help with home repairs or chores for individuals or couples living in their own home who are unable to perform these tasks independently. The range of services and costs varies widely; some local Area Agencies on Aging underwrite the costs. Service groups, such as church youth groups, Scouts, or adult volunteer groups, may also offer this service.

In recent years, some unscrupulous individuals and groups have preyed on older people with home repair scams. Caution your elderly patients about this practice, and help make a wise, informed choice if they need home repairs.

Homemaker services

Help with such activities as light cleaning, cooking, shopping, and laundry is available for a fee for elderly people living at home. This service may be available through the Area Agency on Aging at a reduced cost.

Hospice care

For the terminally ill patient and his family, hospice care can be offered in an institutional or home setting. Medical insurance may cover this service for qualifying patients. Hospice care may also be provided by the pastoral care department of the affiliated hospital, a home health agency, the patient's church, or a parish nurse. Many sponsoring agencies (usually home health agencies) offer bereavement services to grieving family members after the patient's death.

Housing

Housing services are available through a variety of sources. Older adults on a fixed income may qualify for government-subsidized senior housing arrangements, and many communities have a homesharing program through the Area Agency on Aging. Reverse mortgages make it possible for many people on a fixed income to stay in their homes until they die.

Personal care and assisted living homes are an option for some, although they can be expensive and are unregulated. Foster care is another option; the Veterans Administration has a domiciliary care program that is in this category.

Continuing care and life care communities are another housing alternative for people with adequate financial resources. These communities, which require a substantial entrance fee as well as a monthly assessment, offer care on a continuum from independent living to skilled nursing services. This care is guaranteed for life. Many also offer social and recreational activities on site in addition to health promotion and wellness programs. Residents have a degree of autonomy in managing the community.

Legal assistance

Free or low-cost legal services are available for income-qualifying elders through the Older Americans Act. Other community agencies and advocacy groups also provide legal services on a volunteer or low-cost basis. AARP also offers assistance in this area.

Multipurpose senior centers

These centers provide a wide variety of services to active, independent adults in the community. Services may include health screening and health promotion programs, social and recreational programs, tax assistance, educational programs, information and referral services, congregate meals, and transportation. Many of these programs are funded through the Area Agency on Aging.

Nutrition

Nutrition programs provide congregate meals in senior centers, churches, community centers, group housing, and similar settings. In addition to balanced meals, they provide an opportunity for socialization — an important secondary benefit for many older adults. Other programs offer home-delivered meals to homebound clients 5 days a week, usually consisting of a hot meal and a cold meal that can be eaten later in the day. Some programs even offer special diets. Churches and other community groups also provide frozen meals for older people confined to their homes; in some cases, a friendly visitor comes periodically to offer a social link.

Parish nurses

A community resource that doesn't lend itself to categorization is the parish nurse program. Based in the Catholic Church, parish nurses offer holistic nursing services enhanced by a spiritual focus. Older people are the main — but not the only — recipients of this service. Many parish nurse programs are interdenominational and have a case management component.

Psychological counseling

The Older Americans Act provides for psychological help for the elderly through existing community mental health networks, Medicare, and Medicaid. Special day care programs for adults with emotional or mental problems are available in some communities and personal care settings. Such programs offer depressed or mentally impaired older adults a combination of socialization, structured activity, individual and group therapy, and nutritional and recreational services.

Respite care

Respite care provides caregiver relief for a brief, time-limited period. It can be offered in the home, through a day care program, or within a facility. An advantage of care in the home is that the patient is familiar with the physical environment. But finding responsible, caring providers can be difficult. You should counsel families to carefully examine their options before choosing a respite program.

Retirement planning

Retirement planning services may be offered through the Older Americans Act. AARP also offers educational programs on this topic.

Transportation

Disabled older adults may find transportation through public or private sources. Many senior centers, day care centers, and other facilities have their own transportation. Weekly shopping trips and periodic health care appointments may also be in-cluded. In some communities, volunteer transportation may be obtained from church groups, such as Fish and Interfaith, or from neighbors and family.

SELECTED RESOURCES

The following list of national organizations can provide more information on aging and age-related health problems. Consult a telephone directory for state and local agencies.

Government agencies

Administration on Aging
Department of Health and Human Services
330 Independence Ave. SW
Washington, DC 20201

National Association of Area Agencies on Aging
1112 16th St. NW, Suite 100
Washington, DC 20036

National Council on Aging
409 3rd St. SW, Suite 200
Washington, DC 20024

National Institute on Aging
Building 31C, Room 2C06
9000 Rockville Pike
Bethesda, MD 20892

Health organizations

American Association for Geriatric Psychiatry
P.O. Box 376-A
Greenbelt, MD 20768

American Geriatrics Society
770 Lexington Ave., Suite 400
New York, NY 10021

American Health Care Association (Nursing Homes)
1201 L St. NW
Washington, DC 20005-4014

American Nurses Association
600 Maryland Ave. SW
Washington, DC 20024-2571

American Society for Geriatric Dentistry
211 E. Chicago Ave.
Chicago, IL 60611

Gerontological Society of America
1275 K St. NW, Suite 350
Washington, DC 20005-4006

Health Care Organization
Division of Long Term Care
Oak Meadows Bldg., Room 2F5
Baltimore, MD 21207

Health Resources and Services Administration
5600 Fisher Lane, Room 1405
Rockville, MD 20857

National Association for Home Care
519 C St. NE
Washington, DC 20002-5809

National Hospice Organization
1901 N. Moore St., Suite 901
Arlington, VA 22209

National Gerontological Nursing Association
c/o Mosby–Yearbook, Inc.
7250 Parkway Drive, Suite 510
Hanover, MD 21076

Social welfare organizations
American Bar Association
Commission on Legal Problems of the Elderly
1800 M St. NW
Washington, DC 20036

American Association of Retired Persons
601 E St. NW
Washington, DC 20049

Children of Aging Parents
1609 Woodbourne Rd., Suite 302-A
Levittown, PA 19057

Gray Panthers
2025 Pennsylvania Ave. NW, Suite 821
Washington, DC 20006

Institute for Retired Professionals
New School for Social Research
66 W. 12th St.
New York, NY 10011

National Caucus and Center on Black Aged
1424 K St. NW, Suite 500
Washington, DC 20005

National Council on the Aging
600 Maryland Ave. SW, Suite 100 W
Washington, DC 20024

National Institute on Adult Daycare
c/o National Council on the Aging
600 Maryland Ave SW, Suite 100 W
Washington, DC 20024

National Senior Citizens Law Center
1052 W 6th St., Suite 700
Los Angeles, CA 90017

Older Women's League
666 11th St. NW
Washington, DC 20001

Other health and social welfare organizations

Alcoholism
Alcoholics Anonymous World Services
P.O. Box 459 Grand Central Station
New York, NY 10163

Al-Anon Family Group Headquarters
1372 Broadway
New York, NY 10018

Alzheimer's disease

Alzheimer's Association
919 N. Michigan Ave., Suite 1000
Chicago, IL 60657-1676

Alzheimer's Disease Education and Referral Center
P.O. Box 8250
Silver Spring, MD 20907-8250

Arthritis

National Arthritis Foundation
P.O. Box 19000
Atlanta, GA 30326

Cancer

American Cancer Society
1599 Clifton Rd. NE
Atlanta, GA 30329-4251

National Cancer Institute
Office of Communication
9000 Rockville Pike, Room 10A24
Rockville, MD 20892

Hearing problems

Alexander Graham Bell Association for the Deaf
3417 Volta Pl. NW
Washington, DC 20007

National Association of the Deaf
814 Thayer Ave.
Silver Spring, MD 20910

National Hearing Aid Society
20361 Middlebelt Rd.
Livonia, MI 48152

Heart disease

American Heart Association
7320 Greenville Ave.
Dallas, TX 75231

Kidney disorders

National Kidney Foundation
30 E. 33rd St., 11th Floor
New York, NY 10016

Mental health disorders

Mental Disorders of the Aging
Research Branch DCR
5600 Fishers Lane, Room 11C-03
Rockville, MD 20857

National Association of Psychiatric Health Systems
1319 F St. NW, Suite 1000
Washington, DC 20004

National Institute of Mental Health
Public Inquiries
5600 Fishers Lane, Room 7102
Rockville, MD 20857

Nutritional problems

American Dietetic Association
216 W. Jackson Blvd., Suite 800
Chicago, IL 60605-6995

American Society for Parenteral and Enteral Nutrition
8630 Fenton St., Suite 412
Silver Springs, MD 20910-3805

Consumer Nutrition Hotline
(800) 366-1655

Dietitians and Health Care Facilities Consultant
P.O. Box 2067
Pensacola, FL 32513

Gerontological Nutritionists
4103 44th St.
Sacramento, CA 95820

National Association of Meal Programs
206 E. St. NE
Washington, DC 20002

National Association of Nutrition and Aging
Services Programs
2675 44th St. SW, Suite 305
Grand Rapids, MI 49509

National Meals on Wheels Foundation
1133 20th St. NW, Suite 321
Washington, DC 20036

Parkinson's disease
American Parkinson's Disease Association
60 Bay St., Suite 401
Staten Island, NY 10301

National Parkinson's Foundation
Bob Hope Rd.
1501 NW 9th Ave.
Miami, FL 33136

Respiratory disorders
American Lung Association
1740 Broadway
New York, NY 10019

Speech problems
American Speech-Language-Hearing Association
10801 Rockville Pike
Rockville, MD 20852

Stroke
National Stroke Association
8480 E. Orchard Road, Suite 1000
Englewood, CO 80111-5015

Stroke Club International
805 12th Street
Galveston, TX 77550

Vision problems
American Council of the Blind
1155 15th St. NW, Suite 720
Washington, DC 20005

American Foundation for the Blind
15 W. 16th St.
New York, NY 10011

American Printing House for the Blind
P.O. Box 6085
1839 Frankfort Ave.
Louisville, KY 40206

Blinded Veterans Association
477 H St. NW, Suite 800
Washington, DC 20001

National Society to Prevent Blindness
500 E. Remington Rd.
Schaumburg, IL 60173

Selected references

Adams, W., et al. "Alcohol-Related Hospitalizations of Elderly People," *JAMA* 270(10):1222-25, September 8, 1993.

American Academy of Nursing Expert Panel. AAN Working Paper: "Violence as a Nursing Priority: Policy Implications." *Nursing Outlook* 41(2):83-92, 1993.

American Cancer Society Textbook of Clinical Oncology, 2nd ed. Washington, D.C.: Panamerican Health Organization, 1995.

Anderson, M.A., and Braun, J.V. *Caring for the Elderly.* Philadelphia: F.A. Davis Co., 1995.

Anderson, K., and Dimond, M. "The Experience of Bereavement in Older Adults," *Journal of Advanced Nursing* 22(2):308-15, August 1995.

Anetzberger, G.J., et al. "Elder Mistreatment: A Call for Help," *Patient Care* 27(11):93-130, 1993.

Atkinson, R.M., and Ganzini, L. "Substance Abuse," in *The American Psychiatric Press Textbook of Geriatric Neuropsychiatry.* Edited by Coffey, C.E., et al. Washington, D.C.: American Psychiatric Press, Inc., 1994.

Badger, T. "Physical Health Impairment and Depression among Older Adults," *Image: Journal of Nursing Scholarship* 25(4):325-30, Winter 1993.

Bahr, R.T. "Sleep Disturbances," in *Gerontological Nursing.* Edited by Stanley, M., & Beare, P. Philadelphia: F.A. Davis Co., 1994.

Barnea, Z., and Teichman, M. "Substance Misuse and Abuse among the Elderly: Implications for Social Work Intervention," *Journal of Gerontological Social Work* 21(3/4):133-48, August 1994.

Beck, J.C., et al. "Geriatric Assessment: Focus on Function," *Patient Care* 28(4):10-32, February 28, 1994.

Bellville, W.J., et al. "Influence of Age on Pain Relief from Analgesics," *JAMA* 217(13):1835-41, 1971.

Beresford, T.P. "Alcoholism in the Elderly," *International Review of Psychiatry* 5:477-83, 1993.

Berg, S., and Dellasega, C. "The Use of Psychoactive Medication and Cognitive Function in Older Adults," *Journal of Aging and Health* 8(1):136-149, 1996.

Berkow, R. and Abrams, W., eds. *Merck Manual of Geriatrics,* 2nd ed. Rahway, N.J.: Merck and Co., Inc., 1995.

Beyea, S.C., and Nicoll, L.H. "Administering I.M. Injections the Right Way," *American Journal of Nursing* 96(1):34-35, January 1996.

Billig, N. *Growing Older and Wiser.* New York: Lexington Books, 1993.

Bookin, D., ed. *Working with Impaired Elders in the Community: A Guide to the Decision-Making Process and Legal Intervention.* Cleveland: The Federation for Community Planning, 1992.

Brady, R., et al. "Geriatric Falls: Preventive Strategies for the Staff," *Journal of Gerontological Nursing* 19(9):26-32, 1993.

Buffum, M., and Wolfe, N. "Posttraumatic Stress Disorder and the World War II Veteran," *Geriatric Nursing* 16(6):264-270, 1995.

Burke, M., and Walsh, M. *Gerontologic Nursing.* St. Louis: Mosby–Year Book, Inc., 1992.

Burrows, A., et al. "Depression in a Long Term Care Facility: Clinical Features and Discordance between Nursing Assessment and Patient Interviews," *Journal of Amercian Geriatrics Society* 43(10):1118-22, October 1995.

Busby-Whitehead, J. "Exercise in the Elderly," in *Care of the Elderly: Clinical Aspects of Aging,* 4th ed. Edited by Reichel, W. Baltimore: Williams & Wilkins Co., 1995.

Cacace, M., and Williamson, E. "Grieving: The Death of an Adult Child," *Journal of Gerontological Nursing* 16-22, February 1996.

Call, A.C. "A Literature Review: Assessment and Intervention in Elder Abuse," *Journal of Gerontological Nursing* 20(7):25-32, 1994.

Cammer, B.E., et al. "Elder Abuse and Neglect: How to Recognize Warning Signs and Intervene," *Geriatrics* 50(4):47-52, 1995.

Capriotti, T. "Unrecognized Depression in the Elderly: A Nursing Assessment Challenge," *Medsurg Nursing* 4(1):47-54, 1995.

Carnevali, D.L. *Nursing Management for the Elderly,* 3rd ed. Philadelphia: J.B. Lippincott Co., 1992.

Carney, R., et al. "Association of Depression with Reduced Heart Rate Variability in Coronary Artery Disease," *American Journal of Cardiology* 76(8):562-4, September 15, 1995.

Cirone, N. "Diabetes in the Elderly: Part I," *Nursing96* 26(3):34-39, March 1996.

Clinical Practice Guidelines: Depression in Primary Care, Treatment of Major Depression. Rockville, Md.: U.S. Department of Health and Human Services, Public Health Service, Agency for Health Care Policy and Research, 1993.

Clinical Practice Guidelines: Post Stroke Rehabilitation. Rockville, Md.: U.S. Department of Health and Human Services, Public Health Service, Agency for Health Care Policy and Research, 1995.

Clinical Practice Guidelines: Treatment of Pressure Ulcers. Rockville, Md.: U.S. Dept. of Health and Human Services, Public Health Service, Agency for Health Care Policy and Research, 1994.

Clinical Practice Guidelines: Urinary Incontinence in Adults. Rockville, Md.: U.S. Dept. of Health and Human Services, Public Health Service, Agency for Health Care Policy Research, 1992.

"Clinical Practice Recommendations," *Diabetes Care* vol. 16, May 1993.

Clinician's Handbook of Preventive Services. Washington, D.C.: U.S. Department of Health and Human Services, Public Health Service, 1994.

Cohen, C., et al. "Old Problem, Different Approach: Alternatives to Physical Restraints," *Journal of Gerontological Nursing* 22(2):23-29, 1996.

Colley, C.A., and Lucas, L.M. "Polypharmacy: The Cure Becomes the Disease," *Journal of General Internal Medicine* 8(1):278-83, May 1993.

Commodore, D.B. "Falls in the Elderly Population: A Look at Incidence, Risks, Healthcare Costs, and Preventive Strategies," *Rehabilitation Nursing* 20(2):84-88, 1995.

Cooper, J.W. "Drugs that Cause Falls in the Nursing Home," *Nursing Homes* 42(4):45-47, May 1993.

Copel, L.C. *Nurse's Guide to Psychiatric and Mental Health Care.* Springhouse, Pa.: Springhouse Corp., 1996.

Coward, R. "Double Jeopardy — Aging beyond the Country Myth," *Aging Today* 14[5]:7-9, September-October 1993.

Coyne, A.C., et al. "The Relationship between Dementia and Elder Abuse," *American Journal of Psychiatry,* 150(4):643-46, 1993.

Cromwell, S.L. "The Subjective Experience of Forgetfulness among Elders," *Qualitative Health Research* 4(4):444-62, November 1994.

Crook, J.M., et al. "Epidemiological Comparison of Persistent Pain Sufferers in a Group Family Practice and Specialty Pain Clinic," *Pain* 36:49-61, 1989.

Daly, M.P., and Richardson, J.P. "Geriatrics for the Clinician: Nutrition in Old Age," *Maryland Medical Journal* 44(5):377-81, May 1995.

Delfino, D. "Helping the Elderly with Drug Therapy," *Nursing93* 23(2):16, February 1993.

DeLima, G.N. and Hilderbrandt, V. *Geriatric Patient Education Resource Manual,* supplement 3, vol. 1. Gaithersburg, Md.: Aspen Pubs., Inc., 1994.

DeMaagd, G. "High-Risk Drugs in the Elderly Population," *Geriatric Nursing* 16(5):198-206, September-October 1995.

Department of Health and Human Services. "Medicare and Medicaid: Regulations for Long-Term Care Facilities," *Federal Register* 54:5322, 1989.

Deyo, R.A., et al. "A Controlled Trial of Transcutaneous Electrical Nerve Stimulation (TENS) and Exercise for Chronic Low Back Pain," *New England Journal of Medicine* 322(23):1627-34, 1990.

Diagnostic and Statistical Manual of Mental Disorders, 4th ed. Washington, D.C.: American Psychiatric Association, 1994.

Drake, A.C., and Romano, E. "Protect Your Older Patient," *Nursing95* 25(6):34-41, June 1995.

Dunne, F.J. "Misuse of Alcohol or Drugs by Elderly People," *BMJ* 38(5):608-09, March 1994.

Dwyer, J. "Strategies to Detect and Prevent Malnutrition in the Elderly: The Nutrition Screening Initiative," *Nutrition Today* 29(5):14-25, September-October 1994.

Ebersole, P., and Hess, P. *Toward Healthy Aging,* 4th ed. St. Louis: Mosby–Year Book, Inc., 1994.

Egbert, A. "The Older Alcoholic: Recognizing the Subtle Clinical Clues," *Geriatrics* 48(7):63-66, July 1993.

Egbert, A.M., et al. "Randomized Trial of Post-Operative Patient Controlled Analgesia vs Intramuscular Narcotics in Frail Elderly Men," *Archives of Internal Medicine* 150:1897-1903, 1990.

Elaz, F., et al. "Restraint Reduction: Can It Be Achieved?" *The Gerontologist* 34(5):694-99, 1994.

Eliopoulos, C. *Gerontological Nursing,* 3rd ed. Philadelphia: J.B. Lippincott Co., 1993.

Engberg, S., et al. "Self-Care Behaviors of Older Women with Urinary Incontinence," *Journal of Gerontological Nursing* 21(8):7-14, August 1995.

Eppard, J., and Anderson, J. "Emergency Psychiatric Assessment: The Nurse, Psychiatrist, and Counselor Roles during the Process," *Journal of Psychosocial Nursing* 33(10):17-23, 1995.

Faller, N., and Lawrence, K. "Comparing Low-Profile Gastrostomy Tubes," *Nursing93* 26(3):46-47, December 1993.

Farrell, K., and Ganzini, L. "Misdiagnosing Delirium as Depression in Medically Ill Elderly Patients," *Archives of Internal Medicine* 155(22):2459-2464, December 11-25, 1995.

Felten, Beverly Sigl. "Effects of Widowhood on Quality of Life Indicators in Older Adults over the Age of 75," unpublished research, 1991.

Ferguson, J., and Smith, A. "Aggressive Behavior on an Inpatient Geriatric Unit," *Journal of Psychosocial Nursing* 34(3):27-32, 1995.

Ferrell, B.R., et al. "Development and Evaluation of a Pain Education Program," *Cancer* 72:3426-32, 1993.

Ferrell, B.R., et al. "Pain Management for Elderly Cancer Patients at Home," *Cancer* 74:2139-46, 1994.

Finkel, S. "The Nursing Home Patient and Prescribing Psychotherapeutic Drugs," *Nursing Home Medicine* 1(6):6-9, 1993.

Fishman, P. "Healthy People 2000: What Progress toward Better Nutrition?" *Geriatrics* 51(4):38-42, April 1996.

Floyd, J.A. "Another Look at Napping in Older Adults," *Geriatric Nursing* 16:136-38, 1995.

Folstein, M.F., et al. "Mini-Mental State: A Practical Method for Grading the Cognitive State of Patients for the Clinician," *Journal of Psychiatric Research* 12(3):189-98, 1975.

Food Facts For Older Adults. Washington, D.C.: U.S. Department of Agriculture, Human Nutrition Information Service, 1993.

Fuller, K., and Lillquist, D. "Geropsychiatric Public Sector Nursing: Placement Challenges," *Journal of Psychosocial Nursing* 33(8):20-22, 1995.

Fulmer, T.T. "Elder Mistreatment," *Annual Review of Nursing Research,* 12:51-64, 1994.

Galindo, D., and Kaiser, F.E. "Sexual Health after 60," *Patient Care* 29(7):25-38, April 15, 1995.

Galindo-Ciocon, D.J., et al. "Gait Training and Falls in the Elderly," *Journal of Gerontological Nursing* 21(6):10-17, 1995.

Gambert, M. "Substance Abuse in the Elderly," in *Substance Abuse: A Comprehensive Textbook.* Edited by Lowinson, J.H., et al. Baltimore: Williams & Wilkins Co., 1993.

Gambert, S.R., et al. "How Many Drugs Does Your Aged Patient Need?" *Patient Care* 28(6):61-72, March 30, 1994.

Gibson, C.J., et al. "Effectiveness of Bran Supplement on the Bowel Management of Elderly Rehabilitation Patient," *Journal of Gerontological Nursing* 21(10):21-30, 1995.

Giving Drugs by Advanced Techniques. Advanced Skills Series. Springhouse, Pa.: Springhouse Corp., 1993.

Griffiths, H.J., et al. "Total Hip Replacement and Other Orthopedic Hip Procedures," *Radiologic Clinics of North America* 33(2):267-287, 1995.

Gupta, K.L. "Alcoholism in the Elderly: Uncovering a Hidden Problem," *Alcoholism* 93(2):203-07, February 1993.

Haight, B. "Suicide Risk in Frail Elderly People Relocated to Nursing Homes," *Geriatric Nursing* 16(3):104-107, 1995.

Hazzard, W.R., et al. *Principles of Geriatric Medicine and Gerontology,* 3rd ed. New York: McGraw-Hill Book Co., 1994.

Healthy People 2000: National Health Promotion and Disease Prevention Objectives. Washington, D.C.: U.S. Department of Health and Human Services, Public Health Service, 1991.

Hegner, B., and Caldwell, E. *Assisting in Long Term Care.* Albany, N.Y.: Delmar Pubs., 1994.

Hughes, E. "Creating a Functional Environment for Elder Care Facilities," *Geriatric Nursing* 16:172-76, 1995.

Janelli, L.M., et al. "Physical Restraints: Has OBRA Made a Difference?" *Journal of Gerontological Nursing* 20(6):17-21, 1994.

Johnson, V.E. *I'll Quit Tomorrow: A Practical Guide to Alcoholism Treatment.* San Francisco: Harper SF, 1990.

Johnson, B.K. "Older Adults and Sexuality," *Journal of Gerontologic Nursing,* 22(2):6-15, February 1996.

Juergens, S. "Problems with Benzodiazepines in Elderly Patients," *Mayo Clinic Proceedings* 68:818-820, 1993.

Kahn, R., et al. *Medical Management of Insulin-Dependent (Type I) Diabetes,* 2nd ed. Alexandria, Va.: American Diabetes Assoc., 1994.

Kahn, R., et al. *Therapy for Diabetes Mellitus and Related Disorders,* 2nd ed. Alexandria, Va.: American Diabetes Assoc., 1994.

Kamisar, Y. "Active Versus Passive Euthanasia: Why Keep the Distinction?" *Trial* 29(3):32-37, 1993.

Kane, R.L., et al. *Essentials of Clinical Geriatrics,* 3rd ed. New York: McGraw-Hill Book Co., 1994.

Katz, S., et al. "Studies of Illness in the Aged: The Index of ADL, a Standardized Measure of Biological and Psychosocial Function," *JAMA* 185:914, 1963.

Katz, S., et al. "The Index of ADL: A Standardized Measure of Biological and Psychosocial Function," *JAMA* 185:914, 1963.

Kaufmann, M. "Activity-Based Intervention in Nursing Home Settings," in *Functional Performance in Older Adults.* Edited by Bonder, B.R., and Wagner, M.B. New York: F.A. Davis Co., 1994.

Kayser-Jones, J. "Mealtime in Nursing Homes: The Importance of Individualized Care," *Journal of Gerontological Nursing* 22(3):26-31, 1996.

Kolodney, Masters, W.H., and Johnson, V.F. *Textbook on Human Sexuality for Nurses.* Boston: Little, Brown & Co., 1979.

Koroknay, V.J., et al. "Maintaining Ambulation in the Frail Nursing Home Resident: A Nursing Administered Walking Program," *Journal of Gerontological Nursing* 21(11):18-24, 1995.

Lachs, M.S., and Fulmer, T. "Recognizing Elder Abuse and Neglect," *Clinics in Geriatric Medicine* 9(3):665-81, 1993.

Lachs, M.S., and Pillemer, K. "Abuse and Neglect of Elderly Persons," *New England Journal of Medicine,* 332(7):437-43, 1995.

Lay, T. "The Flourishing Problem of Elder Abuse in Our Society," *ACCN* 5(4):507-15, 1994.

Lebowitz, B., et al. "Geriatric Pharmacology," *Psychopharmacology Bulletin* 31(4):641-649, 1995.

Lemieux-Charles, L., et al. "Ethical Issues Faced by Clinician/Managers in Resource-Allocation Decisions," *Hospital & Health Services Administration* 38(2):267-285, Summer 1993.

Luekenotte, A.G. *Gerontologic Nursing.* St. Louis: Mosby–Year Book, Inc., 1996.

Luekenotte, A.G. *Pocket Guide to Gerontologic Assessment,* 2nd ed. St. Louis: Mosby–Year Book, Inc., 1994.

Mahoney, F.I., and Barthel, D.W. "Functional Evaluation: The Barthel Index," *Maryland State Medical Journal* 14(2):61-65, 1965.

Maklebust, J., and Sieggreen, M.Y. *Pressure Ulcers: Guidelines for Prevention and Nursing Management,* 2nd ed. Springhouse, Pa.: Springhouse Corp., 1996.

Mastering Documentation. Springhouse, Pa.: Springhouse Corp., 1995.

Masters, W.H., and Johnson, V.F. *Human Sexual Response.* Boston: Little, Brown, & Co., 1966.

Masters, J. "When Lithium Does Not Help: The Use of Anticonvulsants and Calcium Channel Blockers in the Treatment of Bipolar Disorder in the Older Person," *Geriatric Nursing* 75-78, March-April 1996.

Max, M.B., et al. "Effects of Desipramine, Amitriptyline, and Fluoxetine on Pain in Diabetic Neuropathy," *New England Journal of Medicine* 326(19):1250-56, 1992.

McDowell, B.J., et al. "Successful Treatment Using Behavioral Interventions of Urinary Incontinence in Homebound Older Adults." *Geriatric Nursing* 15(6):303-307, 1994.

McInnes, E., and Powell, J. "Drug and Alcohol Referrals: Are Elderly Substance Abuse Diagnoses and Referrals Being Missed?" *BMJ* 308(12):444-46, February 1994.

Melding, P.S. "Is There Such a Thing as Geriatric Pain?" *Pain* 46:119-21, 1991

Midanik, L., et al. "The Effect of Retirement on Mental Health and Health Behaviors: The Kaiser Permanente Retirement Study," *Journal of Gerontological Psychology* 50(1):S59-S61, January 1995.

Miller, C.A. *Nursing Care of Older Adults: Theory and Practice,* 2nd ed. Philadelphia: J.B. Lippincott Co., 1995.

Mindnich, D., and Hart, B. "Linking Hospital and Community," *Journal of Psychosocial Nursing* 33(1):25-28, 1995.

MNA Human Rights/Ethics Committee Position Statement on Assisted Voluntary Self-Termination. Okemos, Mich.: Michigan Nurses Association, 1994.

Mudd, S.A., et al. "Alcohol Withdrawal and Related Nursing Care in Older Adults," *Journal of Gerontological Nursing* 20(10):17-26, October 1994.

Naylor, M., and Brooten, D. "The Roles and Functions of Clinical Nurse Specialists," *Image: Journal of Nursing Scholarship* 25(1):73-78, Spring 1993.

Noe, C., and Barry, P. "Healthy Guidelines for Cancer Screening and Immunizations," *Geriatrics* 51(1):75-83, January 1996.

Nursing Home Law and Rules. Columbus, Ohio: Ohio Department of Health, 1994.

Nursing Procedures, 2nd ed. Springhouse, Pa.: Springhouse Corp., 1996.

Nutrition and Your Health: Dietary Guidelines for Americans, 4th ed. Washington, D.C.: U.S. Department of Health and Human Services, Public Health Service, 1995.

Nutrition Screening Initiative. Washington, D.C.: U.S. Department of Health and Human Services, 1993.

OBRA-State Operations Manual and Interpretive Guidelines (Government Publication, HCFA-Pub 7, Transmittal No. 274). Washington, D.C.: U.S. Department of Health and Human Services, Health Care Financing Administration, 1995.

Ohio State Medical Association (OSMA) and Ohio Department of Human Services (ODHS). *Ohio Physicians' Elder Abuse Prevention Project-Trust Talk: Break the Silence, Begin the Cure.* Columbus, Ohio: Ohio State Medical Association, 1994.

Parmelee, P.A., et al. "The Relation of Pain to Depression among Institutionalized Aged," *Journal of Gerontology* 64(1):P15-P21, 1991.

Patient Teaching Loose-Leaf Library. Springhouse, Pa.: Springhouse Corp., 1990.

Payne, R. "Transdermal Fentanyl: Suggested Recommendations for Clinical Use," *Journal of Pain and Symptom Management* 7(3)(Suppl.):S40-S44, 1992.

Piper, A., Jr. "Truce on the Battlefield: A Proposal for a Different Approach to Medical Informed Consent," *The Journal of Law, Medicine, and Ethics* 22(4):301-13, 1994.

Polanski, A., and Tatro, S., eds. *Luckmann's Core Principles and Practice of Medical Surgical Nursing.* Philadelphia: W.B. Saunders Co., 1996.

Pope, D. "Music, Noise, and the Human Voice in the Nurse-Patient Environment," *Image: Journal of Nursing Scholarship* 27(4):291-300, Winter 1995.

Portenoy, R.K. "Opioid Therapy for Chronic Noncancer Pain: The Issue Revisited" *American Pain Society Bulletin* 1(4):4-7, 1991.

Portenoy, R.K. "Chronic Opioid Therapy for Persistent Noncancer Pain: Can we Get Past the Bias?" *American Pain Society Bulletin* 1(2):1,4-5, 1991.

Position Statement on Active Euthanasia. Washington, D.C.: American Nurses Association, 1994.

Position Statement on Assisted Suicide. Washington, D.C.: American Nurses Association, 1994.

Preskorn, S. "What Is the Message in the Alphabet Soup of Cytochrome p450 Enzymes?" *Journal of Practical Psychiatry and Behavioral Health* 238, 1995.

Rayome, R.G. "Simple Urodynamic Techniques," *Journal of Wound, Ostomy, and Continence Nurses Society* 22(1): 17-26, 1995.

Reynolds, C.F., et al. "When Depression Strikes the Elderly Patient," *Patient Care* 85-102, February 28, 1994.

Richards, B. "Geropsychiatric Nursing: Present Issues and Future Challenges," *Nursing Clinics of North America* 29(4):49-56, 1994.

Roca, R. "Psychosocial Aspects of Surgical Care in the Elderly Patient," *Surgical Clinics of North America* 74(2):223-243, April 1994.

Rochon, P.A., et al. "Reporting of Age Data in Clinical Trials of Arthritis," *Archives of Internal Medicine* 153:243-48, 1993.

Roe, B. *Clinical Nursing Practice: The Promotion and Management of Continence.* New York: Prentice Hall, 1992.

Rossen, E.K., and Buschmann, M.T. "Mental Illness in Late Life: The Neurobiology of Depression," *Archives of Psychiatric Nursing* 9(3):130-136, June 1995.

Ruiz, B., et al. "The Role of Gerontological Advanced Practice Nurses in Geriatric Care," *Journal of the Amercian Geriatrics Society* 43(9):1061-1064, 1995.

Saslaw, J.S., et al. "Ongoing Collaboration between the Interdisciplinary Team and Community Resources in the Resolution of Abuse of Elderly Patients." Poster session, *Case Western Reserve University Research Day,* November 5, 1995.

Schainen, J.S. "Screening for Polypharmacy in a Nursing Home Care Unit," *Journal of Gerontological Nursing* 20(3):41-44, March 1994.

Schank, M.J., et al. "Parish Nursing: Ministry of Healing," *Geriatric Nursing* 17(1):11-13, 1996.

Schatzberg, A. "Fluoxetine in the Treatment of Comorbid Anxiety and Depression, *Journal of Clinical Psychiatry Monograph* 13(2):2-12, 1995.

Schorling, J.B., et al. "Identifying Problem Drinkers: Lack of Sensitivity of the Two-Question Drinking Test," *American Journal of Medicine* 98(3):232-36, March 1995.

Scope and Standards of Gerontologic Clinical Nursing Practice. Washington, D.C.: American Nurses Association, 1995.

Seltzer, M.L. "The Michigan Alcoholism Screening Test: The Quest for a New Diagnostic Instrument," *American Journal of Psychiatry* 127(12):89-94, June 1971.

Siegler, M. "Defining the Goals of Ethics Consultations: A Necessary Step to Improving Quality," in *Quality Review Bulletin.* Oakbrook Terrace, Ill.: Joint Commission on Accreditation of Healthcare Organizations, January 1992.

Sky, A., and Grossberg, G. "The Use of Psychotropic Medication in the Management of Problem Behaviors in the Patient with Alzheimer's Disease," *Medical Clinics of North America* 78(4):811-821, 1994.

Staab, A.S., and Hodges, L.C. *Essentials of Gerontological Nursing: Adaptation to the Aging Process.* Philadelphia: J.B. Lippincott Co., 1996.

Stanley, M., and Beare, P.G., *Gerontological Nursing,* Philadelphia: F.A. Davis Co., 1995.

Steinberg, R.B., et al. "Acute Toxic Delirium in a Patient Using Transderm Fentanyl," *Anesthesiology and Analgesia* 75:1014-16, 1992.

Stracke, H., et al. "Mexiletine in the Treatment of Diabetic Neuropathy," *Diabetes Care* 15(11):1550-55, 1992.

Sullivan-Marx, E. "Psychological Responses to Physical Restraint Use in Older Adults," *Journal of Psychosocial Nursing* 33(6):20-25, 1995.

Sunderland, T. "Treatment of the Elderly Suffering from Dementia," *Journal of Clinical Psychiatry* 13(1):31-33, 1995.

Switzer, K.H. "Informed Consent for Inserting a CVC," *AJN* 95(6):66-67, 1995.

Tandan, R., et al. "Topical Capsaicin in Painful Diabetic Neuropathy," *Diabetes Care* 15(1):15-18, 1992.

Teaching Aids for Home Care Nurses. Springhouse, Pa.: Springhouse Corp., 1996.

Thibault, J.M., and Maly, R.C. "Recognition and Treatment of Substance Abuse in the Elderly," *Primary Care* 20(1):155-64, March 1993.

Thomas, B.L., "Research Considerations: Guardianship and the Vulnerable Elderly," *Journal of Gerontological Nursing* 20(5):10-16, 1994.

Tideiksaar, R. *Falls in Older Persons: Prevention and Management in Hospitals and Nursing Homes.* Boulder, Colo.: TACTILITICS Inc., 1993.

U.S. Preventive Services Task Force. *Guide to Clinical Preventive Services.* Baltimore: Williams & Wilkins Co., 1989.

Uriri, J.T., and Thatcher-Winger, R. "Health Risk Appraisal and the Older Adult," *Journal of Gerontological Nursing* 21(5):25-31, 1995.

Van Ort, S., and Phillips, L. "Nursing Interventions to Promote Functional Feeding," *Journal of Gerontological Nursing* 21(10): 6-13 (1995).

Vaughn, K., et al. "A Retrospective Study of Patient Falls in a Psychiatric Hospital," *Journal of Psychosocial Nursing* 31(9):37-41, 1993.

Vernon, M., and Bennett, G. "Elder Abuse: The Case for Greater Involvement of Geriatricians," *Age and Aging* 24:177-79, 1995.

Waldman, S.D., and Coombs, D.W. "Selection of Implantable Narcotic Delivery Systems," *Anesthesia Analgesia* 68:377-84, 1989.

Wall, R.T. "Use of Analgesics in the Elderly," *Clinics in Geriatric Medicine* 6(2):345-64, 1990.

Watson, Y.I., et al. "Clock Completion: An Objective Screening Test for Dementia," *Journal of the American Geriatrics Society* 41:1235-40, 1993.

Weiss, K. "Management of Anxiety and Depression Syndromes in the Elderly," *Journal of Clinical Psychiatry* 55(2):5-11, February 1994.

Where to Turn for Help for Older Persons. Washington, D.C.: U.S. Department of Health and Human Services, Administration on Aging, 1988.

Wieder, A.J., and Wolf-Klein, G.P. "When Medications Change, Tell the Caregiver, Too," *Geriatrics* 49(8):48-50, August 1994.

Wold, G. *Basic Geriatric Nursing.* St. Louis: Mosby–Year Book, Inc., 1993.

Yoshikawa, M.D., et al. *Ambulatory Geriatric Care.* St. Louis: Mosby–Year Book, Inc., 1993.

Zullich, S.G., et al. "Impact of Triplicate Prescription Program on Psychotropic Prescribing Patterns in Long-Term Care Facilities," *Annals of Pharmacotherapy* 26:539-45, 1992.

Index